Horse Owner's

VETERINARY

Handbook

This book is not intended as a substitute for the medical advice of veterinarians. Readers should regularly consult a veterinarian in matters relating to their horse's health, and particularly with respect to any symptoms that may require medical attention.

In writing this book, we have described the signs and symptoms that will lead you to a preliminary idea of what is happening with your horse, so you can weigh the severity of the problem. Knowing when to call your veterinarian is very important. Delays can be dangerous.

At the same time, we have sought to provide guidance for the acute or emergency situations that you must handle on your own until you can get veterinary attention for your horse. Life-saving procedures are explained step by step. However, a veterinary handbook is not a substitute for professional care. Advice from a book can never be as helpful or as safe as actual medical advice. No text can replace the interview and the hands-on examination that enables a veterinarian to make a speedy and accurate diagnosis.

However, the knowledge provided in this book will enable you to more effectively cooperate and better understand your interactions with your veterinarian. You'll be more alert to the signs of health problems and better able to describe them. You'll know more about basic care for your horse, and you'll be prepared in an emergency.

Horse Owner's

VETERINARY

Handbook

Third Edition

Tom Gore, DVM
Paula Gore, MT, ASCP, BB
James M. Giffin, MD

Edited by Beth Adelman

636.10896 GORE-T 2008

Gore, Tom.

Horse owner's veterinary
  handbook

WILEY

Wiley Publishing, Inc.

Library Resource Center
Renton Technical College
3000 N.E. 4th Street
Renton, WA 98056

Copyright © 2008 by Howell Book House. All rights reserved.

Howell Book House
Published by Wiley Publishing, Inc., Hoboken, New Jersey

No part of this publication may be reproduced, stored in a retrieval system or transmitted in any form or by any means, electronic, mechanical, photocopying, recording, scanning or otherwise, except as permitted under Sections 107 or 108 of the 1976 United States Copyright Act, without either the prior written permission of the Publisher, or authorization through payment of the appropriate per-copy fee to the Copyright Clearance Center, 222 Rosewood Drive, Danvers, MA 01923, (978) 750-8400, fax (978) 646-8600, or on the web at www.copyright.com. Requests to the Publisher for permission should be addressed to the Legal Department, Wiley Publishing, Inc., 10475 Crosspoint Blvd., Indianapolis, IN 46256, (317) 572-3447, fax (317) 572-4355, or online at http://www.wiley.com/go/permissions.

Wiley, the Wiley Publishing logo, Howell Book House, and related trademarks are trademarks or registered trademarks of John Wiley & Sons, Inc. and/or its affiliates. All other trademarks are the property of their respective owners. Wiley Publishing, Inc. is not associated with any product or vendor mentioned in this book.

The publisher and the author make no representations or warranties with respect to the accuracy or completeness of the contents of this work and specifically disclaim all warranties, including without limitation warranties of fitness for a particular purpose. No warranty may be created or extended by sales or promotional materials. The advice and strategies contained herein may not be suitable for every situation. This work is sold with the understanding that the publisher is not engaged in rendering legal, accounting, or other professional services. If professional assistance is required, the services of a competent professional person should be sought. Neither the publisher nor the author shall be liable for damages arising here from. The fact that an organization or Website is referred to in this work as a citation and/or a potential source of further information does not mean that the author or the publisher endorses the information the organization or Website may provide or recommendations it may make. Further, readers should be aware that Internet Websites listed in this work may have changed or disappeared between when this work was written and when it is read.

For general information on our other products and services or to obtain technical support please contact our Customer Care Department within the U.S. at (800) 762-2974, outside the U.S. at (317) 572-3993 or fax (317) 572-4002.

Wiley also publishes its books in a variety of electronic formats. Some content that appears in print may not be available in electronic books. For more information about Wiley products, please visit our web site at www.wiley.com.

Library of Congress Cataloging-in-Publication Data:
Gore, Tom.
Horse owner's veterinary handbook / Tom Gore, Paula Gore, James M. Giffin ; edited by Beth Adelman. — 3rd ed.
p. cm.
ISBN-13: 978-0-470-12679-0
1. Horses Diseases—Handbooks, manuals, etc. 2. Horses—Handbooks, manuals, etc. I. Gore, Paula, 1956– II. Giffin, James M. III. Giffin, James M. Horse owner's veterinary handbook. IV. Title.
SF951.G45 2008
616.1'0896—dc22
    2008001418

10 9 8 7 6 5 4 3

Third Edition

Cover design by José Almaguer
Book production by Wiley Publishing, Inc. Composition Services

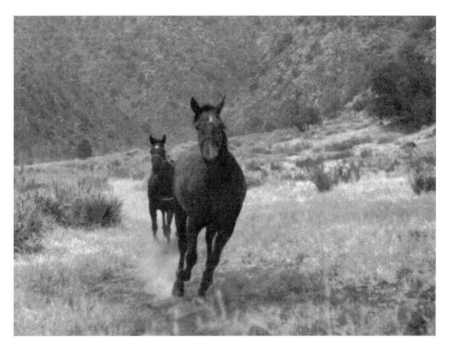

A horse gallops with its lungs,
perseveres with its heart,
and wins with its character.

—Tessio

FINDING IT QUICKLY

A special **Index of Signs and Symptoms** is on the inside of the front cover for fast referral. Consult this index if your horse exhibits any unexplained behavior. It will help you locate the problem.

The detailed **Contents** outlines the organs and body systems that are the sites of disease. If you can locate the problem anatomically, look here first.

The **Index** begins on page 657 and gives you a comprehensive guide to the book's medical information. Where a page number is in bold, it indicates more detailed coverage of the subject.

Cross-references note pertinent supplementary or related information.

A **Glossary** on page 634 defines medical terms used preferentially to best explain the subject or condition. Many of these words are now being used commonly among veterinarians and their clients. Glossary terms are found in italics in the text. (Italics may also be used for emphasis.)

An appendix of **Normal Physiological Data** can be found on page 619.

ACKNOWLEDGMENTS

We are grateful to the numerous researchers, clinicians, and educators whose work served as sources for our information. Some are mentioned here, but there were countless others who inspired us.

We appreciate the time and effort Dr. Tim Holt spent with us so we could understand equine acupuncture—and his great photos.

We would like to express our thanks to the Colorado State University Library and Colorado State University Veterinary Teaching Hospital for the unlimited resources available. A special thanks to our daughter, Katie, who ferried books home for us to use and return in a timely manner, only to have us check them out again—thanks for keeping your good humor.

We extend our sincerest appreciate to Wiley Publishing and Roxanne Cerda, who gave us the opportunity to produce this work, and to Beth Adelman, for not only editing our revision but for keeping us on track. To Shawn Bott, DVM, of Countryside Large Animal Veterinary Service in Greeley, Colorado, our sincerest thanks for the technical advice.

We appreciate the time and efforts of Dr. Lauren Cinagey and Dr. Christina Kobe in the technical review of our book. Different perspectives are invaluable.

We are forever indebted to Dr. Jim Giffin for inviting us to participate to begin with. We will miss his collaboration, his keen mind, and his good eye for detail.

And finally, we dedicate this edition to our mothers. They never held us back, always encouraged us to do our best, and admonished us to "just be careful." We love you, Mom!

—*Tom and Paula Gore*

CONTENTS

INTRODUCTION

Horses have captivated our hearts and imaginations since the beginning of time, when they were immortalized on cave walls. As humans industrialized and technology boomed, horses could have become obsolete to the point of near extinction, and yet their popularity has continued to grow. The equine industry has exploded and the horse enjoys a popularity not previously seen. Today, horses turn up in books and on television and movie screens in surprisingly large numbers.

If you type "great horses" into any Internet search engine, you will get more than 12 million hits. *Merriam-Webster Collegiate Dictionary* defines great "as superior in character or quality." I would add to that definition "ability." No one would dispute the greatness of Secretariat, Citation, and Seabiscuit; anyone watching Barbaro run his last, heart-breaking race would agree his chance at greatness ended too soon. Yet, each of us may have a different definition of what a great horse is to us, not necessarily limited to public fame.

Two decades ago, a red filly was born with a silly lop ear and a crooked front leg. Not the most beautiful horse, Lucy (named after a famous redhead) achieved greatness in our family. Her ear straightened out and her crooked leg never interfered with her abilities (except as a halter horse). Easy to train, she carried me and my unborn son elk hunting one fall, my 8-year-old daughter learned to drive her in competition, my son barrel raced her, she won money team penning, she loved cattle work, and would willingly pack an elk. Lucy had an impressive resume. At a time when she might be considered old, she became some one else's dream come true. As a retired gentleman's first horse, we hope she will again achieve greatness, due to her superior character and dependability.

Our equine companions enrich our lives, and for that alone they deserve the best care. Health care has become increasingly more focused on preventive medicine, and this is no less important for the horse. Advances in medicine have increased our ability to prevent disease and have given us many treatment options. When properly cared for, horses are living longer, more productive lives.

Along with the advances in traditional medicine comes the growing popularity of alternative therapies. With this in mind, in this new, fully updated and expanded edition, we include a new chapter introducing some of the holistic options available. The equine industry is constantly being challenged with newly emerging diseases, and these too have been included in this edition. Not so long ago, West Nile virus was a problem in a few areas of New

York State; now it's reached the West Coast in epidemic proportions, and a vaccine has been developed to help prevent it. The equine industry is constantly challenged with these newly emerging diseases, and this edition reflects the huge amount of research and medical developments that have taken place.

This book is intended as a guide, and we have made every attempt to be as accurate and current as possible. We cannot stress enough how important it is for you to cultivate a relationship with your veterinarian. Your veterinarian will want you to know what you can do yourself as well as what needs prompt professional medical care. Not only will your veterinarian be happy to show you how to give vaccinations, for example, but the equine veterinarian is an important source of information about horse care. This book and your veterinarian are just tools in the horse owner's toolbox, enabling you to give your horse the very best care.

The price of prevention is certainly less expensive than the cost of treatment—and perhaps loss.

—Paula Gore

EMERGENCIES

Emergency care is just that—care applied to a potentially serious condition that must be dealt with immediately. One of the cardinal rules in dealing with any emergency is for you to remain calm. If you panic, you won't be thinking clearly and you will panic your horse. Take a deep breath, quietly reassure your horse, and then do what is necessary. Don't hesitate to ask for help and remember that your horse is relying on you.

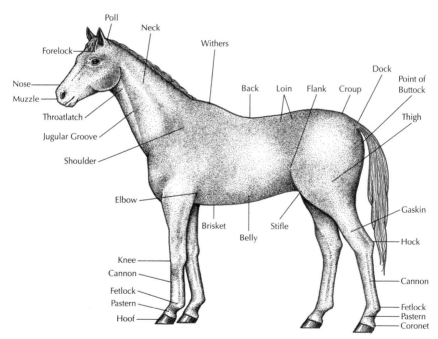

Basic anatomy of the horse.

Handling and Restraint

A horse who is frightened, injured, or in pain is a potential danger to himself and to his handlers. Do not handle or attempt to treat an agitated horse without professional assistance. In most cases, an injured horse will need to be given an intravenous sedative or be tranquilized before treatment can begin.

Most horses should be restrained for routine procedures such as shoeing, applying insecticides, floating the teeth, deworming, and giving injections. When restrained, a well-socialized horse recognizes that he is going to be handled and submits readily to the customary treatment.

The method of restraint will depend on the horse's disposition and spirit, his prior training, the duration of treatment, and whether the procedure is likely to cause pain. In general, it is best to begin with the least severe restraint that will allow examination.

Some specific methods for handling and restraint are discussed in this section.

Head Restraint

Even when a procedure is relatively minor and painless, it is still important to have an assistant restrain the horse's head. The assistant should hold the lead and be prepared to divert the horse's attention. The assistant should stand on the same side as the examiner, to keep the horse from wheeling into or kicking the examiner. Both should be on the left side whenever possible, because horses are used to being handled on the left.

A simple and effective method of restraining the head is to have the assistant hold the horse's muzzle with the left hand and the nape of the neck with the right (as shown in the photo at the top of page 3). To prevent the horse from ducking, the left thumb is inserted beneath the noseband of the halter. This method is useful for procedures such as floating the teeth.

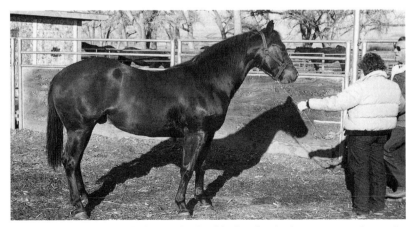

Secure the horse with a halter and a lead before beginning any sort of examination or treatment.

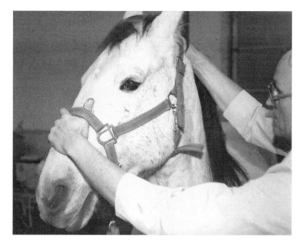

This is a simple way for an assistant to restrain the horse's head for a short procedure, such as giving an injection.

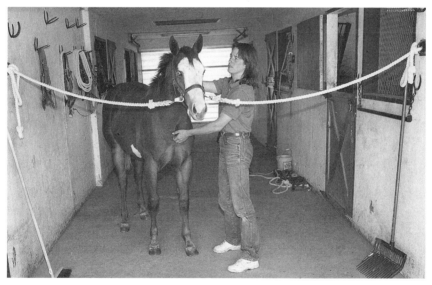

When working alone, it is safer to cross-tie the horse than to tie him to a fence or post.

When an assistant is not available, you can restrain the horse's head by cross-tying the horse between two walls or posts. The tie ropes should be anchored firmly at about the level of the horse's shoulders and snapped onto the halter. Tie the anchored ends with a slipknot for quick release.

Halter and Lead

The first step in dealing with a frightened or difficult horse is to gain control with the halter and lead. Approach the horse from the front while talking in a soothing and familiar manner. Never approach a horse from the rear or out of his line of vision.

If the horse is agitated, take as much time as necessary to gain his confidence. It is best to approach from the left, because horses are used to being handled from that side. Rub the horse on the shoulder or neck for a few moments to establish physical contact and to help calm the horse. Then slip the halter over his nose and tighten the buckle.

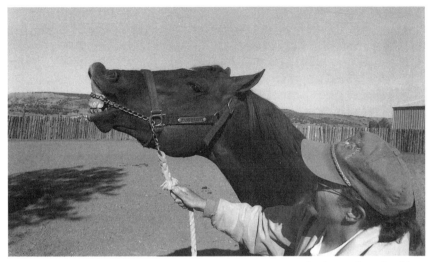

A chain across the gums is an effective restraint and keeps the horse from backing or rearing.

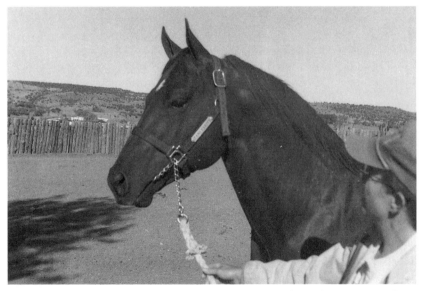

The chain can be placed through the horse's mouth, as shown here, or over the nose.

Always lead from the left side, holding the shank about 18 inches from the halter. Hold the lead firmly but do not wrap it around your hand or thumb; this would be unsafe if the horse decided to pull back or jump away and the lead was wrapped around your hand. When administering treatment, don't tie the lead shank to a fence or post. Many horses restrained in this manner for treatment will sit back forcefully on their haunches, invariably breaking the fence or a piece of tack. If the horse realizes he can escape by force, it will be extremely difficult to tie that horse up in the future. If you are forced to work alone, cross-tie the horse as described in the previous section.

The least aggressive restraint is to pass the lead shank under the horse's chin. This restraint will suffice for most handling situations. However, if the horse rears, do not jerk on the chain as it could cause him to fall over backward.

A chain shank or war bridle should be removed whenever a horse is tied. If the horse becomes upset and pulls back, the bridle or shank will constrict around his head or muzzle and cause serious injury.

Another method that can be used for a horse who refuses to advance on the lead (for example, through a door) is to blindfold the horse and then either lead or back him through the door.

Twitches

Twitches are among the oldest and most widely used methods of restraint. A twitch is thought to stimulate the release of endorphins in a manner similar to acupuncture and to produce sedation comparable in degree to chemical tranquilization.

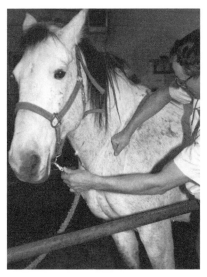

Apply the skin twitch by grasping a fold of skin in front of the shoulder.

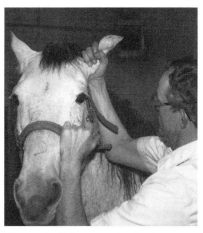

The ear twitch can make the horse head-shy. It should be used only by experienced handlers.

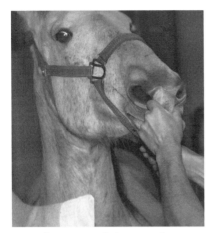 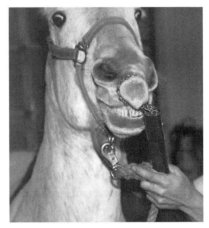

To apply a nose twitch, grasp the horse's upper lip to steady his head . . .

. . . then slip the loop over the horse's nose with the lips folded under.

Some horses should not be twitched. Because of past abuse, they may greatly resent the twitch and even fight it. These horses should be restrained in some other manner.

The skin twitch is applied by grasping a fold of skin just in front of the horse's shoulder. It may provide enough distraction for you to perform short procedures.

The ear twitch is applied by grasping and squeezing the ear with the heel of the hand pressed against the horse's scalp. Slight pressure is exerted

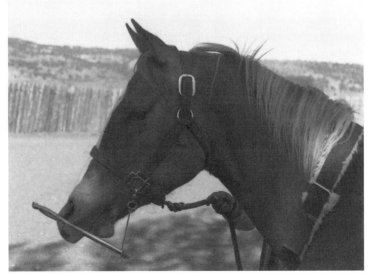

A lip twitch attached to the halter is useful when an assistant is not available.

downward. The major disadvantage of the ear twitch is that it can make the horse head-shy. Therefore, the ear twitch should be used cautiously and only by experienced horsemen.

The nose twitch and the lip twitch are used most often. However, they tend to lose their effectiveness when the skin becomes numb. To delay numbness, the twitch can be applied loosely and tightened as necessary. To apply a nose twitch, first grasp the upper lip between thumb and fingers to steady the head. Slip the loop over the horse's nose with the lip folded under so that the lining of the mouth is not exposed. Tighten the loop by twisting the handle.

The most humane twitch is a lip twitch attached to the halter so that it can't come off during the procedure. This twitch is a simple clamp with a string and a snap attached to the handles. Place your hand through the open twitch, firmly grasp the horse's nose, slide the twitch onto the nose, squeeze the handles together, wrap the string around the handles, and attach the snap to the halter to hold it in place. The lip twitch is especially useful when you are unfamiliar with horse restraints or are obliged to work alone.

Handling the Feet

To pick up the front foot, stand to the side in case the horse strikes out. Slide your hand down the horse's leg while squeezing on either side of the flexor tendon above the fetlock. It may be necessary to push the horse onto the opposite leg while picking up the foot and flexing the joint.

When preparing to pick up a back foot, approach from the side. A horse who resents being approached from behind sometimes (but not always) gives evidence by moving away and taking weight off the leg in preparation for kicking. For safety reasons, do not approach him from the rear.

To pick up the foot, slide your hand along the inside of the leg behind the cannon bone and draw the leg forward, then pull backward. Lift the leg and support it on your thigh. Note that the stifle joint is extended and the hock and toe are held in a flexed position. This helps to restrict voluntary movement of the leg.

When releasing the foot, simply reverse the procedure.

Preventing the Horse from Kicking

If a horse is inclined to kick while undergoing treatment, lifting a front leg will prevent him from doing so because a horse cannot kick with one foot off the ground. The leg can be restrained by tying it up with a rope or strap. The rope or strap should be equipped with a quick-release mechanism in case the horse loses his balance. You'll need a sideline to tie up a back leg.

Hobbling the hocks prevents kicking and allows the horse to bear weight on all four legs. This is important for long procedures or when a *mare* has to support the weight of a mounting *stallion*.

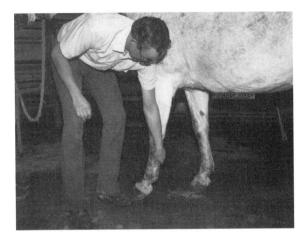

When picking up the front foot, be sure to stand well to the side.

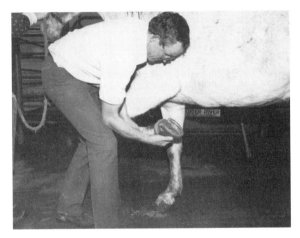

Flex the horse's knee to examine the sole and frog.

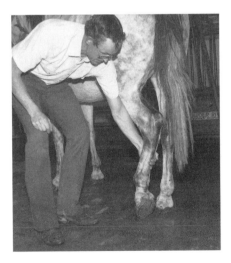

When picking up the back foot, approach the horse from the side. Slide your hand inside the cannon bone and draw the leg forward.

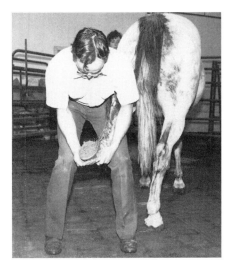

Support the leg on your thigh with the horse's stifle joint extended. This makes it difficult for the horse to pull free.

Stocks

For rectal and vaginal examinations, it is most convenient to restrain the horse in stocks or a *palpation* chute. In addition, stocks are particularly suitable for dental extractions and surgery on a standing horse. A partition at the back of the stock protects the examiner from being kicked. Once in stocks, the horse should be backed up against the partition to prevent him from kicking over the top.

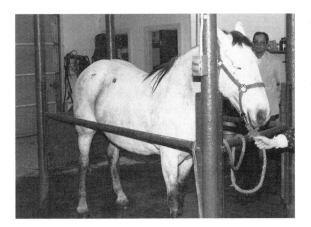

A stock with a kicking partition at the back is a safe restraint for rectal and vaginal examinations.

Tail Restraint

Tying a rope to the tail and pulling it straight back is a useful restraint for rectal and vaginal examinations. The rope should be held by an assistant and not tied to a stationary object.

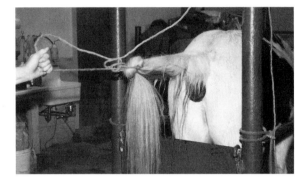

The tail restraint should always be held by an assistant.

Restraining a Foal

Young *foals* who are not halter-broken but are wearing a halter should not be restrained by grasping the halter. These young horses often react by rearing back and falling. This can lead to a brain concussion or a spine fracture. Instead, another kind of tail restraint is a good way to control weanlings who are not halter-broken. (Forced tail flexion should be used with caution in older horses, because coccygeal fractures and nerve injuries may occur.)

Grasp the foal's tail and pull it over the back in an arc while encircling the base of his neck with your other arm. This provides effective immobilization for short procedures, such as passing a stomach tube or giving an injection.

Nursing foals become excessively agitated and difficult to control if separated from their dams. If the foal cannot be approached easily in the paddock or field, mother and foal should both be led into a small enclosure such as a smooth-walled stall. The foal is then cornered and can be easily held with one arm encircling his chest and the other behind the rear legs above the hocks. The tail can be held over the back, as well.

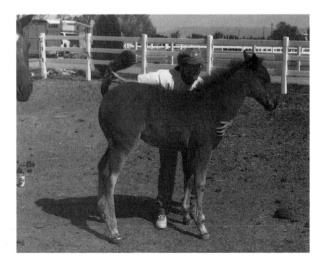

This is the correct method for restraining a foal.

Chemical Restraint

Intravenous sedation is indicated for horses who resist physical restraint, and for those in pain or about to undergo a painful procedure. Intravenous sedation is given by injection into the jugular vein. Depending on the circumstances, your veterinarian may select a drug or drug combination from the following classes.

- Phenothiazines (such as acepromazine) are tranquilizers that act on the central nervous system to produce calming and deep drowsiness. Rarely, they produce extreme anxiety, muscle twitching, dropping of the penis, sweating, and convulsions.

- Narcotics (such as morphine, Demerol, and butorphanol) are painkillers. When used in pain-free horses, they may produce excitation, apprehension, and increased muscular activity. Constipation and urinary retention are possible side effects. Untoward effects can be reversed by giving an antidote.

- Xylazine (Rompun) combines both tranquilization and pain control. It has a good margin of safety and can be used in combination with other drugs for better sedation and anesthesia. It is often the drug of choice for procedures requiring intravenous sedation. Drugs such as detomidine (Dormosedan), romifidine (Sedivet), and other alpha-2 agonists are gaining popularity.

Keep in mind that the effects of tranquilizers and sedatives vary. A horse may still kick or strike even though he seemed to be fully tranquilized. Exercise the same precautions as you would around a horse who is not sedated. Sedated horses should be kept away from *forage* and concentrate until they are fully awake to prevent choking.

For more information on tranquilizers and sedatives, see *Anesthetics and Tranquilizers* (page 588).

Abdominal Pain (Colic)

Sudden, severe pain in the abdomen in the horse is called *colic*. A horse with colic appears anxious and upset, and may kick at his abdomen, roll on his back, kick his feet in the air, break out in a sweat, and strain as if he is trying to pass urine or stool.

Treatment: Colic is a symptom rather than a specific disease. There are a great many diseases associated with signs of colic. Accordingly, a veterinary examination is necessary to determine the nature and seriousness of the problem. For more information, see *Colic* (page 381).

Library Resource Center
Renton Technical College
3000 N.E. 4th Street
Renton, WA 98056

Burns

Burns are caused by fire, electric shocks, skin friction, frostbite, and caustic chemicals. Acids, alkalis, solutions that contain iodine, and petroleum products are the most common causes of chemical burns. Saddle sores, galls, rope burns, and friction injuries are discussed in chapter 4, "The Skin and Coat."

Frostbite usually affects the ears and can lead to a loss of skin and cartilage, leaving a cropped appearance.

Steam, hot water scalds, and flame burns cause damage to the skin and underlying tissue in proportion to the length and intensity of exposure. With a surface burn you will see skin redness, occasional blistering, perhaps slight swelling, and the burn is painful. With deep burns the skin appears white and the hair comes out easily when pulled. Paradoxically, deep burns are not necessarily painful because the nerve endings may have been destroyed. When more than 20 percent of the body surface is involved in a deep burn, the outlook is poor. Fluid losses are excessive and shock will quickly set in.

Treatment: Treat chemical, acid, and alkali burns by flushing copiously with large amounts of lukewarm water. To be effective, this must be done immediately after the exposure.

Apply cold water compresses or ice packs to local burns for 30 minutes to relieve pain. Replace as compresses become warm. Clip away hair and wash gently with a mild soap, such as Ivory. Do not break blisters, because they provide a natural barrier to *infection*. Apply a topical antibiotic ointment such as Furacin, Silvadene cream, or triple antibiotic ointment. Aloe vera cream has medicinal properties and is particularly soothing on mild burns. Do not apply oil, grease, or iodine-containing surgical cleansing solutions, because they are irritating and will increase the depth of the burn and thus the potential for infection.

Burns can be treated by leaving them open to the air, or closed under a bandage or dressing, depending on the location of the injury. Where practical, protect the wound with an outer gauze dressing and change it daily (see *Wounds*, page 32).

Cardiovascular Collapse

Too much stress on the heart can lead to sudden circulatory collapse. In racehorses, the stress is that of maximum physical exertion over a relatively short period of time. In hard-working performance and endurance horses, the stress is less than the maximum but occurs over an extended period of time. The initial signs are those of exhausted horse syndrome (page 13). If the exercise is continued, collapse will follow.

Sudden Collapse

During maximal physical exercise, the cardiac output of a racehorse increases to seven times normal, while the heart rate increases to 200 beats per minute (from a normal 35 to 45 beats per minute at rest). Blood flow through skeletal muscles may be 20 times that of the resting state.

Under such circumstances, the equine heart muscle labors under a sustained deficiency of oxygen, a condition known as *hypoxia*. A switch to *anaerobic* metabolism may sustain the heart for some time, but with continued exertion, a point is eventually reached at which the heart can no longer supply enough oxygen to the muscles. At this point, the heart may decompensate and the horse will collapse.

Cardiac *arrhythmias* are thought to be the immediate cause of sudden cardiovascular decompensation (see *Arrhythmias*, page 318). Contrary to popular belief, horses with arrhythmias usually do not drop dead under the rider. The first indication is an abrupt drop in running speed. This alerts the rider and allows her to pull up and dismount.

The ability of a horse to tolerate cardiovascular stress is directly related to his athletic fitness. Fitness depends on how well the horse has been trained and conditioned. To achieve a high level of conditioning, a horse must be free of health problems, including *anemia*, valvular disease, myocarditis, intestinal *parasites*, bronchitis, and heaves—which compromise the efficiency of the heart and lungs.

Prevention: To prevent sudden cardiovascular collapse in the competition horse, it is important to:

- Screen all horses for cardiac and respiratory diseases.
- Correct any medical problems that may exist.
- Institute a program of graduated exercise, aimed at obtaining maximum athletic fitness.
- Monitor and recognize the immediate signs of exhaustion and rapidly correct dehydration and electrolyte deficits.

Exhausted Horse Syndrome

This syndrome affects performance and endurance horses experiencing submaximal exertion over an extended length of time. After a short period of hard work, the glucose stored by the muscles is depleted. When this happens, energy is generated by switching from glucose metabolism (*aerobic* metabolism) to fat metabolism (anaerobic metabolism). Anaerobic metabolism produces lactic acid and waste products, which accumulate and cause fatigue of heart and skeletal muscles.

The *basal* metabolic rate increases 10 to 20 times during sustained exercise. This generates a tremendous amount of heat that must be dissipated to maintain normal body temperature. Sweating is the chief way of dissipating body heat in the horse. As much as 6 to 12 gallons (22 to 45 l) of sweat can be lost during an endurance ride in hot, humid weather. Sweat contains substantial amounts of calcium, potassium, bicarbonate, sodium, chloride, and magnesium—minerals in the body known collectively as *electrolytes*.

When fluid and electrolyte losses are severe, horses may lose the ability to sweat—even if they have a high rectal temperature (see *Heat Stroke*, page 19).

Recognizing Impending Exhaustion

During endurance races, problems are recognized at veterinary checkpoints or mandatory rest stops. An exhausted horse shows an elevated rectal temperature along with a fast heart rate, flared nostrils, and a rapid breathing rate. If the horse is severely overheated, the breathing rate can actually be greater than the heart rate. *Capillary refill time* is prolonged to greater than three seconds (see *Capillary Refill Time*, pages 315 and 622).

After 15 minutes of rest, the heart rate should drop to less than 70 beats per minute and the breathing rate to less than 40 breaths per minute. If this does not happen, the horse should be rested until it does.

While resting, the exhausted horse may experience muscle cramps, tremors, and stiffness, and be unwilling or unable to move. This condition, called endurance-related *myopathy*, is not the same as the tying-up syndrome, although most of the signs are similar (see *Exertional Myopathy*, page 18).

A badly exhausted horse is apathetic, depressed, weak, unwilling to drink water, and appears *febrile* and dehydrated. He may sweat at a reduced rate or not at all. Such horses should be removed from the race to prevent sudden heart failure or metabolic collapse.

Thumps

This condition, which veterinarians call synchronous diaphragmatic flutter (SDF), occurs in some exhausted horses. Thumps is caused by low blood calcium in association with other electrolyte deficiencies. It is characterized by spasmodic contraction of one or both flanks, forceful enough to be felt or heard by the rider.

The thumps themselves are caused by rapid contractions of the diaphragm in unison with the heartbeat. The diaphragmatic nerves that pass over the heart apparently respond to its electrical field. Thumps should be considered a warning sign and an indication for further veterinary evaluation.

Post-Exhaustion Syndrome

Some severely exhausted horses do not recover after rest. These horses remain depressed, with persistently elevated heart and breathing rates. Liver and kidney failure can occur. This may lead to death. Reports have shown that horses with post-exhaustion syndrome have received phenylbutazone (Butazolidin) or another nonsteroidal anti-inflammatory drug (NSAID) early in the course of exhaustion. Therefore, these drugs should be withheld until the horse is adequately rehydrated.

Treating the Exhausted Horse

Stop all exercise. Move the horse to a cooler environment. As soon as possible, begin to replace fluids and electrolytes. If the horse is unable to drink, replacement solutions should be given, either intravenously or orally by stomach tube. Large volumes (usually several gallons) of a solution that contains electrolytes are required. A suitable oral electrolyte solution can be prepared by adding 1 tablespoon (18 g) of ordinary table salt and 1 tablespoon of Lite salt to 1 gallon (3.8 l) of water. (Lite is half sodium chloride and half potassium chloride. It is available at most grocery stores.)

This solution is high in chloride, the electrolyte lost in the greatest amount in sweat. It does not contain calcium, because large amounts of calcium may cause sudden heart failure. A number of commercial oral rehydrating solutions (containing sodium, potassium, chloride, calcium, bicarbonate, and glucose) are commercially available through your veterinarian or a horse supply store.

Continue administering the electrolyte solution until the horse recovers sufficiently to drink water on his own.

Lower the horse's body temperature as described in *Heat Stroke* (page 19). Thumps will disappear spontaneously with rehydration. A replacement solution containing calcium will expedite this process.

Preventing Exhausted Horse Syndrome

A horse on a long, physically depleting ride needs an average of 1 gallon (3.8 l) of water per hour. Statistics show that horses who drink frequently during an endurance race are much less likely to drop out of the race than those who do not. Consequently, endurance riders condition their horses to drink small amounts of water frequently during training. Accordingly, allow and encourage your horse to drink often. Frequent drinks during any strenuous athletic endeavor enable the horse to alleviate thirst, which is a signal of dehydration. Common sense dictates small, frequent drinks to help cool the equine athlete and prevent dehydration.

Sodium, chloride, potassium, bicarbonate, calcium, and magnesium are lost in the sweat and urine in proportion to the severity of stress, temperature, humidity, and individual sweating characteristics of the horse. To compensate for these losses, it may be advisable to give controlled amounts (perhaps several quarts; 1 quart is roughly 1 liter) of electrolyte-enriched water during the race, even though it may not be needed by all horses. It will not harm the horse as long as fresh water is available and the horse is allowed to drink as much as he wants during rest stops. However, keep in mind that water is far more essential than electrolytes. Do not give electrolyte water as a substitute for fresh water.

It is best not to feed a competition horse before a race, even though some people like to feed hay to an endurance horse at rest stops. Feeding diverts energy to digestion. This energy can be better used in supplying cardiovascular and musculoskeletal needs.

Dehydration

Dehydration is a loss of body fluids. It is not recognized until a 5 percent or greater loss of body weight in water occurs. A loss of 12 to 15 percent of body weight in water is life threatening.

Signs of dehydration include weakness, *depression*, dry mucous membranes (of the mouth and tongue), sunken eyeballs, prolonged *capillary refill time* beyond three seconds, and a heart rate over 60 beats per minute. Circulatory collapse and shock may result in death if not promptly treated.

The degree of dehydration can be estimated by testing skin elasticity. When the skin of the lower chest above the elbow is picked up into a fold, it should spring back into place. In horses with moderate to severe dehydration, the skin stays up in a ridge or returns to its original position very slowly (see *Hydration*, page 623).

Severe dehydration is most often caused by profuse diarrhea, prolonged physical exertion in hot weather, acute gastric dilatation, intestinal obstruction, or *peritonitis*. The dehydration is often complicated by *sepsis*, electrolyte deficit, and acid-base imbalance.

Dehydration also can occur with fever, heat stroke, choking (esophageal blockage), and loss of consciousness (which prevents the horse from drinking).

Treatment: Mild dehydration (for example, due to water deprivation for 24 hours) can be corrected by allowing the horse to drink small quantities of water at frequent intervals. Electrolyte-enriched water, as discussed in *Exhausted Horse Syndrome* (page 13), is indicated when water loss is accompanied by electrolyte loss. Excessive sweating and watery diarrhea are signs of severe electrolyte loss.

Moderate to severe dehydration must be treated by a veterinarian. Corrective replacement solutions containing water and electrolytes can be given by a nasogastric tube, assuming the horse does not have an intestinal problem such as diarrhea or bowel obstruction. The maximum rate of administration by nasogastric tube should not exceed 6 quarts (5.7 l) of fluid every two hours.

Intravenous solutions are commonly given through the jugular vein, although other sites are available if circumstances require. Because the intravenous route allows for the most rapid replacement of fluid, it is the one most preferred to treat severe dehydration and ongoing fluid losses.

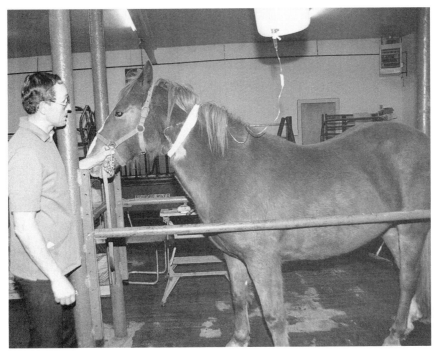

Large volumes of intravenous fluids are needed to correct moderate to severe dehydration.

Electric Shock

Horses who chew on electrical insulation can receive a shock sufficient to cause electrocution. Improperly grounded electric hot walkers are another cause of fatal shock. A horse can also be electrocuted by coming into contact with a pool of water electrified by a downed wire.

Horses are occasionally killed by lightning. A horse does not have to be struck directly to be killed. A tall tree with deep roots and spreading branches can serve as a conduit for a bolt of lightning, conducting electricity through the ground to any animal standing in the immediate vicinity of the tree during a thunderstorm. The same thing can happen when lightning hits ponds and fences or barns and stables that are not protected by lightning rods.

Most lightning strikes are fatal. The singed hair and skin of the dead horse gives evidence of the cause of death.

A horse who survives a major shock will often be knocked unconscious. Upon recovering, the horse may demonstrate signs of brain injury, including dizziness, altered vision, excitability, or paralysis.

Many electrocutions can be prevented. Faulty stable wiring should be replaced. Electric wire that is accessible to horses and rodents should be encased in metal housing. Lightning rods should be attached to all stables and barns. Electric walkers should be grounded. Fence wire connected to wooden posts is not well grounded and will conduct electricity. To ground the fence, replace a wooden post with a metal post every 50 yards. Keep horses out of wet pastures and away from small ponds during thunderstorms.

Exertional Myopathy (The Tying-Up Syndrome and Azoturia)

The tying-up syndrome and *azoturia* represent escalating degrees of the condition called exertional myopathy. Azoturia is the more severe form. Both tend to occur in heavily exercised horses who continue to consume a high-carbohydrate diet even when the exercise is temporarily discontinued. As the activity is resumed, the horse finds it difficult and painful to move. The term "Monday morning disease" was first used to describe this condition, since it was noted that horses who were rested and fed a working ration over the weekend often became stiff and sore when they returned to activity on Monday.

Exertional myopathy is caused by an accumulation in the muscles of a carbohydrate storage compound called glycogen. Glycogen storage occurs to a much greater extent in horses than in other animals, and even more so in horses with exertional myopathy. Excess glycogen accumulates in the muscles. Then, as the horse exercises, muscle glycogen is rapidly broken down to release blood sugar. This produces lactic acid that builds up to levels well beyond that which can be removed by metabolism. Lactic acid damages skeletal muscle and causes the release of muscle enzymes and *myoglobin*. Myoglobin is excreted in the urine and blocks the *nephrons*, causing acute kidney failure.

The tying-up syndrome, which is the milder form, occurs in race and performance horses during the cooling-out period after vigorous exercise. Signs include stiffness, muscle tremors, anxiety, and sometimes sweating. The muscles of the loin and hindquarters, in particular, are tense, hard, and painful. If myoglobin, a protein in heart and skeletal muscles, is found to be present in the urine, the condition becomes azoturia.

Azoturia signs begin 15 to 60 minutes after the beginning of exercise. The horse becomes anxious, sweats profusely, and has a rapid pulse. This is followed almost immediately by a stiffening of all major muscles, accompanied by staggering and wobbliness in the rear. Collapse is possible.

A horse with severe azoturia passes reddish-brown to black urine containing myoglobin pigment. With a mild attack, pigment will be found only on chemical analysis. The presence of myoglobin in the urine confirms the diagnosis and rules out endurance-related myopathy, colic, tetanus, and laminitis.

Signs of exertional myopathy may resemble those of colic. It is important to distinguish between these two conditions, since exercising or even walking a horse with acute exertional myopathy could be fatal.

Treatment: On first suspicion of exertional myopathy, stop all activity and enforce absolute rest. Any degree of activity, even returning to the stall, makes the condition much worse. Speak to the horse calmly to relieve anxiety. Cover the horse with a blanket and obtain veterinary assistance.

Tranquilizers such as acepromazine and pain relievers such as meperidine (Demerol) may be prescribed by your veterinarian to help relieve anxiety and may aid in the removal of lactic acid by improving circulation to the muscles. Oral NSAIDs, particularly naproxen, are especially effective in relieving stiffness and should be continued for several days. DMSO may be used by your veterinarian for its antioxidant properties. If corticosteroids are given, they should be administered only during the first few hours. They should not be used thereafter, because steroids have been implicated in causing attacks of exertional myopathy and can contribute to the development of laminitis.

Severely affected horses are given large volumes of intravenous fluid, along with an oral electrolyte solution, by stomach tube to promote urine flow and protect the kidneys from myoglobin damage. Thiamin and pantothenic acid (both present in the B complex vitamins) facilitate the elimination of lactic acid.

The outlook for recovery is good if the horse remains standing and his pulse returns to normal within 24 hours. It is good if the horse lies down but is able to maintain a *sternal position*. If the horse remains on his side and his pulse does not return to normal within 24 hours, the *prognosis* is guarded. Death can occur from acute kidney failure or the complications of prolonged *recumbency*.

Prevention: A horse who has recovered from exertional myopathy is susceptible to recurrent attacks. In part, these attacks can be prevented by withholding grain during periods of inactivity, maintaining a regular exercise program with at least some exercise each day, and starting all exercise activities slowly and increasing them gradually.

Vitamin E and selenium may prevent recurrent attacks in some horses. Commercial preparations are available. They can be given once a month by injection or can be added in low doses to the horse's feed. In certain geographic areas, your veterinarian may recommend checking your horse's blood level of selenium to avoid toxicity from oversupplementation. The anticonvulsant drug Dilantin has been reported to prevent some recurrences.

Heat Stroke

Heat stroke is an emergency that requires immediate recognition and treatment.

Horses dissipate body heat primarily through sweating. When the humidity is high and air temperature is close to body temperature, cooling by sweating is not an efficient process. The horse then attempts to dissipate heat through rapid air exchange, or panting.

Common situations that predispose horses to overheating include:

• Being transported in hot, poorly ventilated trailers

• Sustained exercise in warm, humid weather

• Being excessively dehydrated as a consequence of water deprivation, extreme exertion, or fever

• Anhydrosis (the inability to sweat in response to exercise or heat production)

Heat stroke begins with symptoms similar those described for *Exhausted Horse Syndrome* (page 13). If these symptoms go unchecked, the thermoregulatory mechanism malfunctions and the horse's body temperature may rise to as high as 115°F (46°C)—well above levels of heat exhaustion. The horse loses his ability to sweat and becomes disoriented and unsteady on his feet. The situation is now critical and the horse may collapse and die at any moment.

Treatment: Rapid cooling must begin at once. While awaiting the veterinarian, move the horse to shade and spray him repeatedly with cold water. Apply ice packs or alcohol sponges to the neck, flanks, and lower extremities. Electric fans are a very effective way of cooling a horse, although they are not always available. Cold water enemas, administered by the veterinarian, produce rapid cooling.

Dehydration is always a factor and should be corrected with large volumes of intravenous fluids containing electrolytes (see *Dehydration*, page 16).

Prevention: Heat stroke can be prevented by limiting the horse's exposure to predisposing situations and by ensuring that hard-working and endurance horses drink frequently during prolonged exercise.

Insect Stings, Spiders, and Scorpions

The stings of bees, wasps, yellow jackets, and ants all cause painful swelling at the site of the sting. If an animal is stung many times, he could go into shock as the result of absorbed toxins. Rarely, a hypersensitivity reaction called anaphylactic shock can occur if the horse was previously exposed to the same toxin (see *Anaphylactic Shock*, page 28).

The bites of black widows spiders, brown recluse spiders, and tarantulas also are toxic to animals. The sign is sharp pain at the site. Later, the horse can develop chills, fever, and labored breathing. An antivenin of equine origin is available to treat the black widow bite. The antibiotic dapsone is recommended to treat brown recluse spider bites. Tarantula bites may require treatment with an antihistamine.

The stings of centipedes and scorpions cause a local reaction and, at times, severe illness. These bites heal slowly. Poisonous scorpions (two species) are found in southern Arizona.

To treat stings and bites:

1. Identify the insect, if possible.
2. Remove any embedded stinger with tweezers, or scrape it out with a credit card (only bees leave their stingers behind).
3. Make a paste of baking soda and water and apply it directly to the sting.
4. Use ice packs to relieve swelling and pain.
5. Apply calamine lotion or Cortaid to relieve itching.

Poisoning

A poison is any substance that is harmful to the body. This includes manufactured products such as medications and cleaning solutions. Animal baits are palatable poisons that encourage ingestion. Horses will readily consume them if given the opportunity. This also makes them an obvious choice for intentional poisoning.

Pastures contain a variety of plants, often unrecognized but potentially toxic. Poisonous substances can also be found in roughages and improperly stored grain and hay. Accidental ingestion of these compounds is the most common cause of poisoning in horses.

The great variety of potentially poisonous plants and forages makes identification difficult, but most farm extension agents and veterinarians will be familiar with the common toxic plants and forages prevalent in your area.

Ingesting plant and forage toxins causes a complete spectrum of toxic symptoms. They include mouth irritation, drooling, tongue paralysis, diarrhea, rapid heart rate, rapid labored breathing, cyanosis, depressed senses, abnormal gait, staggering and loss of balance, limb paralysis, muscle tremors and convulsions, collapse, coma, and death. Some plants can cause sudden death without any warning signs. For more information on specific poisonings, see *Forage Toxicities* (page 427). Feed meant for cattle can also be poisonous to horses.

Medications, when given in an overdose or by the wrong route, may cause death. For this reason, only people who are properly trained should give intravenous medications. Occasionally, a horse will suffer anaphylactic shock (see page 28) when given a drug by injection due to a profound allergy to the drug.

Seizures caused by strychnine and other central nervous system poisons may be mistaken for epilepsy. Immediate veterinary attention is needed in cases of poisoning. In contrast to a poison seizure, epileptic seizures are brief, seldom last more than a minute, and are followed by a quiet period in which the horse appears dazed but is otherwise normal. Seizures caused by poisoning are often continuous or recur within minutes. Between episodes the horse is agitated and sweating, and may exhibit tremors, loss of coordination, weakness, colic, and diarrhea.

General Treatment for Poisoning

If poisoning is suspected, contact your veterinarian at once. If possible, locate the source of the poison and remove it to prevent further contact. Have it with you to answer any questions from the veterinarian. If the horse is down and having difficulty breathing, clear the airway (see *Shock*, page 27).

If your horse ingests an unknown substance, it is important to determine whether that substance is a poison. Most products have labels that list their ingredients, but if the label doesn't tell you the composition and toxicity of the product, call the ASPCA Animal Poison Control Center at (888) 426-4435 for specific information. The Poison Control Center has a staff of licensed veterinarians and board-certified toxicologists on call 24 hours a day, every day of the year. You will be charged a consultation fee of $50 per case, which can be charged to most major credit cards. There is no charge for follow-up calls in critical cases. At your request, they will also contact your veterinarian. You can also log onto www.aspca.org and click on "Animal Poison Control Center" for more information.

In some cases, you can call the emergency room at your local hospital, which may be able to give you information about how to treat the poison. Specific antidotes are available for some poisons, but they cannot be administered unless the poison is known, or at least suspected by the circumstances. Some product labels have phone numbers you can call for safety information about their products.

Signs of acute poisoning appear shortly after ingestion. Residual poison may be present in the horse's stomach. A gastric tube should be passed into the stomach and the contents suctioned and removed. The stomach is then washed out with large volumes of water to remove as much residual poison as possible.

After gastric *lavage*, an activated charcoal slurry is introduced through the stomach tube. The charcoal absorbs chemicals remaining in the stomach and small intestine. To prepare the slurry for an adult horse, mix 1 pound (453 g) of activated charcoal with 2 quarts (2 l) of water; for a foal, mix ½ pound (226 g) of charcoal with 1 quart (1 l) of water.

The next step is to prevent further absorption by eliminating the poison from the digestive tract. This is accomplished by giving a laxative immediately after the charcoal slurry. The two laxatives recommended for this purpose are magnesium sulfate (Epsom salts) and sodium sulfate (Glauber's salt). Sodium sulfate is preferred when used with activated charcoal, but either laxative is acceptable. Both are dissolved in water and given at a rate of 1 pound

(453 g) of laxative per gallon (3.78 l) for a mature horse; or ⅓ pound (150 g) of laxative per ⅓ gallon (1.26 l) for a foal. The laxative can be repeated in 8 to 12 hours.

Mineral oil is a mild laxative and intestinal protectant. It is preferred for some poisonings to prevent the absorption of toxins. The recommended dose is 3 to 4 quarts (3 to 4 l) for a mature horse and 1 pint (½ l) for a foal. Mineral oil must be given by stomach tube.

Large volumes of intravenous fluids are given in most cases of acute poisoning to support circulation, treat shock, and protect the kidneys. A large urine output may assist in eliminating the poison. Corticosteroids are often given for their anti-inflammatory effects. A horse in a coma may benefit from tracheal *intubation* and artificial ventilation during the phase of respiratory depression.

Convulsions caused by poisons are associated with prolonged periods of oxygen deficit and the potential for brain damage. Continuous or recurrent seizures should be controlled with intravenous diazepam (Valium), phenobarbital, pentobarbital, or methocarbamol (Robaxin).

If the horse has a poisonous substance on his skin or coat, wash the area thoroughly with soap and large volumes of water, or give the horse a complete bath in lukewarm water. Even if the substance is not irritating to the skin, it should be removed. Gasoline and oil stains can be removed by soaking the area with mineral or vegetable oil. Work the oil into the coat. Then wash the coat with a mild detergent such as Ivory soap.

Poison Baits

Animal baits containing strychnine, sodium fluoroacetate, arsenic, phosphorus, zinc phosphide, metaldehyde, or other poisons are used in rural areas to control gophers, coyotes, and other animals. In stables and barns they are used to eliminate rodents. These poisons are now being used less frequently because of livestock losses, concerns about persistence in the environment, and the potential to poison companion animals and children.

A variety of toxic signs occur when poison baits are ingested. The signs include hyperexcitability, tremors, loss of coordination, weakness, seizures, coma, respiratory depression, and circulatory collapse. These poisons are extremely toxic and may produce death in a matter of minutes.

Strychnine

This is available commercially as coated pellets dyed purple, red, or green. Signs occur less than two hours after ingestion. The first signs are agitation, excitability, and apprehension. They are followed by intensely painful convulsions with rigid extension of all limbs. The horse arches his neck and is unable to breathe. Any slight stimulation, such as touching the horse or making a loud noise, will trigger a seizure.

Treatment: Treat as described in *General Treatment for Poisoning* (page 22). Intravenous pentobarbital or phenobarbital is given during the first 48 hours to control seizures. Administer oxygen. Maintain a quiet environment and avoid unnecessary handling.

Sodium Fluoroacetate (Compound 1080)

This highly potent rat and gopher poison is often mixed with cereal, bran, and other rat feeds. Signs of poisoning include agitation, profuse sweating, trembling, straining to urinate or defecate, a staggering gait, and terminal convulsions. Because of its rapid action, sudden death without observed signs may be the only indication of poisoning.

Treatment: Treat as described in *General Treatment for Poisoning* (page 22). An antidote (glyceryl monoacetin) is available from chemical supply stores. Intravenous calcium chloride or calcium gluconate may be needed to correct low serum calcium.

Arsenic

This heavy metal is often combined with metaldehyde in slug and snail baits, and may be in ant poisons, weed killers, and insecticides. Arsenic has a very rapid action and a major potential for unintentional poisoning. Fortunately, its use has been greatly curtailed. Death can occur before symptoms are observed. In less acute cases, the signs are severe colic, weakness, trembling, staggering, salivation, diarrhea, and paralysis.

Treatment: Treat as described in *General Treatment for Poisoning* (page 22). A specific antidote (dimercaprol, also called British anti-Lewisite or BAL) is available. It should be given as soon as the diagnosis is suspected.

Metaldehyde

This poison, often combined with arsenic, is used commonly in rat, snail, and slug baits. It looks and tastes like dog food. The contents of the horse's stomach may have an odor of formaldehyde. Signs of toxicity include excitation, drooling and slobbering, uncoordinated gait, muscle tremors, and weakness that progresses to recumbency in a matter of hours. Death is by respiratory failure.

Treatment: Treat as described in *General Treatment for Poisoning* (page 22). Intravenous diazepam (Valium) or pentobarbital is given to control tremors. There is no antidote.

Phosphorus

This chemical is present in rat and cockroach poisons. The horse's breath may have the odor of garlic. The first signs of intoxication are colic and a hemorrhagic diarrhea. These signs may be quickly followed by coma and death.

Alternately, some horses experience a symptom-free interval lasting two to four days, which is then followed by signs of liver and kidney failure.

Treatment: There is no specific antidote. Treat as described in *General Treatment for Poisoning* (page 22).

Zinc Phosphide

This substance is found in rat poisons. Zinc phosphide in the stomach releases phosphine gas, which has the odor of garlic or rotten fish. Intoxication causes rapid, labored breathing, colic, weakness, stumbling, ataxic gait, convulsions, and death within two days.

Treatment: Treat as described in *General Treatment for Poisoning* (page 22). There is no specific antidote, but the stomach should be *lavaged* with 5 percent sodium bicarbonate, which raises the gastric pH and delays the formation of gas.

Rodenticide Anticoagulants

Rat and mouse poisons containing dicumarol-related compounds block the synthesis of vitamin K. Vitamin K is essential for blood clotting; a deficiency of vitamin K results in spontaneous bleeding. There are no signs of poisoning until the horse develops spontaneous bleeding and passes blood in the urine or stool, bleeds from the nose, or hemorrhages beneath the gums and skin. The simultaneous use of nonsteroidal anti-inflammatory drugs such as phenylbutazone may increase the bleeding.

The first-generation anticoagulants (warfarin, pindone) require repeated consumption to produce a hemorrhagic effect. However, the newer and more commonly used second-generation anticoagulants (of the bromadiolone and brodifacoum classes) require just a single exposure.

A closely related condition is dicumerol poisoning. Dicumerol is found in sweet clover contaminated by a mold. Eliminating moldy hay will prevent this problem.

Treatment: Treatment of spontaneous bleeding caused by all anticoagulants involves administering fresh whole blood or frozen plasma in amounts determined by the rate and volume of blood loss. Vitamin K1 is a specific antidote. It is given immediately by subcutaneous injection and repeated at intervals as necessary until the activated clotting time (ACT) returns to normal. Second-generation anticoagulants remain in the horse's system for several weeks and require prolonged observation and treatment.

Insecticides

Insecticides (also discussed in chapter 2, "Parasites") constitute a large group of toxic compounds to which the majority of horses are exposed. They are therefore a potential risk for poisoning.

Organophosphates and Carbamates

These compounds, used extensively in pesticides and dewormers, are the most frequent cause of insecticide poisoning. Organophosphates include dichlorvos, malathion, coumaphos, stirofos, haloxon, and trichlorfon. The most commonly used carbamates are sevin, pyrantel pamoate, and pyrantel tartrate. Organophosphates are a particular problem when topical insecticides are applied to a horse shortly after he has been dewormed with either dichlorvos or trichlorfon. This combination of two sources can result in overdose and toxicity.

Signs of toxicity with organophosphates and carbamates include hyperexcitability, colic with a tucked-up abdomen, muscle tremors, patchy sweating, profuse salivation, diarrhea, and a stiff-legged gait progressing to staggering. Collapse, followed by respiratory failure, is terminal. Seizures do not occur with insecticide poisoning.

The organophosphate haloxon has been shown to produce recurrent laryngeal nerve paralysis in foals. In adults, it produces paralysis of the anus, bladder, and pelvic limbs.

Treatment: Following oral ingestion, remove contents from the stomach by gastric tube and prevent absorption by administering activated charcoal and a sodium or magnesium laxative as described in *General Treatment for Poisoning* (page 22). Hyperexcitability and salivation are controlled with intravenous atropine. Repeat subcutaneously as needed. The specific antidote for organophosphate poisoning is 2-PAM (protopam chloride). It should be given as soon as the diagnosis is suspected. Tranquilizers and morphine should be avoided, since they may exacerbate symptoms.

Chlorinated Hydrocarbons

Chlorinated hydrocarbons, of which the prototype is DDT, are used in field and seed sprays, and as dusts against plant pests. Their use has been curtailed because of persistent toxicity in the environment. Only lindane and methoxychlor are approved for use around livestock.

Chlorinated hydrocarbons are readily inhaled and easily absorbed through the horse's skin. Toxicity can occur from repeated or excessive exposure. Signs of toxicity occur rapidly. They include hyperexcitability with twitching of the face, followed by muscle tremors that begin at the head and progress backward to involve the neck, shoulder, trunk, and rear legs. Seizures and convulsions are followed by respiratory paralysis and death.

Treatment: There is no specific antidote. Following oral ingestion, flush out the stomach and administer activated charcoal followed by mineral oil and a laxative as described in *General Treatment for Poisoning* (page 22). Seizures are controlled with intravenous diazepam (Valium) or pentobarbital. For skin exposure, the coat should be washed thoroughly with soap and water to remove residual insecticide.

Shock

CIRCULATORY SHOCK

Circulatory shock is a state of low blood flow. It is the result of cardiac output that is insufficient to meet the body's needs for oxygen. Adequate cardiac output requires a healthy heart, open blood vessels, and sufficient blood volume to maintain pressure. Any condition that adversely affects one or more of these will produce shock.

The body attempts to compensate for inadequate circulation by increasing the heart rate, constricting the blood vessels in the skin, and maintaining fluid in the circulation by reducing the output of urine. This becomes increasingly difficult when vital organs are not getting enough oxygen to carry on these activities. After a time, shock becomes self-perpetuating. Prolonged shock causes death.

Common causes of shock are dehydration (from profuse diarrhea or excessive sweating), hemorrhage, severe colic, peritonitis, blood-borne infection, heat stroke, snakebite, electrocution, poisoning, and major trauma. Foal *septicemia* is the most common cause of shock in neonates.

Treatment: First, evaluate the horse. Is he breathing? Does he have a heartbeat? What is the extent of his injuries? Is he in shock? If the horse is in shock, summon your veterinarian and proceed as follows:

1. If the horse is unconscious, check to be sure the airway is open. Clear secretions from the mouth with your fingers. Pull out the tongue to prevent it from blocking the airway. If possible, maintain the horse in a position in which the head is level with the body.

2. Allow the horse to assume the most comfortable position. An animal will naturally adopt the least painful position that allows him to breathe.

3. Control bleeding as described for *Wounds* (page 33).

4. To slow the progress of shock:
   - Calm the horse and speak soothingly.
   - When possible, splint or support broken bones before moving the horse.
   - Cover the horse with a coat or blanket to provide warmth. Do not wrap him tightly.

Veterinary treatment involves rapid rehydration with large volumes of intravenous electrolyte solutions to maintain blood pressure and tissue perfusion (blood flow into the tissues). Other steps that may be indicated include administering oxygen, blood transfusions, corticosteroids, antibiotics, and various drugs to support the circulation.

The outlook depends on the cause of the shock and how quickly treatment is initiated.

Anaphylactic Shock

This is an acute hypersensitivity reaction that develops after a horse has been exposed to an *allergen* to which he is highly sensitive. The allergens most frequently involved in anaphylactic reactions are the penicillin antibiotics, vaccines, and the immune serums, such as antivenins. Signs of *anaphylaxis* are produced by histamine and other substances released by mast and basophil cells (which are reactive white blood cells) in response to the challenge of the allergen.

Anaphylaxis can be localized or generalized (*systemic*). For example, a local reaction to an insect bite may consist only of itching and a hivelike swelling around the site of the bite. With a systemic reaction, the itching, swelling, and *hives* become generalized, or appear elsewhere on the body. A severe systemic anaphylactic reaction is accompanied by anxiety, sweating, marked difficulty breathing, diarrhea, a drop in blood pressure, shock, collapse, and, eventually, death.

Treatment: Early recognition of severe anaphylactic shock is essential. Sudden anxiety with difficulty breathing following either a vaccination or the administration of a drug are indications to treat. The specific antidote is epinephrine. Mild reactions are treated with 1 to 2 ml of a 1:1,000 epinephrine solution given intramuscularly (*IM*) or subcutaneously (*SC*). Life-threatening reactions require the immediate administration of 4 to 8 ml of the 1:1,000 epinephrine solution IM or SC, or 3 to 5 ml of the 1:10,000 solution intravenously (*IV*) via the jugular vein over three to five minutes. (Note the different solutions for IM and IV administration.) Repeat epinephrine every 15 minutes as necessary. If time permits, a permanent IV line should be established, as further medications and large volumes of fluid may be necessary to support the circulation.

An injectable corticosteroid (dexamethasone 0.1 mg per pound, 453 g, of body weight) is frequently administered for its anti-allergic effects. An antihistamine such as pyrilamine maleate, at a dose of 0.5 mg per pound by IM or IV injection, is often sufficient for a mild local reaction, and is useful in a severe reaction as a complement to the medications already listed.

Prevention: As a precaution, do not administer a drug or vaccine that has produced any sort of allergic reaction in the past, including hives. Drugs used for treating anaphylactic shock should be available in the medical supplies of all facilities that routinely give injections to horses.

Snake and Lizard Bites

Poisonous and nonpoisonous snakes are widely distributed throughout North America. Snakebites tend to occur during the spring and summer, when snakes are most active. Horses are usually bitten on the nose. In general, the bites of nonpoisonous snakes do not cause swelling and pain. They show teeth marks in the shape of a horseshoe (no fang marks; see the illustration on page 30).

In the United States there are four poisonous species: rattlesnakes, cottonmouth moccasins, copperheads, and coral snakes. The diagnosis of a poisonous snakebite is made by the appearance of the bite, the behavior of the animal, and the identification of the species of snake. (Kill it first, if possible.)

Pit Vipers (Rattlesnakes, Moccasins, Copperheads)

Identify these species by their large arrow-shaped heads, the pits below and between the eyes, their elliptical pupils, and the presence of fangs in the upper jaws. The most dangerous snake for horses is the large rattlesnake commonly found in the western and southwestern United States. It is easily identified by its characteristic rattle.

Pit viper venom produces red blood cell *hemolysis* and destroys tissue by breaking down proteins. It also depresses the heart.

The strike of the rattlesnake, and to a lesser extent that of other pit vipers, causes tissue swelling around the bite. When the horse is bitten on the nose (most common), the swelling may be mistaken for a bee sting or a spider bite. Identification of two puncture wounds in the skin (fang marks) will reveal the true cause.

In a severe case, however, the whole head, including the nose, eyelids, and ears, may be swollen to an extreme degree, giving rise to nasal obstruction and difficulty breathing. A frothy, bloodstained discharge may drain from each nostril.

Signs and symptoms depend on the size and species of snake, the location of the bite, and the amount of toxin absorbed by the horse. Most horses show few signs other than swelling at the site of the bite. With a severe reaction, the horse will become depressed and weak. When death occurs, it is caused by respiratory failure or cardiac arrest.

Coral Snake

The coral snake, found primarily in the Southeast, is an infrequent cause of snakebites. This snake has a retiring nature and lives in a habitat different from that of most horses. Identify the coral snake by its rather small size, small head with a black nose, and vivid body bands of red, yellow, white, and black, with the red and yellow bands always next to each other. The fangs are in the upper jaw.

There is a species of nonpoisonous snake that resembles the coral snake. In this snake, the black bands are bordered by yellow bands on both sides.

The local reaction in the horse is less severe than it is with a pit viper, but the pain is excruciating. Look for the fang marks.

Coral snake venom is neurotoxic (destructive to nerve tissue). Signs include paralysis, convulsions, and coma.

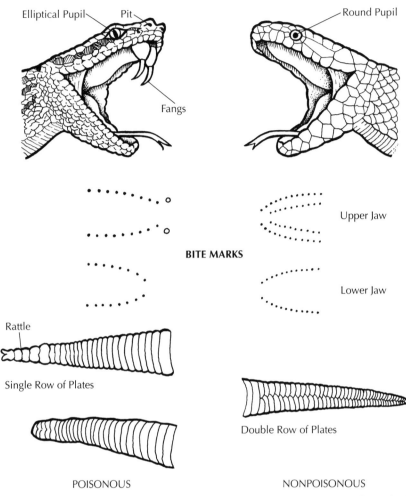

BITE MARKS

Upper Jaw

Lower Jaw

Rattle

Single Row of Plates

Double Row of Plates

POISONOUS

NONPOISONOUS

Characteristics of pit vipers and nonpoisonous snakes. Note the elliptical pupil, pit below the eye, large fangs, characteristic bite, and single row of subcaudal plates on the belly of the pit viper.

Lizards

Two species of poisonous lizard are found in the United States, both in the Southwestern states. They are the Gila monster and the Mexican bearded lizard. The bites of these lizards could be fatal to a horse.

Lizards have a tendency to bite and hold on. If the lizard has a firm hold on the horse, pry open the lizard's jaws with pliers and remove it.

Treating Snake and Lizard Bites

Fortunately, because of the large size of the adult horse, poisonous snake and lizard bites are rarely fatal. Foals are at somewhat greater risk of systemic reactions and death.

The first step is to identify the reptile and look at the bite. If the animal is not poisonous, cleanse and dress the wound as described in *Wounds* (see page 32). If it appears the horse has been bitten by a poisonous snake or lizard, summon your veterinarian and proceed as follows.

1. Restrain the horse. Bites are extremely painful. If the horse is recumbent, treat for shock, see *Shock* (page 27).

2. Keep the horse quiet. Venom spreads rapidly if the horse is active. Excitement, exercise, and struggling all increase the rate of toxin absorption.

3. If the bite is on the leg, apply a constricting bandage (a handkerchief or a strip of cloth) several inches above the bite. You should be able to get a finger beneath the bandage. Loosen the bandage for 5 minutes every hour.

4. Cold water packs can be applied to the bite at 15-minute intervals to reduce swelling. Ice packs, however, cause additional tissue damage and should not be used.

5. Washing the wound may upset the horse and increase venom absorption. Later, under controlled conditions with the horse sedated, the wound should be thoroughly cleansed, irrigated, and disinfected.

6. Incising the fang marks and applying suction in the field is not a practical undertaking for most equine snakebites and may increase the horse's anxiety and struggling. In particular, do not attempt to suck out the venom, as you could absorb the toxin.

Antivenins are available through your veterinarian. They are not always necessary for the adult horse but may be indicated for the foal. To be maximally effective, antivenin must be given within two hours of the bite. Swelling and nasal obstruction respond to corticosteroids. Snake and lizard bites frequently become infected. Antibiotics, tetanus shots, and wound care are important.

Sudden Unexplained Death

A horse may be found dead without obvious explanation. Intentional poisoning comes to mind first. However, most poisonings are accidental and not the result of malicious intent. All unexplained deaths should be investigated in an effort to establish the cause. Measures may need to be taken to protect other animals on the property.

A postmortem examination in the field may disclose the cause of death and thus eliminate the suspicion of poisoning. Diagnostic centers can provide full *necropsy* services to identify the cause of death. If the cause is not readily apparent, samples of blood, urine, stomach contents, and tissue from the kidney, liver, brain, spleen, hair, or hoof should be taken and sent to a laboratory for tissue and chemical analysis. It is also important to send samples of feed, water, weeds in the area, and suspect animal baits. Cost needs to be taken into account when deciding how thoroughly to pursue the investigation, because these studies can be expensive.

The following are some causes of sudden unexplained death, listed in approximate order of frequency.

- Peritonitis caused by acute gastric dilatation and ruptured gastric ulcer, colonic perforation, or intestinal strangulation
- Ingesting poisonous plants
- Forage toxicities, including botulism, moldy corn poisoning, sorghum toxicity, other mycotoxins and molds, blister beetle poisoning, and monensin (commercially known as Coban or Rumensin, this substance is a feed supplement commonly used for cattle and poultry that is toxic to horses)
- Cardiac arrhythmias causing cardiac arrest from unsuspected heart disease
- Ingesting poison baits
- Lightning strikes
- Fatal infections, including anthrax, equine infectious anemia, bacterial diarrhea, rabies, and equine piroplasmosis
- Head and neck trauma caused by falls or running into posts and walls
- Anaphylactic shock caused by insect stings, spider bites, or vaccinations
- Poisonous snakebites

Despite laboratory studies, the exact cause of death may never be determined. The most probable cause of death is then based on circumstantial and laboratory evidence and the clinical judgment of your veterinarian.

Wounds

In caring for wounds, the most important considerations are to first stop the bleeding and then to prevent infection. Be prepared to restrain the horse before you treat the wound (see *Handling and Restraint*, page 2).

Controlling the Bleeding

Bleeding may be arterial (spurting bright red blood from the arteries) or venous (oozing dark red blood from the veins), and sometimes both. Do not wipe a wound that has stopped bleeding. This will dislodge the clot. Do not pour peroxide on a fresh wound. Bleeding will then be difficult to control. In addition, peroxide damages cells and prolongs wound healing.

The two methods used to control bleeding are the pressure dressing and the tourniquet.

Pressure Dressing

The most effective and safest method for controlling bleeding is to apply pressure directly to the wound. If the wound is on the leg, take several pieces of clean bandage material or sterile gauze, place them over the wound, and bandage snugly. Watch for swelling of the limb above and below the pressure dressing. Swelling indicates impaired circulation, in which case the bandage must be loosened or removed.

If material is not available for bandaging, or if the wound is on the body, place a pad on the wound and press firmly. Hold it in place for 15 minutes.

If blood soaks through the bandage or bleeding persists after the pad is removed, apply further pressure (or a tourniquet) and notify your veterinarian. An arterial bleeder may need to be tied off.

Tourniquet

A tourniquet may be required to control a spurting artery. Tourniquets can be used only on the legs and tail to control arterial bleeding that can't be controlled with a pressure dressing. *Tourniquets should never be used if bleeding can be controlled by direct pressure.* Always place the tourniquet above the wound (between the wound and the heart).

Vetwrap, a self-adhesive support wrap, makes a good tourniquet, is easy to apply, and will stay tight. In a life-threatening emergency, a suitable tourniquet can be made from a piece of cloth, belt, tire, or length of gauze. Loop it around the limb, then tighten it by hand or with a stick inserted beneath the loop. Twist the loop until the bleeding stops.

A tourniquet should be loosened every 10 minutes to prevent tissue *hypoxia* (damage due to lack of oxygen) and to check for persistent bleeding. If bleeding has stopped, apply a pressure bandage as described in the previous section. If bleeding continues, let the blood flow for 30 seconds and then retighten the tourniquet for another 10 minutes.

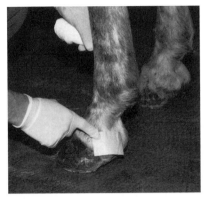

To make a pressure dressing, place sterile pads over the wound.

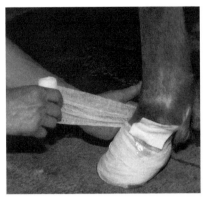

Cover the pads with gauze.

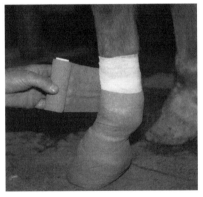

A stretch bandage helps to apply even pressure. It should not be pulled too tight.

Preventing Infection

Horses are more susceptible to tetanus than are most other domestic animals. Accordingly, all horses with wounds should receive tetanus prophylaxis. If the horse has been immunized against tetanus, he should be given a booster shot when he is wounded. If the vaccination history is unknown and the wound is either heavily contaminated or is a deep puncture wound (which is especially tetanus-prone), tetanus toxoid and tetanus *antitoxin* should be given in two different intramuscular locations. For a previously unvaccinated horse (or one whose status is not known), follow with a second tetanus booster in four weeks.

All wounds are contaminated with dirt and bacteria. Proper care will reduce the risk of tetanus and prevent some infections.

To treat extensive wounds and those requiring a cast, the horse will need to be chemically restrained using a local or regional anesthetic, and occasionally a general anesthetic. These wounds should be treated by a veterinarian. Cover the wound with a sterile dressing to prevent further contamination while awaiting veterinary instructions (see *Pressure Dressing*, page 33).

Wound Care

The five steps in wound care are skin preparation, cleansing, debridement, wound closure, and controlling infection.

Skin Preparation

Remove the original protective dressing and clean the area with a sterile surgical scrub solution. The two most commonly used solutions are povidone-iodine 10 percent (Betadine) and chlorhexidine diacetate 2 percent (Nolvasan). In the concentrations provided in the stock solutions, these preparations are irritating to unprotected tissue, so be sure to dilute them, following the manufacturer's recommendations. Scrub the skin around the wound but avoid contact with the open wound.

Then start at the edges of the wound and clip the hair back to prevent long hair from entering the wound.

Note that 3 percent hydrogen peroxide, often recommended as a wound cleanser, has little value as an antiseptic and is extremely toxic to tissues. Do not use it.

Cleansing

The purpose of cleansing is to remove dirt and bacteria. Vigorously scrubbing out a wound with a brush or gauze pad will further traumatize the wound and negate the benefits of cleansing. Wound *lavage* is a nontraumatic and a highly effective method of cleansing a wound. It involves irrigating the wound with copious amounts of irrigating fluid until the tissues are clean and glistening.

Tap water is a suitable and convenient lavage solution. Tap water has a negligible bacterial count and is known to cause less tissue irritation than sterile or distilled water. To provide antibacterial activity, add chlorhexidine or Betadine to the water. Studies show that chlorhexidine has the greater residual antibacterial effect, but either solution is satisfactory when correctly diluted.

To dilute chlorhexidine, add 25 ml of the 2 percent stock solution to 1 liter (about 1 quart) of water, for a 0.05 percent irrigating solution. To dilute povidone-iodine, add 10 ml of the 10 percent stock solution to 1 liter (about 1 quart) of water for a 0.1 percent irrigating solution.

The effectiveness of wound lavage is related to the volume and pressure of the fluid used. A bulb syringe is a low-pressure system and requires correspondingly more fluid to achieve marginally satisfactory wound cleansing. A large syringe with a 19-gauge needle is sufficient to remove a moderate amount of dirt and bacteria. A plastic spray bottle will provide about the same pressure. A home Water-Pik unit (used by people) or a commercial lavage unit provide a high-pressure stream of fluid and are the most effective. A garden hose with a pressure nozzle would also work well as the initial water lavage, followed by one of the devices just mentioned to deliver the antiseptic surgical scrub.

Debridement

Debridement, which follows wound lavage, is the removal of devitalized tissue and any remaining foreign material using tissue forceps (tweezers) and a scalpel. Before starting, put on sterile surgical gloves and be sure all instruments are clean. Devitalized tissue and foreign matter are removed by scalpel dissection. Experience helps to determine the difference between normal and devitalized tissue, and to control bleeding that results from the scalpel dissection.

Wound Closure

The next decision is whether to close the wound or allow it to heal open. Wounds that are sutured and then become infected pose a serious risk of *sepsis*. Infections in open wounds, however, are far less troublesome.

Wounds that have been heavily contaminated are likely to become infected. These wounds should not be sutured. Similarly, wounds older than 12 hours should not be sutured. Suturing should not be done if there are signs

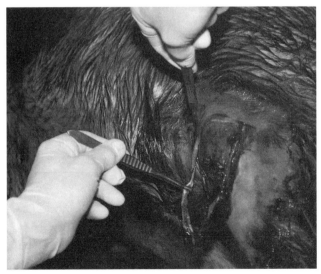

Debridement is the removal of devitalized tissue, which predisposes the wound to infection.

of inflammation in and around the wound, because this indicates impending infection.

Puncture wounds are quite likely to become infected. The external opening should be enlarged to provide drainage, after which the tract should be irrigated with a dilute antiseptic surgical scrub solution. Bites are heavily contaminated puncture wounds. With all animal bites, keep in mind the possibility of rabies. Puncture wounds should not be sutured. Administer tetanus prophylaxis, as described on page 63.

Fresh lacerations on the face are best sutured to prevent infection, minimize scarring, and speed recovery. Small lacerations may not need to be sutured. Lacerations on the leg usually cannot be closed because the skin is too tight and the sutures will pull through.

Occasionally, it is possible to close a wound that has been left open for several days and has developed a bed of clean granulation tissue. These wounds have acquired resistance to infection. Suturing such a wound is called a delayed primary closure.

The length of time that sutures should remain in depends on the location and other characteristics of the wound. Most sutures can be removed within 14 to 21 days, although some may be removed sooner. Follow your veterinarian's instructions.

Extensive, complicated wounds that must be left open should be cared for initially at a veterinary hospital. These wounds are likely to become infected and require intensive management, including daily lavage and debridement in many cases. Skin margins must grow together as open wounds heal, and it may take weeks or months for the skin to close.

Controlling Infection

Small open wounds can be treated at home. Medicate twice daily with a topical antibiotic such as triple antibiotic ointment. Recent evidence suggests that a steroid-antibiotic ointment (started after seven days) may increase the rate of skin closure. The horse should be confined to a clean stall until the surface of the wound has a protective scab. Restrict access to muddy paddocks and pastures until the wound is healed.

Infected wounds with a covering of *pus* will require moist sterile dressings. A number of topical antiseptics are effective in treating superficial wound infections. They include chlorhexidine and Betadine, diluted as described on page 35; furacin topical cream or solution 0.2 percent; silvadene cream 1 percent; and topical antibiotics containing bacitracin, neomycin sulfate, and polymyxin B sulfate. Apply directly to the wound or first place on a gauze pad. Change the dressings once or twice daily to aid in the drainage of pus. Seek immediate medical attention if the drainage is soaking the bandage more than once a day.

Oral and intramuscular antibiotics will not prevent wound infections but are indicated in the presence of *cellulitis* or *abscess* (see *Pyoderma*, page 123).

Most wounds on horses will heal with minimal scarring and a good functional result if the wound does not become infected and if it is protected from fly attacks. Flies seriously complicate the process of wound healing, promote infection, and cause the formation of excessive fibrous tissue in the wound. To protect the horse from flies and other biting insects, see *Controlling External Parasites* (page 63).

Granulation Tissue (Proud Flesh)

Part of the process that occurs during the healing of a wound is the formation of granulation tissue. When the skin surface has been cut, the defect must be filled in before the skin can regrow. Granulation tissue is how this is accomplished.

When the skin is cut, bleeding occurs and clots form. These blood clots reorganize into capillaries. This is the basis for the granulation tissue, but it is very fragile. Easily disrupted, it bleeds; new clots form and new capillaries are laid down on the original capillary bed. Once the skin defect has filled, the granulation tissue begins to contract, thereby reducing the size of the wound. Skin cells migrate over the surface of the granulation tissue to begin producing new skin.

A common condition in horses, proud flesh is an excess or overgrowth of granulation tissue. It is most often found on wounds below the knee or hock. Proud flesh makes it difficult for the skin cells to grow over the cut and often damages the new skin on the periphery of the wound. Proud flesh deteriorates the wound instead of healing it, and so must be discouraged.

Some outdated wound treatments, such as scarlet oil and gentian violet, actually promote and create more granulation tissue. Using bandages continuously may keep the wound site clean, but bandaging has been shown by studies to increase the amount of granulation tissue.

Treatment: If proud flesh production is suspected, seek veterinary advice for diagnosis and treatment. Treating exuberant granulation tissue is a complex issue and will vary from horse to horse.

Applying caustics, such as antimony trichloride, may have a place in treating some cases. Cases have also been treated by freezing the granulation tissue using liquid nitrogen or by applying probes placed in liquid nitrogen. Both the caustic chemicals and applied freezing techniques cause the death of the surface cells of the proud flesh, so their use requires skill and great care to not harm the growth of new skin. Once the proud flesh dies to a level below the surrounding new skin, the skin cells may then advance over the bed of remaining live granulation tissue.

The treatment that many veterinarians favor is surgical removal of the raised bed of exuberant granulation tissue. The portion of proud flesh that is above the adjoining skin level is carefully cut away, which allows the cells of the new skin to advance over the bed of granulation tissue.

Treatment may also involve advanced treatments such as skin grafts or laser treatments. Talk to your veterinarian to arrive at a treatment that is best for your horse.

Bandaging

Wounds may be bandaged or not, depending on their location. Wounds about the head are best left open to facilitate treatment. Many wounds of the upper body are difficult to bandage and do not benefit greatly from being covered. However, bandaging has the advantage of protecting a wound from dirt, manure, and fly attacks. It also restricts movement, compresses skin flaps, eliminates pockets of serum, and keeps the wound edges from pulling apart. Bandaging is most effective for extremity wounds. In fact, all leg and foot wounds should be bandaged.

Unlike a temporary pressure dressing, a foot or leg bandage will remain for some time. It is important to pad the extremity well to prevent the bandage from becoming too tight and shutting off the circulation. Place several sterile Telfa pads over the wound and cover with one or more large pads to completely surround the leg. Wrap the whole thing with an elastic bandage, starting with the hoof and working up the leg. Be sure to overlap as you go. This prevents the skin from forming ridges and becoming pinched beneath the bandage. If this happens, the skin can become devitalized.

Do not cinch the wrap, but roll it around the leg without stretching the fabric. This will prevent the cumulative effect of an elastic bandage becoming too tight. Flex the joints beneath the bandage several times to ensure the bandage is secure, but not so tight as to interfere with the circulation. If there is doubt about the adequacy of circulation, loosen the bandage.

Bandages over clean, healing wounds can be changed every two to three days, but they should be inspected twice daily for signs of circulation problems, excessive pressure, limb swelling, slippage, drainage, or soiling. (If the bandage is soaked, bacteria can wick into the wound.) If any of these conditions are present, replace the bandage. Polyvinyl duct tape can be used to waterproof the bandage.

A draining or infected wound will need to be redressed at least daily. The bandage should be sufficiently bulky to absorb the drainage without soaking through. Disposable diapers can be used for bandages that incorporate the foot.

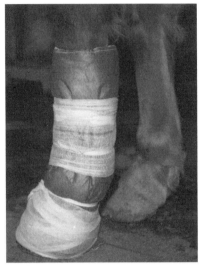

Foot and leg bandage. Cover the entire circumference of the leg with a soft pad and hold in place with a gauze roll.

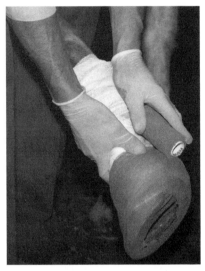

Wrap from bottom to top with an elastic bandage, maintaining even tension without cinching the wrap.

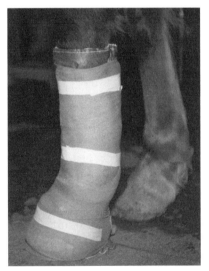

The hoof should be included. This helps to immobilize the joints.

For foot wounds that require prolonged treatment, a protective boot or shoe with a removable treatment plate can be used. Wounds of the sole are discussed in *Foot Wounds* (page 210).

Parasites

2

Parasites, both internal and external, exist wherever there are horses. You can never completely eliminate from your horse's environment all the insects, worms, and arachnids that bite and suck. Although this is inescapable, there is much you can do to keep your horse relatively untroubled by parasites and at the top of her form. In horses, good parasite control goes hand in hand with good health. Control is best accomplished by routine deworming, as described in this chapter, and by implementing environmental practices aimed at reducing parasite populations and limiting your horse's exposure.

Internal Parasites (Worms)

Internal parasites are among the most serious and common health problems affecting the horse. During their passage through the host, worms injure organ systems and create problems that lead to *anemia*, diarrhea, weight loss, poor condition, and general debility. In young animals they can permanently damage the lining of the bowel, creating malabsorption and nutritional deficiencies that interfere with growth and development. Worms can be a predisposing cause in cases of intestinal *colic*.

A complete program for controlling these parasites is described beginning on page 49.

Strongyles

Strongyles number among them some of the most harmful and damaging of all internal parasites of the horse. These parasites are arbitrarily divided into two groups: the large strongyles (also called bloodworms) and the small strongyles. The harmful effects of the large strongyles are much greater than those of the small ones. The larvae of the large strongyles migrate through the horse's circulation and damage blood vessels, while the larvae of the small strongyles remain in the wall of the gut.

The life cycle of the two species is similar, up to a point. Female worms lay eggs that are shed in the feces. Under favorable environmental conditions, the eggs become free-living larvae in one to two weeks. Larvae in grass and *forage* are ingested by grazing horses. This is where the two species diverge.

Large Strongyles

There are three important species but *Strongyles vulgaris* is the most harmful. The *infection* rate may be between 70 and 100 percent of all adult horses. Once ingested, the larvae of S. *vulgaris* penetrate the walls of the intestines and enter the arteries that supply blood to the digestive organs. Damage to the arteries caused by S. *vulgaris* leads to thrombosis (clotting), embolism, and the development of *aneurysms*. The larvae of the other two species migrate to the liver, flanks, tissues around the kidneys, and pancreas.

An *embolus* is a blood clot in a large vessel that breaks off and travels to a small vessel, where it creates a blockage. This blockage is called an embolism. This destroys part of the blood supply to the organ, in this case a segment of bowel. However, perforation is not common in horses because of a remarkable network of cross-connections in the arterial supply to the intestines. These cross-connections compensate for areas of interrupted blood flow. It has been suggested that this collateral circulation is an evolutionary adaptation to millions of years of selective pressure imposed by these parasites.

An *aneurysm* is a saclike enlargement of the artery. Aneurysms have the potential to rupture and cause internal bleeding. This is rare, because aneurysms are filled with clotted blood and fibrous connective tissue. Aneurysms are dangerous primarily because they produce emboli.

Episodes of thrombosis and embolism are the main cause of the colic and abdominal pain that accompanies repeated attacks of strongyles. Arterial *thromboembolism* may be diagnosed by rectal *palpation*, if the *lesion* is within reach. Having lived in the arteries for about five months, the larvae of S. *vulgaris* return to the intestines and develop into adult worms, where they attach by suckers to the walls of the bowel. Microscopic bleeding occurs where the worms attach and reattach. A heavy infection can cause severe anemia. The entire life cycle takes 11 months. Regular deworming is important because parasites are in different stages of growth all the time.

Small Strongyles

Small strongyles are the most common internal parasite in adult horses and occur frequently in *foals*. Larvae penetrate the walls of the intestines, where they encyst. During this stage they cause colic, bleeding, anemia, protein loss, and intestinal malabsorption. In the spring (and during times of stress), larvae rapidly emerge from the gut wall and cause severe diarrhea, chronic weight loss, and unthrifty appearance.

Controlling Strongyles

Controlling strongyles is the number one priority in all deworming programs. The eggs of both small and large strongyles do not appear in the feces for 9 to 12 months after the initial *infestation*. However, it is safe to assume that regardless of fecal exam results, the horse is or will soon be infected.

The arterial stage of *S. vulgaris* is not killed by most dewormers (the avermectins being the exception). Therefore, it is important to eliminate the nonmigrating stages before they penetrate the tissues. This can only be accomplished by using a proven deworming program, as discussed in *Controlling Internal Parasites* (page 49). An occasional treatment does not offer protection and will not prevent the potentially devastating consequences of these parasites. In addition, the life cycles of large and small strongyles vary in length, which is why your horse needs to be dewormed frequently.

Small strongyles have developed resistance to benzimidazole dewormers. Using deworming agents in rotation mitigates this problem. Including ivermectin in all deworming programs is highly recommended.

Ascarids

The harmful species of roundworm is *Parascaris equorum*. This adult worm lives in the small intestines and may grow to 12 inches (30 cm) long. *P. equorum* is the major worm problem in nursing and weanling foals. It occurs rarely, if at all, in horses over 2 years of age.

The female worm produces eggs that are shed in the feces. These eggs are highly resistant to environmental influences and remain infective for months or years. Eggs are taken up by the foal in contaminated feed and water. The eggs hatch in the small intestines and produce larvae that penetrate the walls of the gut. The larvae then migrate through the liver and reach the lungs. Here, they enter the airways and are coughed up and swallowed. Back in the small intestines, they mature into adult worms. The entire process takes about 10 to 12 weeks.

The signs of ascarid infection depend on the burden of parasites and whether a large number of eggs are ingested at one time or a small number over a long time. Under natural circumstances, infection tends to be chronic and ongoing rather than sudden and overwhelming. The major adverse effects of ascarid infection are malnutrition and retarded growth. Severely infected foals fail to thrive and have a rough haircoat and a potbelly. A huge number of worms produces diarrhea.

When larvae are migrating in the lungs, the foal may have a persistent cough or a nasal discharge. Adult worms in the intestines may produce *colic*.

Treatment: Following the administration of a rapid-acting dewormer, such as piperazine, a large mass of dead worms can form a blockage that leads to intestinal obstruction. This can be avoided by using a slow-acting dewormer, such as oxibendazole, and repeating it a second time. For more information, see *Worm Impactions*, page 377.

Prevention: Preventing *ascarids* involves interval deworming, starting at 8 weeks of age and continuing every two months until 1 year of age. *P. equorum* does not develop resistance to dewormers. The same dewormer can be used as often as necessary.

Threadworms

The threadworm of concern in horses is *Strongyloides westeri*, the first intestinal parasite to mature in young foals. The infection is acquired primarily through larvae ingested in the dam's milk. Since foals routinely eat manure, they can also ingest larvae shed in the *mare*'s feces. Larvae mature to adult worms in the small intestines. The entire process takes less than two weeks, and may contribute to increased severity of foal heat diarrhea. By 16 weeks of age, foals develop resistance to threadworms and maintain a minimal infection.

In older horses on pasture, the larvae may also infect the horse by burrowing through the skin, where the larvae are picked up by blood vessels and are carried to the lungs. In the lungs, the larvae access the bronchioles, are coughed up and swallowed by the horse, and attach to the intestines to begin a new life cycle. While in the lungs, the larvae may cause respiratory distress and even hemorrhage. If larvae enter the horse through the skin, dermatitis and irritation may be seen.

In the lungs, the larvae can cause bleeding and respiratory problems. However, the major illness caused by threadworms is mild to moderate diarrhea that often occurs at 9 to 16 days of age—the same time as foal heat diarrhea (see page 555). Characteristically, the foal does not appear ill and suckles normally.

A disease in humans called cutaneous larvae migrans (creeping eruption) can be caused by the larvae of threadworms. As the larvae penetrate the skin, they cause lumps, streaks beneath the skin, and itching. The disease is self-limiting.

Treatment: Threadworm infection should be considered a likely cause of moderate diarrhea in all suckling foals, even though in some cases the diarrhea is due to other causes. A deworming agent that is effective against threadworms, such as oxibendazole or ivermectin, should be administered. If the diarrhea clears up quickly, that suggests threadworms were the cause.

Prevention: Reduce the burden of infestation by removing manure and changing the stall bedding daily. In areas where threadworms are a problem, deworm foals at 3 weeks of age. Also deworm the mare 12 hours postpartum to prevent milk-borne and fecal transmission.

Stomach Bots

This infection is caused by the larval phase of the bot fly. Adult flies are nearly as large as bees. They do not bite, although fly attacks may agitate the horse and cause alarming escape behavior. Since this fly is found in all parts of North America, virtually all horses are infected.

There are three common species of bot fly. They differ only in where they lay their eggs on the horse, and how their larvae reach the stomach.

Gastrophilus intestinalis, the most common bot fly, glues its eggs to the hairs of the horse's chest, shoulders, and forelegs. The eggs hatch quite rapidly in response to an increase in temperature that occurs as the horse licks her legs or brings her warm breath in contact with the eggs. The larvae enter the surface of the tongue and burrow into the muscle, where they remain for one month. Later they molt, are swallowed, and attach themselves to the lining of the stomach.

Eggs of the species *Gastrophilus nasalis* are deposited on hairs beneath the jaw or on the throat (which is why they are called "throat bots"). Eggs hatch into larvae in six days. The larvae find their way into the horse's mouth and burrow into pockets between the molar teeth. Here they undergo a second molt, are swallowed, and attach themselves to the lining of the stomach.

Gastrophilus hemorrhoidalis eggs are deposited on the short hairs of the lips and follow the same sequence. This species is rare.

Bot larvae spend about 10 months attached to the wall of the stomach. In the spring, they release their hold and pass out with the manure. The larvae burrow into the ground and remain in a pupal stage for three to five weeks. Soon after, adult flies emerge.

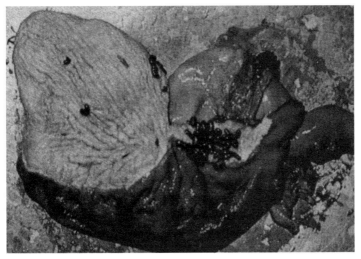

Bot larvae in the stomach of an untreated horse.

Signs of bots vary with the stage of infestation. Larval ulcerations in the mouth can cause pain on eating and lead to weight loss and failure to thrive. A more serious problem is caused by the stomach larvae, which produce colic, ulcers, and, rarely, perforation with fatal peritonitis (see *Gastric Rupture*, page 366).

Treatment: Assume that all untreated horses living in temperate zones are infected with bots. Bot treatment should be given in late fall one month after a killing frost. A second treatment is recommended at the beginning or middle of the bot season, usually in early spring. Organophosphates and ivermectin are the *anthelmintics* of choice. They are effective against both the mouth and stomach stages of bots. Horse feed supplements containing stirofos (an organophosphate) can be given to kill bot larvae in the stomach.

Prevention: Sponging the horse's neck, shoulders, chest, lips, and forelegs once or twice a week with warm water can reduce the number of larvae that enter the mouth. Insecticides containing insect growth regulators (IGRs), when used as directed and applied to these areas, prevent bot eggs on the horse's hair from hatching. This lowers the burden of infection. Also see *Controlling External Parasites* (page 63).

Pinworms (Oxyuris)

Pinworms are common parasites, occurring primarily in stabled horses. They cause intense anal itching. The infected horse backs up against a post or wall and rubs her tail and hindquarters back and forth incessantly. In time the skin on the hindquarters becomes excoriated and the hair is rubbed off, giving the characteristic ratty-looking tail. (Another cause of severe tail itching and hair loss is the tail mange mite; see *Mange*, page 126.)

The adult pinworm lives in the colon. The egg-bearing female migrates through the anus and deposits her eggs on the horse's *perineum*. The eggs are sticky and adhere to fences, bedding, stable walls, and other spots where the

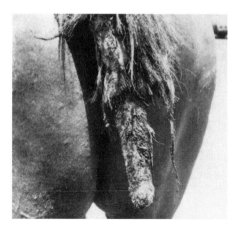

Pinworms are one cause of severe tail *pyoderma*.

horse rubs her bottom. Eggs hatch within one week. Infective larvae drop to the ground, where they contaminate feed. Once ingested, they pass into the colon and develop into adults. The entire life cycle is completed in eight weeks.

While this sequence is typical, pinworms sometimes complete all stages of their life cycle in the horse's large intestines. When this happens, a large burden of adult worms can cause inflammation of the colon and episodes of colic.

Pinworm eggs can be found by applying a clear tape to the perineum and then examining the tape under a microscope.

Treatment: Reduce the burden of infestation by cleaning the anal area with warm, soapy water daily. Use disposable paper towels to avoid transmitting eggs to other horses. Pinworms are sensitive to many of the deworming agents listed in the table on page 52. The anthelmintics used in routine deworming programs will also control pinworms. Horse pinworms cannot be transmitted to people, dogs, or other domestic animals.

Tapeworms

There are three species of tapeworm that infect horses. For many years, tapeworm infections were ignored because tapeworms were not believed to be prevalent in horses, nor were tapeworms thought to cause any serious illnesses in the horse. However, research into colic found that more than one in five cases of spasmodic colic and three out of four ileocecal impactions are found in horses with tapeworm infestations. A blood test that detects an antigen that is specific for a tapeworm protein was then developed. Using this blood test revealed that tapeworm infection rates ranged from 10 percent to 12 percent of all horses on the West Coast, 6 percent east of the Mississippi River, and as high as 95 percent of horses in the Midwest!

Research into tapeworms in horses has also revealed that horses younger than 2 years of age and horses over 15 years appear to have higher rates of tapeworm infections. Current thinking is that middle-age horses may develop a certain degree of immunity to the tapeworm's specific protein antigen, which declines as the horse ages. Another factor is that middle-age horses are in their peak working years and may not be pastured as much, and are therefore less likely to ingest the forage mite that carries tapeworm eggs.

Tapeworms depend on forage mites that live in pasture grass as intermediate hosts for one stage in their life cycle. Eggs are passed in the feces and ingested by the mites. The horse acquires the tapeworm by eating an infected mite while grazing. Adult worms develop in the horse and take up residence in the small and large intestines, where they can grow to 12 inches (30 cm) long. It takes four to eight months to complete the cycle.

The diagnosis is made using a blood or *serology* test, and occasionally by seeing egg cases in manure. Egg cases resemble kernels of rice and are capable of movement.

Treatment: Until recently, there were very few anthelmintics available that effectively treat tapeworm infections. For a number of years, pyrantel pamoate was used in an *off-label* application at twice the normal dosage. Now praziquantel has been approved by the FDA to treat tapeworms in horses. Praziquantel is combined in anthelmintic products with one of the avermectins—moxidectin or ivermectin—and has been shown to be quite effective in removing tapeworms.

Lungworms

Lungworm infection in horses has been related to contact with burros and *donkeys*. These animals appear to be the natural hosts, but they seldom show evidence of infection. In older horses and ponies the disease occurs *sporadically*. Foals, if infected, do not show symptoms.

Adult worms up to 4 inches (10 cm) long live in the lungs and lay eggs in the airways. The eggs are carried by *ciliary* action toward the larynx, where they are swallowed and passed in the feces. Eggs hatch within a matter of hours. The larvae are ingested by the grazing horse, penetrate the wall of the bowel, and are carried to the lungs. Because eggs hatch rapidly, feces should be examined for larvae rather than for eggs. A special technique is required.

The principal signs of lungworm infection are a persistent cough lasting several months, along with labored breathing on exertion and loss of weight and appetite. Wheezes can be heard with a stethoscope. These signs are similar to those of recurrent airway obstruction (*RAO*, page 303), which is far more common than lungworms. Association with donkeys, however, should raise the suspicion of lungworms.

Treatment: The avermectins are effective and should be administered every eight weeks. Separate horses from donkeys or treat donkeys concurrently.

Stomach Worms (Habronema)

There are three species of stomach worms that infect the horse. These small worms live in colonies in the wall of the stomach. Eggs, which are passed in the feces, are picked up by adult stable and house flies that serve as intermediate hosts. Habronema larvae escape from the mouthparts of these flies as they feed on wounds or around moist areas of the horse's body, especially the inner corners of the eyes and the male genitalia. To complete the cycle, the horse must swallow larvae or an infected fly.

In most cases stomach worm infection is asymptomatic. However, a large burden of worms can produce severe gastritis. One species of stomach worm produces tumorlike enlargements in the wall of the stomach. If one of these ruptures, fatal peritonitis ensues. This is rare. The most common problems with habronema are larval attacks directed at the skin (summer sores) and eyes (conjunctivitis).

Treatment: Fly control is important and will reduce the incidence of skin and eye infections. Ivermectin is effective against both the adult worms in the stomach and larvae in wounds and the eyes. A routine deworming program controls stomach worms.

Hairworms (Small Stomach Worms)

The small stomach worm *Trichostrongylus axei* infects cattle and horses. Horses grazed with cattle are more likely to develop an infection. The adult worm is small and slender, measuring less than half an inch (13 mm) long. It lives deep in the walls of the stomach. Severe infestation produces gastritis with ulcers, weight loss, and anemia. The diagnosis is difficult to make because the eggs of hairworms are similar to the eggs of strongyles.

Treatment: Routine deworming with ivermectin every eight weeks controls these worms.

Liver Flukes

Liver flukes are a parasite of ruminants, mostly of sheep and cattle, that may, rarely, infect horses. Liver flukes in horses have been reported in Australia and the United Kingdom. The intermediate hosts are snails found in wet streams and swampy areas. The horse is a dead-end host for these parasites, meaning that the flukes usually do not complete their life cycle in the horse. Because of this, the liver fluke may not develop eggs that can be detected in fecal examinations.

There are reports that liver fluke infestation and damage to your horse's liver may result in occasional diarrhea, loss of weight, anemia, and possibly *jaundice*.

Treatment: There are no parasiticides for liver flukes that are approved for use in horses. Two parasiticides not approved for use in horses that have been tried in Australia and the United Kingdom are oxyclozanide and triclabendazole. Albendazole has been used in the United States to treat liver flukes in cattle, but its use has been strictly regulated by state agriculture departments.

Controlling Internal Parasites

Because internal parasites are so ubiquitous and easily transmitted, it is not possible to rid horses of all internal parasites or to prevent reinfection. You should therefore assume that all horses are infested with worms. Deworming programs are primarily aimed at controlling bots and the large and small strongyles. In young foals, the aim is to control all these parasites, plus ascarids.

Deworming Agents (Anthelmintics)

The table on page 52 shows the currently recommended deworming agents and their effectiveness against common internal parasites. Most deworming agents can be divided into five principal classes according to their chemical structure and mode of action.

1. Benzimidazoles (BZDs)
2. Organophosphates
3. Piperazines
4. Carbamates
5. Avermectins

Benzimidazoles (BZDs) include mebendazole, thiabendazole, cambendazole, fenbendazole, oxfendazole, and oxibendazole. Febantel is a closely related compound that is altered in the horse's body to function as a benzimidazole. The benzimidazoles are highly effective against strongyles and pinworms. All but thiabendazole are excellent against ascarids. The benzimidazoles have a high margin of safety and can be given to foals and pregnant mares after the first trimester. This often makes them the drugs of choice for sick and stressed horses. However, the emergence of small strongyles that are resistant to BZDs has become a significant problem. Oxibendazole is the only BZD currently effective against small strongyles.

Organophosphates are represented by dichlorvos and trichlorfon. Dichlorvos is moderately effective against strongyles. Both are good to excellent against ascarids, pinworms, and bots. Organophosphates should not be used in combination with tranquilizers because of adverse reactions.

Organophosphates may be present in some insecticide preparations used on the horse, such as sprays, powders, or dips. Avoid using topical insecticides containing organophosphates within one to two weeks of deworming with an organophosphate, because there could be a buildup of chemicals resulting in toxicity (see *Poisoning*, page 21).

Organophosphates should not be given to foals under 4 months or to mares past mid-pregnancy.

Piperazine is excellent for ascarids. However, because it is a fast-acting agent, it should be avoided in horses with heavy infestations because of the danger of causing toxicity and worm impactions (see *Ascarids*, page 43).

Carbamates include pyrantel pamoate and pyrantel tartrate. Pyrantel has a wide margin of safety and, like the benzimidazoles, is preferred in foals, late-*gestation* mares, and sick or stressed horses. It is excellent against all the common worm parasites except bots. In addition, it is effective against tapeworms when given at twice the normal dosage. Many strongyle species that develop resistance to BZDs are responsive to pyrantel.

Avermectins, such as ivermectin and moxidectin, have a *broad spectrum* of activity against both internal and insect parasites and are effective against drug-resistant strongyles. The avermectins also kill migrating larvae. Avermectins should be included in all deworming programs because of their unique effectiveness against the tissue stages of large strongyles, ascarids, Onchocerca, and bots.

When choosing a product for its specificity and spectrum of activity, look for the active drugs listed on the label. Preparations containing the same drug carry different names when marketed by different companies. In addition, many proprietary deworming agents on the market include more than one class of drug.

Deworming Your Horse

In general, deworming agents can never be completely effective in ridding a horse of all parasites. There are several reasons. First is the continuing problem of reinfection. As a horse grazes on pasture, she automatically becomes reinfected by ingesting larvae present in grass and forages. Second, most dewormers (with the exception of ivermectin) attack only the adult worms in the intestinal tract. They do not kill and remove encysted larvae and stages migrating in the horse's tissues. This is especially true for strongyles, ascarids, and strongyloides. These larvae escape the drug and thus serve as a basis for further infection. Third, the development of drug-resistant worms is a continuing problem, especially in the case of the small strongyles that have become resistant to the benzimidazoles.

Therefore, to administer an effective deworming program, several important points should be considered.

- Deworm all horses on the premises at the same time. Little is accomplished if some horses are left untreated, since they will contaminate pastures and paddocks used by all.

- Deworm at regular intervals using one of the programs described in the next section. This has the advantage of achieving and maintaining low levels of infestation. It also avoids the danger of killing too many worms at one time and producing a large mass of deteriorating worms that can cause *toxemia* or bowel obstruction.

- The dewormer must be highly effective for the species in question and be used in the correct dosage. Dividing a dose between two horses means that neither receives an adequate dose. If the horse spits out some of the dewormer, many worms will survive and the horse will remain infected.

Deworming Agents

Drug	Bots	Habronemas	Ascarids	Strongyles	Threadworms	Pinworms	Tapeworms	Lungworms
Piperazine Used with BZDs against resistant small strongyles	No effect	No effect	Good	Good	No effect	No effect	No effect	No effect
Organophosphates Do not use past mid-pregnancy; do not use with insecticides or tranquilizers; narrow margin of safety								
Dichlorvos	Excellent	No effect	Good	Fair	No effect	Good	No effect	No effect
Trichlorfon	Excellent	No effect	Excellent	No effect	No effect	Excellent	No effect	No effect
Carbamates Safe and effective								
Pyrantel pamoate	No effect	Excellent	Excellent	Excellent	Excellent	Excellent	Fair	No effect
Pyrantel tartrate	No effect	No effect	Excellent	Excellent	No effect	Excellent	No effect	No effect
Benzimidazoles (BZDs) Do not use during first 3 months of pregnancy; resistant small strongyles an emerging problem								
Thiabendazole	No effect	Good	Fair	Excellent	Fair	Fair	No effect	No effect
Cambendazole	No effect	Excellent	Excellent	Excellent	Excellent	Excellent	No effect	No effect

Drug	Bots	Habronemas	Ascarids	Strongyles	Threadworms	Pinworms	Tapeworms	Lungworms
Mebendazole	No effect	Fair	Excellent	Excellent	Fair	Excellent	No effect	Good
Febendazole	No effect	Fair	Excellent	Excellent	Fair	Excellent	No effect	No effect
Oxfendazole	No effect	Excellent	Excellent	Excellent	Fair	Excellent	No effect	No effect
Oxibendazole	No effect	Excellent	Excellent	Excellent	Excellent	Excellent	No effect	No effect
Febantel (Pro-BZD)	No effect	Excellent	Excellent	Excellent	Good	Excellent	No effect	No effect
Avermectins Kills migrating larvae of most internal parasites; broad spectrum; no resistance								
Ivermectin*	Excellent	Excellent	Excellent	Excellent	Excellent	Excellent	No effect	Excellent
Moxidectin	Excellent	Excellent	Excellent	Excellent	Excellent	Excellent	No effect	Unknown
Praziquantel	No effect	No effect	No effect	No effect	No effect	No effect	Excellent	No effect

*Also effective against the filaria of Onchocerca, larvae of Habronema, and arterial larvae stages of strongyles.

- It is necessary to treat expectant mares to prevent foals from becoming overburdened with parasites shortly after birth. Deworming during pregnancy is discussed in *Care and Feeding During Pregnancy* (page 506).
- Read and understand the labels completely before using any dewormer. Be sure to follow all instructions for preparation and dosage. Above all, *do not overdose*. Anthelmintics are toxic.

Dewormers can be added to the feed, given by drench or stomach tube, or injected by syringe into the back of the horse's mouth (see *How to Give Medications*, page 596).

Deworming Programs

Three programs (interval, strategic, and daily) have proven effective in controlling internal parasites. Each has certain advantages when you are considering variables such as climate, geographic location, number and concentration of horses, convenience, expense, and history of parasite problems in the past. Because of the variables involved, it is important to include your veterinarian in the selection and implementation of the program.

Interval Deworming

Deworming at intervals is common. The standard interval is eight weeks or less, but varies according to local conditions and should be determined by fecal examinations performed every two weeks after a deworming. These examinations disclose the length of time that parasite eggs remain suppressed after treatment. In general, this interval is six to eight weeks in the central United States, with marked increases in fecal egg concentrations thereafter. When fecal egg concentrations rise sooner, choose a shorter deworming interval.

Interval deworming can be performed on a fast or a slow schedule. On a fast schedule, the deworming medication is changed each time it is given. By changing dewormers, the parasites are continually exposed to a new anthelmintic drug, thus preventing the development of resistance to a single drug.

Example of an Adult Fast Interval Deworming Schedule	
Month	**Dewormer**
January	Oxibendazole
March	Pyrantel pamoate
May	Oxibendazole
July	Avermectin
September	Pyrantel pamoate
November	Avermectin

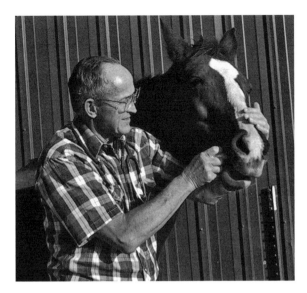

Paste dewormers are easy to give. Insert the syringe through the interdental space and depress the plunger. Many horses look forward to their "treat."

On a slow schedule, the same dewormer is used every two months for one to two years. In theory, drug-resistant worms should emerge when the dewormer is not rotated. In practice, drug-resistant worms do not develop if ivermectin is substituted once or twice every 12 months in place of the selected dewormer. In fact, since resistance to ivermectin has never been demonstrated, ivermectin itself can be used as the selected drug in a slow schedule.

Foals

It is important that selected dewormers be effective against ascarids, strongyles, bots, and threadworms. It is recommended that the first deworming be given at 2 months of age and subsequent treatments be given at two-month intervals thereafter. When the foal reaches 1 year of age, she can be placed on the same program as adult horses living on the premises.

Example of a Foal Interval Deworming Schedule	
Age	**Dewormer**
2 months	Avermectin
4 months	Pyrantel pamoate
6 months	Oxibendazole
8 months	Avermectin
10 months	Pyrantel pamoate
12 months	Oxibendazole

Alternately, ivermectin can be used every two months instead of rotating the drugs. Ivermectin and moxidectin have the broadest spectrum and they are safe.

On farms with threadworm problems, foals should be dewormed at 2 weeks of age with ivermectin, oxibendazole, or pyrantel pamoate. Mares harboring threadworms should be dewormed within 12 hours of *foaling*. This reduces milk-borne transmission and environmental contamination by larvae.

Strategic Deworming

This program is used at certain times of the year when fecal egg counts rise or during key seasons, such as spring and late fall. This program is designed for adult horses living in the north and central United States and Canada, and similar temperate climate zones. It controls parasites while reducing cost, labor, and the likelihood of producing drug-resistant worms.

The first dewormer is given in the spring before adult strongyle egg numbers begin to peak. The result is that there is less egg shedding, and therefore the transmission of worms during the grazing season is significantly reduced. In addition, a dewormer that is effective against bots, such as ivermectin or an organophosphate, should be given in the late fall or early winter, about one month after a hard freeze kills bot flies. Waiting one month ensures that all ingested bot larvae will have had time to reach the stomach. An additional bot treatment in midsummer is recommended.

Example of a Strategic Deworming Program	
Month	**Dewormer**
May	Oxibendazole
July	Avermectin
December	Avermectin

Continuous or Daily Deworming

In this program, the horse is fed pyrantel tartrate (2.64 mg per kilogram of body weight) in alfalfa pellets every day to control the adult intestinal forms of large and small strongyles, ascarids, and pinworms. Pyrantel tartrate does not kill tissue stages of these worms, but when given daily, it does kill larvae before they begin their tissue migration. This has great advantages for elderly and stressed horses, including competitive horses to avoid any loss of performance due to parasites, and in circumstances in which other methods have failed to reduce egg counts and numbers of infective larvae.

One other advantage of daily deworming is that as opposed to other programs, pyrantel tartrate does not have to be given to all horses on the premises to control worms in a single individual. This is advantageous for horses in boarding facilities and for farms where horses come and go frequently.

A potential drawback is the risk that feeding low levels of a dewormer will lead to the development of drug-resistant worms. However, this does not appear to be a problem with pyrantel tartrate, a dewormer to which no parasite has yet developed resistance.

Pyrantel tartrate does not kill bots. Accordingly, a boticide should be administered in midsummer and late fall.

Environmental Control of Internal Parasites

Environmental control of parasites is an integral part of an effective worm management program. To decrease exposure to worm larvae and eggs, implement the following steps:

- Remove manure and old bedding from stalls daily, and at regular intervals from corrals and paddocks. Dispose of it properly. Manure should be composted for one year before being used as fertilizer on pastures.

- Harrow pastures in hot, dry months to break up and spread horse manure.

- Feed hay or grain in cribs or mangers. Avoid feeding horses on the ground. Prevent horse manure from contaminating water troughs.

- Avoid overstocking and overgrazing pastures. Pastures that have been extensively grazed should not be restocked for 4 to 12 months, depending on seasonal influences. Note that larvae are killed rapidly in hot dry climates, less rapidly in cool damp climates, and least rapidly in cold climates.

- New arrivals should be dewormed with ivermectin and quarantined for three weeks before being introduced to resident horses. As soon as possible, put them on the same deworming program as other horses on the premises.

- Perform fecal examinations two or three times a year to monitor the effectiveness of the deworming program. Fecal exams should be performed 14 days after deworming. Horses on an effective deworming program should not be passing parasite eggs at 14 days. On large farms, monitoring 20 percent of the horses provides a representative sample.

External Parasites

Flies, mites, ticks, lice, gnats, and mosquitoes are common external parasites that can irritate and even injure a horse. Many also present a health problem because they carry disease. Most of them are blood-sucking. A heavy infestation can cause dermatitis, failure to thrive, anemia, and, in severe cases, even death.

Flies

All flies pass through four stages of development: egg, larva (or maggot), pupa, and adult. This can occur in a few weeks, but some species take a year to complete their life cycle.

The nonbiting flies (housefly and face fly) feed on secretions from the eyes, nose, and mouth, and on open wounds often produced by the bites of other insects. Bot flies, which lay their eggs on the hair of the horse, have no functional mouth parts and do not bite, as commonly believed. The biting flies (stable fly, horsefly, deer fly, and horn fly) are bloodsuckers, as are most species of the gnat or black fly.

Housefly and Stable Fly

These flies lay eggs in manure piles and decomposed plant debris, including hay and bedding. They feed primarily during the day. At night, they roost on nearby vegetation or on the rafters of barns and stables. These species carry diseases that include equine infectious anemia, anthrax, and summer sores.

Houseflies feed on secretions from the eyes, nose, and mouth. As such, they are capable of transmitting contagious conjunctivitis and eyeworms. The bites of the stable fly produce skin lumps covered by black scabs, which are called external parasitic nodules. These painful nodules are made worse by rubbing and biting at the skin.

For control on the premises, residual insecticide surface sprays, quick-kills using space sprays or foggers, and fly baits are effective.

For control on the horse, use an insecticide hand wash or direct mist spray. Effective chemicals include pyrethrins and piperonyl butoxide. Apply to the

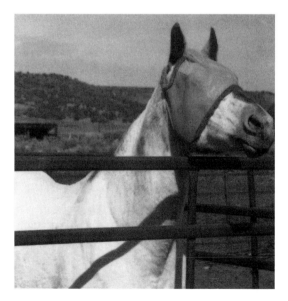

Face masks prevent conjunctivitis caused by flies feeding on eye secretions.

head, neck, chest, withers, and abdomen. To control the stable fly, also apply to the lower body and legs. Repeat the applications at least every other day. Feed supplements containing stirofos can be given to kill fly larvae that hatch in the manure.

Face masks are effective exclusion devices. They are especially useful if the flies are causing conjunctivitis.

Face Fly and Horn Fly

These flies breed only in cow manure and therefore attack horses pastured near cattle. The face fly produces intense irritation as it feeds on mucus secretions from the mouth, nostrils, and eyes. It is a vector for eyeworms and transmits a contagious form of conjunctivitis. Face flies feed for a limited time and are difficult to control.

Face masks are effective exclusion devices. Plastic strips impregnated with an insecticide and fitted to the halter may help protect the face. Better control can be achieved by using an insecticide wipe-on. Apply to the face, muzzle, and around the eyes daily.

The biting horn fly is relatively easy to control with residual insecticide sprays applied at intervals stated on the product label. A light spray to the shoulders, neck, and withers usually is sufficient.

Horsefly and Deer Fly

Horseflies and deer flies are incessant biters. The bites are painful, result in blood loss, open the way to screwworm attacks, and may become infected. In addition, horseflies are the vectors for more than 35 horse diseases, including equine infectious anemia. Vicious attacks can make the horse unmanageable and lead to escape activities such as running and kicking.

These flies lay their eggs in leaves and moist soil around the edges of ponds and ditches and in wooded areas. The breeding source is difficult to control, but stabling is effective because it removes the horse from the fly's locale. Most species of horsefly and deer fly will not enter stables.

Control on the horse is like that described for the stable fly (page 58). The insecticide used should be labeled as effective against the horsefly. Two such insecticides are resmethrin with cyclopropane carboxylate and tetramethrin. Frequent application of a repellent is often the most practical solution.

Blowfly and Screwworm Fly

These flies deposit their eggs in open wounds such as those produced by castration, trauma, and the bites of other insects. The navel stump of the newborn is a favored site. The eggs develop into maggots.

Maintain good wound care, as described in *Wounds* (page 35). Apply a dust or aerosol spray containing coumaphos into and around an open healing wound once a week.

Gnats

There are many species of gnat. The most common bloodsucking species are the buffalo gnat (black fly) and the "no-see-ums" (Culicoides). Some species spread vesicular stomatitis. Black flies secrete a toxin capable of causing cardiac and respiratory *depression*. Swarm attacks have been known to cause death. Breeding sources are so variable that source control is impractical. Peak gnat activity occurs at twilight, at night, and at dawn.

Gnats are highly irritating to horses and initiate head-tossing, ear-twitching, skin-twitching, and incessant biting or rubbing. The ears are favorite sites for attack. Bites caused by gnats ooze serum and form scabs or blisters. The skin may become sensitized by repeated attacks. This leads to dermatitis and hair loss.

To control gnats on the horse, apply insect repellents and insecticides containing pyrethrins with piperonyl butoxide, resmethrin with cyclopropane carboxylate, or tetramethrin daily. Be sure to get the product well spread on the inside edges of both ears. Petroleum jelly, a menthol rub, and Cut-Heal similarly applied are safe to use within the ears to protect the skin. Ear nets are especially useful for protection against gnats. Stabling horses before sunset is helpful.

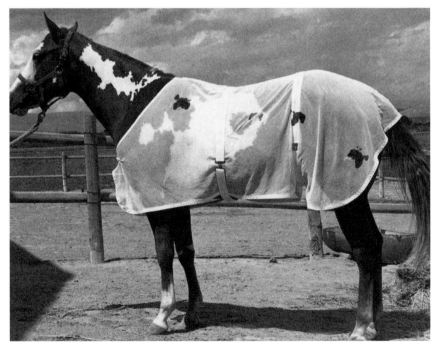

A light nylon covering helps to protect the body from stable flies, houseflies, and other incessant biters.

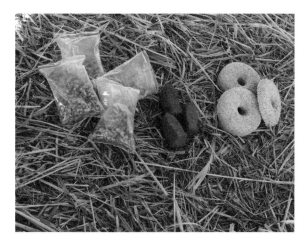

Different varieties of mosquito control are safe to use in your horse's water supply; some are biological and some are chemical, and they come in a variety of forms. It is important to check the label to make sure they are non-toxic to fish and safe for livestock.

Mosquitoes

Mosquitoes are of particular importance because they transmit Eastern, Western, and Venezuelan equine encephalomyelitis, and West Nile virus. Some horses are unusually sensitive to mosquito bites and can develop an allergic dermatitis.

Mosquitoes lay their eggs directly on water. Common breeding grounds include ponds, horse troughs, drainage ditches, and water puddles. Control of breeding areas depends largely on eliminating standing water. Although spraying for mosquitoes by aircraft can be most effective, it is not very practical for the average horse owner. There are many commercial larvicides available that are safe for livestock and are nontoxic to fish. These can simply be added to the water source to eliminate a breeding ground for mosquitoes. The most common active ingredient in these products is *Bacillus thuringiensis ssp. israelensis* or *methoprene*.

The most active mosquito feeding period is the first two hours after sunset. Stabling before sunset and applying repellents and insecticides as described for gnats (page 60) are the most effective forms of control. Since mosquitoes are poor flyers, barn fans may prevent mosquitoes from landing.

Lice

There are two species of lice that infect the horse. Biting lice feed only on skin scales. Sucking lice feed on the horse's blood. When present in large numbers, they can cause severe anemia, weight loss, roughened haircoat, and growth retardation in young horses. Horse lice are species-specific. They are rapidly transmitted from horse to horse but do not attack people.

Adult lice are pale-colored insects about 2 to 3 millimeters long and can be seen by parting the hair in sites of skin involvement. They lay eggs (called nits), which look like white grains of sand attached to the hair shafts. Nits are difficult to brush off. Inspection with a magnifying glass makes identification easy. Mane hair is a good place to look for lice. Adult lice cause intense itching. The most commonly involved sites are the head, face, ears, neck, back (topline), and the area around the base of the tail. As the horse rubs, bites, and scratches at the irritation, there is traumatic loss of hair and scabs and sores develop on the skin. Infestation is more common in winter than in summer.

Lice are sensitive to a number of topical insecticides, including permethrins. Retreat in two weeks to kill new lice hatching from residual eggs. Blankets, halters, saddles, and other accessories may harbor lice or nits. Wash thoroughly or rub on a pesticide solution. Retreat articles in two weeks. The oral dewormer ivermectin kills lice on the horse. The dose is 0.2 mg per kilogram of body weight. Repeat in 14 days.

Chiggers

Chiggers, also called red bugs, are the larvae of a mite that uses birds, reptiles, and rodents as the primary host. In the absence of a natural host, they will attack horses. A heavy infestation causes intense itching, rubbing, and biting, with traumatic skin damage, especially on the head, neck, chest, and legs. Repellents and residual insecticides afford some protection.

Chiggers can be controlled in the pasture using a pesticide wash containing coumaphos or malathion. A single application to the pasture is sufficient. Wait one month before putting your horse back into a chigger-infested pasture.

Ticks

Ticks are found in nearly all parts of the country and are especially prevalent in spring and fall. Horses are most likely to acquire ticks at pasture, after trail rides, and when transported long distances.

The male tick is a small, flat insect about the size of a match head. A "blood" tick is a female tick, about the size of a pea, feeding on the horse. Ticks can be found anywhere on the horse, but many species prefer the ears (see *Ear Ticks*, page 172). Always check the inside and outside of the ear flaps after the horse has been any place ticks might be present.

Horse ticks have a complicated life cycle. Some species use three hosts, including wild and domestic animals and humans. Most ticks remain on the horse throughout their lives, where they feed and mate. It takes about one year to complete the life cycle.

Diseases transmitted by ticks include Lyme disease, equine piroplasmosis, equine ehrlichiosis, and tick-bite paralysis. Tick bites predispose the horse to screwworm attacks. A heavy infestation can cause anemia.

Treatment: Ticks that are not attached to the skin are easily removed with a pair of tweezers. There are also special tick removing devices that are widely available, including Ticked Off, Protick Remedy, and Tick Nipper. Once removed, the tick can be killed by putting it in rubbing alcohol.

You must be careful if you find a tick with its head buried in the skin, because the head may detach and remain behind. Grasp the tick firmly with tweezers or a tick removal device, as close to the horse's body as possible without pinching her skin, and lift it off. A drop of alcohol or nail polish applied to the tick may cause it to release its hold.

Ticks carry diseases dangerous to humans. Accordingly, do not squeeze or crush a tick with your bare fingers. Use the tweezers to place the tick in a jar or plastic dish with a little alcohol, seal it well and dispose of the container in an outdoor garbage can. Don't flush it down the toilet, because the tick will survive the trip and infect another animal. Wash the tweezers thoroughly with hot water and alcohol.

If the head or mouth parts remain embedded in the skin, redness and swelling is likely to occur at the site of the bite. In most cases, this reaction clears up in two to three days. A dab of antibiotic ointment will help prevent most skin infections. However, if it does not—or if the redness seems to be getting worse—consult your veterinarian.

When many ticks are present, apply a topical insecticide (pyrethrin) or administer ivermectin paste as described in *Lice* (page 61). Retreat in seven days.

Prevention: For outdoor control, cut tall grass, weeds, and brush. Treat the premises with an insecticide. Spraying the horse with a garden hose at high pressure after trail rides will remove many ticks before they can attach. Insecticides and repellents labeled as effective against ticks can be applied liberally to the legs and underside to prevent ticks from getting and staying on the horse. Apply before riding in tick-infested areas and again post ride.

Controlling External Parasites

To prevent parasites on the horse, it is necessary to reduce their number by attacking them in the stable and on the premises. It is also helpful to provide insect protection by applying or administering appropriate repellents and insecticides.

Insecticides and Repellents

Pesticides recommended for use on horses and in the barn or stable include pyrethrins (natural and synthetic), organophosphates, organochlorides, insect growth regulators, synergists, and repellents. In addition, the oral deworming agent ivermectin can be used to kill lice, mites, and ticks feeding on the skin of the horse. Whatever product you use, it is important to follow the product directions and be aware that adverse reactions may occur when several products are used together.

Pyrethrin, a natural extract of the African chrysanthemum flower, kills quickly but has little residual activity because it is rapidly degraded in the environment by ultraviolet light. Pyrethrin has a low potential for toxicity and is considered among the safest of insecticides. It is found in many shampoos, sprays, dusts, dips, foggers, and premise sprays.

Pyrethroids are synthetic compounds that resemble pyrethrin in structure but are more stable in sunlight and therefore have longer residual activity. Permethrin is a commonly used synergized pyrethrin. That means the insecticidal effects of natural and synthetic pyrethrins are enhanced and amplified when combined with piperonyl butoxide and N-octyl bicycloheptene dicarbomide, which work by inhibiting the insect's own enzymes.

Organophosphate insecticides are unstable and do not persist long in the environment. They are among the most toxic to mammals. Coumaphos, malathion, stirofos, and dichlorvas (DDVP) are incorporated into products for use on horses. To avoid toxicity, it is important to use them exactly as directed by the manufacturer.

Insect growth regulators (IGRs), such as methoprene (PreCor) and fenoxycarb, are hormonelike compounds that prevent larvae from developing into adults. They do not affect the cocoon or adult stages. Both are degraded by sunlight and are therefore used mainly for indoor treatment. Methoprene is used in foggers and premise sprays alone or in combination with pyrethrins or organophosphates to kill both eggs and adults.

Synergists are compounds such as piperonyl butoxide and MGK 264 that can act alone but are frequently are added to commercial insecticide preparations to enhance the total effectiveness of the product.

Repellents keep bugs away but do not kill them. In many cases, using repellents is the easiest and most convenient way of offering protection from fly species and mosquitoes. Butoxypolypropylene glycol (BPG) and dipropyl isochinchomeronate are examples of repellents commonly used on horses. To be effective, repellents must be applied at least once a day.

Control on Horses

A number of insecticides are safe and effective for use on horses and aid in the control of external parasites. To be effective, some insecticides must be applied daily during peak insect season. However, too-frequent application can lead to toxicity. For this reason, the pyrethrins and permethrins, having the widest margin of safety, are often the best choices for frequent application.

Topical insecticides can be applied using one of several methods, including hand washing the horse with a sponge, misting or spraying, and dusting or powdering. To ensure safety and effectiveness, follow the manufacturer's recommendations for preparation, dosage, and route of administration.

Some horse dewormers contain chemicals similar to those found in topical insecticides. Using one of these shortly after deworming could lead to a toxic accumulation. As a precaution, do not use a topical insecticide of the same class as the dewormer within two weeks of deworming.

With most topical insecticides, the effects are transient. Daily application will be necessary to maintain protection. An exception is a product with a pour-on application of a long-lasting permethrin, which lasts up to a week with a single application. Poridon is one brand of this product. It is a thick, viscous material that hardens to a flexible film. It contains an ingredient that causes the insecticide to migrate out of the film and move down the coat from one hair to the next. Eventually, a large area of the coat is covered with the product. Apply 3 to 4 ounces (90 to 120 ml) down the middle of the horse's back from the poll to the base of the tail. The product can be applied on the face as a bead line from the forehead to the nose (avoid contact with the eyes), and as a line down the front or back of the legs. This product works especially well during the bot fly season. It is effective against all species of flies, mosquitoes, and Culicoides gnats. It will not discolor the hair or irritate the skin. It is not absorbed through the skin and is safe to use on pregnant mares. Specific insect parasites and how to control them are discussed in *External Parasites* (page 57).

Premise Control

This can be accomplished by mechanical methods such as barn fans (which help prevent flying insects from landing on the horses) or chemical methods. One mechanical method used in stables, barns, and indoor enclosures is the electronic bug-killer. Since flies roost at night, the bug-killer is only effective against mosquitoes and gnats. The apparatus must be installed carefully and placed out of reach of horses. Flypaper strips attract and capture flies. However, they usually do not significantly affect the fly population.

Manure attracts flies and is an excellent breeding ground for insect parasites. *A well-planned manure disposal system is essential.* If manure must be stockpiled before being taken away, store it well away from horse facilities.

Chemical control methods are effective and should be used routinely. Many chemical companies provide insecticide products for use in stables and barns. Study the label to determine the product's effectiveness and safety. To ensure effective control, prepare and apply the product according to the instructions on the label. Do not use insecticide products on horses unless they are specifically recommended for that purpose. Many of these products

Compounds Commonly Used to Control External Parasites

Compound	Action	Application	Deer fly, horsefly	Lice	Stable fly, horn fly, house flies	Screwfly	Tick	Chigger	Blowfly	Gnat	Mosquito
Butoxypolypropylene glycol (BPG)	Repellant	Topical repellant	No	No	No	No	No	No	No	No	No
Coumaphos	Insecticide	Topical repellant	No	No	No	Yes (both fly and larvae)	No	No	Yes, both fly and larvae	No	No
Dipropyl isochinchomeronate	Repellant	Topical repellant	No	No	No	No	No	No	No	No	No
IGRs Stirofos (Raybon)	Prevents larvae from hatching	Must be fed and passed through the feces	No	No	Yes	No	No	No	No	Yes	No
Methoprene	Prevents larvae from hatching	In feed or lick, or added to water sources	No	No	No	No	No	No	No	No	Yes
B. thuringiensis	Prevents larvae from hatching	Added to water sources	No	No	No	No	No	No	No	No	Yes
Ivermectin	Insecticide	Oral	No	Yes	No	No	Yes	No	No	No	No
Malathion	Insecticide	Pasture spray	No	No	No	No	No	Yes	No	No	No
Pyrethrins with piperonyl butoxide	Insecticide	Topical repellant	No	No	Yes	No	Yes	No	No	No	Yes
Resmethrine with cyclopropane Permethrin Cymectrin	Insecticide	Topical repellant	Yes	Yes	Yes	Yes	No	No	No	Yes	Yes

should not be inhaled, ingested, or come in contact with the skin and eyes. Familiarize yourself with the signs of insecticide toxicity and be prepared to treat accordingly (see *Insecticide Poisoning,* page 25).

The major insect problem in horse stables and barns is flies. For fly control, residual insecticide surface sprays provide long-term killing action. Permethrin and cypermethrin sprays kill stable flies for six to eight weeks. Space sprays provide a quick knockdown. They can be sprayed directly on resting flies or used as mists or fogs. Try to time the spray or fog with the daily pattern of fly activity. These products are sprayed to the point of drip run-off on surfaces where flies roost. Remove all horses before spraying.

Pyrethrins and permethrins are used in space sprays, which are applied in closed-in areas. Remove all horses before spraying.

Dichlorvos (0.46 percent granules) is a fly bait that can be sprinkled on the ground or on wet sacking. One pound (453 g) added to 1 gallon (3.8 l) of water makes a liquid spray. Other fly baits are commercially available but can be extremely toxic to horses and must be used with caution to prevent accidental ingestion.

Stirofos is an organophosphate insecticide present in certain commercial larvicides, including Endrol and Equitrol. When added daily to the horse's feed, stirofos kills horsefly and stable fly larvae hatching in the manure. It does not control horn or face fly larvae, which develop only in fresh cow manure. If the horse is a finicky eater, start by feeding her small amounts and build up to the amount recommended on the label.

Fly predators are tiny parasitic wasps that do not sting or bite, so they aren't a pest themselves. They attack immature forms of flies, including the house fly, horn fly, and stable fly, where these flies breed, usually on or near manure. For fly predators to be effective, several conditions must be met:

- Fly predators must be released ahead of the first fly hatch.
- Flies reproduce nine times faster than the fly predators, so the fly predators must be supplemented every three or four weeks during the warm months for good fly control.
- Do not combine a predator program with indiscriminate pesticide spraying, because the fly predators are susceptible and will be killed. However, repellants on the horse, baits, and traps, and the use of selective area spraying, is encouraged.
- The whole farm must be treated, and not just the areas the horse frequents.

No program can give 100 percent fly control, but good manure control and a combination of treatments and controls can greatly reduce the fly population on your property.

3

INFECTIOUS DISEASES

Infectious diseases are caused by bacteria, viruses, protozoans, fungi, and rickettsia, all of which invade the body of a susceptible host and cause illness. Most infectious diseases are transmitted from one animal to another by contact with infected urine, feces, and other bodily secretions or by inhaling *pathogen*-laden droplets in the air. A few are sexually transmitted. Others are acquired by contact with spores or bacteria in the soil, which get into the body through the respiratory tract or a break in the skin. A number of infectious diseases are transmitted by insects and ticks; a few are blood-borne and can be transmitted by poor husbandry techniques.

Although pathogens exist everywhere in the environment, only a few cause *infection*. Fewer still are contagious. Many infectious diseases are species-specific. For example, a dog cannot catch a disease that is specific to a horse, and vice versa. In a few instances, a disease is *zoonotic*, meaning it can be passed to humans from animals, or to animals from humans.

Many infectious agents are able to survive for long periods outside the host animal. This knowledge is important in determining how to contain the spread of infection. For many diseases, the best way to prevent them is by vaccination and environmental management. Immunity and vaccinations are discussed at the end of this chapter.

Bacterial Diseases

Bacteria are single-celled microorganisms. Although some are beneficial to the body, many are noted for their ability to cause disease. Bacteria may also release *exotoxins* or *endotoxins* into the body. Exotoxins are toxic proteins produced by the bacteria and released into their environment. Endotoxins are part of the outer cell wall of bacteria and are released when the cell membranes rupture.

Salmonellosis

Salmonellosis is the most common cause of infectious diarrhea in the adult horse and an important cause of *septicemia* in *foals*. For a discussion of salmonella bacterial *enteritis* in newborns, see page 557. This is a zoonotic disease.

Many species of salmonella are infectious to horses, although the majority of cases are caused by *Salmonella typhimurium* and *Salmonella newport*. Salmonella are remarkably resistant to environmental factors and remain alive for months or years in soil and manure. Adult horses become infected by ingesting bacteria present in feed and water. Once the number of bacteria in the environment reaches a critical threshold, outbreaks of infection occur and may reach epidemic proportions. The seriousness of the illness is related to the size of the bacterial population. With a small number of bacteria, infection may be asymptomatic.

Adult salmonellosis occurs as an acute illness and as a chronic intermittent diarrhea. Horses who recover can later become symptomatic or can be asymptomatic carriers.

The acute diarrhea is called enteric salmonellosis. This is a severe inflammation of the small and large colon, often complicated by toxicity related to the absorption of bacterial *endotoxins*. The onset is sudden, with high fever and *colic* and a foul-smelling, watery, green to brown diarrhea. The horse becomes intensely ill and rapidly dehydrates. Death can occur within twelve hours. There are atypical cases in which the only symptoms are fever, colic, and mild diarrhea.

Stressed horses are most susceptible to enteric salmonellosis. Common stresses include hard training, deworming, pregnancy, overcrowding, hot weather, illness, surgery (especially in the abdomen), prolonged transport during which food and water are withheld, and antibiotics that alter the intestinal flora.

Horses who recover from the diarrhea may shed salmonella in their manure for several weeks or longer. These asymptomatic shedders generally pass small numbers of bacteria and do not appear to pose a threat to healthy horses. Many adult horses become carriers and do not show clinical signs or become contagious until a stressful situation arises.

There are also chronic long-term bacteria shedders. Some of them suffer from chronic intermittent diarrhea and pass watery or "cow pie" stools. Episodes of diarrhea are usually triggered by stress. During such episodes, these symptomatic shedders pose a threat to other horses.

Salmonella are difficult to recover on stool examination. At least five negative stool *cultures* are required to exclude the diagnosis. In horses with chronic diarrhea, at least fifteen negative stool cultures are required. Tissue culture of the colon obtained by rectal *biopsy* is more accurate and should be used along with multiple stool cultures to diagnose chronic diarrhea.

Treatment: Salmonella rapidly develop resistance to antibiotics, which renders antibiotic treatment to control the diarrhea largely ineffective. However, antibiotic therapy can be useful to prevent septicemia in a severely ill horse. Endoserum, an *antiserum* that contains high levels of anti-endotoxin antibodies, can be given intravenously and has been shown to provide some protection against the effects of the endotoxin.

The most important objective in treating infectious diarrhea is to correct the deleterious effects of dehydration and electrolyte and protein losses. This is accomplished with intravenous electrolyte solutions and plasma. Large volumes are often required.

The anti-inflammatory drug flunixin meglumine (Banamine) is also given to mitigate the effects of the endotoxin. DMSO is used for its antioxidant effects. Both drugs are given intravenously.

Prevention: Isolate infected horses in an area distant from other horses. All personnel who come in contact with infected horses should wear rubber gloves, outer protective clothing, and rubber boots, which should be left in the isolation area. Wash your hands thoroughly with disinfectant soap. Change out of your protective outer clothing and boots before leaving the isolation area. Extreme care must be taken to avoid contaminating food intended for people. *Salmonella typhimurium* is a leading cause of epidemic outbreaks of food poisoning. It is estimated that several thousand people are hospitalized and nearly a thousand people die in the United States of salmonella food poisoning each year.

To control the spread of bacteria, thoroughly clean and disinfect the isolation area. Remove all manure and organic material. Clean barns and stalls with a hot steam spray or use an iodine-based disinfectant. A solution containing phenol (carbolic acid), such as Kerol disinfectant, or an aldehyde solution can be effective, provided that all organic material is first removed from the premises.

Contaminated pastures should not be used by horses for one year.

Proliferative Enteropathy

Proliferative enteropathy is an infectious disease of foals and weanlings caused by the bacteria *Lawsonia intracellularis*. It is transmissible between animals and causes severe weight loss and diarrhea. See *Proliferative Enteropathy* (page 558) for more information.

Strangles

Strangles is a severe acute upper respiratory and throat infection caused by the bacteria *Streptococcus equi* subspecies *equi*. The disease is named for the noise the horse makes when there is an exceptional amount of *purulent* discharge in the nose and nasopharynx. Strangles is transmitted from one horse to another by infective secretions and by contaminated feed, watering troughs, stalls, and horse equipment. In newborns, *Streptococcus equi* subspecies *equi* is a cause of foal septicemia.

Strangles generally occurs in horses 1 to 5 years of age. Symptoms appear two to six days after exposure. The illness begins with a nasal (and sometimes eye) discharge; at first it is watery and mucuslike, and later becomes thick, yellow, and purulent. This is accompanied by a dry, painful cough. The horse may have a fever up to 104°F (40°C).

During the next 10 to 14 days, an untreated horse develops large, swollen, tender lymph nodes high in the neck behind the lower jaw (submandibular adenopathy) and at the back of the throat (retropharyngeal adenopathy). Swallowing is painful. The horse often stands with his head held down and his neck stretched out.

After a few days, the lymph nodes in the neck soften, break down, and discharge a thick, creamy *pus*. The fever breaks and the horse begins to feel better. The draining neck wounds heal slowly with scarring.

Occasionally, an *abscessed* lymph node in the retropharyngeal area drains internally and infects the guttural pouches and sinuses. From these sites, the horse may repeatedly inhale infected secretions, resulting in bronchopneumonia.

Signs that the guttural pouch may be infected include difficult and painful swallowing, shortness of breath, a purulent nasal discharge, and excessive salivation. A retropharyngeal abscess may damage the nerves at the back of the pharynx, paralyzing the swallowing muscles or the muscles of the face and ears. The diagnosis of retropharyngeal abscess is made by soft tissue X-rays of the neck, by *endoscopy*, and by *ultrasound*.

A well-recognized complication of *Streptococcus equi* infection is the spread (via the bloodstream) of bacteria to other parts of the body, particularly to the lymph nodes of the intestines, and also to the liver, kidneys, spleen, heart, and brain. This syndrome is called bastard strangles. It is characterized by weight loss, episodes of *colic*, and a general decline in health despite treatment.

Purpura hemorrhagica, an uncommon sequel to strangles, is characterized by a purplish discoloration of the mucous membranes caused by capillary bleeding. The bleeding appears one to three weeks after the onset of illness. It is accompanied by labored breathing and swelling of the head, belly, and limbs. The mortality rate varies.

Treatment: Strangles must be treated by a veterinarian. It is important to confirm the diagnosis. This is done by taking smears and cultures of infected discharges. Encourage draining of abscessed lymph nodes by applying warm Epsom salt poultices. Abscesses that do not drain on their own should be drained surgically when they are fluid-filled and soft.

Horses with strangles should be isolated from other horses and kept in a warm, dry stall. Good nursing care is important. Wrap their legs. Feed a soft diet such as soaked pellets or chopped wet hay. Fresh water should be available at all times and the horse should be encouraged to drink. Clean the nostrils to remove thick secretions.

Penicillin is effective against *Streptococcus equi*, but the timing of antibiotic administration is important. In the early stages, before the lymph nodes enlarge, high doses of penicillin G procaine will stop the disease. However, when antibiotics are started after the lymph nodes enlarge (a condition called *lymphadenopathy*), they appear to delay drainage and may even cause an abscess to drain internally. However, in a severely ill horse, high doses of penicillin G procaine should be given regardless of whether lymphadenopathy has developed, and should be continued throughout the course of the illness, including at least five days beyond the development of the last abscess.

Bastard strangles and purpura hemorrhagica require hospitalization and intensive veterinary management. Purpura hemorrhagica may be treated with corticosteroids administered with intravenous fluids.

Prevention: Strict hygiene is important. *Streptococcus equi* bacteria can remain infective for up to one year. Scrub and disinfect or steam-sterilize the premises as described in *Salmonellosis* (page 69).

A vaccine against strangles is available, but its usefulness is questionable. The immunity that follows vaccination (as well as the immunity that follows natural infection) is short-lived. Outbreaks of strangles have occurred on farms where horses have been vaccinated in strict accordance with the manufacturer's directions. Furthermore, vaccines have been associated with abscess at the injection site, as well as fever and other reactions. The M-protein vaccines,

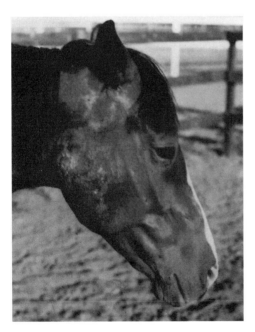

Abscesses in the submandibular area are typical of strangles.

which are derived from a certain protein on the cell of the *Streptococcus* bacterium, appear to cause the fewest reactions. There is also a live attenuated vaccine that can be given *intranasally*.

Vaccination is currently recommended on farms where strangles is *endemic*, and for horses visiting such farms. It is especially important to protect newborn foals. This is accomplished by vaccinating mares in late pregnancy and foals beginning at 8 weeks of age (see the table on page 103).

Clostridial Infections

Several species of Clostridia produce disease in horses. They are also all zoonotic. The bacteria or their spores are found in soil contaminated by horse and cow manure and are present in the intestinal tracts of most animals, where they do not normally cause illness.

All clostridial species produce powerful exotoxins. These lethal toxins are responsible for the major effects of the illness. Botulism, caused by *Clostridium botulinum*, is discussed on page 431.

Tetanus (Lockjaw)

This disease affects almost all animals, including humans. It is caused by *Clostridium tetani*; it is not contagious. Horses are more susceptible to tetanus than are other domestic animals because horses have less natural immunity and are subject to many types of injuries that enable the bacteria to thrive. There is considerable variation in the signs and symptoms of equine tetanus. Death is not inevitable. Some horses experience a mild illness and recover with treatment.

Tetanus infections occur in wounds where the oxygen content is low. The ideal environment is a deep puncture wound that has sealed over. The rusty nail injury is the classic example, but any cut or injury can serve as an entry portal. Wounds of castration and docking are quite prone to tetanus infection, as are wounds of the soles of the feet. Bacteria in infected wounds produce a potent neurotoxin that is transmitted along nerves and ascends to the spinal cord. The toxin is also absorbed locally and carried by the bloodstream to the brain.

Symptoms of tetanus can appear as early as one week after injury, but may be delayed for several weeks. There will be a wound, but often it is difficult to locate. Early signs include colic and vague stiffness. They are followed by spasms in the jaw, neck, hind limbs, and the muscles around the wound. A characteristic sign is the appearance of a film over the inner third of the eyes—*protrusion* of the third eyelid. This sign, when present along with the other signs described, is considered diagnostic of tetanus. The protrusion is best seen when the horse is excited or is tapped under the chin.

As the disease worsens, the horse develops labored breathing. Stiffness develops in the front and rear legs, causing the horse to adopt a sawhorse stance with his neck stretched out and his head extended. The tail is held out stiffly (known as pump-handle tail), the ears are erect, and the nostrils are flared. He has great difficulty in backing or turning. The jaw muscles contract so that the horse is unable to open his mouth or swallow (which is where the name "lockjaw" originated). Food and water dribble from the mouth. In the final stage the horse goes down, assumes an arched appearance, and dies of respiratory paralysis. This sequence is characteristic of fatal tetanus. However, not all horses progress to *recumbency*.

Treatment: Early surgical treatment of the wound is critical in stopping the progress of the disease. This involves opening the wound widely, removing all devitalized tissue, irrigating thoroughly, injecting penicillin into the wound, and leaving the wound open for effective drainage. High doses of intravenous penicillin are routinely used. Tetanus *antitoxin*, tranquilizers, muscle relaxants, intravenous fluids, and skilled nursing in a veterinary hospital alter the course for the better. If the horse survives more than seven days, the outlook for recovery is good.

Prevention: Cleanse and dress all fresh wounds as described in *Wounds* (page 35). This will prevent most cases of tetanus.

Immunize all foals and adult horses as described in the table on page 100. (Also see *Special Circumstances*, page 99, for when to use tetanus antitoxin as a preventive.) To heighten immunity and maximize protection for the newborn foal, pregnant mares should be given a tetanus booster three to six weeks before *foaling*.

Malignant Edema (Gas Gangrene)

Malignant *edema* is a rare, frequently fatal soft tissue infection caused by *Clostridium septicum*. Like tetanus, malignant edema occurs in unclean wounds, particularly those caused by sharp objects. Common sites are cuts about the feet and legs. In these areas there is less muscle and more connective tissue, which appears to favor the spread of the infection. It also occurs in wounds of castration. It has been known to follow intramuscular injections.

Signs appear within one to two days. There is pronounced swelling and sometimes gas in the tissues. A blood-tinged, gelatinous fluid oozes from the wound.

Other signs of malignant edema are caused by absorption of exotoxins. These signs include high fever, *depression*, progressive swelling of the head or legs, difficulty breathing, and death.

Treatment: Early surgical treatment of the wound, as described for *Tetanus* (page 73), is essential. Antibiotics are routinely used. Intravenous fluids, steroids, and blood transfusions may be indicated to limit the spread of the infection and to treat *shock* and septicemia.

Prevention: Prevention of the disease is like that described for *Ulcerative Lymphangitis* (page 76).

Intestinal Clostridiosis (Perfrigens)

Intestinal clostridiosis is a severe, often fatal, acute colitis caused by the bacteria *Clostridium perfringens*, normally present in small numbers in the colon of healthy horses. The symptoms are like those of enteric salmonellosis, colitis X, and Potomac horse fever. It is difficult to tell these four diseases apart.

Signs and symptoms of intestinal clostridiosis are caused by an exotoxin produced by the bacteria. The onset is sudden, with pronounced listlessness and apathy, high fever, rapid pulse, and explosive diarrhea that is watery, dark, and foul-smelling. The horse moves with difficulty and usually lies down. Shock and dehydration are important early signs. Tremendous quantities of fluid and *electrolytes* are lost in the diarrhea.

Treatment: Immediately notify your veterinarian if your horse has large-volume diarrhea. A stool smear may reveal high numbers of *Clostridium perfringens*. This helps make an early diagnosis. In any case, cultures should be taken to identify conclusively the cause of the diarrhea. Large volumes of intravenous fluid therapy are essential. Penicillin in high doses is effective when started before shock and collapse.

Flunixin meglumine (Banamine) has anti-exotoxic and anti-endotoic effects that reduce inflammation. *Clostridium perfringens* antitoxins for types C and D are available, although most cases of intestinal clostridiosis are caused by type A. Maintain strict hygienic precautions to prevent human exposure.

Prevention: Long-term use of the antibiotic tetracycline has been associated with some cases of intestinal clostridiosis. Tetracycline should not be used for prolonged periods if another suitable antibiotic is available.

Colitis X

Colitis X is a toxic disease of the cecum and large colon that produces severe, watery diarrhea and *shock*. It occurs in adult horses and is usually fatal.

It has been suggested that colitis X is a form of intestinal clostridiosis or salmonellosis in which bacteria, for reasons unknown, cannot be cultured. A stressful event (surgery, hard training, transport, or deworming), or the administration of the antibiotics lincomycin or tetracycline, often precedes the outbreak of diarrhea. However, colitis X can occur in horses who have not been stressed and who are in all other respects entirely healthy.

Signs include sudden pain in the abdomen accompanied by an explosive, watery, and sometimes bloody diarrhea. Shock and collapse occur rapidly. The horse often dies in a matter of hours.

Colitis X is almost impossible to tell apart from the other causes of acute infectious colitis (salmonellosis, intestinal clostridiosis, or Potomac horse fever).

Treatment: In many cases, the colitis occurs so rapidly that treatment is not possible. With early diagnosis, the horse's life may be saved by intensive intravenous fluid therapy, antibiotics, and other supportive measures, as discussed in the treatment section of *Intestinal Clostridiosis* (see page 75).

Lyme Disease (Borreliosis)

Borreliosis is caused by a bacteria called *Borrelia burgdorferi* and affects horses, humans, and many other animals. The bacteria require an intermediate rodent host, either the white-footed mouse, the California kangaroo rat, or the dusky-footed wood rat. Many species of immature ticks feed on these rodents and acquire the bacteria. After the ticks develop into adults, they feed on large mammals. The bacteria are then transmitted to these mammals by the ticks' saliva.

Infection in the horse spreads slowly. Symptoms may not appear for weeks or months. Occasionally, arthritis characterized by intermittent pain and muscle wasting, may affect one or more joints. These signs often suggest an injury rather than an infectious disease. Rarely, the bacteria infect the brain or an eye, causing encephalitis or *uveitis*.

The diagnosis is made by detecting serum antibodies to *Borrelia burgdorferi*. A rise in the serum *antibody* level over several weeks is considered indicative of recent exposure.

Treatment: Tetracycline antibiotics appear to be the most effective treatment in horses. Early treatment gives the best results. Unfortunately, the diagnosis is often delayed. The borreliosis bacteria attach closely to the horse's body cells; metronidazole (another antibiotic) may be effective in these encysted cases.

Prevention: Keeping ticks off your horse is the best prevention. If possible, remove horses from brushy pastures in the spring and fall, when ticks are most active. Check your horse regularly by feeling his entire body with your hands for bumps (ticks) attached to the skin. Remove ticks as described in *Ticks* (see page 62). Spraying the horse with a garden hose at high pressure after trail rides will remove many ticks before they attach. Insecticides and repellents labeled as effective against ticks can be applied liberally to the legs and underside to prevent ticks from getting and staying on the horse. Apply the product before riding in tick-infested areas and then again after the post-ride spray.

Ulcerative Lymphangitis (Pigeon Fever)

Ulcerative lymphangitis is an infection of the lymphatic system of the legs. It is caused by the bacteria *Corynebacterium pseudotuberculosis*. Ulcerative lymphangitis is found in all conditions but especially where horses are crowded with poor sanitation. It is also spread by several species of flies.

Bacteria gain entrance through cuts or abrasions in the skin. The first sign is swelling in the lower half of the leg. The hind limbs are more often affected. Abscesses occur beneath the skin along the lymphatic channels. These abscesses open and discharge a thin, bloody fluid that later becomes thick and yellow. A few horses develop internal infection of the organs. As the abscesses heal, new ones develop above the old ones. Lymphatic channels along the course of the leg become thick and cordlike. Often the limb appears to be healed but later breaks open with new nodules and draining sores.

Although lymphangitis is seldom fatal, scarring of the lymphatic channels can lead to permanent restriction of the flow of lymph fluid.

A variation called pigeon fever was first reported in California and has spread to the southwestern states. The horse develops an abscess over the sternum or occasionally in the groin. The infection is thought to be spread by ticks, horseflies, and perhaps other insects.

The diagnosis of ulcerative lymphangitis can be confirmed by *ultrasonography* of internal organs or a culture of wound discharge. Ulcerative lymphangitis should be distinguished from sporotrichosis and glanders.

Glanders, one of the oldest zoonotic diseases known in horses, has been largely eradicated. Rare cases do occur. It is caused by the bacteria *Burkholderia mallei*. The cutaneous form of glanders produces lymphangitis and abscesses beneath the skin that closely resemble those of ulcerative lymphangitis. Glanders also attacks the lungs and the membranes of the nose. It is highly infectious, nearly always fatal, presents a serious hazard to human health, and is considered a potential agent of bioterrorism. As such, your veterinarian is required to report the disease to the animal health authorities.

Treatment: Isolate infected horses. Your veterinarian will direct treatment, which includes antibiotics, surgical drainage, and wound irrigation, but the best treatment must be determined for each individual. Other measures include poultices, dressings, anti-inflammatory drugs for pain and leg swelling, and physical therapy. Relapse is common, but some cases heal without scarring and restriction.

Prevention: Horses should be kept in clean, dry stalls. Use only clean curry combs and brushes. Remove nails and other sharp objects in stalls and paddocks. Treat skin injuries promptly to prevent infection (see *Wounds*, page 32). Observe suitable antiseptic precautions when handling and caring for infected wounds and dressings to prevent both human exposure and spreading the disease to other horses. Disinfect the stable or isolation area as described for *Salmonellosis* (page 69). A good fly control program (see *Flies*, page 63) is very important in preventing the spread of the disease.

Brucellosis

This disease is caused by the bacteria *Brucella abortus*. It is now quite rare in the United States and Canada, due to successful efforts to eradicate the disease in cattle. However, it remains a problem in Mexico and the Caribbean. Horses become infected by ingesting contaminated feed or water, or by direct penetration of the bacteria through the mucous membranes.

Equine brucellosis is difficult to recognize because of its nonspecific symptoms. They include intermittent fever, change in attitude, muscle stiffness, and reluctance to move. Tendons, muscles, bones, and joints can become infected. Serum agglutination *assays* (a diagnostic blood test using paired samples taken two weeks apart) will show a rising antibody level to *Brucella abortus*, indicating exposure.

Two conditions associated with *Brucella abortus* are fistulous withers and poll evil. Both occur when bacteria gain entrance through a break in the skin, causing a deep-seated infection characterized by the formation of one or more draining sinus tracts or fistulas (abnormal passages to the outside of the body) that discharge *pus*. The tracts close spontaneously or with treatment but are likely to recur.

Poll evil affects the poll of the head just behind the ears. The disease first presents as a swelling on one or both sides of the poll. There may be a history of a blow, such as striking the back of the head against the top of a door. Involvement of the neck ligament causes intense pain when the horse moves his head.

Fistulous withers involves the bursal sac overlying the first thoracic vertebral spines. The initiating event may be pressure at the withers from a badly fitting saddle or harness. Extensive involvement can lead to *osteomyelitis* of the vertebrae.

Not all cases of poll evil and fistulous withers are caused by *Brucella abortus*. The bacteria *Streptococcus zooepidemicus* and *Actinomyces bovis* may be found alone or combined with *Brucella abortus* in some cases. In addition, the hair-like worm *parasite Onchocerca cervicalis* (see *Ventral Midline Dermatitis*, page 121) has been implicated in the early stages of fistulous withers and poll evil.

Treatment: In cases of proven *Brucella abortus* infection, the horse should be quarantined to prevent contact with other horses and humans. Brucellosis causes undulant fever in humans, so infected discharges should be handled with extreme caution. If the condition becomes chronic, wide surgical removal of devitalized and infected tissue is required for a permanent cure.

Poll evil and fistulous withers are difficult to treat because of their deep-seated nature. Antibiotics are effective in the early stages but have limited use when the condition becomes chronic with draining sinuses. Ivermectin is given to limit or eliminate potential *Onchocerca* involvement.

Prevention: Keep horses away from infected cattle. Horses should not be allowed into pastures used by such cattle for at least three months.

Tuberculosis

The tubercle bacillus infects humans and all domestic animals. There has been a steady decline in equine tuberculosis with control and eradication of the disease in livestock. Horses apparently possess some natural resistance.

Tuberculosis is not an obvious respiratory infection in horses. Bacteria gain entrance through the digestive tract and infect the lymph nodes of the intestines. Later, they progress to the bloodstream and involve the liver, lungs, bones, and other organs.

Early diagnosis is difficult because of the nonspecific signs—the principal one being chronic, progressive weight loss. Fever, cough, and rapid breathing occur late in the disease. Diagnosis is confirmed by biopsy or by culturing the tubercle bacillus from infected discharges. Skin tests for tuberculosis are not reliable in horses.

Treatment: The development of new antibiotics have increased successful treatment. There has not been any known case of the spread of tuberculosis from horses to humans.

Anthrax

Anthrax is a highly contagious, rapidly fatal disease that affects nearly all animals, including humans. The disease is caused by *Bacillus anthracis*, a bacterium that forms spores that can remain dormant in the soil for up to 50 years. Horses acquire the disease by grazing on infected pastures. The bacteria enter through abrasions in the mouth or by direct passage through the intestinal tract.

The first indications of acute anthrax are high fever and colic and the appearance of hot, swollen areas on the neck, throat, and belly. Symptoms progress to rapid breathing, stupor, staggering gait, coma, and death. Bloody discharges occur from the body orifices, particularly from the rectum. Sudden, unexplained death should alert you to the possibility of anthrax.

The diagnosis is suspected because of the characteristic signs and symptoms, especially a bloody discharge with swelling at the throat. It is more likely to be suspected in areas where anthrax is endemic. Microscopic examination of a blood sample may show the characteristic bacteria in the blood.

Treatment: A horse exposed to anthrax should be isolated and treated with penicillin at the first sign of fever (temperature 1°F above normal). Because of rapid progression, death often occurs before treatment can be started. Penicillin, when given early in the illness, may prove effective.

Prevention: Quarantine infected horses. Anthrax is a distinct hazard to human health. Great care must be exercised in handling sick horses.

Public health measures require that carcasses of animals killed by anthrax be burned or buried in lime. Pastures, paddocks, stalls, and other contaminated areas should be disinfected with a 10 percent formaldehyde solution.

Horses living in anthrax-endemic areas can be protected by a vaccination program, on advice from your veterinarian. Side effects of vaccination, including local inflammation at the injection site and fever, are common. Do not administer antibiotics within one week of vaccination, as this may interfere with the efficacy of the vaccine.

Viral Diseases

Viruses are disease-causing *organisms* that are even more basic than cells. They are simply packages of protein.

Rabies

Rabies is a fatal disease that occurs in nearly all warm-blooded animals, although rarely in rodents. Rabies in dogs and cats has been greatly reduced by mass vaccination. The usual source of infection for horses is a bite from an infected skunk, fox, bat, or raccoon. Other wild animals serve as a reservoir for the disease and account for sporadic cases. Any wild animal who allows you to approach it without running from you is acting abnormally. Rabies should be suspected. *Do not pet, handle, or give first aid to such an animal.*

The rabies virus is present in infected saliva and generally enters at the site of a bite. However, saliva on an open wound or mucous membrane also constitutes exposure to rabies. The average incubation period after exposure in horses is three weeks to three months, but may be as long as six months. The virus travels to the brain along nerve networks. The farther the bite is from the brain, the longer the incubation period. The virus then travels back along nerves to the mouth, where it enters the saliva and the animal can transmit the disease.

Signs of rabies in horses vary and often suggest some other neurological disorder or infectious disease. For the most part, many signs of rabies are nonspecific, which is why it poses such a great risk for human exposure. Horses seldom exhibit the furious form of rabies and "go mad" and attack people. However, unprovoked excitement and crashing about are possible signs and make the horse extremely dangerous.

Horses typically suffer from the paralytic form of rabies. The signs of paralytic rabies include apathy and disinterest in surroundings, weakness, staggering, difficulty swallowing, frothy salivation, inability to drink, and various degrees of lameness and limb paralysis. Thrashing convulsions and coma occur before death.

A distinguishing feature of equine rabies is its rapid course. Death generally occurs within five days of the onset of symptoms. Accordingly, any rapidly fatal illness accompanied by weakness or paralysis suggests the possibility of rabies.

Treatment: There is no effective treatment for rabies. A horse who has been exposed to rabies—and particularly if he was bitten by an animal suspected of having rabies—should be placed in strict isolation. This holds true even if the horse is known to be vaccinated for rabies. Notify your veterinarian, who is required to report the incident to the state health authorities. If the attacking animal was a domestic dog or cat, a protocol for impounding and observing the animal should be initiated through your veterinarian.

When the biting animal is captured and confined, observation will determine its state of health. If the animal was either killed at the time of the attack or dies subsequently during confinement, its brain should be removed and sent to a laboratory equipped to diagnose rabies from antibody studies. The only definitive way to diagnose rabies is by *necropsy*. If the attacking animal was a wild animal who escaped, there is no way to prove it was not rabid. In that case, post-exposure treatment should be given to the immunized horse.

Post-exposure treatment depends on the immune status of the horse. If the horse was previously vaccinated against rabies, give a rabies booster now. If the horse was never vaccinated against rabies and has had exposure, consult your veterinarian about whether a vaccination series now would serve any purpose.

If it is proven that the attacking animal had rabies, any exposed unvaccinated horse should be immediately euthanized. If rabies exposure is not conclusively established, the horse should be quarantined and observed for six months. If symptoms develop, the horse must be euthanized.

Prevention: Rabies can be prevented by vaccination. There are several vaccines approved by the U.S. Department of Agriculture. A single annual vaccination is required. Rabies vaccination is not generally recommended for breeding mares. Because this disease is rare in horses, vaccination is suggested only in areas where rabies is endemic—although experts disagree, and some believe rabies vaccine should be administered routinely due to the effectiveness of the vaccine and the severity of the disease. Consult your veterinarian or local health department for information on local rabies incidence and vaccination recommendations.

Preventive vaccines are available for high-risk groups of humans, including veterinarians, animal handlers, cave explorers, and laboratory workers.

Equine Viral Encephalomyelitis (Sleeping Sickness)

The most common mosquito-transmitted infectious diseases that attack the central nervous system of horses are Eastern equine encephalomyelitis, Western equine encephalomyelitis, Venezuelan equine encephalomyelitis, West Nile virus, and Japanese encephalitis. Eastern equine encephalomyelitis is the most virulent, with fatality rates of 70 to 90 percent. Western equine encephalomyelitis is the least virulent, with fatality rates of 20 to 50 percent.

Eastern equine encephalomyelitis occurs along the Eastern seaboard of North America, the Gulf Coast, and around the Great Lakes. It also occurs in Alberta, Canada, and Central and South America. Western equine encephalomyelitis occurs in the United States, commonly from the Mississippi Valley westward. It also occurs in Mexico and in Central and South America.

Venezuelan equine encephalomyelitis was first described in Colombia. It subsequently migrated through Mexico into Texas and is now endemic in South and Central America, Mexico, and the West Indies. West Nile virus first appeared in New York State in 1999 and has spread westward across North America.

These viruses are transmitted by the bite of a mosquito, which must first feed on an infected bird or rodent. Contact with infected horses is not a zoonotic problem because people, like horses, acquire the disease from the bite of an infected mosquito. Outbreaks in horses actually serve as a warning, since they usually precede signs of human illness by two to three weeks. Cases occur in humans each year and a small percentage are fatal.

The horse is considered a dead-end host for the virus of Western equine encephalomyelitis; that is, once a horse becomes infected, the levels of virus in his blood are too low for further mosquito transmission. This often happens with Eastern equine encephalomyelitis and with West Nile virus, as well. However, with Venezuelan equine encephalomyelitis, the levels of virus in the horse's blood are high enough to infect feeding mosquitoes, making horses a reservoir for infection.

Equine viral encephalomyelitis begins one to three weeks after a mosquito bite and generally lasts 5 to 14 days. Signs and symptoms of all five diseases are similar. (For more information on West Nile virus, see page 83.) The first indication is a high fever, which lasts one to two days and may go unnoticed. This is followed by the onset of acute encephalitis. Signs of brain inflammation include compulsive walking and circling, loss of coordination, and apparent blindness. The horse may crash into walls and fences.

Later, the horse becomes extremely depressed and oblivious to his surroundings, standing with his head held low, tongue hanging out, and ears and lips drooping. The stage is called "sleeping sickness" because of the characteristic nodding of the head as if the horse is going to sleep.

Spinal cord inflammation (*myelitis*) produces a staggering gait, weakness, and muscle twitching. The final stage is paralysis. The horse sinks to the ground, develops seizures, and is unable to breathe.

Some horses who recover may have impaired vision, permanent muscle weakness, and a behavior disorder or a learning disability.

Suspicion of equine encephalomyelitis is based on the appearance and *condition* of the horse, his geographic location, occurrence during the mosquito season, and knowledge of other cases in the area. A serologic blood *titer* (which measures the concentration of antibodies in the blood) with a result greater than four times normal is highly suggestive of equine encephalomyelitis. Isolation of the virus from the blood or brain is diagnostic.

Treatment: It is directed at supporting the horse through the acute phase of the illness. Intensive nursing is critical for a successful outcome. Confine the horse to prevent self-injury. Wrap his legs. Provide free access to water.

Anti-inflammatory drugs may be prescribed by your veterinarian for fever and muscle pain. Diazepam (Valium) or barbiturates such as phenobarbital are used for seizure control. Antibiotics are used only to treat secondary bacterial infections. Steroids may be of benefit.

Feed a palatable semi-liquid diet such as 1 to 2 pounds (453 to 907 g) of alfalfa pellets per 100 pounds (45 kg) of body weight per day, soaked in water to form a thick slurry. If necessary, administer feed and water by stomach tube. Intravenous fluid supplements may be required.

If the horse goes down, the outlook is poor. Good nursing care involves rolling the horse several times a day to prevent both pressure sores and the muscle wasting associated with prolonged recumbency. Well-padded bedding is essential. Maintain the horse in the *sternal position*, if possible. An in-dwelling catheter can be used to empty the bladder and keep the horse clean and dry.

Prevention: Encephalomyelitis can be prevented by vaccination. The available vaccines are all effective. Eastern equine encephalomyelitis and Western equine encephalomyelitis are combined as a single injection; West Nile virus is a separate vaccination. Both are recommended for all horses. Annual boosters should be given in the spring at least one month before the mosquito season begins. In areas where there are mosquitoes all year long, give a booster every three to six months. Vaccinate pregnant mares with inactivated vaccine three to six weeks before foaling.

An outbreak of Venezuelan equine encephalomyelitis in the United States has not been reported since 1971. Accordingly, Venezuelan equine encephalomyelitis vaccine is no longer widely used in the United States, but may be a good idea in endemic areas, including Texas and the Southwest, or in competition horses who may be traveling to endemic areas.

Control mosquitoes as described in *Mosquitoes* (page 61).

West Nile Virus

West Nile virus is caused by a member of the flavivirus group of viruses and spread by the bite of an infected mosquito—most often the northern house mosquito (*Culex pipiens*). Mosquitoes first become exposed to the virus when they feed on infected birds. Once the mosquito is infected, it may transmit the virus to people or to other animals when it bites them.

Following transmission by an infected mosquito, West Nile virus multiplies in the horse's blood system, crosses the blood brain barrier, and infects the brain. The virus interferes with normal central nervous system functioning and causes inflammation of the brain. The incubation period is usually 5 to 15 days.

Not all horses become clinically ill. In those who do become clinical, the signs include loss of appetite and depression, loss of coordination, muscle weakness, and muscle trembling. Many are recumbent and have trouble rising. Occasionally infected horses may have a fever, droopy lip or muzzle twitching, grinding of teeth, head pressing, aimless wandering, convulsions, inability to swallow, circling, hyperexcitability, and rarely blindness.

People cannot get West Nile virus from infected horses, and horses do not pass it on to other horses. However, mosquitoes can transmit the disease to humans in the area if they first bite infected horses.

Treatment: Treatment is limited to supportive care using *NSAIDs*, steroids, and DMSO. Sometimes IV therapy with mannitol may relieve swelling around the brain. There are a number of serum products that claim to have a therapeutic effect against West Nile virus. Check with your veterinarian to be sure the serum product is licensed specifically to treat West Nile virus. (Currently, there are only two acceptable licensing authorities for serum products in the United States: the Food and Drug Administration Center for Veterinary Medicine and the State of California.) Your veterinarian will determine the best treatment(s).

Prevention: There are two vaccinations available: a killed virus and a recombinant DNA vaccine. For vaccination information, see the table on page 160. Horses vaccinated against Eastern, Western, and Venezuelan equine encephalitis are not protected against West Nile virus.

Mosquito control is of paramount importance. Mosquitoes lay their eggs in standing water. Water tanks and automatic waterers are prime sources of mosquito larvae, as are pet water dishes and any source of standing water. Water must be changed frequently or a commercial larvicide may be added. For more on mosquito control, see *Mosquitoes*, page 61.

Equine Viral Respiratory Diseases

Viral respiratory diseases are highly contagious, often serious illnesses of horses. They spread rapidly and are transmitted by airborne inhalation and contact with the respiratory secretions of infected or recently infected individuals. To contain the spread of these illnesses, it is important to isolate infected horses during the contagious period, which lasts four to six weeks after infection, and to use good hygiene in handling and caring for sick horses.

Signs and symptoms are so similar that it is difficult to tell these diseases apart without special laboratory tests. The results of such tests are not always available to veterinarians in time to be of use in planning treatment, and so the tests are not usually performed.

Respiratory viruses attack the airways and disrupt the protective blanket of *mucus* that lines the trachea and the bronchi. This leads to a cough, which persists for several weeks after the initial attack. Secondary bacterial infections are common.

Uncomplicated viral respiratory illnesses should not be treated with antibiotics or combinations containing antibiotics and steroids. Antibiotics often reduce the population of protective bacteria in the upper respiratory tract, allowing virulent bacteria to proliferate. Steroids are immunosuppressive and may lower a horse's natural resistance to the virus and make the disease worse.

Antibiotics are reserved for treating secondary bacterial infections. As a rule, if fever persists more than five days and is accompanied by a *mucopurulent* nasal discharge (a snotty nose), antibiotics are justified. Cultures from tracheal washings, which provide a bacterial diagnosis, are preferred before antibiotics are prescribed.

Equine Influenza

This contagious illness is caused by two species of myxovirus, which can be subdivided into several strains, each capable of causing rapidly developing outbreaks of respiratory disease. These viruses attack the lining of the entire respiratory system, including the lower respiratory tract, where complications can lead to pneumonia. Young and old horses are most susceptible.

After a short incubation period, the disease begins with a high fever that lasts about three days. A characteristic feature of influenza is the dry, hacking cough that later becomes moist and productive. This is accompanied by a clear or mucoid nasal discharge. The cough usually persists for several weeks, even though the actual illness lasts three to seven days. Other signs include runny eyes, loss of appetite, apathy, and muscle stiffness.

Influenza is a relatively mild infection, but secondary complications may occur, the most common being bacterial rhinitis. The nasal discharge becomes thick and puslike, and the horse's breathing is noisy. A persistent fever and labored respiration may be signs of the onset of pneumonia.

Treatment: Isolate the horse to prevent the spread of the disease. Stall rest is important. The stall should be dry and well-ventilated. Closing a stable (to keep it warm) will invariably increase respiratory symptoms. If the stable is cold, apply a horse blanket. Wrap the legs. Provide clean water and a palatable diet free-choice. NSAIDs are used to control fever and muscle stiffness. Antiviral drugs may decrease the severity and duration of equine influenza.

Restrict exercise until the cough disappears. The horse should be rested at least three weeks and perhaps longer. A rapid return to exercise and training is associated with relapse and chronic bronchitis.

Prevention: Vaccinations will prevent influenza infections or reduce their severity. However, immunity to influenza following vaccination or recovery from a natural infection is short-lived, seldom persisting for more than a year. In addition, epidemics may be caused by new virus strains. Accordingly, vaccines may have to be modified from time to time to provide the best coverage. Current vaccines contain myxovirus strains A-1 and A-2.

For these reasons, most veterinarians recommend frequent vaccination. Although the manufacturers of the vaccines recommend annual boosters, they simply do not provide adequate protection for the majority of horses. The recommended flu immunization schedule for foals and adult horses is shown in the table on page 100. This schedule assumes that a newborn foal is protected during the first five months of life by passive antibodies acquired from his mother's *colostrum*. If the dam was not vaccinated, these antibodies are lacking and influenza vaccine should be administered to the foal at 1, 2, and 3 months of age (a three-dose primary series), and then every three months until maturity.

Rhinopneumonitis

Equine herpesvirus, which causes rhinopneumonitis, is the most common cause of respiratory illness in foals, weanlings, and yearlings. It is highly contagious and spreads rapidly throughout a farm, often following the arrival of a new horse carrying the virus. The two strains seen most often are EHV-1 and EHV-4.

The principal sign is a copious nasal discharge, which becomes *mucoid* and puslike if the horse develops a secondary infection. Foals may develop a dry cough that persists for two to three weeks. Severe or fatal foal pneumonia is the major complication of rhinopneumonitis.

In pregnant mares, EHV-1 produces *abortions* late in pregnancy throughout a farm. These "abortion storms" can affect the majority of pregnant mares on the premises. The abortions occur weeks or months after exposure to the virus. Occasionally, instead of aborting, the mare delivers a foal with pneumonia who dies within the first week of life.

A neurological form of EHV-1 occurs in mature horses and in mares who have aborted. Signs include staggering gait, loss of coordination, and various forms of paralysis (see *Equine Herpes Myeloencephalitis*, page 356).

Treatment: It is like that for *Equine Influenza* (see page 85).

Prevention: Immunity following vaccination and natural infection is short-lived. Frequent vaccinations are required to maintain resistance. It is most important to protect foals, yearlings, *stallions*, and broodmares. The suggested immunization schedule is shown in the table on page 103. If the dam was not vaccinated, these antibodies are lacking and the vaccine should be administered to the foal at 1, 2, and 3 months of age (a three-dose primary series), and then every three months until maturity.

Rhinopneumonitis vaccines containing EHV-4 are preferable for foals, weanlings, yearlings, and pleasure horses, since the majority of respiratory infections are caused by EHV-4. Broodmares should continue to be vaccinated with EHV-1, the strain responsible for nearly all recorded abortions.

Vaccines are available that combine two inactivated strains of influenza (A-1 and A-2) with EHV-4. This combination may be especially suitable for foals.

Adenovirus and Rhinovirus

Adenoviruses produce mild respiratory illnesses in young horses. However, this virus group is a common cause of serious illness and death in neonatal foals who lack maternal antibodies (see *Lack of Colostrum*, page 549). In foals of Arabian or part Arabian ancestry suffering from combined immunodeficiency syndrome (CID), adenovirus infection is fatal. Thus, adenoviruses appear to be opportunistic invaders, causing serious illness only in foals who lack normal immunity.

Rhinoviruses are highly contagious but generally produce few symptoms. The horse may have a fever, runny nose, conjunctivitis, cough, and occasionally a sore throat.

Treatment: There is no specific treatment, other than rest and good nursing care.

Prevention: There are no vaccines available to prevent adenovirus or rhinovirus infections. Isolating infected horses may be helpful to prevent the spread in other members of the herd.

Equine Viral Arteritis

Most horses are exposed to equine viral arteritis, but only a few develop symptoms. The disease gets its name from the injury it causes to the walls of small arteries. Small bleeding points, called petechial hemorrhages, appear on the mucous membranes inside the nostrils and on the conjunctiva that covers the whites of the eyes. Conjunctivitis and red swelling about the eyes can be taken as a sign of generalized arteritis.

The primary mode of transmission for equine viral arteritis is sexual contact, with susceptible mares bred to stallions who are carriers. Secondary transmission occurs with virus shedding into the respiratory tract. There is a difference in the *seropositivity* of different breeds: 24 percent of Standardbreds are positive for equine viral arteritis, 93 percent of Austrian Warmbloods are positive, 1.6 percent of American Quarterhorses, and 6 percent of Thoroughbred horses.

The acute respiratory illness produced by equine viral arteritis is like that of equine influenza. Typically, fluid accumulates in the abdominal wall, *scrotum*, sheath, and hind limbs. Other signs include apathy, loss of appetite, colic, diarrhea, and dehydration.

A major problem associated with equine viral arteritis is viral abortion, discussed in *Abortion* (page 507).

Treatment: Treatment of respiratory illness is like that described for *Equine Influenza* (page 85). Immunity after illness is lifelong.

Prevention: It is important to prevent stallions from becoming carriers. A vaccine that protects breeding stock should be considered in areas where equine viral arteritis is endemic. The immunity is rapid and lasts three to four years. Note that vaccination produces *seroconversion*. This could complicate the interpretation of tests required for exporting the horse. In some states, vaccination requires prior approval from the state veterinarian. Vaccinate mares and stallions (one dose) three weeks before breeding. Do not vaccinate mares during pregnancy. Although immunity lasts three to four years, current recommendations call for annual boosters.

Equine Infectious Anemia (Swamp Fever)

Equine infectious anemia (EIA) is a retrovirus infection transmitted in blood, saliva, urine, milk, and body secretions. Bloodsucking flies and other biting insects are the usual vectors for transmission. However, the virus can also be spread by blood transfusions and unsterile syringes, and can cross the placenta and infect the foal. EIA is potentially a sexually transmitted disease, as well.

The frequency of EIA in North America has been significantly lowered by control measures introduced in the mid-1970s. The disease is now infrequent.

EIA-positive horses remain infected for life and thus present a continuing hazard to other horses. Risk of transmission is greatest when the carrier horse is acutely ill or in a state of relapse, at which time virus blood levels are high enough to infect feeding insects.

EIA should be suspected in any horse with periodic fever and *anemia*. It can be confirmed by a positive Coggins (AGID, agar gel immunodiffusion) or *ELISA* blood test. Three distinct types of illness are described, but symptoms overlap.

Acute illness is characterized by high fever, severe anemia, weakness, swelling of the lower abdomen and legs, weak pulse, and irregular heartbeat. The anemia is due to the rapid breakdown and destruction of red blood cells. The mortality rate is high. Sudden death may be the first sign.

Subacute illness progresses more slowly and is less severe. It is characterized by recurrent fever, weight loss, anemia, and swelling of the lower chest and abdominal wall, penile sheath, scrotum, and legs. An enlarged spleen is often felt on rectal examination. The horse may be *jaundiced*.

Chronic illness is characterized by recurrent fever and anemia. The horse tires easily, weight loss is apparent, and he is unsuitable for work. A relapse with reversion to acute or subacute illness is possible weeks, months, or even years after the original attack.

EIA is a rare cause of abortion. Abortion can occur at any time during pregnancy, caused by a relapse when the virus enters the blood. The majority of sick mares abort. However, a few give birth to healthy, unaffected foals.

Treatment: It is directed at supporting the horse with blood transfusions and good nursing care. Treatment should only be attempted after consulting your veterinarian, due to the risk of infecting other horses. Steroids are contraindicated because they increase the potential for relapse. There is no effective treatment to clear the carrier state.

Prevention: Regulations require that all horses who test positive for EIA must be reported by the testing laboratory to federal authorities. The owner of the horse is given the option of euthanizing the horse, branding and quarantining him at least 200 yards from other horses for life, or shipping the horse to a recognized research facility.

Even though the disease is infrequent, outbreaks of EIA continue to occur. Accordingly, it is wise to isolate visiting mares and new horses until a negative test can be obtained.

Vesicular Stomatitis

Vesicular stomatitis is a contagious viral disease affecting cattle, horses, and swine. It is transmitted by bloodsucking black flies, sand flies, and possibly other biting insects, and by contact with contaminated tack and equipment.

There is a short incubation period, followed by fever and listlessness. Small blisterlike blebs containing clear fluid (*vesicles*) then appear on the mucous membranes of the mouth and tongue, in the nose, and on the coronary bands of the feet. As the disease progresses, the blisters swell and break, leaving raw, painful *ulcers*. Some of the *lesions* on the udders, on the *prepuce*, underneath the abdomen, and on the muzzle may crust over. These crusts are infective. Infected horses generally drool copiously, refuse to eat and drink, and may show signs of lameness.

Vesicular stomatitis can be transmitted from infected horses to people. In humans, vesicular stomatitis causes blisters in the mouth and flulike symptoms including fever, muscle aches, headaches, and malaise.

All vesicles contain live virus. To prevent illness, wear rubber gloves and avoid direct contact when handling sick animals.

Treatment: Notify your veterinarian. Infected horses must be quarantined. Treat stomatitis as described in *Stomatitis* (see page 179). Most horses recover from the virus in one to two weeks, but occasionally the vesicles become infected and require antibiotics.

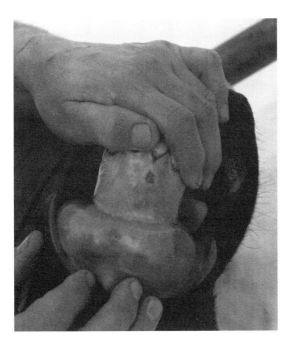

This ulcer on the gum is similar to a late stage of vesicular stomatitis.

Prevention: Insect control helps prevent further transmission (see *Controlling External Parasites*, page 63). Avoid close contact with horses from areas where the disease has recently been diagnosed. Do not share feed or water buckets between horses.

A vaccine has been developed. Its use in endemic areas is regulated by state animal health and USDA authorities.

African Horse Sickness

Relatively unknown a few years ago, African horse sickness (AHS) is an emerging disease that may have a significant impact on the horse community. The mortality rate in horses is 70 to 95 percent; in *mules* it is about 50 percent and in *donkeys* it is around 10 percent. Currently, AHS is a truly African disease that is endemic in the central tropical regions of that continent, from where it spreads regularly to Southern Africa and occasionally to Northern Africa.

Caused by an orbivirus, the usual mode of transmission is *Culicoides spp.*, gnats, although occasionally mosquitoes and ticks can carry it. Moist, mild conditions and warm temperatures favor the presence of insect vectors. There is concern that AHS could spread into Europe and from there to other continents.

The incubation period for AHS is usually 7 to 14 days, but may be as short as 2 days. The signs and symptoms are rather vague, and include fever and malaise, sometimes with cardiac involvement that may have some *edema*, and sometimes respiratory involvement with coughing. There are a variety of other diseases this could be confused with, including anthrax, equine infectious anemia, equine viral arteritis, and equine encephalitis. There are three serological tests—ELISA, complement fixation, and immunoblotting—available to confirm the diagnosis. However, death often occurs before a diagnosis can be made.

Treatment: There is no efficient treatment for African horse sickness. Affected horses should be euthanized and their cadavers destroyed to prevent gnats from feeding and infecting other horses.

Prevention: The insects responsible for spreading AHS must be controlled with an adequate insecticide program. Vaccines are available and may be given at your veterinarian's discretion, if the disease spreads.

Rickettsial Diseases

Rickettsia are disease-causing parasites (about the size of bacteria) that are carried by fleas, ticks, mites, and lice. The rickettsia live within cells. The majority are maintained in nature by a cycle that involves an insect vector, a permanent host, and an animal reservoir.

Equine Granulocytic Ehrlichiosis

Equine granulocytic ehrlichiosis (EGE) is a noncontagious disease of horses caused by *Anaplasma phagocytophilum*. This rickettsia is transmitted to the horse by a tick bite. The disease was first identified in northern California, where it is still most often found. It has been found to affect horses throughout the United States, Canada, Brazil, and Europe.

In horses younger than 3 years of age, the disease is mild and always includes fever. Other signs include listlessness, loss of appetite, jaundice, slight swelling of the legs, and muscle stiffness. In horses over 3 years, these symptoms are more pronounced. The horse is reluctant to move and experiences marked swelling of the legs, particularly the hind limbs. A staggering gait with loss of coordination is characteristic.

EGE should be suspected when a *febrile* illness occurs during tick season in an endemic area, such as northern California. Blood smears taken within the first three to four days of illness may show inclusion bodies in white blood cells; these inclusion bodies signify the presence of rickettsia. The best diagnostic test is the highly sensitive PCR (polymerase chain reaction) test.

Treatment: The antibiotic oxytetracycline is highly effective against rickettsia and should be given for 7 to 14 days. Improvement begins almost at once. Confine an *ataxic* horse to prevent self-injury. Wrap the legs to reduce swelling. Cortisone may be of benefit. To prevent relapse, complete the full course of antibiotic therapy and rest the horse for three weeks.

Prevention: Control ticks as described in *Controlling External Parasites* (see page 63). Inspect your horse after riding in tick-infested areas. Rickettsial infections can be prevented if ticks are removed within the first two to three hours.

Potomac Horse Fever

Potomac horse fever is a noncontagious disease of horses that occurs in mid to late summer and is caused by *Neorickettsia risticii*. This organism is transmitted to horses who graze and drink near freshwater streams. The organism has been found in caddis flies, flukes, and snails in endemic areas. Mayflies are also implicated as part of the life cycle, and when these and the caddis flies swarm and then die under barn lights or on pasture, there is a much greater risk of infection. Research is ongoing, but many authorities believe the horse is infected by drinking water or swallowing caddis flies that contain the organism. Originally identified in Maryland, Potomac horse fever has now been found in most of the United States and in Canada, South America, India, and northern Europe.

The horse may develop symptoms one to three weeks after ingesting the rickettsia. Not all infected horses exhibit symptoms of the disease. Those horses who become sick start with depression and loss of appetite, then have high fever, followed by moderate to severe diarrhea. Pregnant mares will abort the fetus in two to three months, regardless of how severe the symptoms were. Many infected horses progress to severe dehydration, *toxemia*, and laminitis.

The disease can be confused with salmonellosis or clostridial diarrheas. Diagnosis is made based on seasonal occurrence, typical symptoms, and a rapid PCR (polymerase chain reaction) test, using either blood or diarrheic feces.

Treatment: Treatment is usually successful when oxytetracycline (an antibiotic) is given very early in the disease and continued for three to five days. Flunixin meglumine (Banamine), an anti-inflammatory drug, can help reduce the effects of the toxins that get into the bloodstream from the inflamed intestinal tract. Intravenous fluids containing added potassium, magnesium, and calcium are used to combat the fluid losses in severe cases of diarrhea. No matter how quickly treatment is initiated, a pregnant mare will likely abort.

Prevention: There are vaccines that will prevent most symptoms of the disease. Discuss with your veterinarian which vaccine appears to be most effective in your area, and whether routine vaccination is advised. In known endemic areas, horses should not be allowed access to natural water sources from mid to late summer.

Systemic Fungal Diseases

Fungi are a large family that includes mushrooms. They live in soil and organic material. Many types of fungi spread via airborne spores. Fungus spores, which resist heat and can live for long periods without water, gain entrance to the body through the respiratory tract or a break in the skin.

Fungal diseases can be divided into two categories. The first are fungi that affect only the skin or mucous membranes. (These are discussed in chapter 4, "The Skin and Coat.") In the second category, the fungus is widespread and involves the liver,lungs, brain, and other organs, in which case the disease is *systemic*.

Fortunately, systemic fungal diseases are not common in horses. When present, they tend to occur in chronically ill or immunosuppressed individuals. Prolonged treatment with steroids and/or antibiotics can change a horse's pattern of resistance and allow a fungus infection to become established. Infrequently, a healthy, robust horse develops a systemic fungal infection.

Systemic fungal infections do not respond to conventional antibiotics and require intensive veterinary management. The drug of choice for most systemic fungal infections is amphotericin B. This drug requires close monitoring due to its potential for kidney toxicity. When a fungal infection becomes systemic, *euthanasia* is often recommended.

Fungal infections are not contagious in the usual sense, but can be transmitted to humans via puncture wounds or direct contact with open sores. Good hygiene is important when handling and caring for a horse with any fungal infection.

Histoplasmosis

This disease is caused by a fungus found in the central United States near the Great Lakes, the Appalachian Mountains, and the valleys of the Mississippi, Ohio, and St. Lawrence rivers. Spores are found in soil contaminated by the dung of migratory birds and starlings. Most infected horses suffer only a mild respiratory illness. However, on rare occasions, the disease can become systemic. The signs include chronic cough, recurrent bouts of pneumonia, difficulty breathing, and loss of weight and muscle substance.

A definitive diagnosis of histoplasmosis is often very difficult to obtain. Tests using a polymerase chain reaction hold the most promise of providing a specific diagnosis.

Treatment: Treatment for severely affected horses is possible, but must be continued for many months. This disease has been treated successfully.

Prevention: This is best accomplished by keeping wild and domestic birds out of stalls and barns.

Coccidioidomycosis

This is a mild respiratory infection which, on rare occasions, can become systemic and spread to all organs of the body. It is found in dry, dusty parts of the southwestern United States and in California. Serologic blood tests are available that may help to make the diagnosis.

Treatment: Medications such as itaconazole and fluconazole have been used to treat systemic infections. Supportive care is similar to that for encephalitis (see page 354).

Aspergillosis

This disease is acquired by inhaling spores found in damp hay. It generally occurs in stabled horses. It can be prevented by stable cleanliness. The signs are those of pneumonia that does not respond to treatment. The horse may suffer a chronic wasting disease similar to that of histoplasmosis (see page 93).

Treatment: Medications such as itaconazole and fluconazole have been used to treat systemic infections. Supportive care is similar to that for encephalitis (see page 354).

Cryptococcosis

This disease is acquired by inhalation. The fungus grows well in bird dung, in particular the droppings of pigeons and bats. Infection begins in the nasal passages and extends to the lower respiratory tract, where it causes pneumonia.

Treatment: Amphotericin B, in conjunction with flucytosine or fluconazole, is the treatment for cryptococcosis.

Prevention: Avoid stabling horses in enclosures that house pigeons, other birds, and bats.

Protozoan Diseases

Protozoans are one-celled organisms that are invisible to the naked eye but are easily seen under the microscope. Protozoan diseases are not common in horses. Equine protozoal *myeloencephalitis* is an inflammation of the brain and spinal cord caused by a protozoan that migrates randomly through the central nervous system. It is discussed on page 354. Dourine is a fatal sexually transmitted disease that is present in some less developed countries but eradicated in the United States. There are also two protozoan species that cause diarrhea in young horses. Both are discussed in chapter 18, "Pediatrics."

Equine Piroplasmosis (Babesiosis)

This is a protozoan infection transmitted by a tropical horse tick. The disease is endemic to southeastern Florida, Texas, Mexico, and Central and South America. The protozoan attacks red blood cells, causing a rapid *hemolysis* with severe anemia and *hemoglobinuria.* Infected horses develop high fever, swollen limbs, weakness, rapid pulse, pale gums, and swelling of the eyelids and face. Death can occur in one to two days. Horses who recover may be carriers for several years.

The protozoan can be seen microscopically in red blood cells. This establishes the diagnosis.

Treatment: Drugs are available to treat the illness and eliminate the carrier state. Discuss treatment options with your veterinarian. The disease is best prevented by controlling ticks, as described in *Controlling External Parasites* (page 63).

Antibodies and Immunity

An animal who is immune to a specific *pathogen* has natural proteins in his system called *antibodies* that attack and destroy that pathogen before it can cause disease.

When a horse becomes ill with an infectious disease, his immune system makes antibodies against that particular pathogen. These antibodies protect the horse against reinfection. The horse has now acquired active immunity. Active immunity is self-perpetuating; the horse continues to make antibodies after the disease has gone away. Any time the horse is exposed to that particular pathogen, his immune system will produce more antibodies. The duration of active immunity varies, depending on the pathogen and the horse.

Active immunity also can be induced by vaccination. The horse is exposed to heat-killed pathogens, live or attenuated (*antigens* that have been treated to make them less infectious) pathogens rendered incapable of causing disease, or toxins and pathogen products that will also stimulate a response by the horse's immune system. As with natural exposure, vaccination stimulates the production of antibodies that are specific for the particular pathogen in the vaccine. However, unlike natural exposure, the duration of protection may be limited. Accordingly, to maintain high levels of protection, booster vaccines are recommended. How frequently a horse will need boosters depends on the antigen used, number of exposures to the pathogens, the horse's own immune response, and the type of vaccination used. Vaccination schedules need to be customized for each individual horse.

Vaccinations may not be successful in all horses. Rundown, malnourished, debilitated horses may not be capable of responding to a disease challenge by developing antibodies or building immunity. Such horses should not be vaccinated at that time, but should be vaccinated when they're in better health. Immunosuppressive drugs, such as cortisone and *chemotherapy* agents, depress the immune system and also prevent the body from making antibodies.

Another type of immunity is called passive. Passive immunity is passed from one animal to another. In many species, including humans, the infant is born with antibodies and *immunoglobulins* obtained while in the uterus. However, in horses antibodies are not passed across the placenta. The foal is born without immunity to disease and can acquire antibodies only by ingesting their mother's *colostrum* during the first 18 hours, when antibodies are free to cross the intestinal mucosal barrier. By 24 hours, this barrier closes and antibodies are no longer absorbed.

The length of passive protection depends on the antibody level in the blood of the mare at the time of foaling. A mare vaccinated within three months of foaling has the highest levels, and her antibodies will protect her foal for 16 weeks. Of course, if the mare was not vaccinated against a particular disease, her foal will receive no protection.

Passive antibodies can bind up or neutralize vaccine antigens, rendering them less effective. This is one reason why vaccinations do not always produce solid immunity in very young foals. Revaccination at 3 months of age is recommended for all foals vaccinated shortly after birth.

Another method of providing passive immunity is to inject a horse with serum from another horse who has a high level of type-specific antibody. Tetanus antitoxin is an example of such an immune serum.

Vaccinations

There are many vaccines currently available for use in horses, and they use several different technologies to convey immunity. Inactivated or *killed vaccine* products are just that—the vaccine contains units of the target organism that has been killed by some manufacturing process. The dead organism will not replicate in a horse, so it is incapable of causing disease. Instead, this type of vaccine relies on surface antigens, along with immune stimulants called adjuvants, to stimulate an immune response. Modified live vaccines (*MLV*) use an actual live organism that has been modified during the manufacturing process so that it can replicate in the animal's body but will not cause disease. As a general rule, modified live vaccines produce a longer lasting immunity to the desired disease, but killed vaccines may stimulate a faster response by the body.

In addition to the active components of the vaccine, many vaccines contain an adjuvant that is added to stimulate a reaction and, to a certain degree, inflammation, which causes a quick and active response by the horse's body. Sometimes a horse may have a severe reaction to the adjuvant or to the disease organism itself. This is discussed in *Adverse Reactions* (see page 98).

Recombinant vaccines are among the newest products in the rapidly emerging biotechnology market. They do not use an adjuvant. The technology relies on the ability to splice gene-sized fragments of DNA from one organism (a virus or bacteria) and to deliver these fragments to another organism (the horse), where they stimulate immunity to the disease. Recombinant vaccines deliver specific antigen material on a cellular level without the risk of vaccination reactions associated with adjuvants or with giving the entire disease-causing organism. There are a handful of recombinant vaccines available for horses as this book is being written, including one for equine influenza. More are likely to be developed soon.

Most equine vaccines are administered deep into the horse's muscle (intramuscularly), but some are given by inserting a small plastic tube into the horse's nose and injecting the vaccine into the nasal passages (intranasally). While not conclusive, there is some evidence that intranasal vaccines work better than intramuscular vaccines in preventing respiratory infections, because the nasal cavity or pharynx are where the bacteria or virus enters the respiratory system.

Core and Noncore Vaccines

The veterinary community has divided vaccines into two main categories: core and noncore. Core vaccines are those that should be given to all horses on a regular schedule. These vaccines include Eastern, Western, and West Nile encephalomyelitis vaccines, and tetanus toxoid.

Noncore vaccines are vaccines that only some horses need, depending on factors such as the environment in which the horse is kept, the prevalence of diseases in certain geographic areas, and possibly, restrictions for breeding stock. Environmental considerations include a boarding stable or frequent exposure to other horses at shows or county fairs. These vaccinations usually include strangles, equine influenza, and rhinopneumonitis. Geographic locations may indicate the need for rabies vaccinations or *Clostridium botulinum* toxin. Noncore vaccinations with breeding considerations include rhinopneumonitis and equine viral arteritis.

Combination Vaccines

Many of the core vaccines can be purchased as a combination product that includes several disease preventives. These are called multivalent vaccines. The most common is the Eastern and Western encephalomyelitis vaccine combined with tetanus toxoid. This vaccine may also be referred to as a three-way vaccine. Combined with equine influenza, it is called a four-way. A five-way or a five-in-one vaccine usually contains tetanus, Eastern and Western encephalomyelitis, influenza, and rhinopneumonitis. However, it is important to note that not all multivalent vaccines contain the same combinations of antigens. In other words, a three-way vaccine may protect against the three diseases just mentioned, or it may protect against some other combination of three diseases. Always make sure you know exactly which vaccinations you are giving your horse.

You must also familiarize yourself with the needs of horses in your area and discuss with your veterinarian which products need to be administered to your horse. Then, you must read the label of the vaccine you have chosen to make sure it contains the desired vaccines.

Most of the combination vaccines available for horses are reliable and safe, and they will protect your horse from disease. The efficacy of these products is well established. Currently, however, there is a lot of debate about whether these combination products should be used, because they may be more likely to cause adverse reactions or to overwhelm the horse's immune system. Although adverse vaccine reactions do occur, they are limited to a very small percentage of the horse world. It is the authors' opinion that a healthy horse who can perform to your expectations is greatly preferable to a sick, disabled, or even a dead horse. All of these points should be discussed with your veterinarian to protect your friend and companion.

Why Vaccines Sometimes Fail

Vaccines are usually very effective in preventing serious illnesses. However, not every vaccine is 100 percent effective 100 percent of the time. The causes of vaccination failure vary, because not all vaccines are the same. Some vaccines may be able to protect just 70 percent of all horses vaccinated, but in the face of a large, severe epidemic in your area, it is much more effective and cost efficient to protect 70 percent of the horse population than it would be to treat 95 percent of the horses for the disease.

Some causes of vaccination failure can be attributed to improper technique (giving the vaccine just under the skin rather than deep into the muscle), improper storage (allowing the vaccine to get warm or exposing it to direct sunlight), or administering the vaccine to a horse whose immune system is already stressed by another disease or poor nutrition. A horse who has already been exposed to the disease he is being vaccinated against will not have the necessary time to develop antibodies against the disease before he becomes sick.

Another reason for failure in very young animals is that the mare may have passed protective antibodies to the disease through her colostrum, and this will block effective stimulation of immunity to the vaccine by the foal's immune system.

There is no doubt that some vaccines may appear to be expensive, and thus there is a temptation to divide one dose of vaccine between two horses. However, each vaccine dose is formulated to provide the best possible immune response for one individual. Dividing the single dose into two doses can result in neither animal being protected and both horses becoming ill.

If you wish to administer vaccinations yourself, it is important to learn the proper techniques from your veterinarian. Most veterinarians are willing to instruct you, to ensure that you are proficient in proper technique, understand the different methods of administering vaccines, and understand how to read and follow the instructions that come with the vaccine. You should also make sure you understand when and how often to administer boosters.

You should review the instructions provided with the vaccine every time you give a vaccination to avoid administering it inappropriately. Some diseases may be transmitted from horse to horse if you use the same needle to administer vaccines to more than one horse. For this reason, you must use a fresh sterile needle for each horse. Some vaccines are administered intranasally, using a special device. You will also need to review the techniques and instructions for administering those vaccines.

Adverse Reactions

When learning how to administer vaccinations properly, you also need to discuss with your veterinarian what to do in case of a vaccination reaction. Most vaccine reactions are a local response by the horse's body to the adjuvant or some other component of the vaccine. This is evidenced by heat and swelling at the site of the injection within a few days after the vaccination is given. This type of reaction is usually not life-threatening and disappears within several days.

Some local reactions are painful enough that a horse may refuse to eat or exercise. Nonsteroidal anti-inflammatory agents may be needed. Occasionally, poor injection techniques may cause an abscess, particularly if clean procedures are not used when giving the injection. The affected area will have to be drained, and antibiotics may be required. Usually, this situation causes a vaccine failure, and the vaccinations should be repeated after the site has completely healed.

The most severe form of a vaccination reaction is *anaphylaxis*. This occurs in a very few individuals whose body reacts immediately and powerfully to the antigens in the vaccine. This is a very serious condition in which the horse's blood pressure drops suddenly and he has severe breathing difficulties. The horse may collapse and even die.

Anaphylaxis can occur within minutes or up to a few hours after the vaccination has been administered. This is why it is important to keep an eye on a horse immediately after vaccination. Treatment must be given quickly. Usually, this consists of giving epinephrine and antihistamines by injection. Sometimes a corticosteroid may also be given. You should have these treatments on hand and have already discussed the drugs' use and manner of administration with your veterinarian.

Special Circumstances for Foals

Tetanus is a major concern for newborn and suckling foals. The vaccination schedule for foals who acquire passive immunity from their mothers is shown in the table on page 100. In the circumstance in which the mare was not vaccinated against tetanus, the foal should receive both tetanus antitoxin and tetanus toxoid within the first 24 hours of life. To complete the initial series, give a tetanus toxoid at 4 weeks and 4 months of age.

Tetanus antitoxin is no longer routinely given to newborn foals because of the potential for serum hepatitis. In fact, tetanus antitoxin is contraindicated in all immunized horses whose vaccination series is current. The two indications for tetanus antitoxin are a tetanus-prone wound occurring in either an unvaccinated horse or one in whom the vaccination status is unknown. In these individuals, administer tetanus antitoxin and tetanus toxoid at two different intramuscular injection sites. Follow in one month with a second tetanus toxoid.

Early immunization for rhinopneumonitis and influenza is recommended for foals whose mothers were never immunized, since these foals do not have passive immunity against these diseases. Foals should be immunized at 1, 2, and 3 months of age, and then given boosters every three months until they are mature.

If a primary vaccination series begins in an older horse, follow the same immunization schedule shown for foals and weanlings in the table on page 100.

Vaccination Guidelines for Horses

This suggested vaccination schedule is provided by the American Association of Equine Practitioners and is based on generally accepted veterinary practices. These guidelines are neither regulations nor directives for all situations, and should not be interpreted as such. Discuss this information with your veterinarian, and use this information, coupled with available products, to arrive together at a determination of the best professional care for your horse. As with all medications, read the label and product insert before administering any vaccine.

Vaccine	Foals and Weanlings	Yearlings	Performance Horses	Pleasure Horses	Broodmares[1]	Comments
West Nile virus	From unvaccinated mare: First dose at 3 to 4 months; second dose 1 month later; third dose at 6 months in endemic areas; From vaccinated mare: first dose at 5 months; second dose 6 weeks later	Annual booster, prior to expected risk; vaccinate semiannually or more frequently (every 4 months), depending on risk	Annual booster, prior to expected risk; vaccinate semiannually or more frequently (every 4 months), depending on risk	Annual booster, prior to expected risk; vaccinate semiannually or more frequently (every 4 months), depending on risk	Annual booster, 4 to 6 weeks prepartum	Annual booster is after primary series. In endemic areas, booster as required or warranted due to local conditions and disease risk.
Tetanus	From unvaccinated mare: first dose at 3 to 5 months; second dose at 6 to 7 months; From vaccinated mare: first dose at 6 months; second dose at 7 months; third dose at 8 to 9 months	Annual booster	Annual booster	Annual booster	Annual booster, 4 to 6 weeks prepartum	Booster at the time of a penetrating injury or surgery if the last booster was not administered within 6 months.

Vaccine	Foals and Weanlings	Yearlings	Performance Horses	Pleasure Horses	Broodmares[1]	Comments
Encephalomyelitis (EEE, WEE, VEE)[2]	EEE (in high-risk areas): first dose at 3 to 4 months; second dose at 4 to 5 months; third dose at 5 to 6 months; WEE, EEE (in low-risk areas), and VEE from unvaccinated mare: first dose at 3 to 4 months; second dose at 4 to 5 months; third dose at 5 to 6 months; WEE, EEE (in low-risk areas), and VEE from vaccinated mare: first dose at 6 months; second dose at 7 months; third dose at 8 months	Annual booster, spring	Annual booster, spring	Annual booster, spring	Annual booster, 4 to 6 weeks prepartum	In endemic areas, booster EEE and WEE every 6 months. VEE is only needed when there is a threat of exposure. However, VEE may only be available as a combination vaccine with EEE and WEE.

continued

Vaccination Guidelines for Horses (continued)

Vaccine	Foals and Weanlings	Yearlings	Performance Horses	Pleasure Horses	Broodmares[1]	Comments
Influenza	Inactivated injectable from unvaccinated mare: first dose at 6 months; second dose at 7 months; third dose at 8 months; then at 3-month intervals; Inactivated injectable from vaccinated mare: first dose at 9 months; second dose at 10 months; third dose at 11 to 12 months; then at 3-month intervals	Booster every 3 to 4 months	Booster every 3 to 4 months	Annual booster, with added boosters prior to likely exposure	At least semi-annual boosters, 4 to 6 weeks prepartum	A series of at least three doses is recommended for primary immunization of foals. Use inactivated vaccine for prepartum booster.
	Intranasal modified live virus: first dose at 11 months (has been safely administered to foals less than 11 months)	Booster every 6 months	Booster every 6 months	Booster every 6 months	Booster annually and before breeding; not recommended for pregnant mares until more data are available	If the first dose is administered to foals less than 11 months of age, administer a second dose at or after 11 months.

Vaccine	Foals and Weanlings	Yearlings	Performance Horses	Pleasure Horses	Broodmares[1]	Comments
Rhinopneumononitis (EHV-1 and EHV-4)[3]	First dose at 4 to 6 months; Second dose at 5 to 7 months; Third dose at 6 to 8 months; Then at 3-month intervals	Booster every 3 to 4 months, up to annually	Booster every 3 to 4 months, up to annually	Semiannual booster is optional	Booster at fifth, seventh, and ninth month of gestation with inactivated EHV-1/EHV-4 combovaccine; Optional dose at third month of gestation	Vaccinating mares before breeding and 4 to 6 weeks prepartum is suggested. Breeding stallions should be vaccinated before the breeding season and semiannually.
Strangles	Injectable: first dose at 4 to 6 months; second dose at 5 to 7 months; third dose at 7 to 8 months (depending on the product used); fourth dose at 12 months; Intranasal: first dose at 6 to 9 months; second dose 3 weeks later	Semiannual booster	Semiannual booster is optional if risk is high	Semiannual booster is optional if risk is high	Semiannual booster with 1 dose of inactivated M-protein vaccine, 4 to 6 weeks prepartum	Vaccines containing M-protein extract may be less reactive than whole-cell vaccines. Use when endemic conditions exist or risk is high. Foals as young as 6 weeks of age may safely receive the intranasal product. A third dose should be administered 2 to 4 weeks before weaning.

continued

Vaccination Guidelines for Horses (continued)

Vaccine	Foals and Weanlings	Yearlings	Performance Horses	Pleasure Horses	Broodmares[1]	Comments
Rabies	From unvaccinated mare: first dose at 3 to 4 months; second dose at 12 months; From vaccinated mare: first dose at 6 months; second dose at 7 months; third dose at 12 months	Annual booster	Annual booster	Annual booster	Annual booster, before breeding	Vaccination is recommended in endemic areas. Do not use modified live virus vaccines in horses.
Potomac horse fever	First dose at 5 to 6 months; Second dose at 6 to 7 months	Semiannual booster	Semiannual booster	Semiannual booster	Semiannual booster, with 1 dose 4 to 6 weeks prepartum	Booster May to June in endemic areas.
Botulism	From unvaccinated mare: see comments; From vaccinated mare: 3-dose series of toxoid at 30-day intervals, starting at 2 to 3 months of age	Consult your veterinarian	Consult your veterinarian	Consult your veterinarian	Initial 3-dose series at 30-day intervals, with the last dose 4 to 6 weeks prepartum; Annually thereafter, 4 to 6 weeks prepartum	Only in endemic areas. A third dose administered 4 to 6 weeks after the second dose may improve the response of foals to primary immunization. Foals from unvaccinated mares may benefit from toxoid at 2, 4, and 8 weeks of age; transfusion of plasma from a vaccinated horse or antitoxin. Efficacy of all three needs further study.

Vaccine	Foals and Weanlings	Yearlings	Performance Horses	Pleasure Horses	Broodmares[1]	Comments
Equine viral arteritis						
Annual booster	Annual booster for to be breeding stallions: one dose at 6 to 12 months	Intact colts intended for colts intended to be breeding stallions	for colts intended to be breeding stallions	Annual booster for colts intended to be breeding stallions	Annual booster for seronegative, open mares before breeding to carrier stallions; Isolate mares for 21 days after breeding to carrier stallion	Annual booster breeding stallions and teasers, 28 days before the start of breeding season. Virus may be shed in semen for up to 21 days. Vaccinated mares do not develop clinical signs, even though they become transiently infected and may shed virus for a short time.
Rotavirus A	Little value to vaccinate a foal because there is insufficient time to develop antibodies to protect during this susceptible age	Not applicable	Not applicable	Not applicable	Vaccinate mares in eighth, ninth, and tenth month of gestation, each pregnancy.	Passive transfer of colostral antibodies aids in preventing rotaviral diarrhea in foals. Check concentrations of immunoglobulins in foals to be sure there is no failure of passive transfer.

[1]Schedules for stallions should be consistent with the vaccination program of the adult horse population on the farm and modified according to risk.
[2]EEE=eastern equine encephalomyelitis, WEE=western equine encephalomyelitis, VEE=Venezuelan equine encephalomyelitis
[3]EHV-1 and EHV-4=equine herpesvirus

4

THE SKIN AND COAT

Skin is a barrier that keeps out bacteria and other foreign agents. It is involved in the synthesis of essential vitamins. It provides sensation to the surface of the body. It gives form to the body and insulates the horse against extremes of heat and cold.

The skin of the horse is remarkably strong and sensitive. Despite its apparent toughness, however, it is easily damaged by cinches, girths, and horse tack, and by rough handling with the wrong type of grooming equipment. Once the surface of the skin is broken or disturbed by trauma or a skin disorder, the condition tends to spread rapidly and becomes a major problem to the horse and her owner.

The outer skin layer is the epidermis. It is a *scaly* layer that varies in thickness on different parts of the horse's body. It is thinnest over the muzzle, around the lips, in the skin creases of the groin, and beneath the front legs. In these areas it is most easily traumatized.

The epidermis is modified to form hornlike growths on the legs called chestnuts and ergots. Chestnuts are located on the front legs above the knees and on the back legs below the hocks. Contrary to popular belief, they do not represent the vestiges of missing digits. Ergots are found at the back of the fetlocks. Their size varies among different breeds. In some horses they are hidden by long hair feathers.

The next layer inward is the *dermis*. The dermis gives rise to the skin appendages, which are the sweat glands, sebaceous glands, and hair *follicles*. Sweat glands are present everywhere on the body except the legs, and are most numerous behind the ears, on the neck, and on the chest and flanks. Sweat is alkaline and salty, and it produces the horse's characteristic odor.

Sebaceous glands open directly on the skin and discharge an oily or waxy substance called sebum. Sebum coats the hair, waterproofs the coat, and causes the individual hairs to lie flat. It also gives the coat its luster or shine. Frequent brushing and grooming increase the secretion of sebum and make the coat "bloom."

Hair follicles are present everywhere except beneath the tail, around the genitalia, and on the inside of the thighs.

106

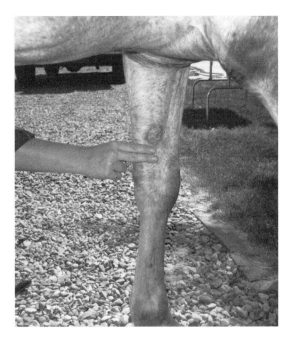

Chestnuts, like human fingerprints, are unique to each horse. They can be used for accurate and permanent identification.

Beneath the skin is a layer of fat that insulates against extremes of temperature. Wasting diseases with a loss of subcutaneous fat cause the skin to become dry and hidebound, especially over the ribs.

The horse's outer haircoat is composed of long, heavy guard hairs. Tiny muscles called piloerectors connect to the roots of the guard hairs. When these muscles contract, they make the hairs stand out, thus trapping warm air and providing better insulation in cold weather.

Beneath the outer coat is a dense, thick undercoat. The undercoat is shed in spring and fall. At such times, the horse should be groomed vigorously to remove dead hair.

Additionally, the horse has hair of a different quality that is not shed. This is the hair of the eyelashes, mane, and tail, and the tactile hair of the muzzle.

A condition called patchy shedding may occur in the spring. Some horses shed large patches of hair all at once, producing bare areas 8 to 10 inches (20 to 25 cm) in diameter. The skin is perfectly normal. There is no itching, but the condition may be mistaken for a fungus and the horse might be treated for ringworm. A similar loss of hair can occur several days after a high fever. Seasonal shedding in horses is not associated with matting and clumping. Mats, clumps, and a disordered appearance suggest a fungal *infection*.

Hirsutism is excessive growth of the haircoat. This condition is most common in senior horses and those with Cushing's disease. A growth on the pituitary gland is another cause. Hirsute hair is exceptionally long and coarse and often becomes matted and curly.

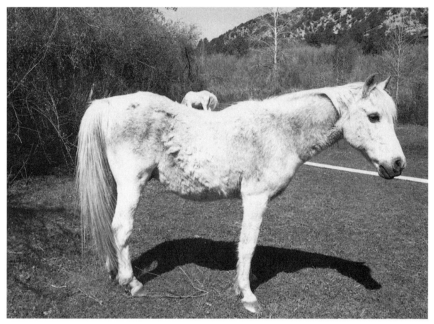

Patchy shedding is normal in the spring.

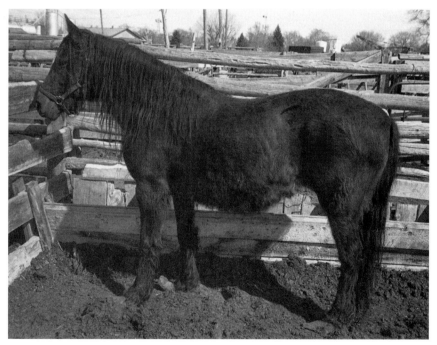

An old, malnourished mare with chronic laminitis and a hirsute coat.

The color of a horse's coat is determined by cells at the roots of hair follicles, called *melanin* granules. The specific color is mediated by variations in the density and distribution of these granules, which are controlled by complex genetic influences that are not fully understood in horses. A saddle sore or girth gall can damage the melanin layer and result in an area of *depigmentation*, seen as a spot of white hair. Leg wraps and bandages can also cause this damage when they are placed too tight.

How to Avoid Coat and Skin Problems

The appearance of the coat is a good indication of the health of the horse. The coat of a horse in good health is smooth, fine, and glossy. The coat of a horse in ill health is dry, coarse, "staring," and lacks the luster and shine imparted by the skin oils.

Grooming

Brushing your horse a few minutes each day will help keep her free of skin and hair problems. Brushing removes dirt and debris and also stimulates sebum production. Horses at pasture usually cannot be groomed daily, but they still should have their feet cleaned and their coat brushed at regular intervals.

Grooming should be a pleasurable experience for both you and the horse. Be aware of sensitive and ticklish areas and groom them gently. This gives you an excellent opportunity to examine the outside of the horse for any abnormalities or conditions that weren't previously there. Grooming tools that are especially useful are listed here. Your choice of tools will depend on the character and condition of the horse's coat.

- **Body brush.** This is a fine, soft brush used over the entire body. It is the principal tool in grooming. Brushes with natural bristles produce less static and broken hair than those with nylon bristles.
- **Curry comb.** Rubber and metal combs are available. Rubber combs are less likely to injure the skin. Metal combs are best reserved for removing hair from grooming brushes. Combs are useful in grooming horses with long, thick coats. They are also good for loosening dirt and removing loose hair when the horse is shedding. Use the curry comb firmly but gently in small circles over the neck and body. Do not use a curry comb about the head or below the knees and hocks.
- **Dandy brush.** This coarser brush is used on the lower legs to remove mud. It also can be used to brush out the mane and tail.
- **Sweat scraper.** This is a flexible strip or curved solid piece of metal used for scraping off moisture after exercise or bathing. It helps speed up the drying process before grooming.

- **Drying towel.** A drying towel can be made from an old blanket cut into sections 2 to 3 feet (60 to 90 cm) square. Wool is best for absorbing moisture. Cotton or burlap can be used to dry and polish the coat.
- **Grooming cloth.** This is a dry cloth used to wipe off the head, nostrils, and base of the tail, and to apply hair conditioners.
- **Hoof pick.** This is a small metal pick used for cleaning the frog and sole.

A horse should be groomed before and after a workout. Remove dirt and surface debris from the skin, taking extra care in the saddle area (the girth, back, and withers). This helps to prevent any injuries from the equipment rubbing against dirty skin.

Starting at the head, wipe the face, eyes, nostrils, earflaps, and dock with a soft, clean cloth. If these areas are especially dirty, a moist sponge works well; just take care not to get any water in the horse's eyes or ears. Only a soft brush should be used on the face and ears. Always brush in the direction of the hair growth.

Systematically work your way from front to back, top to bottom. While standing on one side of the horse, begin brushing using the body brush. Begin at the neck and work down the front of the chest and the side of the shoulder. Brush the foreleg, back, belly, loin, croup, and hind leg. A curry comb works well to remove mud, and then follow with the body brush. The brush strokes should be in the direction of the hair growth, with a slight flipping at the end of the stroke to flick the remaining dust free from the haircoat. Do not use the curry comb below the knee; a coarse dandy brush is good for removing stubborn mud and dirt from the lower leg. Cross to the other side of the horse and repeat the routine.

The mane and tail can be brushed with a dandy brush or a wire pin brush. Be sure and stand to one side while brushing the tail in case the horse kicks out.

Finally, clean the feet with a hoof pick. Start at the frog and work toward the toe, stroking away from you. For more details, see *Hoof Care* (page 202).

After a workout, the horse should be walked and cooled before grooming. At this time, water may be offered if the horse is thirsty. Using the sweat scraper, scrape off the surface moisture and rub the horse down with a drying towel. Once dry, a soft brush may be used to remove dried sweat and to replace the hair in its natural position. Once again, pick the hooves out to make sure the horse hasn't picked up any stones during the ride, and at this time a hoof dressing may be applied, if desired.

A thorough grooming not only keeps the horse's skin in good health but also feels good to the horse and is a reward for work well done.

Bathing

How frequently you should bathe your horse depends on how you ride her and the condition of her coat. Avoid bathing a horse in cold weather. Chilling lowers the horse's resistance to infection and predisposes her to respiratory diseases.

Horses shed in the spring and fall. A bath helps to remove loose hair, plant matter, and dirt. Exhibition horses are bathed in preparation for horse shows. If you plan to show, it is a good idea to get your horse used to the bath routine. When bathing your horse, use the same systematic approach as described for grooming.

Too much bathing removes skin oils and leaves the coat dull and dry. Shampoos remove dirt, but also remove skin oils that protect the hair and give the coat its sheen. A good horse shampoo should effectively remove dirt but be mild enough to preserve the natural skin oils. Commercial shampoo and hair conditioners are available. These products are protein-based natural moisturizers and are designed to coat the hair shaft much the way sebum does.

Wet the horse with lukewarm water and use a body sponge to apply the shampoo. After soaping thoroughly, rinse the horse well to remove all residual soap from the coat and skin. Remove excess moisture with the sweat scraper and towel the horse vigorously. Cover the horse with a blanket and walk her until she is dry.

The best results are obtained when shampoos are used infrequently, the coat is rinsed thoroughly to remove all soap residue, and the coat is brushed frequently between baths. Rinsing the horse with plain water after a workout helps remove the salty sweat residue and is not hard on the haircoat.

SPECIAL BATH PROBLEMS
Skunk Oil

Commercial skunk deodorizers are available. Skunk oil can also be removed from your horse's coat by soaking the affected areas in the following solution:

> 1 pint (500 ml) hydrogen peroxide
>
> 1 pound (454 g) baking soda (not baking powder)
>
> A couple of squirts of any dishwashing liquid mixed in 1 gallon (3.8 l) of water

These ingredients, in their separate packages, are easy to store in a plastic bucket until they're needed. The recipe must be mixed and used within one hour, and will explode if kept in a covered container. This formula is safe to use around horses, pets, and humans. However, be very careful with this mixture, because hydrogen peroxide can blind your horse if it gets into her eyes. There is a possibility that the solution will bleach the hair through its oxidation effect, so black hair may turn brown or gray until the hair grows back out.

Tar and Paint

Trim away as much hair as you can that contains the tar, oil, or paint. Soak the affected spots in vegetable oil and leave overnight. In the morning, remove the oil with soap and water. If the substance is on the hoof, use a clean cloth to apply nail polish remover and follow it with a good rinsing. Do not use petroleum solvents such as gasoline, kerosene, or turpentine, as they are extremely harmful to the skin and feet.

Cleaning the Sheath

The sheath is a double fold of skin surrounding the penis. There is a pocket within the glans penis above the *urethra* called the urethral diverticulum. Smegma can build up within the sheath, causing irritation and swelling of the sheath and penis. A heavy accumulation of smegma in the urethral diverticulum (called a "bean") can compress the urethra and interfere with the passage of urine.

Male horses should have their sheaths cleaned at least once every six months. For a complete sheath cleaning, many times the horse will require sedation. Males with white skin, such as Pintos and Appaloosas, are especially prone to smegma formation and skin *cancer* on the sheath, and may need to have their sheaths cleaned more often. Cleaning gives you the opportunity to closely examine the sheath. Before cleaning the sheath and penis, the horse should be restrained (see *Handling and Restraint*, page 2). Ivory soap in warm water makes a good wash solution. Do not use preparations that contain iodine such as Betadine, antibacterial soaps, or antiseptic soaps such as chlorhexidine, because they can be extremely irritating to the *prepuce* and penis.

Soap your hand well, then use your fingers to loosen and gently remove an accumulation of smegma in the folds of the skin sheath. **Use caution:** Some horses kick! As the penis extends, wash it in the same manner. If there is an accumulation of smegma in the urethral diverticulum, manually evert the diverticulum and clean the recess. Rinse thoroughly with plain water to remove all soapy residue. Be aware of any unusual appearance, swelling, or irritation on the sheath. If you see any, have a veterinarian take a look because this is a common location for cancer.

The Mane and Tail

Pulling the mane and tail is done to thin and even out hair for the sake of appearance. Mane and tail length are generally determined by breed standards.

Grasp only a few hairs at a time and slide your hand up close to the roots, then give a quick jerk. Work the longest hairs on the underside first. Scissors should not be used to shape the tail, as this will give a poor appearance. Occasionally the mane is "roached" or clipped, either for cosmetic reasons or to prevent snarling.

Body clipping is done to prepare a horse for show, or to facilitate the cooling-down process after strenuous workouts. A clipped horse chills easily and must be protected from the cold. This involves housing the horse in a heated facility, or, in less inclement weather, keeping her blanketed.

Blanketing

Horse blankets are used to keep the coat clean for exhibition purposes after a bath, to protect the horse from flies and biting insects, and to provide additional warmth for a sick horse. It is a good idea to blanket a horse while traveling in a horse trailer. This prevents chilling and protects the skin from injury.

Some horse owners like to blanket a horse throughout the winter because this seems to prevent excessive growth of the hair, induces earlier spring shedding, and produces a better-looking show coat. However, blanketing decreases a horse's adaptation to cold weather and thus may not be advisable in some circumstances (see *Cold Weather Care and Feeding*, page 419).

Be sure the blanket fits properly so that it won't slip and frighten the horse. Blankets should be worn only when a horse is stalled or can be easily observed in a paddock. It is not safe to turn a horse out to pasture wearing a blanket. If the horse will be exposed to rain, the blanket should be waterproof.

Cleaning Tack

Grooming equipment and horse tack should be cleaned and disinfected from time to time to prevent the spread of skin diseases. Several commercial tack washes are available. If possible, keep separate tack for each horse.

Leather apparel should be cleaned with saddle soap and protected against cracks and drying with a good leather oil such as neatsfoot oil. Regularly check the reins, cinch straps, and stirrup straps and repair or replace components that show wear.

Sorting Out Skin Problems

Diagnosing a skin disease can be difficult. The picture is often clouded by the presence of wounds, insect bites, and secondary trauma caused by rubbing and biting at the skin. The horse's history becomes important in deciding what caused the initial insult. Considerations such as age, sex, breed, change in activity or diet, contact with other animals, emotional state, exposure to skin irritants, and environmental influences then become important determinants.

The tables on pages 114–117 serve as an introduction to skin disorders and suggest where to look to find the cause of a problem. To facilitate identification, some skin ailments are listed in more than one table. For conditions caused by *parasites*, you'll find more information in chapter 2, "Parasites."

A horse who repeatedly rubs up against fences, posts, stalls, and other objects, or bites and scratches at her skin, has an itchy skin disorder. To determine the cause, consult the first table, Itchy Skin Disorders, on page 114.

In another group of conditions, hair loss is the principal sign. These diseases do not cause the horse much discomfort—at least not at first—but you will notice patchy hair loss from specific parts of the body. Usually these patches are circular and about 1 to 2 inches (25 to 50 mm) in diameter. Scabs and skin flakes are sometimes present. To determine the possible cause, see the second table, Disorders with Hair Loss, on page 115.

When a horse has a painful skin condition, you will see *pus* and other signs of infection on or beneath the skin. Often the skin becomes abraded and infected as a result of rubbing and scratching. In that case, you must treat both the itchy skin disorder and the secondarily infected skin. The common types of skin infection, also called *pyoderma*, are listed in the third table, Skin Infections (Pyoderma), on page 116.

During the course of grooming your horse, you may discover a lump, a bump, or a growth on or beneath the skin. To learn what it might be, consult the fourth table, Lumps, Bumps, and Growths on or Beneath the Skin, on page 117.

Itchy Skin Disorders

Insect bites: A common cause of itching in the fly season. You will see bumps, blisters, scabs, crusty areas, and occasionally hair loss where insects bite.

Queensland itch (culicoides dermatitis): The most common insect bite allergy in horses. Caused by gnats. Signs include *excoriations*, crusts, scabs, and intense itching with hair broken and rubbed off.

Ventral midline dermatitis: Caused by the migrating phase of a hairlike worm transmitted by gnats. Produces moist, crusty, shallow ulcerations, typically centered along the midline on the undersurface of the abdomen but sometimes on the face and eyelids. Hair is lost around the ulcerations.

Hives: Round, raised *wheals* scattered over the body with hair sticking out in patches. Swelling of the face or eyelids is a possibility. Usually caused by inhaled allergens, occasionally by allergens in the feed.

Irritant contact dermatitis: Red bumps with crusting and hair loss. Found around the muzzle, feet, legs, saddle girth, and other areas that are in contact with irritants. Healed skin may turn white (depigmentation).

Allergic contact dermatitis: Same as irritant contact dermatitis, but requires repeated or continuous contact with allergen (such as horse tack or a rubber bit). Dermatitis may spread beyond the area of contact.

Pemphigus foliaceus: A rare condition caused by an allergic response to a substance in the horse's own skin. Initially produces blisters, scabs, and scaly skin. Later, ulcerations appear with oozing serum and crusting.

Mange: An intensely itchy skin disorder caused by mites. Red lumps are followed by scabs, crusts, and patches of hair loss found all over the body, but especially on the poll, mane, tail, and legs. Mites in ear canals cause head-shaking. Hair is lost due to rubbing.

Chiggers: Intensely itchy skin caused by the larvae of mites. Traumatized skin is found about head, neck, chest, and legs. Seasonal and regional in chigger-infested pastures.

Lice: Intense itching caused by 2 to 3 mm pale insects found around the head and face, ears, topline, and base of tail. Hair is rubbed off, skin is excoriated.

Photosensitivity reaction: Requires exposure to sunlight. Skin shows redness, swelling, and weeping of serum. The outer skin may peel as in sunburn. Usually confined to white or lightly pigmented and hairless areas.

Summer sores (Habronema): Caused by the larvae of stomach worms deposited in open wounds and sores. Occurs only in the fly season. Suspect this when a clean wound or sore suddenly enlarges and becomes covered with a reddish-yellow tissue that bleeds easily.

Pinworms: Intense itching and tail rubbing, primarily in weanlings and young horses. "Ratty" look to the tail.

Disorders with Hair Loss

Patchy shedding: Normal type of shedding. Produces bare patches up to 10 inches (25 cm) in diameter. Skin is healthy and hair grows back in three weeks.

Ringworm: Highly contagious skin fungus. Usually occurs in fall and winter. Commonly located in the saddle girth area. Scaly, crusty, or red circular patches with central hair loss are typical. May see matted clumps of hair that fall out easily.

Seborrhea: A flaky, scaly condition that looks like dandruff. Usually symmetrical. Bare, circular patches occur where crusts peel off. May resemble ringworm.

Rain scalds: A fungal infection that occurs in rainy weather. Characterized by tufts of matted hair that look like large drops of water. Tufts come out, leaving bare patches about 1 inch (25 mm) in diameter. May resemble ringworm. Skin often becomes infected.

Irritant contact dermatitis: Red bumps with crusting and hair loss. Found around the muzzle, feet, legs, saddle girth, and other areas that are in contact with irritants. Healed skin may turn white (depigmentation).

Allergic contact dermatitis: Same irritant as contact dermatitis, but requires repeated or continuous contact with allergen (such as horse tack or a rubber bit). Dermatitis may spread beyond the area of contact.

Tail pyoderma: Furunculosis and *abscesses* occur on the skin of the tail from self-mutilation. The tail is severely abraded. Look for an underlying itchy skin problem, such as tail mites or pinworms.

Selenium toxicity: Loss of hair from the mane and tail (bob-tail disease). Cracks in hoof wall may cause severe lameness. (Discussed in chapter 15, "Nutrition and Feeding.")

Lymphoma: One or more subcutaneous masses or nodules resembling hives; seen in the form that invades the skin (rather than the internal forms).

Skin Infections (Pyoderma)

Cellulitis and abscess: Painful, hot, inflamed skin or pockets of pus beneath the skin. Look for an underlying cause (itchy skin disorder, foreign body, skin wound). One or more abscesses beneath the jaw suggests strangles.

Folliculitis (summer rash): Hair-pore infection that occurs in the saddle area in hot weather.

Furunculosis: A deep-seated hair-pore infection with draining sinus tracts to the skin.

Tail pyoderma: Furunculosis and abscesses that occur on the skin of the tail from self-mutilation. The tail is severely abraded. Look for an underlying itchy skin problem, such as tail mites or pinworms.

Ulcerative lymphangitis: Begins in extremity wounds with swelling of the leg and the appearance of abscesses along the lymphatic channels. The abscesses open and drain pus. (Discussed in chapter 3, "Infectious Diseases.")

Malignant *edema*: Begins in dirty wounds about the legs and face. A soft, hot, painful swelling that progresses rapidly and produces a toxic form of gas gangrene. (Discussed in chapter 3, "Infectious Diseases.")

Poll-evil: A deep-seated infection at the poll, characterized by swelling on one or both sides of the poll, then the formation of one or more draining sinus tracts to the skin. (Discussed in chapter 3, "Infectious Diseases.")

Fistulous withers: The same as poll-evil, but occurs at the withers.

Rain scalds: A fungal infection that occurs in rainy weather. Characterized by tufts of matted hair that look like large drops of water. Tufts come out, leaving bare patches about 1 inch (25 mm) in diameter. May resemble ringworm. Skin often becomes infected.

Sporotrichosis: A draining sore or *ulcer* at the site of a puncture wound, usually on the leg. Nodules appear along the lymphatic channels, ulcerate, discharge pus, and heal slowly. Caused by a fungus.

Grease heel (mud fever): An infection at the back of the fetlocks and/or the heels, characterized by a greasy *exudate* that mats the hair. Proceeds to cellulitis and ulceration. Grapelike clusters may appear.

Summer sores (Habronema): Caused by the larvae of stomach worms deposited in open wounds and sores. Occurs only in the fly season. Suspect this when a clean wound or sore suddenly enlarges and becomes covered with a reddish-yellow tissue that bleeds easily.

Ventral midline dermatitis (onchocerciasis): Caused by the migrating phase of a hairlike worm transmitted by gnats. Produces moist, crusty, shallow ulcerations, typically centered along the midline on the undersurface of the abdomen but sometimes on the face. Hair is lost around the ulcerations.

Lumps, Bumps, and Growths On or Beneath the Skin

Warts (papillomas): Smooth, raised, flesh-colored bumps on the muzzle and lips of young horses. Usually disappear spontaneously in three months.

Sarcoid: The most common tumor in horses. Takes a variety of shapes. May be flat with hair loss, ulcerated, or cauliflower. Found around the eyes and anywhere on the body. Affects horses of all ages.

Tender knots: Frequently found at the site of an injection. Resolves spontaneously. Often painful.

Cattle grubs: Painful nodules beneath the skin, found at the withers, neck, and back, caused by larvae beneath the skin. May have a breathing hole in the skin.

Squamous cell carcinoma: A hard, flat, or ulcerating growth found on older horses of the lightly pigmented breeds, especially in hairless areas exposed to sunlight. Most common on the face and genitalia. Does not heal.

Melanoma: A dark brown to black nodular growth, usually on the underside of the tail; sometimes about the vulva, anus, male genitalia, eyes, or mouth. Commonly found on old gray horses.

Phycomycosis: A deep-seated fungal infection that often occurs at the site of a cut, usually on the leg but sometimes on the head and abdomen. A fast-growing bulbous mass of grayish-pink tissue that discharges infected material through numerous sinus tracts.

Lymphoma: A mass or nodule beneath the skin. Occasionally, the overlying skin becomes ulcerated with a loss of hair.

Abnormal Sweating
ANHIDROSIS (ABSENCE OF SWEATING)

Anhidrosis is loss of the ability to sweat in response to exercise or increased body temperature. Sweating is influenced by the adrenal hormone epinephrine. When released into the bloodstream, epinephrine acts directly on certain receptors in sweat glands, causing them to secrete. The reason why horses with anhidrosis do not sweat when stimulated is not known. One theory is that epinephrine receptors become less sensitive to the effects of the epinephrine. Hair follicles that do not sweat become plugged by dried sebum. This is a contributing factor.

Anhidrosis occurs primarily in horses living in hot, humid climates, particularly in Florida and along the Gulf Coast. It also occurs in horses following relocation from a temperate climate to a subtropical climate. Performance horses, especially racehorses, are most often affected, but pleasure horses also suffer from this condition.

Anhidrosis may be partial or complete, and the onset can be sudden or gradual. Sudden signs appear in hot weather after exercise. The affected horse has a fast pulse, high fever, dry skin, and rapid, labored breathing with flared nostrils at rest. These horses are called "breathers." Unless failure to sweat is noted by the owner, the horse may be treated (mistakenly) for a respiratory infection.

Horses with gradual onset exhibit poor exercise tolerance, a loss of weight and condition, a dry, rough haircoat, and patchy hair loss initially over the face. With long-standing disease, the skin becomes dry, scaly, and excoriated over the body.

The diagnosis of anhidrosis can be established by injecting a patch of skin with epinephrine or terbutaline sulfate. A normal horse drips sweat from the patch within 30 minutes. A horse with anhidrosis either does not sweat from the patch or sweats only when the injected dose is greatly increased.

Treatment: There is no specific treatment to restore sweating. Some horses with temporary anhidrosis apparently adapt or revert to a normal sweating pattern when moved to a cooler climate. If this is not an acceptable alternative, provide fan-cooled or air-conditioned facilities during the summer, and exercise the horse judiciously in warm weather to prevent overheating.

Avoid supplementing the horse's ration with grain and concentrates. Adding 4 ounces (113 g) of Lite (low-sodium) salt to the evening ration is beneficial. Horses with anhidrosis are at increased risk for heat stroke and should be monitored accordingly. See *Heat Stroke* (page 19).

Hyperhidrosis (Excessive Sweating)

Excessive sweating has many causes. It should be thought of as a symptom rather than a specific disease.

Horses can break out in a "cold" or "hot" sweat. Cold, clammy sweating is seen when a horse is stressed or in pain. The temperature drop is due to blood being shunted away from the skin. A hot sweat is due to increased flow of blood through the skin. It has the specific purpose of cooling the horse. Hot sweats are seen after exercise and also occur with high fever. Heavy sweating after a light workout suggests a lack of condition.

Profuse sweating occurs after the administration of certain drugs, such as epinephrine and acepromazine. It is also characteristic of tetanus, encephalomyelitis, and epinephrine-secreting tumors of the adrenal gland.

Patchy sweating over the neck, shoulders, and rib cage is seen with organophosphate insecticide poisoning.

Allergies

An allergic reaction is caused by a foreign protein (*allergen*) that invades the horse's immune system and triggers the release of histamine and other substances that result in self-injury. This is called a hypersensitivity reaction.

Before a horse can become sensitized to an allergen in the environment, she must have been exposed to it at least once before. In the allergic horse, repeat exposure to allergens such as pollens, molds, grasses and weeds, insect bites, certain feeds, and drugs trigger a reaction typified by itching, hives, occasional sneezing, coughing, and tearing. The skin and respiratory tract are the targets for allergic symptoms in horses.

There are two kinds of hypersensitivity reaction. The immediate type occurs shortly after exposure, while the delayed type occurs hours or days later. Insect bites are examples of both types; there can be an immediate or a delayed response. Anaphylactic shock (see page 28) is a life-threatening hypersensitivity reaction of the immediate type.

Hives (Urticaria)

Hives is the appearance of round, raised wheals on the skin, ranging in size from less than 1 inch (25 mm) to several inches in diameter. The hair sticks out in patches over parts of the body. There may be swelling of the face or eyelids. These wheals, which are not painful, pit with pressure. The horse may or may not itch.

Episodes of hives that come and go and last only a few hours are usually caused by inhaled allergens or, less commonly, by allergens in the feed. Inhaled allergens known to cause hives in horses include the down of bird feathers; pollens of numerous trees, bushes, plants, and weeds; grass and grass seeds; and dust, rusts, and molds.

Vaccinations and injected drugs are occasional causes of hives. Insect bites can but usually do not produce hives.

Treatment: Horses with hives usually recover spontaneously without treatment. Your veterinarian may consider a course of short-acting corticosteroids and antihistamines if this is the first episode.

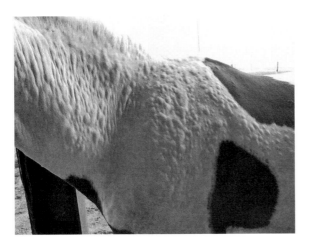

Severe hives of unknown origin; they did resolve after a course of short-acting corticosteroids.

With recurrent hives, attempt to identify the offending allergen and eliminate it from the horse's environment. It is always a challenge to identify the specific *antigens* to which the horse is allergic. A good allergy management program involves a detailed patient history, an assessment of the horse's environment, and a comprehensive clinical examination. Intradermal skin testing is the one way to identify an inhaled allergen. There are *ELISA* blood tests that can test for up to 70 different allergens, including weed, tree, and grass pollens, molds, mites, insects, Culicoides, and feed ingredients. This test can be customized for the airborne pollens that are native to your region.

Successfully avoiding airborne pollens may not be practical. A course of desensitizing injections may be effective in this situation.

When a food allergy is suspected, first take the horse off all sweet feeds and supplements. If this does not prevent recurrence, switch to pellets or alfalfa hay.

Contact and Allergic Contact Dermatitis

These two conditions are discussed together because they produce similar skin reactions. Both are caused by contact with a chemical. Although all horses who come into contact with an irritating chemical will develop a skin irritation, only horses who are allergic to a chemical will develop a hypersensitivity response.

A contact dermatitis of either type causes itchy red bumps and fluid-filled blisters that become crusted and sometimes secondarily infected. Hair is lost in the area of inflamed skin. The healed skin becomes thicker, rougher, and darker.

Contact dermatitis occurs around the muzzle, lower legs, feet, and in sites (like the saddle area) having contact with horse tack.

Common irritants are acids and alkalis, insecticides, detergents, solvents, soaps, and petroleum by-products such as creosote and tar.

Common allergens include dyes and preservatives in horse gear; chemicals in topical insecticides and horse liniments; and various plants including poison ivy and poison oak. Rubber bits can cause reactions around the mouth. The site of the reaction frequently indicates the cause of the dermatitis.

Treatment: Identify the skin allergen by removing the horse from all possible exposure for one to two weeks. If the problem clears, re-expose the horse to the suspected allergen. If the dermatitis returns, the diagnosis is established. Once the allergen is known, prevent further exposure.

When an irritating chemical has made contact with the skin, wash gently with warm water to remove all residue. Treat any secondary skin infection with a topical antibiotic such as nitrofurazone or triple antibiotic ointment.

Ventral Midline Dermatitis (Onchocerciasis)

Ventral midline dermatitis is a skin disease caused by the filarial phase of the hairlike worm *Onchocerca cervicalis*. The adult worm lives in the connective tissue of the horse's neck. The majority of horses in the United States are infected, but only a few develop dermatitis. It is believed that the skin response is due to an allergic reaction to the dying microfilaria.

The filaria migrate under the skin and settle primarily on the midline of the abdomen from the chest to the groin, especially around the umbilicus. Other sites are the withers, face, eyelids, and legs. At these sites, the parasites produce an itchy skin disorder with redness, moist shallow ulcerations, crusting and scaling, and patchy hair loss. Affected areas up to 10 inches (25 cm) in diameter can develop. Scarring and loss of skin pigmentation follow.

These open sores attract Culicoides gnats and other flying insects. Gnats feeding on the open sores pick up filaria and introduce them to a new host. Biting flies and other insects exacerbate the skin disorder and create *pyoderma*.

The *Onchocerca cervicalis* filaria are capable of penetrating the eye and producing *uveitis*, a leading cause of blindness in horses (see page 162).

Treatment: Ivermectin paste is completely effective in ridding the horse of filaria within two to three weeks. Minor reactions can occur with its use. Veterinary supervision is advised.

Adult worms are not affected by deworming agents and therefore serve as a reservoir for recurrent infection. To keep the skin free of disease, ivermectin must be repeated at four-month intervals. A deworming program incorporating ivermectin, as described on page 54, will effectively control onchocerciasis.

Summer Sores

Summer sores are caused by the larvae of stomach worms (Habronema). These larvae are deposited by stable and horse flies as they feed around moist areas on the body, especially the sheath of the penis and corners of the eyes. Larvae also are deposited in open wounds.

Summer sores at the corners of the eyes and on the penis often assume a growthlike (granulomatous) appearance, resembling a sarcoid or squamous cell carcinoma. A skin *biopsy* is the best way to make the diagnosis.

An open wound or sore in the fly season that suddenly enlarges, ulcerates, and becomes covered with reddish-yellow tissue that bleeds easily should be suspected of being a summer sore. Over the raised round surface of the wound is a gritty, greasy-looking exudate containing rice-sized, yellow, calcified dead larvae.

Summer sores may heal, only to break out again next season. This suggests that a hypersensitivity reaction related to the presence of adult stomach worms is a factor in some cases. Horses with summer sores are nearly always heavily parasitized by Habronema. There is severe itching.

Treatment: In the beginning stages, summer sores respond well to ivermectin paste, which is effective against both the adult worms in the stomach and the larvae in the wound. The inclusion of ivermectin in a deworming program will reduce the frequency of summer sores.

Skin preparations containing organophosphate insecticides, wettable powders, and antibiotics can be applied beneath dressings or massaged into larger open sores with good results. Your veterinarian can provide you with a suitable prescription.

Insect Bite Allergies

Flies, mites, ticks, lice, gnats, and mosquitoes are insect parasites that can irritate and injure the horse. Most of them are bloodsucking. The mouth parts of the biting flies, in particular, tear the skin and do considerable physical damage. Hypersensitivity reactions will occur if the horse is allergic to a substance in the saliva of the insect. For more information, see *External Parasites* (page 57).

Culicoides Dermatitis

Also called Queensland itch or summer eczema, this is a seasonal recurring skin disorder caused by the bites of Culicoides gnats, also called midges, no-see-ums, or sand flies. It is the most common insect bite allergy in horses. The saliva of these gnats contains a protein that causes an intense allergic reaction characterized by severe itching. Hair is broken and matted, particularly around the mane, poll, and tail. Hair loss occurs in these areas. The skin shows excoriations, crusts, and scabs. Secondary bacterial infection is common. Thickening of skin and loss of hair pigmentation are later developments.

Although Culicoides hypersensitivity is the most common cause of mane and tail rubbing, the stable fly, horn fly, and black fly also produce an allergic dermatitis difficult to distinguish from Queensland itch. In some cases, more than one insect may be involved.

Treatment: Topical corticosteroid preparations help reduce skin inflammation and the allergic reaction. In severe cases, a short course of steroids may have to be given by mouth or injection. Consult your veterinarian. Treat secondary pyoderma as described in *Pyoderma* (page 123).

Prevention: Culicoides gnats feed primarily at dusk, night, and dawn. To prevent exposure, stable the horse before dusk. Gnats are reluctant to enter barns. Culicoides do not fly well against air currents, so a fan in the doorway, directed away from the stables, may help. The Culicoides gnat breeds in stagnant water and can fly only about 440 to 880 yards (402 to 804 m). Eliminating stagnant water within these flight limits effectively controls the gnat population.

Many topical insecticides do not repel gnats. Poridon, however, is effective against gnats as well as flies and mosquitoes. One application lasts seven days. Apply as directed by the manufacturer.

Pyoderma

Pyoderma means pus in the skin. It is caused by infections, inflammations, and/or any abnormal growth such as a tumor. Most commonly, pyoderma refers to a bacterial infection of the skin that drains pus. Many cases are the result of self-mutilation. When a horse rubs or bites at a persistent irritant, the skin becomes infected. The infection arises only because another itchy skin disorder was present first. Always look for another skin disorder before concluding that pyoderma is the only problem.

The skin infection can manifest in a variety of forms, including:

- **Cellulitis** is an infection of the deep layer of the skin. Most cases are caused by puncture wounds, scratches, and lacerations. Horses are particularly prone to such injuries. Many wound infections can be prevented by proper early treatment of wounds, as described in *Wounds* (page 32). Signs of cellulitis include pain (tenderness to pressure), warmth (the skin feels hotter than normal), firmness (not as soft as normal), and change in color (skin appears redder than normal). As infection spreads out from a wound, you may feel tender cords, which are swollen lymphatic channels. Regional lymph nodes may enlarge. This is a stage beyond cellulitis and is characterized by ulcerative lymphangitis (page 76) and malignant edema (page 74).

- **Abscess** is a localized pocket of pus. Pimples, *pustules*, furuncles, and *boils* are examples of small skin abscesses. An abscess is usually not fixed and firm, and feels like fluid under pressure.

- **Folliculitis** (summer rash) is an infection of the hair pores. It is nearly always caused by a *Staphylococcus* bacterium. It tends to occur in hot weather as a consequence of excessive sweating and friction to the skin from ill-fitting tack. Small pimples appear, usually at points of contact in the saddle or harness areas. These pimples enlarge and form pustules. The pustules rupture and exude pus. Crusts form and the hair becomes matted. Folliculitis can be prevented by good hygiene, including brushing and cleaning the skin and coat after workouts and using clean, dry blankets beneath saddles.

- **Furunculosis** is a deep-seated hair-pore infection with draining sinus tracts and patchy hair loss. It is a progressive form of folliculitis and is more difficult to treat.

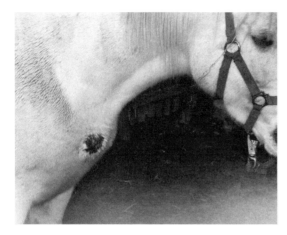

This horse has cellulitis and furunculosis of the skin of the chest wall, the result of a neglected wire cut.

- **Tail pyoderma** begins as an itchy skin disorder caused by mange mites or pinworms. As the horse scratches, rubs, and abrades the skin of her tail, a secondary staph infection occurs and pustules develop. The ailment is complicated by furunculosis and by abscesses that rupture and drain in an unending cycle. Hair is lost on the top of the tail. Treatment is most difficult.

General Treatment of Pyoderma

Any underlying itchy skin disorder should be treated to eliminate rubbing, biting, and self-mutilation. Localize the skin infection by clipping away the hair and applying warm soaks for 15 minutes, three times a day. Saline soaks, made by adding 1 cup (290 g) of Epsom salts to 1 gallon (3.8 l) of warm water, make a good poultice. Daily Betadine scrubs help loosen scabs and promote cleanliness. Topical antibiotics, such as nitrofurazone or triple antibiotic ointment, should be applied two to three times a day. If the horse does not show improvement with these over-the-counter medications, consulting with your veterinarian will provide the best treatment for your horse.

Pimples, pustules, furuncles, boils, and other small abscesses that do not drain spontaneously should be lanced with a sterile needle or a scalpel. Abscesses may be *cultured* to identify the bacteria and to determine appropriate antibiotics. If a cavity is present, flush with a dilute antiseptic surgical scrub (see *Wounds*, page 35). Keep the skin open and draining until the cavity heals from below.

Foreign bodies beneath the skin, such as splinters, must be removed with forceps, as they are a continuing source of infection.

Oral or injectable antibiotics are used in treating wound infections, cellulitis, abscesses, furunculosis, and tail pyoderma. Most skin bacteria respond well to penicillin, oxytetracycline, or trimethoprim-sulfadiazine. Those that do not respond promptly should be cultured and an antibiotic selected based on sensitivity tests.

Grease Heel (Scratches, Mud Fever)

Grease heel is an infection of the skin at the back of the pastern and heel. It occurs most commonly in breeds that have long fetlock hair. Two other predisposing factors are trauma to the skin and wet, muddy footing.

Grit on track surfaces, rough stubble in fields, or bites of chigger mites often cause the initial scratches or breaks in the skin, which become infected by a variety of bacteria, especially *Staphylococcus*. The result is a painful pyoderma in which a greasy exudate of serum accumulates and mats the long hairs. Swelling, hair loss, and ulceration occur as the disease progresses. The horse may become painfully lame and exhibit a stringhaltlike gait. Occasionally, heaps of granulation tissue produce grapelike clusters. The skin cracks and exudes a foul odor.

Treatment: Clip the hair and apply saline soaks and Betadine scrubs, as described in *General Treatment of Pyoderma* (page 124).

In mild cases, apply zinc oxide paste or calamine lotion to dry up the skin. Treat irritated or infected skin by applying an antibiotic-corticosteroid ointment such as Corticosporin. Dress and cover the area with an ace bandage. Use standing wraps or polo wraps. Absorbent dressing may also be used if there is drainage. You should see improvement rather quickly. If not, consult your veterinarian. Oral or injectable antibiotics are needed to treat cellulitis. Grapelike growths should be burned off or removed surgically.

Prevention: Stable horses in clean surroundings with dry bedding. Keep the hair at the heels and pasterns short. Always clean the feet after exercise.

Pemphigus Foliaceus

This is an uncommon scaling and crusting *autoimmune* skin disease caused by the development of antibodies to a substance present in the horse's own skin. Half the cases occur in Appaloosas.

The disease begins with the development of small blisters on the lower body. The blisters rupture and form scabs and scaly skin. Fever, listlessness, and swelling of the legs and the male genitalia are common. In time, the process becomes generalized.

The diagnosis is made by taking a skin biopsy.

Treatment: Steroids can arrest the disease. *Foals* and yearlings may stay in *remission* when the dosage is tapered and discontinued. Older horses tend to relapse and require lifetime treatment. Anticancer drugs that suppress the immune response may be of value.

Mange

Mange is an intensely itchy skin disease caused by tiny spiderlike insects called mites. Mites live on the surface of the skin or in tunnels a few millimeters beneath the skin. Females deposit eggs in burrows or beneath scabs. Eggs hatch in about four days. Mites reach maturity soon thereafter and live only one to two weeks. The whole cycle takes only 15 to 20 days.

There are four species of mites that infect the horse.

- **Sarcoptic mite,** the cause of scabies, burrows beneath the skin of the head, ears, neck, chest, flank, and abdomen. Small red bumps appear around the burrows. As the horse rubs, paws, and bites at the skin to relieve the irritation, the resulting trauma produces further skin injury with crusts, weeping serum, loss of hair, and thickening of the skin. Secondary bacterial infection is common and complicates the picture. Sarcoptic mange is highly contagious and is easily transmitted to people.

- **Psoroptic mite,** also called the tail mite, produces lumps and patches of hair loss over the poll, mane, and tail. It is not transferable to humans. This mite has been eradicated from horses in the United States.

- **Chorioptic mite** causes leg or foot mange. It is found below the hocks and knees. These mites live on the surface of the skin and produce scabs, crusts, and patches of hair loss. The disease may be difficult to distinguish from grease heel.

Ringworm and summer sores may look like mange, but can be distinguished by examining skin scabs and scrapings under a microscope; or, in difficult cases, by taking a skin biopsy to look for mites.

Treatment: Horses with mange should be isolated or quarantined to prevent transmission to other horses. Be sure to keep their tack separated, as well.

Mange should be treated by a veterinarian. Treating sarcoptic, chorioptic, and psoroptic mange involves the use of topical insecticides. A thorough dipping or high-pressure spray application is required to saturate the skin. While washing, dislodge scabs with a stiff brush. Several applications at seven- to ten-day intervals are required. There is little information on the use of ivermectin for treating mange mites in horses, but available reports suggest that the drug may be effective in the usual recommended dosage. There is no satisfactory treatment for demodectic mange in horses.

Dermatophilosis (Rain Scalds, Rain Rot)

Rain scalds is a skin infection caused by the bacteria *Dermatophilus congolensis*. The organism is activated by moisture. Most horses with rain scalds have been exposed to wet, soggy pastures during a period of heavy rainfall immediately before the appearance of skin disease.

The organism is opportunistic and enters through breaks in the skin. Biting fly attacks or grooming with a stiff brush or metal comb often initiate such injuries. In addition, wet skin is more easily abraded than dry skin, and thus is more susceptible to infection.

Rain scalds first appear as pus sticking to tufts of matted hair, giving a characteristic "paintbrush" appearance. The tufts come out, leaving cup-like crusts over the back, rump, saddle area, head, neck, and hind legs. Beneath the adherent crusts is a collection of pus.

In longhaired horses, the scalds may spread and join to form large confluent areas of matted hair and crusts. In shorthaired horses, the scalds usually remain smaller and occur as bumps covered with scabs. Secondary staph infection is common.

Rain scalds can be mistaken for ringworm, and vice versa. Smears taken from the underside of a scab or crust often show the characteristic bacteria. Cultures confirm the diagnosis.

Treatment: Stable the horse in a dry facility and provide dry footing. Clip away hair and apply an antiseptic soak or shampoo (Betadine or chlorhexidine) daily for seven days, then weekly until the skin is healed. It is important to remove scabs with a brush and mild soap. However, if this is too painful or causes bleeding, continue the soaks until the scabs separate easily.

D. congolensis is sensitive to most antibiotics. Topical agents work well. A 0.25 percent chloramphenicol solution is quite effective. Apply daily for five to seven days. Oral or injectable antibiotics (oxytetracycline or penicillin) are indicated for severe or widespread involvement. If staph is suspected, obtain a culture and sensitivity test, because many staph species are resistant to penicillin.

Fungus Infections
RINGWORM

Ringworm is not a worm but a fungus that lives on the surface of the skin. There are five kinds of ringworm in horses. They all cause patchy hair loss.

Ringworm gets its name from its appearance: a rapidly spreading circle with hair loss at the center and a red ring at the margin. Within the circle, the skin becomes scabby and sometimes raw. These circular crusty patches usually are 1 to 2 inches (25 to 50 mm) in diameter, but may become larger.

Ringworm can occur anywhere on the horse's body, but is most common in the saddle area, where it is known as girth itch. Other common sites are the face and neck. One type of ringworm produces matted or clumped hair that falls out in large clumps.

The disease is transmitted among horses by contact with contaminated saddles, blankets, and grooming equipment. Humans, especially children, can pick up ringworm from horses.

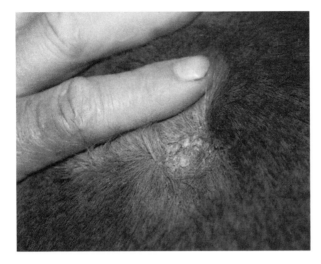

Ringworm is visible as a crusty patch with hair loss, about half an inch (13 mm) in diameter.

When the diagnosis is in doubt, it can be confirmed by microscopic examination of skin scrapings or by fungal cultures.

Treatment: Most cases disappear spontaneously in one to four months. To reduce the spread and shorten the illness, clip away the infected hair at the margins of the ringworm patch and bathe the skin with Betadine soap to remove dead scales. Small patches can be treated with tolnaftate (Tinactin), miconazole, or clotrimazole; all are available without a prescription. With extensive involvement, your veterinarian may prescribe griseofulvin. This drug should not be used on pregnant *mares*.

Prevention: To prevent transmission, disinfect grooming equipment, tack, and apparel with a bleach solution.

Phycomycosis

Phycomycosis is a deep-seated skin infection caused by a funguslike microorganism called *Pythium*. It was originally thought to be caused by leeches, and a *Pythium* infection is still sometimes called "leeches." Many cases occur in low prairie land along the Gulf of Mexico, and also have been reported in Papua New Guinea, Indonesia, Australia, Brazil, Columbia, Costa Rica, Argentina, Greece, Egypt, France, and Japan.

The organism lives in water or moist, decaying vegetation and gains entrance through wounds such as wire cuts. In a very short time, the horse develops a swollen mass of devitalized tissue that is gray or yellow and from which numerous sinus tracts discharge plugs of infected material. Bleeding may occur from the tissue surface. These masses, usually found on the lower legs and sometimes actually encircling them, can grow up to 10 inches (25 cm) in diameter. A horse may have two or more of these exuberant growths on various parts of her body. The organism spreads rapidly to regional lymph nodes and occasionally into the abdomen.

Diagnosis requires a biopsy, culture, and polymerase chain reaction blood test. An infected horse cannot transmit the disease to people or other horses.

Treatment: Only early treatment can cure the horse. The best results are obtained with a combination of immunotherapy and surgery. Immunotherapy involves giving the horse a vaccine prepared from cultures of the *Pythium* organism. At least three vaccinations are required. While waiting for the mass to get smaller, apply Betadine soaks twice daily. This helps prevent secondary bacterial infection.

Only small phycomycosis masses respond to vaccination alone. Most masses must be surgically excised after they have ceased to regress. Multiple operations may be necessary. *Prognosis* is poor.

Sporotrichosis

This disease is caused by *Sporothrix schenckii*, a yeastlike fungus present on vegetation, particularly on the thorns of roses and on plants that have sharp spicules, or needlelike projections. It affects horses worldwide.

A draining sore develops at the site of a puncture wound. This usually occurs on the leg but sometimes on the upper body. Nodules appear beneath the skin along the course of the lymphatic system. The nodules ulcerate, discharge pus, crust over, and heal slowly.

The disease may resemble ulcerative lymphangitis (see page 76). The diagnosis is made by taking a sample of wound discharge for fungus culture or a specimen of infected tissue for fluorescent *antibody* testing.

Treatment: The frequent application of warm packs is highly beneficial, because the fungus is particularly sensitive to heat. Sporotrichosis often

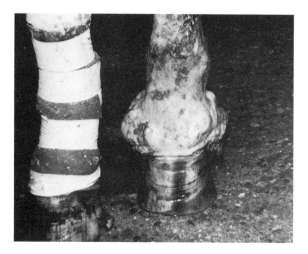

The swollen mass of tissue with draining sinus tracts that is characteristic of phycomycosis.

responds to oral iodine therapy when given for several weeks. To prevent relapse, continue treatment four weeks beyond healing. In horses who relapse or do not respond to this treatment, various drugs used to treat human fungus diseases can be tried under close veterinary supervision.

Sporotrichosis can be transmitted to people. Use disposable rubber gloves and hygienic techniques when handling infected material.

Seborrhea

Seborrhea is a flaky, scaly disease of the skin. It is not an itchy skin disorder, and secondary bacterial infection is not always a problem. Seborrhea is classified as either primary or secondary. Either form may be dry or oily.

Primary seborrhea is rare. It is localized to the mane, tail, and front of the cannon of the hind limbs. Primary seborrhea is sometimes called "stud crud," even though it is not limited to intact males.

Secondary seborrhea is known to be associated with skin infection, nutritional deficiencies, liver disease, intestinal malabsorption, vitamin A deficiency, sex hormone imbalances, and autoimmune skin diseases.

Dry seborrhea is characterized by scaling and flaking that looks much like dandruff. The skin is relatively healthy.

Oily seborrhea scales are held together by sebum, forming thick, yellowish-brown crusts. As the crusts peel off, you may see bare patches of skin up to 8 inches (20 cm) in diameter. With longstanding involvement, the skin becomes thickened and inelastic and the horse generally loses weight and condition.

Seborrhea can resemble ringworm or mange, because all three skin diseases are characterized by patchy hair loss.

Treatment: Secondary seborrhea may clear up when the underlying cause is treated. Primary seborrhea is incurable but can be managed with topical medications.

For dry seborrhea, clip the coat regularly and use a product that contains sulfa or sulfur, a salicylic acid shampoo, or a keratolytic product such as Kerasolv to keep the skin free of flakes. Benzoyl peroxide and sebum-dissolving shampoos help to loosen scales in cases of oily seborrhea.

Small patches can be treated with tolnaftate (Tinactin), miconazole, or clotrimazole; all are available without a prescription. Pragmatar ointment, available from your veterinarian, can be applied to individual skin spots. Topical and oral antibiotics are indicated when there is secondary bacterial infection. Your veterinarian will be able to suggest a treatment best suited for your horse.

Environmental and Traumatic Skin Disorders

PHOTOSENSITIVITY REACTION

Photosensitivity is an abnormal reaction of the skin when exposed to the ultraviolet rays in sunlight. Unlike sunburn, photosensitivity does not require excessive or prolonged exposure. (Sunburn does occur in horses, but usually only in those with white or light-colored skin.)

A horse becomes photosensitive only after a photodynamic chemical is deposited on or within her skin. A photodynamic chemical absorbs ultraviolet energy and transfers it to the dermis. The process is restricted to the hairless, white, or lightly pigmented parts of the body, such as the muzzle, ears, lips, vulva, udder, and coronary bands. The result is a skin reaction characterized by redness, swelling, itching, and weeping of serum. The outer layer of skin may peel as in sunburn. Later, the skin becomes thickened and fissured. Secondary pyoderma often complicates the picture.

Feedstuffs can contain photodynamic chemicals. The major photosensitizing agent in horses is phylloerythrin, a product formed by the breakdown of chlorophyll in the intestines. Normally, phylloerythrin is destroyed by the liver, but in horses with liver disease, toxic levels may reach the skin. This occurs in about 25 percent of horses with liver disease.

Plants that produce photosensitizing chemicals that can be acquired either by direct skin contact or through ingestion include St. John's wort, buckwheat, perennial rye grass, whiteheads, rape (causing a condition known as rape scald), burr trefoil (causing trefoil dermatitis), alfalfa, and many others.

Drugs may cause photosensitivity, especially the phenothiazines (used to treat behavior disorders) and tetracycline antibiotics.

Involvement of the muzzle and lower legs suggests skin contact with pasture plants. A local skin reaction following application of a topical preparation suggests a photosensitizer in the preparation. Involvement of multiple sites suggests a photosensitizer in the feed.

Treatment: Identify and remove the photodynamic agent, if possible. This may require feed analysis, liver function tests, blood work, and investigation of the pasture. Secondarily infected skin is treated as described in *General Treatment of Pyoderma* (page 124).

Based on experience, try the following steps.

- Switch to a new feed.
- Bathe the horse and rinse thoroughly to remove any photosensitizing chemicals.
- Stop all drugs, especially topical ones.

- Keep the horse out of the sun for two weeks.
- Treat with glucocortocoids as needed to reduce inflammation.
- Topical corticosteroids can help to relieve itching.

Friction and Pressure Sores

A poorly fitting or improperly padded saddle can cause a pressure sore, also called a **saddle sore** or a sitfast. Skin injuries also occur as a consequence of ill-fitting bridles and harnesses. The rubbed and chafed areas become swollen, bare, and tender to pressure. With continued trauma, these friction sores become infected.

Galls, also caused by ill-fitting equipment (especially saddles), are painful, swollen pockets of serum that develop either under the skin or beneath the deeper connective fascia. Subfascial galls, which are extremely painful, are found most often on the withers.

Rope burns are friction burns, and may involve the full thickness of the skin.

Treatment: Following an acute injury, apply ice packs several times a day for two to three days. This helps reduce pain and swelling. Apply zinc oxide salve to raw areas to dry and protect the skin. For deep wounds, such as those produced by rope burns, clip the hair, cleanse the area with Betadine, and apply a topical antibiotic such as nitrofurazone or triple antibiotic ointment. Cover with a sterile dressing. Rest the horse.

Galls beneath the skin usually resolve in 7 to 10 days, but subfascial galls take considerably longer. If the horse must be used at saddle, protect the site with an extra blanket or a foam pad. Cut the pad out around the gall or saddle sore to relieve direct pressure.

Rope burns usually occur with ropes made of nylon and hemp. Cotton, which is less likely to produce a burn, is better for tying and picketing. A spray such as Granulex hastens healing.

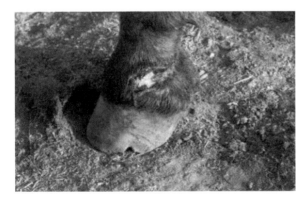

Rope burn caused by improper tying and the horse getting her foot over the lead rope.

Hereditary Equine Regional Dermal Asthenia

Hereditary equine regional dermal asthenia (HERDA), also known as hyper-elastosis cutis, is a genetic skin disease found predominately in the American Quarter Horse, and is prevalent in a particular line of cutting horses. Recent research has implicated horses related to the stud Poco Bueno and his grand-son Doc O' Lena as carriers. The *gene* is *recessive*, which means offspring must receive a carrier gene from both parents to be affected.

HERDA is a structural defect of the skin. Skin is composed of three layers: the outer layer, or epidermis; the middle layer, or dermis; and the inner layer, or sub cutis. In horses with HERDA, the connective tissue, primarily made up of collagen and fibrin, is damaged and breaks with any external stress, causing the skin layers to separate.

The condition appears at about the time a horse would be saddle broke. The act of saddling precipitates the breakdown of the skin. The outer layer of skin splits or separates from the deeper layer or tears off completely. New damage occurs with each trauma to the skin. The sores are slow to heal and rarely without disfiguring scars.

Diagnosis of this genetic disease is a combination of pedigree evaluation, clinical signs, and skin biopsy.

Treatment: Most horses affected live two to four years. They cannot be ridden and should not be bred. These horses are frequently euthanized. The destructive aspect of the skin disorder leaves these horses affected with a very high incidence of infection due to the loss of skin integrity.

Prevention: Genetic testing has been developed to help breeders and veterinarians identify carriers of this disease.

Tumors and Cancers

A *tumor* is any sort of lump, bump, growth, or swelling, such as an abscess. Tumors that are true growths are called neoplasms. *Benign* neoplasms grow slowly and are surrounded by a capsule. They do not invade and destroy tissue, nor do they spread to other areas. They are cured by surgical removal, provided that all the tumor is removed.

Malignant neoplasms are cancers (also called carcinomas, *sarcomas*, and lymphomas, depending upon the cell type). Cancers tend to enlarge rapidly. They are not *encapsulated*. When on the surface, they often bleed. They have the potential to spread via the bloodstream and lymphatic system to remote parts of the body. This is called *metastasizing*.

Cancer is graded according to the degree of malignancy. Low-grade cancers continue to grow locally and attain a large size. They metastasize late in the course of the illness. High-grade cancers metastasize early, when the primary focus is still quite small or is barely detectable.

Tumors are evaluated in the following manner: Suppose a horse has a solid lump on or beneath the skin. It could be benign or malignant. A decision is made to *biopsy* the lump. During this surgery, the lump, or part of the lump, is removed and sent to a pathologist. A veterinary pathologist is a doctor who has been trained to make a diagnosis by visual inspection of tissue under a microscope. An experienced pathologist can tell if the cells present have the characteristics of cancer. He or she can often provide additional information regarding the degree of malignancy. This makes the diagnosis and, in many cases, suggests the best course of treatment.

Neoplasms in the Horse

The majority of neoplasms in horses are visible as ulcerations or growths on or beneath the skin. *Sarcoid* is the most common growth in horses. Next in frequency are squamous cell carcinoma and melanoma. Suspect one of these when there is visible growth of a skin tumor, ulceration of the skin with bleeding, a sore that does not heal, or a nodular brown to black growth in an old gray horse.

Internal cancers are not common in horses. Lymphoma occurs most frequently, followed by stomach cancer. Neoplasms of the ovary, both benign and malignant, occur in the mare's reproductive tract. Benign fibroid growths of the uterus also occur. Less frequent sites of cancer in the horse are the oral cavity and nasopharynx, kidney, adrenal gland, pituitary gland, bladder, liver, colon, bone, and udder.

The effectiveness of any form of treatment depends upon early recognition. Early-stage cancers have a higher cure rate than do late-stage cancers. This holds true for all types of cancer. Unfortunately, most internal cancers are asymptomatic and therefore are not detected until they are quite large, at which time treatment generally is not possible. Occasionally, an ovarian or abdominal neoplasm will be detected unexpectedly during rectal examination performed for some other reason.

The best opportunity for preventing and curing cancer in horses rests in identifying and treating surface tumors.

Benign Surface Tumors

Sarcoids (Blood Warts)

Sarcoids are unique to horses and are the most common surface tumors. They usually occur in horses younger than 4 years, and are most often found on the legs, abdomen, head, and around the eyes. Sarcoids range in size from less than 1 inch (25 mm) up to several inches in diameter. A horse with one sarcoid has a one-in-three chance of developing more.

Sarcoids vary in appearance. Some are rough and wartlike. Others are red growths that resemble granulation tissue or proud flesh. Still others are slightly raised nodules. The nodular type is common about the ears and eyelids. An uncommon type is flat and hairless, and resembles a patch of ringworm.

Equine sarcoid has been found by DNA studies to be caused by the cattle wart virus (bovine papilloma virus Types 1 and 2). Possible modes of transmission include direct contact, the airborne route, and an insect vector. Since sarcoids occur at sites of prior trauma, the virus may be introduced through cuts and wounds.

Although sarcoids do not spread to distant parts of the body, these tumors are locally aggressive and have a high recurrence rate after surgical removal (50 percent within six months).

Treatment: The topical paste fluorouracil (XXterra) has been used successfully on sarcoids. *Cryotherapy* (freezing), often preceded by surgical debulking to reduce the size of the tumor, is another treatment. In this process, liquid nitrogen is sprayed onto the surface of the tumor, or nitrogen-cooled probes are inserted directly into the tumor. The tissue is destroyed by rapid freezing and thawing. Immune therapy, in which a commercially prepared vaccine such as EqStim is injected directly into the tumor, also has been used with success.

Surgical *excision* is an option when the entire tumor, including a surrounding margin of normal tissue, can be removed. This may be difficult or impossible in some locations, especially around the eye. When excision is incomplete, the tumor will recur and be most difficult to treat thereafter.

Chemotherapy using cysplatin injected directly into the tumor has a cure rate of 93 percent when used alone. When combined with surgical removal of the tumor, the success rate goes up to 97 percent.

Radiation therapy with radioactive implants is another treatment option for recurrent sarcoids.

Warts and Papillomas

Warts in horses are skin papillomas caused by a virus. Papillomas begin as smooth, raised, flesh-colored lumps that later become gray and horny. They tend to occur in groups on the muzzle and lips of young horses. They also are found scattered on the ears, eyelids, lower legs, and penis.

Treatment: Warts that become irritated and start to bleed can be removed by cryosurgery or chemical cautery (the application of acid). In time, the horse develops immunity to the papilloma virus, resulting in spontaneous regression usually within three to six months.

Cattle Grubs

Cattle grubs, about the size of a bumblebee, are the larvae of the warbles or heel fly. This fly, which lays its eggs on the hair of the legs of cattle, may accidentally

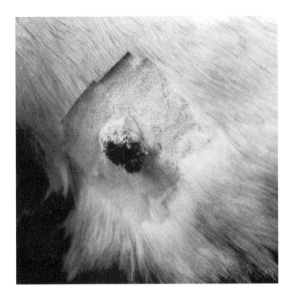

A wartlike sarcoid on the neck.

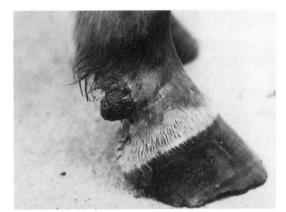

A fleshy sarcoid that developed four months after a wire cut to the pastern.

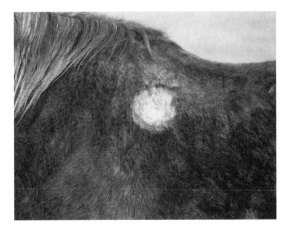

A flat sarcoid resembling a clipped patch of hair with small, grayish, wartlike bumps.

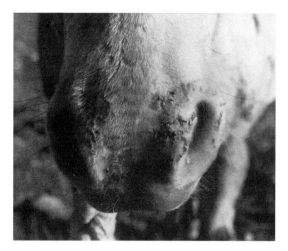

Skin papillomas on the muzzle of a young horse.

attack horses pastured with cattle. The eggs hatch into larvae, which then penetrate the skin and make their way beneath it to settle at the withers, neck, and back. While migrating, it is possible for larvae to penetrate the horse's brain and cause parasitic *myeloencephalitis*. This is rare.

Usually not more than one or two grubs encyst in the horse's tissue. Nodules develop around each grub, and there is a breathing hole in the skin. The resulting lumps are painful and sore and may interfere with the use of a saddle.

Most grubs fail to develop completely and are killed by the host. They become calcified and cause a permanent nodule called a hypoderma nodule.

Treatment: Mature grubs that have not calcified are best treated by enlarging the breathing hole with a scalpel and removing the grub with tweezers. Ivermectin in the usual dosage kills migrating larvae. Insecticides and fly control, as discussed *External Parasites* (page 63), provides control. Avoid pasturing horses close to cattle.

Lumps and Bumps

Other benign tumors can also occur in the horse.

Lipomas are smooth, round or oblong growths made up of mature fat cells surrounded by a fibrous capsule that sets it apart from the surrounding fat. Lipomas grow slowly and may eventually be several inches in diameter. Surgical removal is indicated for cosmetic reasons or to rule out cancer.

Hematomas are a collection of blood beneath the skin, caused by a blow or contusion. Small hematomas disappear spontaneously. Large ones may need to be opened and drained.

Tender knots at the site of injection are often present for a few days in horses that have been given their vaccinations. It seldom requires treatment. On rare occasions, the injection site becomes infected and an abscess develops.

Sebaceous cysts (wens) are uncommon. A sebaceous cyst is made of a thick capsule that surrounds a lump of cheesy material called keratin. It may grow to 1 inch (25 cm) or more in size. Eventually, it is likely to become infected. Most cysts should be removed.

MALIGNANT SURFACE TUMORS
Squamous Cell Carcinoma

This common skin cancer tends to occur in older horses with light skin. It can be found anywhere on the body but is most common in the genital and eye regions. Skin in these areas contains less pigment and therefore absorbs more ultraviolet radiation, which damages the skin and predisposes it to malignant change.

Squamous cell carcinoma begins as a wartlike growth or a flat ulcer with a yellow, infected-looking base. As it grows, it becomes firm, nodular, and fleshy, and bleeds easily. It metastasizes only at an advanced stage and then usually to the nearest lymph nodes.

A sore on the penis or sheath that looks like squamous cell carcinoma may be a summer sore. A skin biopsy is the best way to make the diagnosis.

Squamous cell carcinomas arising from the eyelids, the nictitating membranes, and conjunctiva are discussed in chapter 5, "The Eyes."

Treatment: Any growth in an area of light skin pigmentation should be considered a squamous cell carcinoma until proven otherwise. These tumors are best treated by wide local excision, if this can be done without damaging vital structures. Radiation therapy, which involves implanting radon probes into the cancer, is useful in reducing the size of the tumor and making it easier to remove. Other successful forms of treatment include cryotherapy (as described for the treatment of sarcoids, page 135). Use of 5-fluorouricil cream ointment and laser surgery have also shown some success.

Melanoma

Melanoma is the most significant tumor in horses. This skin tumor occurs almost exclusively in white and gray horses. In fact, most old gray horses, if they live long enough, will develop one or more of these tumors.

Melanomas are gray or black dome-shaped, hairless, nodular growths about 1 inch (25 cm) in size when first discovered. They are found frequently at the root of the tail and in the *perianal* region, including the anus, vulva, and male genitalia, and less frequently on the head and limbs.

Although melanomas appear benign and may remain inactive for many years, once they begin to grow, they spread rapidly. Distant metastases to vital organs are common.

Treatment: All melanomas (except those in the genital and perineal areas) should be removed surgically. Cryotherapy and immune therapy can be considered for larger melanomas and for those in which surgery is difficult.

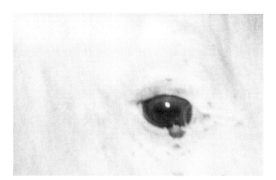

A melanoma arising from the lower eyelid.

Perineal melanomas have a low metastatic rate and are removed only if they interfere with urination and defecation. There is no effective treatment for metastatic disease.

Lymphoma

This is the most common internal cancer in horses. It develops in lymph nodes or in organs that have lymphoid tissue, including the liver, spleen, and lungs. Lymphoma affects horses of all ages. The cause is unknown. The disease is divided somewhat arbitrarily into specific types according to the primary site of involvement; however, there is considerable overlap.

In the intestinal form, there is loss of appetite and weight, mild *colic*, and accumulation of subcutaneous fluid in the lower chest and in the abdomen. A mass may be detected by rectal exam.

In the thoracic (mediastinal) form, there is lung congestion with fluid accumulation in the chest cavity (pleural effusion). Involvement of the larynx or nasal cavity may cause respiratory obstruction.

In the cutaneous (skin) form, you may see one or more subcutaneous nodules or multiple bumps resembling hives, usually found on the bridge of the nose, *perineum*, neck, and elsewhere. These nodules may appear, disappear, and then reappear over an extended period.

A diagnosis of lymphoma is made by removing an enlarged lymph node or biopsying a palpable tumor. If the mass is inaccessible to biopsy, a bone marrow biopsy may be positive. Chest or abdominal fluid, if present, can be withdrawn and sent for *cytology*. Blood tests usually are not diagnostic.

Treatment: There is no effective treatment for lymphoma, although temporary improvement may be achieved using corticosteroids. The cutaneous form may be present for years without causing the horse a problem.

THE EYES

5

The eye is an organ with several parts, all of which are uniquely adapted to meet the special needs of the horse. The large, clear part of the front of the eye is the *cornea*. Surrounding the cornea is the *sclera*, or white of the eye, a narrow rim between the eyelids much less conspicuous in the horse than it is in people. The sclera surrounds and supports the entire eyeball.

The thin pinkish membrane that covers the white of the eye is called the conjunctiva. It also covers the back of the eyelids. This surface layer contains many nerve endings and is highly sensitive.

The horse's upper and lower eyelids are composed of sheets of cartilage covered on the outside by skin. They don't make contact with the surface of the eye because there is a thin layer of tears between them.

The horse has a third eyelid, or *nictitating membrane*, normally not conspicuous but located at the inside corner of the eye. The third eyelid has an important cleansing and lubricating function. The third eyelid is attached to the fat cushion at the back of the eyeball. Accordingly, when the eyeball is drawn back into the orbit, the third eyelid moves upward and covers the eye.

On the upper eyelid are four rows of stiff eyelashes that cross in a trellis fashion. The lower lid generally has only a few straggly hairs, but there is an inherited tendency for some horses to have stiff lashes on their lower eyelids. These hairs can scratch the surface of the eye.

Tears are secreted by the *lacrimal gland*, which is rather large in the horse—2 to 3 inches (5 to 7.5 cm) in diameter. Each lacrimal gland is located in a depression just beneath the supraorbital ridge, a bony arch at the upper part of the eye socket. Tears are carried to the surface of the eye by small ducts that open at the back of the upper eyelids.

The opening at the center of the eye is the pupil. It is surrounded by a circular or elliptical layer of pigmented muscle called the iris that opens and closes the pupil. In young horses the pupil is round. In horses over 5 years of age, it gradually assumes an elliptical shape with a long horizontal axis.

The color of the eyes is due to a pigment in the iris. The usual color is deep hazel or brown with no white visible around the edges. (Appaloosas often have a visible white ring of sclera around the iris.) Occasionally a horse will

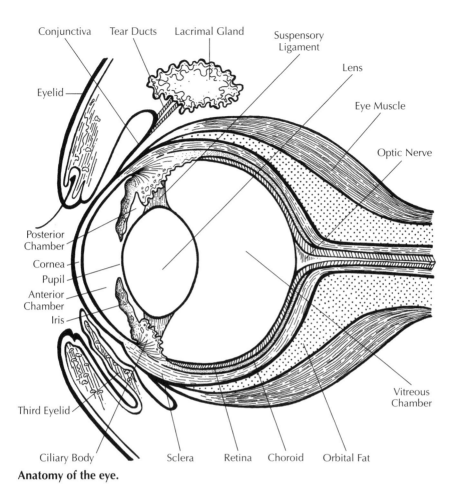

Anatomy of the eye.

have blue eyes. This is often associated with white body spots; the Paint is an example.

The inner eye has three chambers. The anterior chamber is found between the cornea and the iris. It is filled with a clear fluid. The small posterior chamber lies behind the iris and in front of the lens. The large vitreous chamber, which contains a clear jelly, supports the lens from behind and holds the retina in place against the back of the eyeball.

A horse's lens is more spherical and larger than ours. It is contained within a thin capsule and is attached to the inner surface of the eyeball by a series of fine strands called the suspensory ligaments. The suspensory ligaments attach to the *ciliary body*, a structure composed of muscle, connective tissue, and blood vessels. The ciliary body produces the clear fluid in the front part of the eye.

Light enters the eye by first passing through the cornea and the anterior chamber and then through the pupil and the lens. The pupil expands and contracts according to the brightness of the light. Light then travels through the vitreous chamber and is received by the *retina*. The retina is a layer of photoreceptor cells at the back of the eye that converts light into nerve impulses that pass via the optic nerve to the brain.

Immediately behind the retina, and within the choroid (a layer of blood vessels that nourish the retina), is a special layer of cells called the *tapetum lucidum*. This layer acts like a mirror, reflecting light back onto the retina and producing a double exposure of the photoreceptor cells, enhancing the horse's ability to see in low light. It is this layer of cells that makes it seem as if a horse's eyes shine in the dark.

Field of Vision

The shape of a horse's eyeball is quite different from that of most other animals. Whereas in humans the eyeball is roughly spherical, a horse's eyeball is somewhat flattened from front to back. As a result, the distance from the cornea to the retina is not the same in all parts of the eye. The focal length is a few millimeters longer in the upper part of the eye and a few millimeters shorter in the lower part. This produces what is called a ramped retina. It has important implications.

The human eye focuses on objects at varying distances through the action of the ciliary muscles, which change the shape of the lens. But in horses the ciliary muscles are poorly developed. A horse cannot easily change the curvature of his lens (a process called accommodation) to bring objects into focus. Instead, he accommodates by using the lower part of his retina to see objects at a distance and the upper part (with the longer focal length) to see objects close by.

To use the lower part of his retina to see objects at a distance, a horse raises his head and brings both eyes together to look straight ahead. The muscles that assist in this process also raise the ears and prick them forward. Accordingly, when a horse is looking at something in the distance, he stands with his head held high and his ears pricked forward.

The opposite occurs when he is accommodating for near vision. The horse lowers his head and relaxes his eye muscles, which allows the eyes to diverge.

A horse has a wide field of vision (approximately 350 degrees) and can see far out to each side and well behind. However, the binocular visual field is small. Both eyes can be brought together to focus on a single object only in a rather limited field in front (about 65 degrees). At other times the horse sees a different picture with each eye.

There are two blind spots: one about 4 to 5 feet (1.2 to 1.5 m) in front of the horse, where his vision is blocked by his long muzzle; and one directly behind the horse. The horse cannot see the blind spot in front of him unless he lowers his head. When a horse gallops up to a jump, for example, the jump will suddenly enter his blind spot. A rider must be prepared to loosen the reins and let the horse lower his head. Otherwise, the horse may fail to see the jump or refuse to take it. Likewise, a handler should never approach directly behind the horse, who might kick out at what he can hear but cannot see.

A number of investigators have concluded that perhaps a third of all horses are myopic or nearsighted (which means they have trouble focusing on objects at a distance). A small percentage seem to be farsighted (which means they have trouble focusing on objects nearby). Wild horses appear to be farsighted. From this it has been suggested that domestication and breeding practices may have increased the frequency of myopia in the horse.

The Eye Exam

The eye is surrounded by a thick layer of muscle, highly developed in the horse, called the *orbicularis oculi*. As the horse shuts his eyes, this muscle closes down tightly. This makes it difficult to lift up or roll out the eyelids when inspecting the eye for an injury or foreign body. Because of the difficulty in examining the eye, a thorough eye examination in the horse always requires veterinary assistance.

When your veterinarian examines your horse's eyes, they may use a variety of tests. The vet may check for a menace response, which means the horse moves his head away from a perceived threat. The vet may also check for a dazzle response, which is a contraction of the pupil in response to sudden bright light, and do a maze test. (See *Testing for Vision*, page 167, for more on basic vision tests.)

If an *infection* is suspected, care must begin immediately—it cannot wait the 48 hours for bacteria *culture* and sensitivity tests. A *cytology* test, in which the veterinarian looks at a sample of cells, yields immediate results; the vet may see lymph cells, signifying an *immune-mediated* response, fungus, bacteria, or neutrophils (a type of white blood cell).

Tear production may be measured using a small piece of absorbent material called a Schirmer tear test strip. This strip is placed inside the lower eyelid, and over a measured period of time (usually a minute), the tears soak and migrate up the strip, causing a change in color. The wet area is measured and compared to normal values. Abnormal tear production associated with a red eye and copious discharge can occur with several diseases, including keratoconjunctivitis sicca.

Ophthalmoscopy is an examination of the back part of the eyeball (the fundus), which includes the retina, the optic disc, the choroids, and the blood vessels. The ophthalmoscope consists of a mirror that reflects light into the eye and a series of lenses to help focus the view.

Fluorescein stain drops can be placed onto the surface of the eye to check the protective layer of epithelial cells, called the *epithelium*, that cover the cornea. Lack of a cornea epithelium suggests an eye ulcer.

A tonometry test measures intraocular pressure—the pressure inside the eye. This test is used to check for glaucoma.

A complete eye exam, including ophthalmoscopy, should be included as part of a prepurchase or soundness exam. Horses with chronic equine recurrent *uveitis* may have few obvious clinical signs of disease and yet have significant retinal degeneration. Therefore, any horse with retinal degeneration must be suspected of having equine recurrent uveitis and is a likely candidate for future vision problems (see *Uveitis*, page 161).

A new *foal* exam includes checking the eyes to look for *congenital*, inherited, and acquired disorders. For example, microthalmos or small eye globe can be a result of uterine infection but is also seen congenitally in some Thoroughbred horses. *Entropion* is a rolling of the lower lid in against the eye, seen accompanying dehydration, malnutrition, and prematurity. This can be repaired to prevent corneal ulceration. The foal's eyes should also be examined for subconjunctival and retinal hemorrhages. The signs of *jaundice*, indicated by yellow discoloration of the whites of the eyes, might indicate neonatal isoerythrolysis. The exam should also check for birth trauma, corneal ulcers, Horner's syndrome, and tetany. The nasolacrimal system (the tear duct that drains tears to the nose) should be checked for proper functioning. Cataracts can be congenital in foals, and are inheritable in Belgians and Thoroughbreds. Morgan horses have a type of nonprogressive cataract. Cataracts and lens luxations (displacement of the lens from its normal position) are associated with anterior segment dysgenesis in the Rocky Mountain Horse.

If Your Horse Has an Eye Problem

Your horse has an eye problem if there is matter in the eye, the eye waters, the eye is swollen, the nictitating membrane is visible, or the horse blinks, squints, or gives other evidence that the eye is painful. Eye injuries tend to progress more rapidly in the horse than they do in most other animals, and are more likely to be associated with loss of vision. For this reason, any problem associated with the eye is considered an emergency. There are certain things you can look for to determine the need to call your veterinarian, as described in the next section.

Signs of Eye Ailments

Diseases of the eye are accompanied by a number of signs and symptoms. Pain is one of the most serious. *A horse with a painful eye needs prompt veterinary attention.*

- **Painful eye.** Signs of pain include excessive tearing, squinting (closing down the eye), tenderness to touch, and avoiding light. The nictitating membrane may protrude in response to pain. The usual causes of painful eye are injuries to the cornea (abrasion or a foreign body) and disorders affecting the inner eye, especially uveitis.

- **Eye discharge.** The type of discharge helps define its cause. A watery or mucuslike discharge without redness and pain indicates a problem with the tear drainage system (see *The Tearing Mechanism,* page 157). Any discharge accompanied by a painful eye should alert you to the possibility of cornea or inner eye involvement. A discharge from both eyes suggests conjunctivitis or, if the horse also has fever and other signs of illness, a viral respiratory disease or strangles.

- **Red eye.** Redness of the eye is caused by an increase in the number and size of the vessels in the conjunctiva and nictitating membrane. In addition, the eyelids and conjunctiva may appear puffy and/or swollen. Conjunctivitis is the most common cause of a pink or red eye, but diseases of the cornea (ulcers, *keratitis*) and uveitis can also produce a red eye.

- **Cloudy eye.** Loss of clarity or transparency of the surface of the eye indicates an eyeball injury, a disease of the cornea, or an inner eye disorder such as uveitis or cataract. When the cornea is entirely opaque, the owner might think the horse has a blind eye, but this is not necessarily so. A cloudy eye should receive immediate professional attention.

- **Irritation of the lids.** Conditions that cause swelling, crusting, itching, or hair loss are discussed in *The Eyelids* (page 147).

- **Hard or soft eye.** Changes in eye pressure are caused by disorders of the inner eye. The pupil may become fixed and unable to dilate or constrict. A hard eye with a dilated pupil indicates glaucoma. A soft eye with a small pupil indicates inflammation of the inner structures of the eye (uveitis).

- **Abnormal eye movements.** Eyes that focus in different directions or jerk back and forth are discussed in *The Eyeball* (page 155).

- **Color change.** A change in the color of the eye may indicate the *cancers* known as melanoma or squamous cell carcinoma. A yellowish tint to the sclera could be jaundice. The eye may also turn red if there is bleeding inside the eye or white to yellow if there is inflammation or infection inside the eye.

- **Film over the eye.** An opaque or whitish film that moves out over the surface of the eyeball from the inside corner of the eye is a protruded nictitating membrane. This condition is discussed in *The Eyelids* (page 147).

- **Bulging or sunken eye.** A bulging eye occurs with glaucoma, tumors, and abscesses behind the globe, and with an eye out of its socket. A sunken eye occurs with dehydration, weight loss, and eye pain. In a horse with tetanus, the third eyelid will cover the eye, making it appear sunken. Abnormal positions of the eye are discussed in *The Eyeball* (page 155).

Medicating the Eyes

Disorders of the eyelids and conjunctiva can frequently be treated using appropriate ointments or drops. Ointments and drops must be applied several times a day. *Only use preparations specifically labeled for ophthalmic use.* Check to be sure the medication is not out of date. How to apply eye ointments and drops is illustrated in the photos below. The horse may need to be restrained (see *Handling and Restraint*, page 2). Do not use medications left over from one horse to treat another. You may transfer infections, and some conditions may be made worse by using the wrong medication.

A variety of medications are used in the eyes. Some are used to constrict or dilate the pupil; others to treat infections. Corticosteroid preparations should be used only under veterinary supervision. You should *not* use them to treat

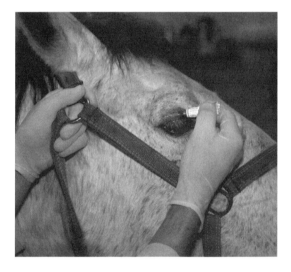

To apply ointment, run a ribbon of medication along the border of the upper eyelid. As the horse blinks, the medication will dissolve and coat the surface of the eyeball.

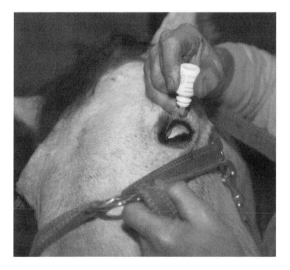

Eyedrops, which are applied directly to the surface of the eyeball, are more difficult to use because horses are eye shy and will attempt to jerk away. Draw up on the skin above the eye to widen the opening.

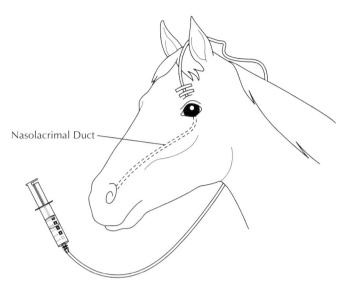

Nasolacrimal Duct

An indwelling catheter makes it easier to medicate the eye. The catheter is inserted through the skin into the conjunctival sac, then comes back out through the skin and is knotted on the outside of the skin. The catheter can be connected to a pump for continuous infusion.

injuries that may involve the cornea. Prolonged administration of antibiotics and corticosteroids may lead to fungal infections.

Do not neglect minor eye ailments. If you do not see improvement in 24 hours, consult your veterinarian. Serious eye disorders require intensive treatment. Your veterinarian may decide to instill the end of a sterile silastic tube into the subpalpebral space beneath the upper eyelid. The other end of the tube is taped to the forehead, poll, and withers. This permits eye medication to be given easily and safely and at times specified by your veterinarian. The procedure is particularly useful when the eyelids have to be sutured together to protect an injured eye. The system can be coupled to a small pump for continuous infusion. This is called a subpalpebral lavage or infusion catheter.

Long-acting preparations are occasionally injected beneath the conjunctiva. The procedure is often combined with the use of topical ointments or drops.

The intravenous route is the best choice for serious, deep inflammations and those that pose a major threat to the eye.

The Eyelids
BLEPHAROSPASM (SEVERE SQUINTING)

Severe squinting is a tight shutting of the eye in response to the presence of an eye irritant or a foreign body in the eye. The reflex spasm of the eye muscles may cause the eyelids to roll in against the cornea. Having once rolled in,

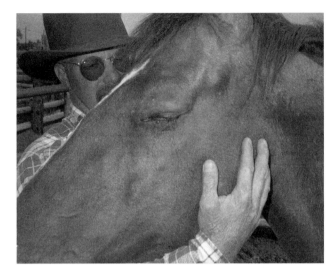

Severe squinting with a tightly shut eye, in this case caused by a painful corneal abrasion.

the rough margins of the lids rub against the eyeball, causing further pain, spasm, and sometimes further injury.

Painful eye disorders, such as corneal ulcers and uveitis, can also cause reflex spasm of the eye muscles.

Treatment: A topical anesthetic ointment can be applied to temporarily relieve the pain and break the cycle. This works only for surface irritants. (Anesthetics may be harmful to the cornea, and your veterinarian may opt for anti-inflammatory medications instead.) Relief is permanent when the irritant, often a foreign body, can be found and removed. Painful inner eye ailments do not respond to topical anesthetics.

Film over the Eye

The third eyelid, or nictitating membrane, is not normally seen but may become visible in response to illness or injury. When the nictitating membrane is visible over the lower inner corner of the eye, it is said to be protruding. Any painful eye illness causing spasm of the muscles around the eye can cause the eyeball to retract back into its socket and the third eyelid to protrude. Tearing and squinting will accompany this situation.

When both eyes are retracted and the third eyelid is visible in both eyes, the condition may be due to tetanus. However, any chronic illness or state of malnutrition that causes the horse to lose weight or become dehydrated (reducing the size of the fat pads at the back of the eyes) can be associated with the appearance of this film across the eyes.

Treatment: A veterinary examination is necessary to determine the cause of the problem.

Puffy Eyelids

Sudden swelling of the eyelids and conjunctiva may be caused by an allergic reaction. Insect bites, inhaled irritants, allergens in medications, and trauma are the most common causes. The conjunctiva and eyelids are fluid-filled, puffy, and soft. The puffy eyes may be accompanied by *hives* in which the hair stands out in little patches over the body.

Treatment: Simple cases are treated with an eye preparation that contains a corticosteroid, such as Corticosporin. This problem is generally of short duration and improves when the allergic agent is removed. If trauma is suspected, there may be corneal damage and your veterinarian should definitely be involved.

Blepharitis (Inflamed Eyelids)

Blepharitis can be recognized by the thick, reddened, and inflamed appearance of the eyelids. Occasionally, there are crusts and hair loss. It tends to occur in younger horses as a result of contact with irritating plants and weeds. It can also be caused by mange mites and ringworm. Horses who lack pigment in the skin of the eyelids may suffer from solar blepharitis.

Blepharitis caused by bacterial infection of the eyelids is not common. A purulent discharge with crusting and matter on the lids suggests this condition. The discharge should be cultured by your veterinarian.

A special type of blepharitis and conjunctivitis is caused by the larvae of Habronema stomach worms. These larvae are deposited by stable flies as they feed around moist areas on the body, including the lid margins and the corners of the eyes. Yellow, slightly raised, gritty nodules and open sores develop in the skin of the upper and lower eyelids, and occasionally on the third eyelid and the surface of the conjunctiva. Penetration of the eye can lead to keratitis or corneal ulcer.

Treatment: Identify and treat any underlying skin disease or allergic reaction that may be contributing to the blepharitis (see *Allergies*, page 118). An antibiotic-corticosteroid eye ointment, such as Neocortef or Corticosporin, helps to reduce swelling and inflammation. However, do not use steroid products without first consulting your veterinarian, because in some cases they can cause further damage. If the condition does not respond in 24 hours, consult your veterinarian.

Bacterial blepharitis is treated with a topical antibiotic ointment such as Neosporin (which contains no steroid). Applying warm packs may be helpful. Severe cases require oral antibiotics.

Tattooing the eyelids is the best treatment for solar blepharitis.

Habronema infection is treated with topical corticosteroids and injection of steroids into the nodules. Ivermectin is used to eliminate the larvae (see *Summer Sores*, page 121).

Trichiasis (Eyelash Irritation)

Aberrant eyelashes on the upper or lower eyelids can rub on the cornea, producing irritation and injury. Most misdirected eyelashes are the result of an improperly healed laceration of the eyelid. Foals may be born with this condition.

Treatment: The offending hair should be removed by electrolysis or surgery.

On occasion, the dock of a long-maned horse will fall in against the eye and cause similar irritation. These hairs should be removed by clipping or in some cases by plucking.

Entropion (Eyelid Rolled Inward)

When an eyelid rolls inward, it irritates and damages the surface of the eye. Most cases are due to scarring of the eyelid after an injury or infection. Entropion can also occur in newborn foals as a birth defect.

Treatment: Surgical correction is indicated in adult horses. In newborn foals, it is usually possible to gently evert the eyelids back to their normal position. If this can be done, the procedure should be repeated several times during the first few days of life. Once a routine of lid manipulation has been established, the condition generally corrects itself in a few weeks. Eye medications is used to prevent infection.

Ectropion (Eyelid Rolled Outward)

When the lower eyelid rolls out, it exposes the eye to irritation. Most cases are due to improperly healed eyelid lacerations.

Treatment: Plastic surgery is necessary to tighten the lid and protect the eye.

Eyelid Lacerations

The eyelids may be lacerated by barbed wire, nails, or other objects. Lacerations at the margin of an eyelid can affect the appearance and function of the eye.

Treatment: Surgical repair is advisable for most eyelid injuries. The earlier the repair, the better the result. A local nerve block and intravenous sedation, or a general anesthetic, is required. Antibiotics are given for seven days after the repair to prevent infection.

Tumors

Benign and malignant tumors occur on the eyelids and on the nictitating membrane. Squamous cell carcinoma is the most common malignant tumor. It usually occurs in older horses who lack pigment on their eyelids. Appaloosas

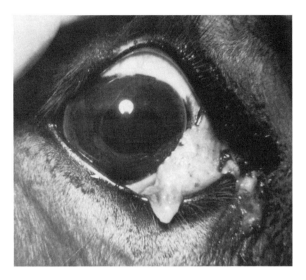

Squamous cell carcinoma of the nictitating membrane.

appear to be at higher risk. These tumors tend to grow slowly and invade the eye. Finally, they spread to lymph nodes in the neck or chest.

Sarcoids are benign tumors of younger horses that occur frequently in the head and eyelid areas. They are caused by a virus. These tumors either grow internally and invade the eye, or externally and break through the skin. They are difficult to treat and tend to recur after removal.

Other tumors occasionally seen are skin papillomas, melanomas, and lymphosarcomas. Melanomas are common in old gray horses. Iris melanomas are usually benign, but the horse will develop glaucoma in the affected eye.

Treatment: All growths of the eyelids should be removed at an early stage. For more information, see *Tumors and Cancers*, page 133.

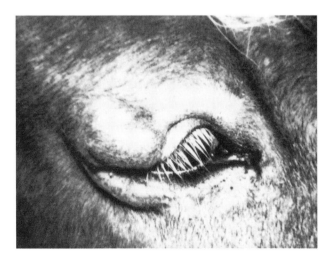

A nodular sarcoid beneath the skin of the upper eyelid.

The treatment of squamous carcinoma involves surgical *excision*, radiation therapy, and freezing, often in combination. Sarcoids are treated by surgery, *cryotherapy*, laser destruction, and immunotherapy, often in combination. Immunotherapy involves injecting a commercial extract containing a bacterial cell wall antigen directly into the tumor. *Chemotherapy* (cisplatin) has been effective for both sarcoid and squamous cell carcinomas, with a success rate of 87 percent for sarcoids and 65 percent for squamous cell carcinoma after one year.

Foreign Bodies and Chemicals in the Eye

Foreign bodies (dust, grass seed, dirt, and specks of vegetable matter) can become trapped behind the eyelids and the nictitating membrane. They can also enter and block the nasolacrimal duct system. Signs of a foreign body include tearing and watering of the eye, along with blinking and squinting. The third membrane may protrude in response to pain. Suspect a foreign irritant when the horse suddenly shows signs of a painful eye.

Chemicals that may commonly irritate the eye include insecticide sprays, detergents, alcohol, antiseptics, and petroleum products.

Thorns and splinters can become imbedded in the cornea or penetrate the anterior chamber. Secondary infection by bacteria or fungi is possible.

Treatment: If you know the eye has been exposed to a chemical, flush the eye repeatedly using a syringe filled with tap water. Due to the associated eye muscle spasm, it may be difficult to adequately flush the eye without a regional eye block and topical anesthetic.

All foreign bodies must be removed as soon as possible. If you are able to see a foreign body on the surface of the eye, you may be able to flush it out by squeezing and gently wiping with a wet ball of cotton. Or you can use a moist swab; the foreign body may adhere to it.

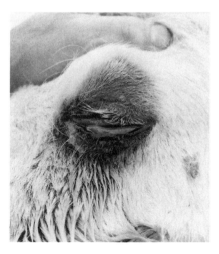

Severe tearing, squinting, and conjunctivitis caused by a foreign body behind the third eyelid.

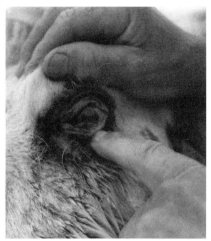

The lids are retracted to examine the eye and the recesses behind the eyelids.

In many cases, *blepharospasm* and swelling of the conjunctiva will make it difficult to examine the eye. The horse will need to be sedated by your veterinarian, after which the orbicularis muscle surrounding the eye can be blocked by an injection and anesthetic drops applied to the eye. The foreign body usually can be identified and removed using blunt-nosed forceps or vigorous flushing.

Thorns and splinters that have penetrated the surface of the cornea require eye surgery and intensive aftercare to prevent complications.

The Outer Eye
CONJUNCTIVITIS (RED EYE)

Conjunctivitis is an inflammation of the conjunctiva, the membrane covering the back of the eyelids and the surface of the eyeball up to the cornea. It is one of the most common eye problems of horses.

Signs of conjunctivitis include red eyes, swollen eyelids, and a sticky, purulent discharge at the corners of the eyes. Conjunctivitis is not painful. When a red eye is accompanied by evidence of pain, such as squinting, tenderness to touch, and *protrusion* of the third eyelid, suspect a serious ailment involving the cornea or inner eye and consult your veterinarian.

Conjunctivitis in horses may be serous or purulent.

Serous conjunctivitis is a mild condition in which the membrane looks reddened and somewhat swollen. The discharge is clear and watery. The usual causes are physical irritants to the eye, such as dust, weeds, flies, sprays, and various allergens including those in topical medications.

Serous conjunctivitis often accompanies equine viral respiratory diseases and viral arteritis. Rarely, it is caused by the *parasite Thelazia lacrimalis*. This is a small white worm, less than 1 inch (25 mm) long, which lives in the space behind the eyelids. These worms must be removed to clear up the problem.

The larvae of Habronema also infect the conjunctiva, as discussed in *Blepharitis* (page 149).

A contagious type of conjunctivitis occurs in foals and occasionally older horses. It appears to be transmitted by house and face flies feeding around the corners of the eyes. A herpesvirus may be the cause. The conjunctivitis generally disappears on its own in about two weeks.

The larvae of neck threadworms may invade the conjunctiva. Signs are inflammation of the eye along the upper rim of the cornea. A secondary keratitis may occur. Treatment is discussed in *Ventral Midline Dermatitis* (page 121).

Purulent conjunctivitis often begins as a serous conjunctivitis that later becomes infected by bacteria. The discharge is then sticky and contains *pus* and mucus. Strangles and equine viral arteritis may cause purulent conjunctivitis. A bacterium called *Moraxella bovis* has been implicated in some cases of conjunctivitis in horses. An overlooked foreign body in the conjunctiva or cornea is another cause.

Treatment: Mild irritating forms of conjunctivitis can be treated with an antibiotic ophthalmic ointment such as Gentamicin or Neosporin. The allergic variety responds well to a corticosteroid preparation (such as Neocortef or Corticosporin). Apply ointments three to four times a day for seven to ten

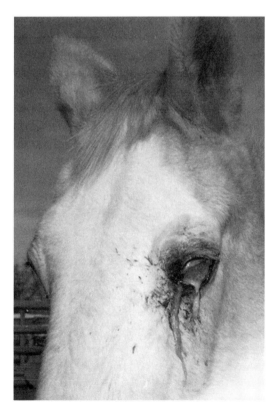

This horse has purulent conjunctivitis. Note the sticky discharge of mucus and pus.

days. You should expect to see improvement within 24 hours. If not, consult your veterinarian. Discontinue a steroid preparation if there are any signs of pain in the eye or if the eye worsens under treatment.

Bacterial conjunctivitis that does not respond to topical antibiotics indicates a resistant bacterium, a foreign body, or an injury to the cornea. Veterinary attention is required.

Dermoid Cyst

A dermoid cyst is a congenital growth that occurs near the corner of the eye. It has a flat, rough surface from which a few short hairs may grow. There is considerable discomfort, with tearing and squinting when the horse blinks his eye. Corneal involvement is possible; this interferes with vision.

Treatment: The dermoid is not a malignant tumor but should be removed because of the discomfort it causes the horse.

The Eyeball

Despite the very large size of the horse's globe, eye injuries are not common. This is due in part to a heavy framework of bone that surrounds the orbit. Furthermore, the eyeball is recessed in a cushion of fat capable of being compressed and then moving up into a bony recess called the supraorbital fossa. When pressure is applied to the eyeball, it moves backward into the space occupied by the fat cushion and is protected from a blow that might otherwise cause it to rupture.

Exophthalmos (Bulging Eye)

In a horse with this condition, swelling of the tissue behind the eye pushes the eyeball forward and causes it to bulge and appear more prominent. Major protrusion prevents the horse from closing his eyelids. The nictitating membrane is often visible.

Blows that fracture the eye socket cause a sudden buildup of blood or fluid behind the eye. Trailer accidents, horse fights, and running into foreign objects are the most common causes of orbital trauma.

Infections that spread to the eyeball from the sinus or the upper teeth also can cause the eye to bulge. This type of infection is called orbital *cellulitis*. It is an extremely painful condition of sudden onset, accompanied by fever, heat, redness, swelling of the eyelids, and a purulent discharge from the eye. It usually responds to high levels of intravenous antibiotics, although the infection sometimes localizes to form an abscess behind the eyeball (called a *retrobulbar abscess*).

Glaucoma may result in increased size of the eye and protrusion.

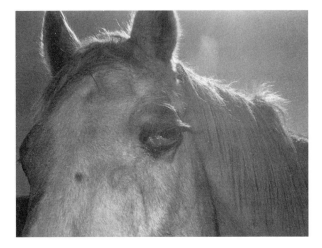

Note the protrusion of the third eyelid in this horse with exophthalmos.

Tumors in the space behind the eyeball are a rare cause of protrusion. Tumors are slow-growing and relatively painless. A variety of benign and malignant growths can occur.

Treatment: All cases of *exophthalmos* are extremely serious and may cause loss of vision. They require immediate veterinary attention. Ultrasound examination of the eye and orbit may prove helpful in detecting masses behind the eyeball. Drugs can be given to reduce the swelling produced by trauma. Surgery may be necessary to replace bone fragments or drain a collection of blood or pus, either behind the eye or within an infected sinus. It may be necessary to temporarily suture the eyelids over a bulging eyeball to protect it from injury and keep it from drying out.

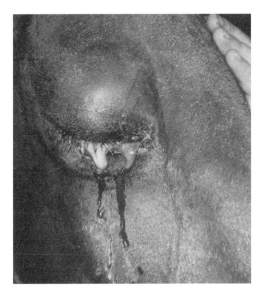

The bulging eye and purulent discharge are characteristic of orbital cellulitis.

Enophthalmos (Sunken Eye)

A sunken eye often develops after a severe eye injury or infection that damages the inner structures of the eye. The eye becomes smaller and sinks into its orbit. When an eye recedes, the nictitating membrane will be visible at the lower inner corner of the eye.

Damage to nerves in the neck can result in a condition called Horner's syndrome. The signs of Horner's syndrome include a sunken eyeball, along with a small pupil, slight drooping of the upper eyelid, and an elevated third eyelid. A guttural pouch infection is one cause of Horner's syndrome.

An abnormally small eyeball may be seen in newborn foals as a result of a congenital defect. It is often accompanied by cataracts.

Treatment: Treatment of the sunken eye is directed by the underlying cause of the problem.

Strabismus (Cross-eyed Gaze)

Strabismus is caused by paralysis of one of the eye muscles. The result is that the eyeball cannot move in a particular direction. This rare condition occurs principally in Appaloosas as a congenital defect. In nearly all cases, one or both eyes are rolled in toward the nose. Because of the abnormal visual axis, these horses stumble and exhibit a nervous temperament.

Treatment: The muscles can be operated on so that the horse will have a more normal field of vision and subsequent improvement in movement and behavior.

The Tearing Mechanism

Tears serve two functions: They cleanse and lubricate the surface of the eye, and they contain immune substances that help to prevent eye infections. A normal accumulation of tears is removed by evaporation. Excess tears are pooled near the inner corner of the eyes and carried by the nasolacrimal ducts down to the nose. The openings of these ducts can be seen near the front of each nasal passage by holding open the nostrils.

Blocked Tear Duct (Watery Eye)

Suspect a blockage in one of the nasolacrimal ducts if the horse has a *unilateral* watery or mucuslike discharge that overflows the eyelids and runs down the side of the face. This condition can be distinguished from conjunctivitis and diseases of the cornea and inner eye by the absence of pain and redness. The eye discharge of equine viral respiratory disease usually is *bilateral* and is accompanied by nasal discharge and other signs of illness.

Most obstructions in a nasolacrimal duct occur where the duct opens into the floor of the nasal cavity. Stones, foreign bodies such as grass seeds, infections, and tumors are possible causes. A rare cause of obstruction is the eyeworm *Thelazia lacrimalis*, discussed in *Conjunctivitis* (page 153).

A blockage high in the duct system is usually caused by an eyelid injury or a tumor of the conjunctiva or the nictitating membrane.

Treatment: To see if the drainage system is open, the pool of tears is stained with fluorescein dye. If the dye appears at the nostril, the tear duct is open. If not, the nasolacrimal system can be flushed via the opening in the nasal cavity using a syringe and small catheter. The flushing often removes the blockage and opens the duct.

Dacryocystitis is an infection of the nasolacrimal duct. It frequently leads to scarring and ductal obstruction. In this situation, your veterinarian may elect to pass a catheter through the duct and leave it in place until healing occurs. Antibiotics and corticosteroids are used to treat the infection and promote healing.

Keratoconjunctivitis Sicca (Dry Eye)

Dry eye is rare in horses. It is caused by the absence of tears. Instead of the bright, glistening sheen seen in the normal eye, the dry eye presents a dull, lackluster appearance. There is a thick, stringy discharge that is difficult to clear away. Later, as the eye becomes infected, puslike discharge may complicate the picture.

Tears are produced by the lacrimal gland and are carried to the eye by small ducts that open at the back of the upper eyelids. Infection followed by *atrophy* of the lacrimal gland can lead to absent tear production and dry eye. Scarring of the eyelids from severe blepharitis or chronic purulent conjunctivitis can also interfere with tear delivery. Rarely, some medications may cause dry eye.

Treatment: It is directed at reestablishing the flow of tears. It may be possible to do this with drugs. Chronic eye infections should be treated and resolved.

The Cornea

The large, clear part of the front of the eye is the cornea. It is covered by a protective layer of epithelial cells called the epithelium. Most corneal diseases begin with an injury to this protective layer. The cornea of the horse is more sensitive to injury than that of humans and most other animals. Consequently, healing is slower and ulcers on the cornea are more apt to result in complications.

Corneal Abrasion

Corneal scratches and abrasions are caused by tail-swishing; branch scratches; and foreign bodies such as stones, awns (bristlelike fibers), and foodstuffs that injure the surface of the globe. Scratches on the cornea are extremely painful and are accompanied by excessive tearing, squinting, tenderness to touch, and avoidance of light. The third eyelid may be visible.

With a severe abrasion, the surface of the cornea immediately surrounding the injury becomes swollen, giving it a cloudy or hazy look.

Treatment: Healing of a small corneal abrasion takes place in 24 to 48 hours by a process in which the epithelium thins and slides over a small defect. Larger and deeper abrasions require careful cleansing; loose cells around the edges of the abrasion must be removed to promote healing. This is done with a cotton-tip applicator after appropriate sedation and application of anesthetic drops to the eye. A corneal abrasion will not heal if a foreign body is imbedded in the cornea or beneath the eyelid.

For all but mild abrasions, veterinary examination is necessary to evaluate and treat the eye injury to prevent the development of corneal ulcer, keratitis, or secondary uveitis.

Corneal Ulcer

Corneal ulcers follow injuries to the cornea that progress rather than heal. Ulcers that do not heal promptly often become infected. Large ulcers may be visible to the naked eye. They appear as dull spots or depressions on the surface of the cornea. Most ulcers, however, are best seen after the eye has been stained with fluorescein.

The most serious complication of ulcers or keratitis is a melting corneal ulcer, in which the stroma (the supporting framework of the eye) quickly melts away. This is a dire emergency and requires immediate treatment if the eye is to be saved.

Treatment: Corneal ulcers are dangerous and must receive prompt veterinary attention. Early treatment is vital to avoid serious complications or even loss of the eye. Corneal scrapings examined under the microscope will show if the *ulcer* is infected.

Uncomplicated small surface ulcers respond to topical ophthalmic antibiotic ointment applied four times a day. Atropine ointment is used to dilate the pupil and relieve intraocular pressure.

Deep or infected ulcers require intensive antibiotic therapy by subconjunctival injection, subpalpebral infusion, or the intravenous route. Cultures are taken by corneal scraping and antibiotics selected according to the results of sensitivity tests. The eyelids may have to be sutured together to protect the eye and keep it from drying out. Soft contact lenses also have been used for this purpose. Eye surgery to create a flap of conjunctiva to cover the ulcer may be required in difficult cases.

Melting ulcers require intense medical and surgical attention. If they are not stopped, the entire corneal surface could disintegrate. Anti-collagenases are used to stop the melting. Frequently this involves putting the serum from the horse's own blood on the surface of the eye to stop the degeneration of the corneal surface. Antibiotics are used as a preventive to avoid a secondary infection. A *systemic* anti-inflammatory, such as phenylbutazone or banamine, is used to manage pain.

White spots on the cornea may persist after healing from any ulcer. If these scars are large enough to interfere with vision, they can be removed surgically.

Special care should be taken with a horse who is being treated for a corneal ulcer. It is helpful to keep the horse in a darkened stall and limit exercise. Hay should be fed from the ground, not in an elevated feeder. A face net is useful to protect the eyes from flies and the bedding should be sprinkled with water to hold the dust down.

Prevention: All painful eye disorders should receive immediate veterinary attention. In particular, foreign bodies should be removed as soon as possible to prevent corneal damage.

Corticosteroids, which are incorporated into many eye preparations used for treating conjunctivitis and inflamed eyelids, should not be put into an eye if you suspect the horse has a corneal injury. This may lead to a rupture of the cornea.

Keratitis (Cloudy Eye)

Keratitis is an inflammation of the cornea. This occurs primarily when the protective surface epithelium is lost following a corneal injury, and secondarily as a corneal response to an inner eye inflammatory process such as glaucoma or uveitis. Keratitis is an extremely painful condition accompanied by excessive tearing, squinting, and aversion to light. It should not be confused with conjunctivitis, which is characterized by a watery or mucoid discharge with little or no pain.

Superficial (surface) keratitis is recognized by loss of transparency of the cornea, which at first appears dull, later hazy, then cloudy and covered by a bluish-white film. A cataract also produces an opaque eye, but this is a disease of the lens and not the cornea; also, cataracts are not painful.

Ulcerative keratitis occurs when a corneal injury becomes complicated by infection. A *purulent* discharge runs from the eye. There are signs of pain in the eye. A number of bacteria may cause this type of keratitis. Cultures and appropriate antibiotics are indicated.

Fungal keratitis is not uncommon in the horse, especially if the eye has been treated for some time with antibiotics, corticosteroids, or both. Potentially infective fungal organisms are present in the horse's environment in abundance, particularly in straw bedding and hay.

Treatment: Corneal scrapings and microscopic exam will disclose active inflammatory cells, bacteria, or fungi. Treatment is similar to that described for corneal ulcer (see page 159).

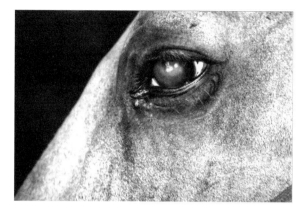

This cloudy eye needs prompt veterinary attention!

The Inner Eye
UVEITIS (EQUINE RECURRENT UVEITIS, MOON BLINDNESS)

The uveal tract is composed of the inner pigmented structures of the eye, which are the iris, the ciliary body, and the *choroid*. Inflammation of one or all of these structures is called uveitis. Because of secondary involvement of the cornea, lens, and retina, bouts of recurrent uveitis will eventually lead to permanent blindness.

Uveitis is one of the most common inner eye disorders of horses and the leading cause of blindness. It has been estimated that 10 percent of horses suffer from this condition. Uveitis may be chronic or acute.

The signs of acute uveitis are a red, painful eye with squinting and occasionally tearing. The eye often appears cloudy or "blind." Other important findings are a small contracted pupil, and a tender soft-feeling eyeball, noted on pressing gently over the closed eye.

The condition most likely to be confused with acute uveitis is a corneal injury. In either case, veterinary examination and treatment are essential.

Once a diagnosis of uveitis has been made, the next step is determining its cause. Infected corneal injuries can spread into the anterior chamber and involve the uveal tract, producing a bacterial uveitis. Signs of surface eye infection and corneal damage will be apparent on ophthalmic examination. However, in most cases of acute uveitis, the cornea is clear, indicating a primary inflammation of the deeper structures.

Signs of chronic uveitis are less pronounced and may be mainly behavioral. Equine eyesight evolved to detect predators, and, consequently, any change in vision can cause anxiety in a horse. If the horse starts acting spooky, bumping into things, or seems reluctant to enter dim areas (including the horse trailer), these could be indications that an eye exam is in order. Head tossing may indicate photophobia (light intolerance), which can also occur with uveitis.

By far, the most common known causes of uveitis are leptospirosis and onchocerciasis. Infrequent causes are strangles, viral arteritis, and toxoplasmosis. Leptospirosis is an infectious bacterial disease caused by spirochetes that infect cattle, sheep, wild animals, rats, cats, and humans. They gain entrance through a break in the skin or through the digestive tract when the horse ingests food or water contaminated by infected urine, particularly that of rodents. Acute uveitis can occur at the same time as acute leptospirosis, but typically it appears months or years after the acute infection. Evidence suggests that the uveitis is not the result of active spirochete infection, but instead is caused by an immune hypersensitivity response in which the inner eye structures react to foreign proteins released by the destroyed spirochetes.

Onchocerciasis is caused by a small threadlike worm that lives in the connective tissues of the neck. Adult worms produce microfilariae that migrate beneath the skin to the sternal midline area, where they cause an ulcerative skin condition. During the course of migration beneath the skin, some microfilariae enter the eyelids and progress to the inner chambers of the eye. Like leptospirosis, the intraocular inflammation is caused by an immune-mediated response to dying microorganisms within the eye. About half of all horses with skin involvement have eye involvement. Treatment of onchocerciasis is discussed in *Ventral Midline Dermitits* (page 121).

Both leptospirosis and onchocerciasis produce bouts of equine recurrent uveitis (ERU), also known as moon blindness or periodic ophthalmia. Since this "blindness" was observed to come and go periodically, it was thought by cowboys to be controlled by the phases of the moon. During an episode of ERU, the eye is cloudy and vision is diminished. These episodes will eventually lead to permanent blindness.

The diagnosis of ERU is based on a comprehensive veterinary examination of the eye, including opthalmography, complete blood count, blood chemistry profile, and *assays* for leptospirosis and toxoplasma. Serologic assays have more value in the early stages of the disease; their value diminishes once the disease process is established. Early identification and treatment is important to shorten treatment and minimize the damage.

Appaloosas seem to be most commonly affected and seem to suffer the most severe forms of ERU. There are also geographic areas strongly associated with ERU, including New York State, because of exposure to leptospirosis.

Treatment: Treatment is directed at preserving vision and reducing inner eye inflammation and recurring episodes. Topical steroids and atropine are used to break adhesions between the iris and the lens, supplemented with NSAIDs (usually flunixin meglumine). Systemic antibiotics are given if this is the first outbreak and the leptospira are still present, but they are not usually given for recurrent episodes because of the autoimmune nature of ERU.

Initially, the drugs will be given at maximum doses. As the inflammation is controlled, doses are stepped down gradually until the lowest maintenance dose is achieved. Treatment is continued until the eye examination reveals a stable condition. Because ERU is often recurrent, the horse should be closely monitored for signs of reactivation, which is an indication to restart treatment.

If control cannot be established or the episodes increase in frequency or intensity, surgery may be indicated. Still considered experimental, the cyclosporine implant appears to have great promise as an effective treatment option. Cyclosporine is an immunosuppressive agent, and is surgically implanted just under the sclera, where the medication is absorbed for up to a year. There are a few complications associated with the implant, and it is only for horses who have not already developed any permanent complications from ERU, such as cataracts or scarring.

Vitrectomy is a surgical procedure more commonly practiced in Europe. It has not gained popularity in North America. The vitreous, a normally clear gel-like fluid, fills the center of the eye, making up two-thirds of the eye's volume. This gel is removed (vitrectomy) to clear inflammatory cells, scar tissue, and any other cellular debris that may obscure light from reaching the retina. After the procedure, the eye will secrete fluid to replace the vitreous.

Deworming preparations that kill larvae of onchocerciasis should not be given if there is active inflammation, but may be considered during a quiescent stage. Eye complications are possible in a horse with a history of ERU. Consult your veterinarian before deworming the horse.

Cataracts

A cataract is a loss of the normal transparency of the lens of the eye. Any spot on the lens that is opaque, regardless of its size, is technically a cataract. To determine if a horse has a cataract, it is necessary for a veterinarian to dilate the eyes and perform an ophthalmologic examination.

Cataracts in horses fall into one of three general categories: congenital cataracts, acquired cataracts that are secondary to eye injuries and uveitis (see page 161), and those related to old age (*senile* cataracts).

Congenital cataracts may be inherited, although this is often difficult to establish. Belgians, Thoroughbreds, and Morgan horses appear to have a higher incidence. Some congenital cataracts follow eye inflammations that occur in the uterus or shortly after birth. Congenital cataracts generally are noted at about 2 weeks of age, but may not be discovered until much later. These cataracts are not progressive and in some cases do not significantly interfere with vision.

Acquired cataracts are common following eye wounds that perforate the front of the eye and involve the lens. These cataracts are permanent and are often progressive. Equine recurrent uveitis is the most common cause of acquired cataracts in the horse. Because of the intraocular inflammation and subsequent scarring caused by the uveitis, blindness often results even though the cataract itself is not progressive.

Senile cataracts do occur in the aging horse but are not common. As horses grow older, there is a normal process of aging of the eyes. New fibers, continually forming on the surface of the lens throughout life, push toward the center. The lens also loses water as it ages. These changes lead to the formation of a bluish haze seen on the lens behind the cornea in horses over 20 years of age. Usually this does not interfere with vision and does not need to be treated. This condition, called nuclear sclerosis, is often thought to be a cataract but actually is not.

Treatment: A cataract needs to be treated only if it impairs vision. Blindness can be corrected by removing the lens (cataract extraction). While this restores vision, there is some loss of visual acuity because the lens is not present to focus light on the retina. (So, unlike in humans with cataracts, the removed lens is not replaced with a plastic lens.) The operation is usually reserved for individuals with cataracts in both eyes and who are otherwise good candidates for eye surgery. Horses with cataracts secondary to uveitis are not good candidates. The best candidates are young horses with congenital cataracts and otherwise normal eyes. Foals who have cataract surgery should be operated on as young as possible.

Glaucoma

Glaucoma is an increase in fluid pressure within the eyeball. It is rare in horses. When present, it usually is due to equine recurrent uveitis or displacement of the lens.

An eye suffering from glaucoma is extremely tender and has a fixed and blank look, which is due to the hazy and steamy appearance of the cornea and the dilated pupil. Tearing, squinting, and protrusion of the third eyelid occur in response to pain. When you press gently on the closed eye with your finger, the affected eye feels harder than the normal one. When glaucoma has been present for some time, the increased intraocular pressure will cause the eye to bulge. Some permanent vision usually is lost before the disease is discovered.

Measurement of intraocular pressure using an instrument placed on the surface of the eye, and inspection of the interior of the eye, are needed to make a diagnosis.

Treatment: In some cases, your veterinarian may recommend drugs to reduce pressure within the eye. Topical corticosteroids such as phenylbutazone or flunixin, carbonic anhydrase inhibitors, dichlorphenamide, acetazolamine, prostaglandins, pilocarpine, and atropine may be beneficial. It is extremely important to follow your veterinarian's instructions exactly. Other treatment options that may be used include surgery using a diode laser and inserting shunts to drain fluid and relieve pressure. Removing the lens early in the course of the disease may help maintain vision and reverse glaucoma. A horse with unmanageable glaucoma may need to have his eye removed.

Displacement of the Lens

When the ligaments holding the lens in place are disrupted, the lens may be displaced forward into the anterior chamber or back into the vitreous chamber. Trauma to the eye, a severe blow to the head, uveitis, glaucoma, and spontaneous displacement owing to poorly developed ligaments are all possible causes of lens displacement.

A displaced lens can cause glaucoma, and glaucoma can cause a displaced lens. It is often difficult to tell which disease came first. A displaced lens is prone to cataract formation.

Treatment: Removal of the lens early on can maintain vision and reverse glaucoma.

Retinal Diseases

The retina is a thin, delicate membrane that lines the back of the eye and is an extension of the optic nerve. It is supported and nourished by the choroid, a layer of vascular tissue behind the retina. In a horse with retinal disease, the eye loses some or all of its capacity to perceive light.

There are many types of retinal disease that can affect horses. These are the most common.

Night Blindness

This disease is due to a defect in the photoreceptor cells called rods. Rods are especially sensitive to light. Their failure to perform results in impaired vision that becomes noticeable at dusk. Daylight vision is unaffected. Night blindness usually occurs in Appaloosas, but not exclusively. It appears to be inherited as a *recessive* trait.

Affected horses often injure themselves repeatedly if left out at night, and should be stalled in a lighted barn.

Treatment: Severe vitamin A deficiency (for more than one year) has been reported to cause night blindness. Dietary supplementation may restore night vision. Because the condition appears to have genetic component, horses with night blindness should not be bred.

Chorioretinitis

In horses with this condition, inflammation of the retina and its supporting vascular layer is followed by scarring and destruction of retinal tissue. The optic nerve is often involved. The most common cause of chorioretinitis is equine recurrent uveitis (page 161).

A type of chorioretinitis can occur after locoweed poisoning.

Optic nerve atrophy has been described as a sequel to severe blood loss, but for reasons unknown this occurs several months after the bleeding episode.

Trauma to the eyeball, and conditions causing a bulging eye (see page 155), are other causes of optic nerve atrophy. Atrophy results in irreversible blindness.

Treatment: When the cause is equine recurrent uveitis, treatment is directed at that condition (see page 162). If the cause is locoweed poisoning, the horse must be removed from the pasture (see *Locoweed Poisoning*, page 429). Treatment of the eye consists of topical anti-inflammatory medications to suppress the inflammatory response.

Retinal Detachment

In horses with this condition, the retina becomes partly or totally detached from the back of the eye. Most cases are the result of recurrent uveitis, in which scar tissue pulls the retina loose from its attachments. Others are related to chorioretinitis or severe head trauma. In horses, most detached retinas are of the nearly total type, resulting in sudden and complete blindness.

Treatment: There is no treatment for complete retinal detachment. With partial detachment, diuretics and anti-inflammatory drugs may help to preserve some vision.

Anterior Segment Dysgenesis

Anterior segment dysgenesis (ASD) is a congenital ophthalmic abnormality caused by a dominant *gene* found in some Rocky Mountain Horses, Mountain Pleasure Horses, Kentucky Mountain Saddle Horses, and Miniature Horses. It is not a degenerative eye disease, but a genetic defect associated with the popular chocolate coat color and flaxen mane and tail.

Horses with ASD have trouble in the front (anterior) part of the eye, which does not develop normally. In some cases, there is also abnormal development in the back (posterior) part of the eye. The most common findings in horses with ASD are cysts and *lesions*. Some horses with ASD suffer no loss of vision; some will be born blind or go blind later in life. Because this is a genetic condition, a veterinary ophthalmologist should be consulted to check all breeding stock.

Treatment: Cataract surgery is the only option. With otherwise healthy foals less than 6 months old who have no accompanying uveitis or ocular problems, *prognosis* is fair. In adult horses, the surgical outcome is poor, with less than a 50 percent success rate.

The Blind Horse

All conditions that prevent light from getting into the eye will impair a horse's vision. Diseases of the cornea (keratitis) and the lens (cataract) fall into this category, as do inflammations of the deep structures of the eye (such as glaucoma or uveitis). Diseases that destroy the retina invariably produce blindness.

Encephalitis and brain trauma produce blindness when the optic nerve or the sight center of the brain has been affected. This is not common.

Most cases of blindness will not be evident on general observation of the eye itself. Ophthalmologic tests are required to make a specific diagnosis.

Testing for Vision

There are signs that a horse is not seeing as well as he should. For example, horses with severely impaired vision often appear uncertain in their movements, step high with great caution, stumble, or tread on objects they usually avoid. Blind horses tend to move their ears constantly and thus may appear unusually alert. Those with partial vision may tilt their heads in an awkward position in order to see better. Occasionally a blind horse will show few if any signs.

Bringing your hand up quickly toward the side of a horse's face to elicit a blink reflex is not a good test for eyesight; there is considerable variation in results, even among sighted horses. In addition, a blind horse may blink if the surface of his eye detects the air current (called the menace response).

A better test for sight is to cover one eye with a blinder and toss cotton balls or gauze pads into the horse's field of vision to see if he follows the object with the uncovered eye.

An obstacle course made of barrels and hay bales can be used to test for vision. First take your horse through the course without blinders. Then cover each eye separately and repeat the experiment. Keep a loose shank. Visually handicapped horses become frightened and may injure themselves if led through the course on a tight lead (known as a maze test).

The loss of one eye is a significant handicap, although many gentle horses with one good eye are able to perform as trail horses and engage in activities that do not require total vision, when guided by an experienced rider. Keep in mind, however, that a visually imperfect horse may spook at any time. Therefore, a small child or an inexperienced rider would not be suitable for a horse with restricted vision. In addition, for the safety of both horse and rider, horses with a visual handicap should not be used for barrel racing, track racing, running, or jumping.

After a diagnosis of total blindness has been made, it does not mean the end of the horse's life. The reality is that most horses, even those with normal eyesight, do not really see very well. They rely to a large degree on their senses of hearing and smell. These senses take over and actually become more acute. This makes it possible for them to get around, sometimes almost normally. However, when confined, a blind horse should always be kept in a familiar enclosure.

6

THE EARS

The horse has a well-developed sense of hearing, enabling her to detect predators and to communicate with the herd. With large mobile ears, which can move independently, the horse can collect sound from different directions without moving her body.

The ear is divided into three parts. The outer ear is composed of the earflap (*pinna*) and the ear canal (external auditory canal). The middle ear is made up of the eardrum (*tympanic membrane*) and the *ossicles*, which are made of three bones. The inner ear contains the labyrinth, the *cochlea*, and the auditory nerve.

The pinna is the visible cuplike part of the external ear that funnels sound waves to the eardrum. Made of cartilage, a type of dense connective tissue, it is controlled by ten muscles that enable the horse to rotate her ears 180 degrees. A horse will usually rotate her ear toward a sound rather than turn her head. Horses also use their ears to convey visual signals such as friendship, acceptance, irritation, dominance, and submission. For example, pricked ears are typical of an alert, interested, or startled animal, while ears pinned back are a threat signal.

The skin on the outside of the pinna is covered with hair and, like the rest of the coat, is susceptible to the same skin diseases. There is also hair on the inside of the earflap. Here it is longer, coarser, and directed outward, helping to keep foreign material out of the ear canal.

Sound, which is actually air vibrations, is collected by the pinna and directed down the external auditory canal to the eardrum, which vibrates. Vibrations of the eardrum are transmitted via a chain of three tiny bones, collectively called the ossicles, to the bony canals of the inner ear, called the *labyrinth*. Within this bony labyrinth is a system of fluid-filled tubes in which waves are created by movements of the ossicles. The waves are transformed into nerve impulses, which are then conducted by the *auditory nerve* to the hearing center of the brain.

The tympanic membrane separates the outer ear from the middle ear and is connected to the ossicles. The middle ear is an air-filled cavity that connects

The structure of the ear.

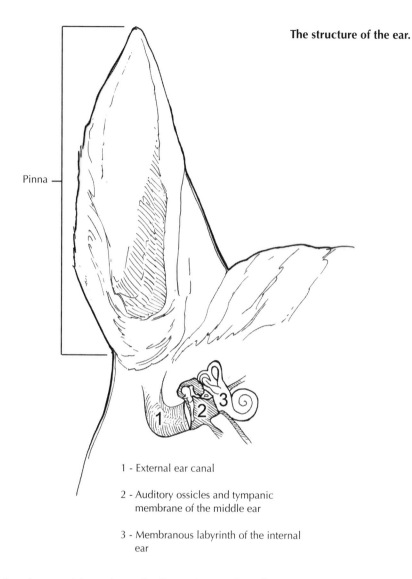

Pinna

1 - External ear canal

2 - Auditory ossicles and tympanic
    membrane of the middle ear

3 - Membranous labyrinth of the internal
    ear

to the pharynx (throat) via the Eustachian tube, allowing for pressure adjust-
ment between the middle and outer ear.

The horse is unique in that she has two large sacs connected to the
Eustachian tube known as the guttural pouches. Located between the pharynx and the skull, they are very close to vital nerves and arteries. A condition
called guttural pouch mycosis, which is a fungal *infection*, can be life threatening if these nerves or blood vessels are affected.

The inner ear consists of a complicated labyrinth of channels that are filled
with fluid. These channels are lined with thousands of sensory cells that signal both the auditory nerve and the vestibular nerve. Hearing and balance are
both influenced here.

You can take advantage of the horse's sensitive hearing by speaking quietly and using your voice as a training aid. Also keep in mind that the horse has two blind spots, immediately in front and directly behind her. Speaking softy to a horse as you work around her will help her know exactly where you are at all times.

Ear Care

The deep recesses of the horse's ears do not need to be cleaned. However, as part of a thorough grooming, it is a good idea to wipe the inside of the pinna gently with a damp cloth to remove dirt and flakes of loose skin.

Do not use soaps, oils, ether, or alcohol on the inside of the earflaps. These substances are extremely painful and can cause severe skin irritation and possibly infection.

Ear medications are applied by spray or dauber. A dauber is a ball of soft material on a stem. An irrigating syringe can also be used to apply medications.

When applying medication into the deep recesses of the ear, there is a distinct possibility of damaging the auditory canal or tympanic membrane. This procedure, if necessary, should be first demonstrated by your veterinarian.

The Pinna
Bites and Lacerations

Bites, lacerations, and puncture wounds of the earflap are not common. Bites, as from other horses, often produce crush injuries with severe swelling. They are prone to infection. Puncture wounds may be complicated by abscesses.

Treatment: Large lacerations, and those involving the cartilage and the margins of the ear, require veterinary attention. Surgical repair will help prevent scarring and deformity.

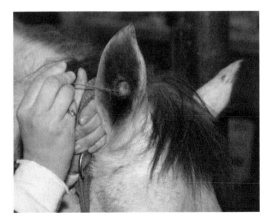

A dauber can be used to medicate the recesses of the external ear. Do not push it down into the ear canal.

Fly-Bite Dermatitis

Buffalo gnats, biting midges, and Culicoides gnats attack the horse's body, especially the ears. The bites of these blood-sucking insects ooze serum and form blisters and scabs that bleed easily when traumatized. A severe dermatitis with hair loss may ensue.

Treatment: Gently cleanse the bites to remove crusted blood. Apply a topical antibiotic ointment, as recommended by your veterinarian. Over-the-counter hydrocortisone creams are effective in calming the inflammation process.

Prevention: The best way to deal with this problem is to prevent fly exposure. Gnats tend to feed in the early morning and the evening. If possible, keep the horse inside during these hours to minimize exposure. Ear nets can be used to protect the ears. Insect control is discussed further in *External Parasites* (page 57).

Ear Plaques

Ear plaques are smooth, raised areas of *depigmentation* seen on the inside of the earflaps. At one time, they were thought to be caused by a fungus. Under the microscope, an ear plaque looks like a type of flat wart. There is evidence to suggest that the wartlike skin changes are the result of chronic irritation caused by the bites of black flies. Although they remain for life, they do not become malignant.

Treatment: These plaques do not appear to bother the horse, since they are neither itchy nor painful. Consequently, they do not need any treatment.

Tumors

The earflap is constantly exposed to ultraviolet radiation from the sun, but it is also well protected by a dense coat of hair. Accordingly, skin *cancer* is not as common as one might expect.

Benign and malignant tumors can occur on the earflap. The most common benign tumor is the *sarcoid*. Melanoma and squamous cell carcinoma are the most common locally invasive growths. Melanomas tend to occur in gray or white horses. They are rare in darker horses.

Treatment: For more information, see *Tumors and Cancers* (page 133).

The Ear Canal
Foreign Bodies in the Ear Canal

Foreign bodies in the ear canal are rare. The coarse hair on the inside of the earflap forms a barrier and prevents foreign objects from entering the deep

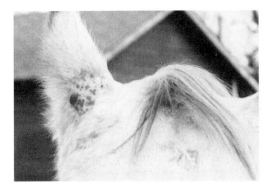

This locally invasive melanoma has been present for many years.

recesses. The most common foreign body is the ear tick, discussed in the next section. Splinters of wood and plant material may also work their way into the ear canal. Signs are head shaking, ear twitching, a head tilt toward the affected side, and rubbing at the ear. A persistent foreign body can lead to an ear canal infection.

Treatment: The ear canal is highly sensitive and horses will resist efforts to explore and probe it. Do not attempt to do this yourself. Your veterinarian will usually need to sedate the horse before examining the ear canal. Foreign bodies are removed with a long alligator forceps.

Ear Ticks

Several species of ticks live in the ear canals of horses. The major ones are the spinous ear tick, the tropical horse tick, the Gulf Coast tick, and the Lone Star tick. In the case of the spinous ear tick, only the larvae and nymphs are parasitic.

Ear ticks burrow deep in the external auditory canal and are not affected by topical insecticides applied to the body. Signs are like those of a foreign body in the ear. An infected bite can lead to an ear canal infection, a perforation of the eardrum, or meningitis.

Treatment: Ticks found on the skin of the horse's earflap should be removed as described in *Ticks* (page 62).

The ear should be examined and treated only after the horse has been sedated by a veterinarian. Ticks in the ear canals are killed by instilling an insecticide aerosol, dust, or smear (pyrethroids are best) into the deep recesses of both ears. The oral deworming agent ivermectin has been used with variable success to kill ticks.

Otitis Externa (Ear Canal Infection)

Ear canal infections are not common in horses. Signs are head shaking, tenderness to touch, holding the painful side down, redness and swelling of the ear folds, a purulent ear discharge, and a bad odor.

A tick or foreign body in the ear is the most common cause of *otitis* externa. Earflap infections can spread to the ear canals. Attempts to examine the ear by poking objects into it can damage the delicate tissues and precipitate otitis externa. A blockage of the ear canal produced by a tumor is a rare cause of ear canal infection.

Treatment: The ear canal should be examined only by a veterinarian. Cleaning the ear is the most important step in treating otitis externa, and cleaning requires sedation and restraint. After the ear has been cleaned, an antibiotic corticosteroid ear preparation (such as Panalog) should be instilled twice daily until the ear is healed. With a severe infection, the ear may need to be cleaned more than once; your veterinarian can demonstrate the proper technique to use so that you do not injure the eardrum.

The Middle and Inner Ear

The vestibular apparatus is a complex system of the ear and nerves that is responsible for the horse's balance as well as perpetually sensing the horse's location and posture both at rest and while she is moving.

Labyrinthitis (Vestibular Disease)

Infections of the middle and inner ear (otitis media and otitis interna) can be recognized by signs of *labyrinthitis*, an inflammation of the labyrinth. The labyrinth is a complex organ similar to a gyroscope. Its purpose is to synchronize the movements of each eye so they both work together, and maintain the horse's posture, balance, and coordination.

A horse with labyrinthitis, will often assume an abnormal posture with a head tilt toward the affected side. Dizziness, incoordination, and loss of balance are evident in the staggering gait, turning and circling toward the affected side, and tendency to lean against walls and fences for support. The horse may exhibit rapid jerking movements of the eyeballs, a condition called *nystagmus*.

The fascial nerve that serves the muscles that control facial expression passes through the middle ear and may be involved in middle ear infections. Paralysis of this nerve causes drooping of the ear, lip, and upper eyelid on the affected side. In addition, the horse is unable to close her eye on the affected side, which can result in the surface of the eye becoming excessively dry.

The usual cause of inflammation of the labyrinth is a bacterial infection of the middle and/or inner ear. The infection ascends through the auditory tube into the middle ear from an infection in the nasopharynx or guttural pouches. Blood-borne spread from a remote site of infection is possible. Encephalitis, meningitis, and ryegrass staggers can produce signs of labyrinthitis. These signs can also occur with brain tumors, antibiotic-induced damage to the auditory nerves, antifreeze poisoning, and a condition called *idiopathic* vestibular syndrome. This syndrome is thought to be caused by a virus. It usually corrects itself spontaneously in one to three weeks.

Vestibular syndrome is characterized by a set of signs seen following a blow to the poll, with hemorrhaging around the brain stem (see *Head Trauma*, page 348). Signs include circling, nystagmus, incoordination, and head tilt.

Treatment: The treatment of labyrinthitis is directed at the primary disease. Bacterial infections require high-dose antibiotic therapy, as prescribed by your veterinarian. The horse should be confined to a quiet, well-bedded stall. A dry eye is treated with drops, ointments, and occasionally by temporarily suturing closed the eyelid.

Horses who recover from labyrinthitis may always exhibit head-bobbing or a coarse tremor of the head, evident during eating or drinking. They are prone to episodes of imbalance and may pose a hazard when used for sport or pleasure.

Deafness

Deafness is seldom a problem because a horse can compensate for a hearing loss by relying on her other senses, particularly her eyesight. Accordingly, signs of deafness are subtle and may go unnoticed for some time.

A horse's ability to hear can be judged by her actions and how she uses her ears. A horse who hears well rotates her ears toward the source of the sound and may turn her head to look. Lack of attentiveness and quiet ears are two indications that the horse is not hearing as well as she should. One way to test this is to approach the horse from outside its field of vision and make a sudden noise. A horse with good hearing will spook or startle. Do not stand directly behind the horse in case she has no trouble hearing and kicks out when spooked.

Loss of hearing can be caused by a middle ear infection (both sides), a head injury, a brain inflammation (encephalitis), and by certain drugs and poisons. In particular, the antibiotics gentamicin, streptomycin, neomycin, and kanamycin can damage the auditory nerves when used for a prolonged period.

THE MOUTH

7

The oral cavity is bounded on the front and sides by the lips and cheeks, above by the hard and soft palate, and below by the tongue and the muscles of the floor of the mouth. Four pairs of salivary glands drain into the mouth.

The horse's mouth is remarkably well-adapted to a life of continuous grazing. The prehensile lips are designed to grasp and hold vegetation, while the sharp incisor teeth form an efficient cutting mechanism. The rough surfaces of the cheek teeth (the premolars and molars) grind down plant material and separate the energy portion from the fiber.

Signs of Mouth Problems

A horse with a painful mouth will change his eating behavior. Eating slowly is common but often owners do not notice the change. Many horses with pain on one side of the mouth will tilt their heads and chew on the other side. A horse with a tender mouth eats selectively, dropping feed that is too coarse. With a very sensitive mouth, the horse may stop eating altogether. Weight loss occurs rapidly once a horse stops eating. A horse with a painful mouth often won't drink cold water, either.

A young horse with a painful mouth may object to bridle training, throw his head, and bleed from the mouth after being ridden with a snaffle bit. Blood may be found in the feed box.

Quidding means spitting out or dropping feed after it has been shifted back and forth from one side of the mouth to the other. This is a sign of painful chewing or the inability to chew properly.

Some horses avoid chewing by bolting their feed. Improper chewing results in feed not being properly ground and therefore not adequately digested. Accordingly, horses with chronic mouth pain lose weight and are prone to *colic* and constipation. This syndrome tends to occur in older horses. It also increases the frequency of choking and large colon impactions.

Common causes of painful chewing include:

- Lacerations of the cheeks, gums, and tongue caused by sharp points on cheek teeth or by dental caps and other teething problems
- Infected and abscessed teeth
- Mouth *infections* such as stomatitis

Drooling is an important sign of mouth infection. The saliva is tenacious, is stained brown, and has a fetid odor.

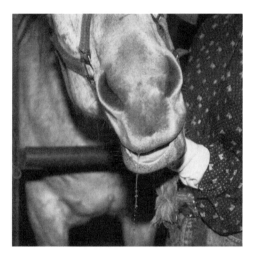

Drooling indicates a mouth infection or paralysis of the swallowing mechanism.

A clear salivary discharge indicates the inability to swallow saliva, caused by a blockage or paralysis of the swallowing mechanism. Drooling saliva also occurs when the horse is being given tranquilizers. A peculiar type of slobbering is caused by the mycotoxin of a fungus present in contaminated *legume* hay. It disappears when the hay is removed.

Lolling is a condition in which the tongue is paralyzed and hangs limply from the mouth between the incisors or protrudes from the side of the mouth through the interdental space. Tongue paralysis occurs with botulism (*forage* poisoning), *encephalitis*, meningitis, rabies, and lead poisoning. Yellow star thistle, Russian knapweed, and ergot poisoning also cause tongue paralysis.

Swelling of the face and a discharge from one nostril indicate a maxillary sinusitis caused by the infected root of an upper molar.

How to Examine the Mouth

Most mouth disorders will become evident by careful examination of the lips, teeth, palate, throat, and soft tissues of the face and neck. Many horses can be examined with minimal restraint. However, a horse with a painful mouth may resist examination and require restraint or tranquilization.

To examine the lips, gums, and incisor teeth, raise the horse's upper lip with one hand while drawing down the lower lip with the other. Healthy gums are firm. In nonpigmented areas the color is pink. Pale gums are a sign of ill health (possibly parasites or *anemia*). Bluish-gray gums (*cyanosis*) indicate low oxygen caused by respiratory or circulatory failure. Yellow gums indicate *jaundice*.

The state of the circulation can be judged by *capillary refill time*—how long it takes the gums to pink up after they have been pressed firmly with a finger. The area you pressed will turn white. When you take your finger away, a pink color should return to the blanched area within two seconds. A delay in capillary refill of three seconds or longer indicates dehydration or shock.

Before opening your horse's mouth to complete the examination, handle him about the head until he relaxes. Then insert the fingers of one hand

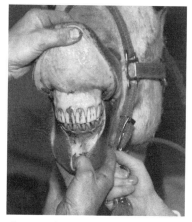

The mouth exam. Draw the lips apart to see the gums and incisors.

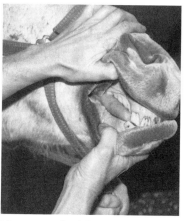

The tongue is visible in the interdental space.

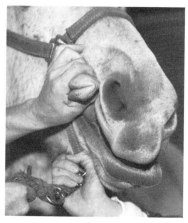

Grasp the tongue and pull it out.

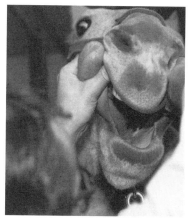

Maintain traction on the tongue. The horse will open his mouth for the examination.

through the interdental space between the incisors and cheek teeth, grasp the tongue and pull it out. The horse will automatically open his mouth and keep it open as long as you maintain a firm hold on the tongue. With the mouth open, you will be able to see the molars, tongue, and palate. Because the soft palate is dropped when the mouth is open, you will not be able to see the nasopharynx (the area of the pharynx that is above the soft palate). This area will need to be examined by your veterinarian using nasopharyngeal endoscopy.

Problems in the Mouth

Lacerations of the Mouth, Lips, and Tongue

The soft tissues of the mouth are common sites for cuts. Most are caused by neglected teeth; others by nails, wire fences, or foreign bodies. Tongue lacerations are usually associated with rough handling and harsh bits. Minor cuts heal rapidly.

Treatment: Bleeding can be controlled by applying pressure to the cut with clean gauze or a piece of linen. Consider suturing when the laceration is large, ragged, or deep; when bleeding resumes after pressure is removed; when the tongue is badly cut; or when lip lacerations involve the borders of the mouth.

A horse with a mouth injury should be switched to a soft diet, such as chopped wet hay or soaked pellets, until he is fully healed. Extensive wounds may require cross-tying and feeding through a nasogastric tube.

Foreign Bodies in the Mouth

Foreign bodies in the mouth may include foxtail weeds, bearded barley, wire, wood splinters, and wood sticks or corncobs lodged in the dental arch. Small plant awns, burrs, and splinters can become embedded on the surface of the tongue. Owing to the natural curiosity of horses, porcupine quills can become imbedded in the face, nose, lips, oral cavity, and skin.

Suspect a foreign body if your horse shakes his head, refuses to eat, and drools. When a foreign body has been present for some time, there will be an offensive mouth odor.

Treatment: Obtain a good light source and, if the horse will cooperate, gently open his mouth. If you can see the foreign body, you may be able to remove it with your fingers. However, many horses with a painful mouth resist handling and require veterinary sedation.

For porcupine quills, use a surgical hemostat or needle-nose pliers to grasp each quill near the skin and draw it straight out in the long axis of the quill. If the quill breaks off, a piece will be left behind. This may result in a deep-seated infection. Veterinary sedation is usually necessary before quills can be removed from the mouth.

STOMATITIS (SORE MOUTH)

A horse with stomatitis drools, refuses to eat, drinks more water than usual, is mouth-shy, and has an offensive mouth odor. The mucous membranes are reddened, swollen, tender, and often have blisters or a tenacious *exudate*.

Specific causes of stomatitis include infected teeth, foreign bodies in the mouth, equine viral infectious diseases (such as rhinopneumonitis or viral arteritis), photosensitivity reactions, prolonged use of phenylbutazone (Butazolidin) or antibiotics, blister beetle poisoning, and alkaloid plant toxicity.

Vesicular stomatitis is a common contagious viral disease that produces blisterlike *vesicles* on the mucous membranes of the lips and tongue, and on the coronary bands of the feet (see *Vesicular Stomatitis*, page 89).

Treatment: Treatment is directed at correcting the underlying cause of the problem, relieving mouth discomfort, and promoting appetite. Rinse the mouth twice daily with either a 3 percent hydrogen peroxide solution (diluted with water 1:10), a 10 percent Betadine solution (diluted 1:10), a 1 percent potassium permanganate solution, or a chlorhexidine solution such as Nolvasan.

Anti-inflammatory drugs reduce pain and swelling. Antibiotics are indicated for secondary bacterial infection. Eliminate coarse hay; feed soft mashes and chopped wet hay.

GROWTHS IN THE MOUTH

Tumors in the mouth are not common. Growths that ulcerate and exude a bad odor are usually malignant. Squamous cell carcinoma is the most common type. It is found most often on the lips, tongue, and gums. Other malignant tumors include fibrosarcoma, melanoma, and lymphoma.

Benign tumors that occur in and around the mouth include *sarcoids*, papillomas, lampas, cysts, neoplasms of dental origin, and granulomas.

Papillomas (warts) are caused by a virus that is different from the one that causes warts on the skin. Warts in the mouth disappear spontaneously.

Lampas is a swelling of the hard palate just behind the front teeth. It occurs, and then the permanent incisors erupt at 3 to 4 years of age. This hard mass forms a ridge that can project below the level of the upper teeth and cause eating problems. Although scraping the palate with a sharp knife and rubbing salt into the wound have traditionally been used to treat this problem, they are not effective. Feed the horse a soft, moist ration to encourage eating. The lampas will disappear spontaneously.

A ranula (honey cyst) is a smooth, rounded salivary gland swelling in the floor of the mouth on one side of the tongue. When a needle is put into the cyst, a thick, mucuslike, honey-colored material runs out. This often brings about a cure without surgery. This procedure should only be done by a veterinarian with the horse under sedation.

The Teeth

The horse has 24 deciduous (temporary or milk) teeth and 44 permanent (adult) teeth in a male or 40 permanent teeth in a female. The variation is because male horses have four canine teeth. Some *mares* can also have canines.

The top surface or crown of the tooth is covered by a hard substance called enamel. Enamel is impervious to bacteria and acids. Beneath the enamel is a softer material called dentin, and beneath the dentin is the pulp or center of

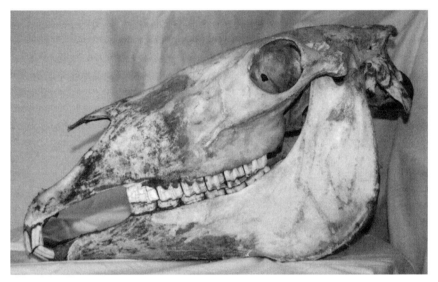

The horse's skull.

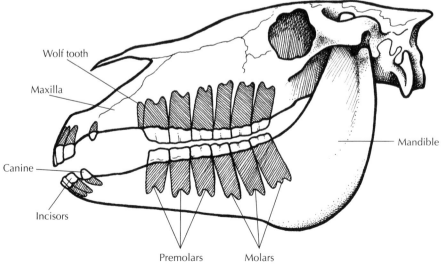

The position of the teeth in the skull.

the tooth. The pulp contains blood vessels and nerves. If the tooth cracks, exposing the pulp, the tooth decays rapidly and the root dies.

The root of each tooth is covered by a substance called cementum that attaches the tooth to the periodontal membrane and thus to the bony socket. The tooth is weakest and most susceptible to periodontal disease and tooth decay at this juncture with the periodontal membrane.

The teeth of horses are very long, with up to 4 inches (10 cm) embedded in the bone of the upper and lower jaws. The teeth of horses erupt continually throughout life at about the same rate as they are worn down by grinding. As each tooth emerges, it is ground and shaped by the opposing tooth.

The nature of the horse's diet and intestinal tract requires that all food must be thoroughly ground between the premolars and molars before being swallowed. If the food is not adequately ground, the horse will not receive the full nutritional benefit and will lose weight and condition.

In the process of grinding, the horse moves his jaws both up and down and from side to side. In a normal horse, the dental arcades (the rows of molars and premolars) of the upper and lower jaws are not in exact alignment along the sides, as they are in people. The arcade of the upper jaw overlaps that of the lower jaw along the sides by about 30 degrees. The effect of the circular grinding action, plus the overlapping arcades, creates uneven tooth wear—specifically, the development of sharp enamel points on the tongue side of the

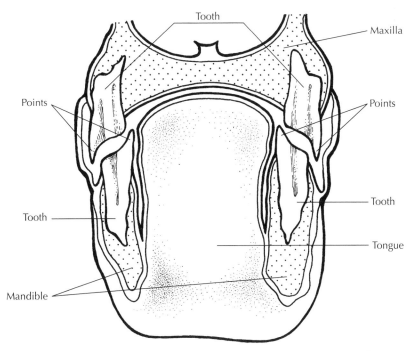

The overlapping upper jaw allows sharp enamel points to develop where the cheek teeth fail to make contact.

lower jaw and the cheek side of the upper jaw. You can test this by sliding your fingers along the spaces between the cheeks and the teeth, feeling for points on the premolars and molars on the upper arcade. When these points are prominent, they interfere with proper chewing and become a source of irritation to the soft tissues of the mouth.

These enamel points should be removed regularly by filing with a long-handled rasp. This filing, called floating the teeth, should be limited to the points of the teeth and should not involve the enamel on the grinding surfaces. For more information, see *Taking Care of Your Horse's Teeth* (page 186).

DECIDUOUS TEETH

Foals are born toothless but begin to acquire teeth within the first week of life. The first to appear are the central incisors. There are two in the upper jaw and two in the lower jaw.

All three premolars erupt at 2 weeks of age. The second incisors appear at 1 month and the third incisors at 6 to 9 months. At about 9 months of age, a foal has a complete set of 24 deciduous teeth.

PERMANENT TEETH

The first permanent molars appear at 9 to 12 months of age. The second molars erupt at 2 years. At 2.5 years, the central deciduous incisors are expelled and replaced by permanent incisors. Also at this time, the first and second premolars make their appearance. The first premolars, commonly called wolf teeth, are usually found only in the upper jaw; if they are present in the lower jaw, they are quite small and needlelike.

At 3 years of age, the third premolars erupt (although the lower ones may erupt 6 months earlier). At 3.5 years, the lateral incisors and the third molars are present. At 4.5 years, the horse has his corner incisors, fourth premolars, and canine teeth. The canine teeth are usually present by then in the male but are absent or rudimentary in the mare.

By 5 years of age, the horse has a complete set of 40 to 44 permanent teeth. (See *Teething Problems*, page 191, for information on possible problems during this process.)

AGING A HORSE BY HIS TEETH

The age at which the permanent teeth erupt is quite constant. In summary, the central incisors erupt at 2.5 years, the lateral incisors erupt at 3.5 years, and the corner incisors erupt at 4.5 years. This sequence, along with the presence or absence of canine teeth in the male, can be used to accurately determine the age of a horse up to 5 years.

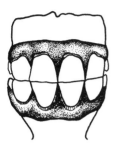
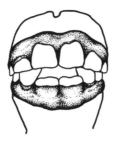
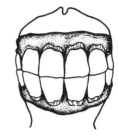
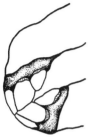
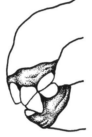
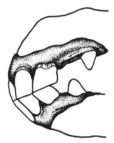

One year of age. The foal has a complete set of deciduous (temporary) teeth.

Two and one-half years. The central incisors are replaced by adult incisors.

Five years. The horse has complete set of adult incisors.

Aging a young horse, showing the characteristic appearance of the incisors up to 5 years of age.

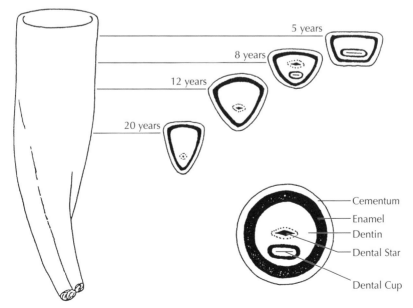

5 years

8 years

12 years

20 years

Cementum
Enamel
Dentin
Dental Star
Dental Cup

Aging the horse from 6 to 21 years. As the incisor teeth wear with age, the dental cups gradually disappear and the teeth become triangular.

With experience, it is possible to determine a horse's age up to 30 years with reasonable accuracy by looking at the dental cups, changes in the shape of the teeth and jaws, and the appearance of *Galvayne's groove*.

Dental cups are hollow depressions present in new teeth. As a consequence of bacterial action on retained food particles, these hollows become dark-stained. As the edges of the cups wear down through age and use, the depressions become shallower and eventually disappear, leaving a white surface with a small, dark central pit called a dental star. The order in which the dental cups disappear from the incisor teeth can be used to age the horse.

Disappearance of the cups and changes in the shape of the teeth follow a generally predictable pattern. The lower incisors also wear about three years faster than the upper incisors.

- **6 years:** The lower central incisors are worn smooth, with shallow cups in the lower lateral incisors.
- **7 years:** The lower lateral incisors are also worn smooth. The lower central and lateral incisors begin to assume a more oval appearance.
- **8 years:** The lower corner incisors are now worn smooth.
- **9 years:** The upper central incisors are smooth, with shallow cups in the upper lateral incisors.
- **10 years:** The upper lateral incisors are now worn smooth. The central and lateral incisors appear somewhat oval.
- **11 years:** The cups of all incisors are worn smooth. Thus, at 11 years of age, a horse is "smooth-mouthed" (referring to the incisors).
- **15 years:** The lower incisors appear shorter than the upper incisors when viewed from the front. All teeth show a distinct dark round dental star in their centers.
- **21 years:** The angle of the jaw is distinctly oblique. There is considerable space between the teeth. The lower incisors may be worn nearly to the gums.

Galvayne's groove can be used to judge the age of horses from 10 to 30 years. This is a groove on the surface of only the two upper corner incisors. It first appears at the gum line at 10 years of age. It works its way downward year by year as the tooth continues to wear. At 15 years, the line is halfway down the tooth. At 20 years, the line is present the full length of the tooth. It then begins to recede from the gum, so that at 25 years it is present in the lower half of the tooth, and is completely gone by age 30.

As the horse advances in age, there is a tendency for the incisors to protrude outward against the lips, creating a jaw and tooth angle that is more oblique. In addition, the gums shrink or recede. The teeth thus appear longer and more exposed when viewed from the side, giving rise to the expression "getting long in the tooth."

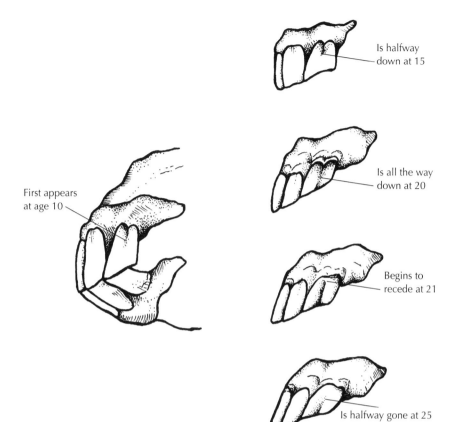

Is halfway down at 15

Is all the way down at 20

First appears at age 10

Begins to recede at 21

Is halfway gone at 25 and disappears at 30

Galvayne's groove can be used to estimate the age of older horses.

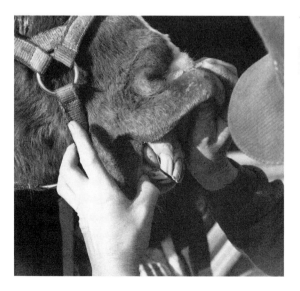

This horse was said to be 12 years old, but judging by Galvayne's groove, the horse is closer to 22.

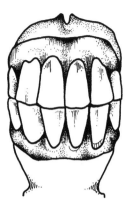

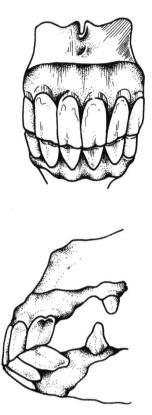

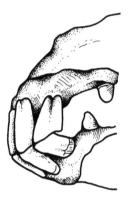

Ten years. The angle of the jaw and teeth is more oblique. The corner incisors are in full contact.

Twenty years. The angulation of the jaw is distinctly oblique. All teeth show wear, especially the lower incisors.

As the horse grows older, age-related changes occur in the shape of the teeth and jaws.

Taking Care of Your Horse's Teeth

Routine dental care can add ten years to your horse's life and increase the efficiency of his feed, thereby improving his performance. Your horse's teeth are continually growing and changing. The foods horses eat—hay, grass, and grains—contain silica, a very abrasive substance that causes the tooth surface to wear down. This wear does not occur evenly, which causes the sharp points that can cut and ulcerate the cheeks.

It is important to check your horse's teeth regularly (see *How to Examine the Mouth*, page 176). In addition, your horse should have a dental veterinary examination every six months until age 2 years, and then annually. With

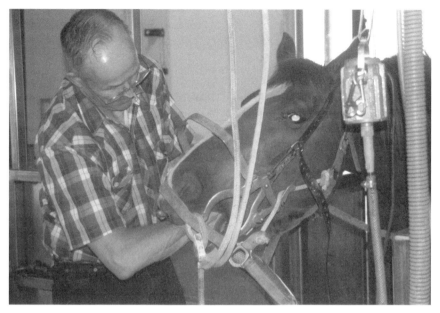

Feeling for points on the molars. The teeth should be checked every six months, especially in young horses.

a little simple observation of the horse, how he eats, his weight and condition, and the smell of his breath, you can determine if a veterinarian's dental examination is needed more often. A thorough oral exam requires the use of a full-mouth speculum and is usually done with the horse under mild sedation.

Dental practitioners are formally schooled in the art of equine dentistry, their main work is to equilibrate and balance the teeth of the horse by cutting, burring, and filing the sharp points of the tooth crown. Often your veterinarian can work together with a dental technician to the benefit of your horse.

Dental examinations are particularly important in young horses, as their teeth wear faster and form extremely sharp enamel ridges. In addition, young horses may have problems associated with caps or impacted adult teeth (see *Teething Problems*, page 191). Most dental problems can be treated successfully if they are identified before tooth disease and abnormal wear patterns become fixed and irreversible. A dental chart similar to one a dentist for humans uses shows what alterations have been made to the horse's teeth. An example can be seen on page 188.

Older horses may have loose teeth. However, they do not always fall out by themselves because the teeth are so tightly packed together. The teeth of older horses should be examined every three months, and any loose teeth should be removed to relieve discomfort and prevent dental infection.

EQUINE DENTAL EVALUATION AND MAINTENANCE CHART

Date: _____

Client: _____

Address: _____

_____ Date: _____

Horse: _____ Ages: _____

Barn: _____ Stall Number: _____

Occlusion before dental work: _____

Occlusion after dental work: _____

Lateral excursion before dental work: _____

Lateral excursion after dental work: _____

Anterior / posterior movement of mandible before dental work: _____

Anterior / posterior movement of mandible after dental work: _____

History / Use / Bitting: _____

Soft tissue damage: _____

Comments: _____

Office Call	
Farm Call	
IV Fee	
Dormosedan	
Torbugesis	
Xylazine	
Yohimbine	
Other	
TOTAL	

General Oral Condition

Incision	Canines	Wolf Teeth	Premolars & Molars
			Near Side Far Side
Caps	None	Extract	Float
Fragments	Male	Normal	Burr
Extract	Female	Lingual	Caps
Realign	Cut	Anterior	Bit-seats
Cut	Buff	Aberrant	Hooks
Burr	Remove tartar	Fragment	Ramps
Overjet / Overbite	Normal	Non-erupted	Table angle
Underjet / Underbite	Fractured	Blind	Balance
Table angle	Location	Upper / Lower	Rims
Other	Other	Other	Waves
			Fractured
			Stepped
Charges: _____	Charges: _____	Charges: _____	Impacted
			Protuberant teeth
			Periodontal disease
Call Back Date and Reason: _____			Malocclision
			Supernumary teeth
_____			Other
Comments: _____			Sub Total: _____
_____			TOTAL Charges: _____

FLOATING THE TEETH

Floating (rasping or filing) the teeth is done routinely once a year after a horse reaches 18 months of age. The purpose of floating is to control the sharp edges and points present on the cheek side of the upper premolars and molars and on the tongue side of the lower premolars and molars. Floating is also used to correct minor abnormalities of wear, such as lowering a tooth that has grown too long.

The filing is done with a long-handled rasp with a carbide-chip blade. The procedure is not painful to the horse and can generally be performed with minimal restraint. These points should be removed with a few strokes of the rasp.

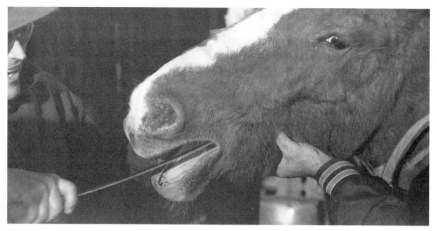

Floating the teeth is not painful, but it does require an assistant to restrain the horse's head.

The same results can also be obtained using power tools. These enable dental procedures to be done more quickly, which increases the horse's comfort level and enables the practitioner to correct more significant problems. However, a greater skill level is necessary to prevent damage to the horse's mouth.

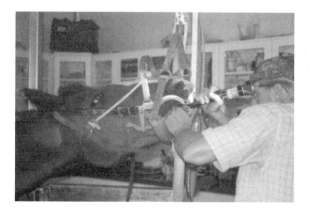

The power float, head sling, and speculum allow dental work to be accomplished efficiently.

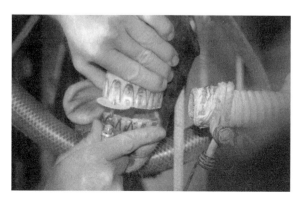

This power tool has a special cutting disk that creates a smooth, level bite for the incisors.

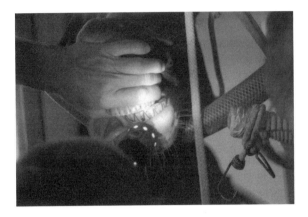

Checking the dental alignment after the work is done.

OTHER DENTAL PROCEDURES

Most dental procedures are not painful because the sensitive structures of the teeth are located deep in the tooth. Accordingly, teeth can be filed, chiseled, or cut to a desired length using special dental instruments under physical restraint or sedation. Tranquilization is needed for some cutting procedures that produce a loud noise when the tooth is snapped, since this could startle the horse.

Dental caps and wolf teeth can be removed with bone cutters, dental elevators, and forceps. Badly infected teeth or split teeth can sometimes be removed with long-handled forceps.

When the root is embedded in bone or the extraction is otherwise complicated, the dental procedure is usually done under a general anesthetic. Some teeth, because of their location, cannot be extracted through the mouth and will need to be repulsed. Repulsion involves making an incision in the skin overlying the tooth, drilling a hole in the bone to the base of the tooth, and then driving the tooth out from its socket with a dental punch and a mallet. This procedure is not without some danger of damaging an adjacent tooth or fracturing the jaw.

Following dental extraction, withhold hay for several days and provide mash or ground feed. After a tooth has been extracted, the opposite tooth will become too long and a step mouth (see page 195) may develop. The horse will require maintenance dentistry to float the opposing tooth every six months.

SPECIAL PROBLEMS OF MINIATURE HORSES

Miniature horses have increased in popularity for horse lovers everywhere. These small horses are often less than 28 inches (71 cm) in height and have presented unique problems in equine dentistry. These dental issues include teeth that do not erupt through the gums (maleruptions), teeth that do not align properly (malocclusion), and teeth that do not develop normally (malformation).

The miniature horse perhaps benefits most from dental examinations at an early age, as a *prophylactic* measure, to address the potential hazards of malocclusions, maleruptions, and malformations as early as possible. Early oral intervention will prolong the miniature horse's life by increasing the efficiency by which he chews, processes, and metabolizes his feed.

Dental Problems
TEETHING PROBLEMS

The teething process in the horse occurs over a long period of time. It generally begins at about 9 to 12 months of age and is completed by 5 years of age. During that time, many things can go wrong.

Dental Caps

Dental caps are deciduous cheek teeth that remain attached to the chewing surfaces of the permanent teeth after they have erupted. These caps are extremely sharp and may cut the cheek or tongue and interfere with eating. Occasionally, a cap becomes partially detached and rotates out to the side, where it damages the cheek and deforms the face.

Treatment: Dental caps, whether loose or not, should be removed once the adult teeth have emerged from the gum line.

Retained Incisors

Retained deciduous incisors are similar to dental caps except that the retained incisors are in front of the permanent incisors.

Treatment: In most cases, the deciduous teeth are loose and can be removed with dental forceps. If this is not possible, extraction is necessary to ensure a correct bite.

Supernumerary Teeth

This uncommon problem is due to splitting of the tooth bud. When that happens, the horse may grow one or two extra teeth (incisors or cheek teeth). Rarely, a horse will have an entire extra row of teeth. Dental crowding can result in tooth overgrowth and gaps between teeth that result in gum infection and tooth decay.

Treatment: Extra teeth that injure the gums or cheeks can be filed or trimmed with dental cutters. Occasionally, extraction will be necessary. A loose supernumerary tooth should be removed.

Absent Teeth

Absent teeth are fairly common. They occur when a tooth bud fails to develop normally.

Treatment: Unless there is a problem with the horse's bite, no treatment is necessary.

Impacted Teeth

Impacted teeth tend to occur in horses with a foreshortened upper or lower jaw (see *Malocclusion,* page 193). These horses have insufficient room for the teeth to erupt normally. This forces the tooth to remain in the jaw bone, creating inflammation and even swelling of the bone. Some cases are associated with dental caps (see page 191).

Treatment: If an impacted tooth becomes infected, it should be extracted. Treating retained dental caps will prevent some cases.

Wolf Teeth

Wolf teeth are vestiges of the first premolars, and are very rare in the lower jaw. In the upper jaw, wolf teeth are common and are the only remnant of the first premolar, which sometimes does not exist at all.

If a horse has wolf teeth, they are almost always removed. Delay in the eruption and displacement of the wolf teeth by the second premolars can cause abnormal alignment, with sharp points lacerating the lining of the cheeks and tongue. Even wolf teeth that do not erupt often need to be removed, because they have short roots that enable them to move easily and this is irritating to the horse's mouth.

Treatment: Wolf teeth may interfere with the bit, irritate the horse's mouth, and be a handicap in training, which is why some owners ask for them to be removed. Extraction is best done at 18 to 24 months of age.

Canine Teeth

Canine teeth (sometimes called tusks) are large curved teeth found in the interdental spaces of male horses. In females, they are either missing or are very small. Canine teeth are often confused with wolf teeth. When the canine teeth erupt between 4 and 5 years of age, the gum surrounding the tooth can become sensitive to the bit. A canine tooth that fails to erupt may cause a cyst in the gum.

Treatment: Canine teeth that become long and sharp and interfere with the bridle should be rasped down.

Hooks

Long, sharp points may develop on the first cheek tooth, the second premolars, and the last lower molars. This may be due to a preexisting malocclusion problem. The long sharp points can lacerate the gums and cause pain on chewing.

Treatment: Small hooks can be filed. Large hooks are also removed using power equipment. The horse should be adequately restrained or tranquilized for the procedure.

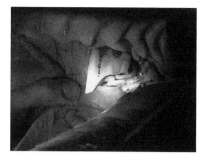

Hooks on the molars and premolars of a mature horse.

Split or Broken Teeth

A fractured tooth may be of no consequence, especially when the fracture does not extend below the gum line. However, if the tooth is broken very short or is lost, the opposing tooth will not be ground down and may become long enough to interfere with chewing.

Treatment: The unopposed tooth should be rasped every four months to prevent mouth injury. If damage to the broken or split tooth involves the root or surrounding bone, the tooth should be removed.

MALOCCLUSION (INCORRECT BITE)

The bite is determined by seeing how the upper and lower incisors meet in front. If a horse has a normal bite, the incisor teeth will meet edge to edge. An incorrect bite is one in which the incisors meet in some other alignment. This results in malocclusion.

Most *congenital* malocclusion problems are apparent during the first weeks of life. Severe malocclusion may lead to mouth infections, poor chewing, and impaired digestion. This can compromise growth and development.

Treatment involves periodically rasping the teeth to remove points and hooks in an attempt to maintain a normal alignment. Placing the horse on hard feed, such as pellets or unprocessed grain, may prolong the need for repeated treatments. Because malocclusions have a hereditary basis, horses with such deformities should not be bred.

Overshot Jaw (Parrot Mouth)

This is the most common malocclusion. In a horse with this deformity, the lower jaw is shorter than the upper jaw. In consequence, the upper incisors overhang the lower ones. Because the upper incisors are unopposed, they grow long like rabbit teeth.

When the malocclusion is restricted to the front teeth, it may not cause a problem. However, if the molars are also out of alignment, they will not be ground down and will form hooks and sharp points. These hooks may interfere with the bit and cause considerable pain.

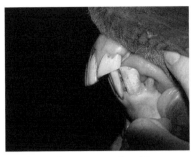

This horse has an overshot bite.

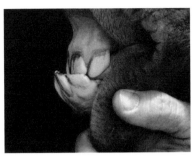

This horse has an undershot bite.

If detected at an early age (less than 6 months), parrot mouth can be treated by applying wire tension bands from the upper incisors to the first maxillary cheek teeth in an attempt to slow the rate of growth of the upper jaw. These braces can be left in place for several months, but should be carefully monitored for adverse effects, such as infection, impaction, and ulceration.

Undershot Jaw (Sow Mouth)

This is the reverse of an overshot jaw—the lower jaw is longer than the upper, and the lower incisors project beyond the uppers like a Bulldog. It is less common than parrot mouth. The horse may have trouble grazing or "nipping" grass.

Shear Mouth

In normal horses, the upper arcade is always wider than the lower arcade. In a horse with shear mouth this discrepancy is exaggerated. This produces long, extremely sharp shearing edges on the cheek teeth. An acquired type of shear mouth occurs in old horses who develop age-related changes involving the shape of the mandible.

ABNORMAL WEAR PATTERNS

Abnormal chewing patterns can produce abnormalities of tooth wear. It has also been suggested that in susceptible horses, some teeth may be innately softer than others and therefore do not offer equal resistance to wear and use. Regardless of the cause, these abnormalities tend to get worse with time. In the early stages, they cause subtle performance problems such as interfering with the bit. As the problem worsens, the horse develops painful chewing, quidding, and weight loss. Whole grain may be seen in the feces.

Wave Mouth

This usually occurs in ponies and older horses and results in an abnormal undulating surface to the teeth when viewed from the side. The crests and troughs created by the wave pattern allow some teeth to become too long; others opposing them are ground down to the gum line. Mouth and gum injuries are common.

Treatment: Mild cases may respond to floating the teeth at frequent intervals. In more severe cases, an attempt should be made to even the arcades by rasping, using motorized equipment.

Step Mouth

In horses with this disorder, there is an abrupt change in the height of adjacent premolars and molars. In many cases, a lost tooth leaves a space that permits an opposing tooth to grow out without meeting resistance. A retained dental cap is another cause of step mouth. Step mouth is a serious problem, because affected horses have great difficulty chewing and digesting their feed.

Treatment: Treatment involves rasping the elongated molars, using motorized equipment, at six-month intervals.

Smooth Mouth

This is caused by equal wear of both the enamel and dentin and produces an absolutely smooth surface on the cheek teeth instead of the normal rough grinding surface. In young horses, it is caused by a defect in the composition and structure of the teeth. In very old horses, it occurs when the teeth are worn down to the roots.

When the cheek teeth are worn absolutely smooth, the horse cannot grind his feed. These horses experience significant weight loss and suffer from digestive ailments such as colic, constipation, and malabsorption. Whole grain may be seen in the feces.

Treatment: Young horses who have been improperly floated may, with time, reestablish normal grinding surfaces. In all other cases, there is no effective treatment except to feed soft mashes, chopped wet hay, or a pelleted feed.

PERIODONTAL DISEASE

The periodontium consists of the gingiva (gum), the alveolar bone (the socket in which the tooth sits), the periodontal ligament (which anchors the tooth in the socket), and the cementum (the outer layer of the tooth). Horses do not develop cavities in the crowns of their teeth as people do. Instead, dental infection begins near the root of the tooth at the junction of the cementum and the periodontal membrane.

Periodontal disease in horses is an inflammation of the tissue and structures around the tooth. It may be painful, and is probably the most common cause of premature tooth loss in adult horses. Periodontal disease predominantly affects the cheek teeth, rarely the incisors. The gums may be involved in the process but are seldom a predisposing cause.

The primary cause of periodontal disease in the horse is the misalignment, or malocclusion, of the cheek teeth. This may be a result of the aging of the horse, improper alignment of cheek teeth caused by genetics, or normal wearing down of the teeth. These predisposing factors may cause abnormal chewing of feed, abnormal wear of teeth surfaces, malocclusion of the teeth, and gaps between the teeth where food may be trapped.

With normal chewing, the horse's mouth is fairly self-cleaning; feed does not accumulate on or around the teeth. When trapped feed packs down between the teeth, it starts to decompose and undergoes bacterial fermentation. The gum will recede and form a pocket. The pocket continues to ferment and the infection progresses toward the tooth root. If this process is not checked, it will continue until the periodontal ligament is destroyed and the tooth will loosen in the socket. Abscesses may occur as a result of periodontal disease (see *Abscessed Tooth*, below).

Signs of periodontal disease may include some or none of these: bad breath, losing weight, dropping feed (quidding), performance problems, or the horse just not seeming "right." A thorough oral exam by your veterinarian is necessary to detect periodontal disease. The cheek teeth, where most periodontal disease occurs, are not easily viewed without specialized equipment.

Treatment: The cause or causes of the periodontal disease must be addressed. Restoring the normal flat contour of the molars is a key step, as is removing impacted feed material from between the teeth. These treatments alone often restore the cheek arcade to normal function, thus eliminating the periodontal disease.

Sometimes an oral rinse of 0.1 percent chlorhexidine solution may be used to control bacterial growth after the entrapped forage is removed. If a tooth appears to be beyond help and the periodontal disease has progressed over a long period of time, the tooth may have to be extracted. This will require frequent check-ups to prevent overgrowth of the opposing tooth.

Antibiotics are seldom required. If antibiotics are indicated, periodontal pockets can be filled with a special antibiotic polymer such as the gel doxycycline (Doxirobe). The polymer prevents the pocket from filling back up with impacted feed material and the antibiotic is slowly released.

There are high-pressure irrigation systems available that use a baking soda and disinfectant slurry. These machines, similar to those used in human and small animal dentistry, also contain high- and low-speed drills, air, and water delivery, sonic scaler, and suction.

Abscessed Tooth

Abscessed teeth are caused by periodontal disease. A special situation involves the cheek teeth in the upper jaw. The roots of these teeth (primarily the first molars) are embedded in the maxillary sinuses. Consequently, root infections of these teeth commonly cause bacterial sinusitis and a *purulent*, foul-smelling, persistent discharge through one nostril (see *Sinusitis*, page 290). A fistula may develop between the oral and nasal cavities.

Treatment: It is necessary to extract the tooth to cure the infection. Antibiotics may be given at the discretion of the veterinarian.

The Feet

8

The foot refers to the hoof and all its internal structures. Most causes of lameness are found in the foot. An understanding of the anatomy and physiology of the hoof is necessary to correctly identify these causes.

A comparison can be made between the bones of the human wrist and hand and the bones of the lower foreleg of the horse. The knee or carpal joint in the horse corresponds to the human wrist. Everything below the horse's knee represents bones of the human hand. Humans have five metacarpal bones, but horses have only three (the second, third, and fourth metacarpals). These bones are called the cannon and splint bones.

The fetlock joint is the same as a human knuckle joint. Everything below the fetlock joint corresponds to the human finger. In essence, the horse has developed a conformation that places all of her weight on a column of bones comparable to the human finger.

The first bone in the human finger is called the proximal phalanx. In the horse the proximal phalanx is also called the long pastern bone. The next bone in the human finger, the middle phalanx, is the short pastern bone in the horse. And the last bone, or distal phalanx, is called the coffin bone (it is buried in the foot).

There are two joints in the human finger. The first, or proximal interphalangeal joint, corresponds to the pastern joint in the horse. The second, or distal interphalangeal joint, corresponds to the coffin joint.

To continue the comparison with the human finger, imagine that the fingernail extends all around the finger like a thimble. In this analogy, the outer insensitive lamina of the horny hoof is like the fingernail. The bed from which the nail is formed corresponds to the inner sensitive lamina of the horse's hoof.

The coffin bone is shaped like the hoof. It is a hard, spongy bone with many perforations for vessels and nerves to pass through the bone and supply the sensitive structures surrounding it. On each side of the coffin bone are grooves that serve as lines of attachment for the lateral cartilages. These are thin plates that slope up and end above the coronary band. They can be felt beneath the skin at the heel and help to shape the bulbs.

The navicular is a wedge-shaped bone at the back of the coffin joint. It is enclosed by the wings of the coffin bone. The navicular bone serves as a pulley or fulcrum for the deep digital flexor tendon.

For information on how to examine the feet and hooves, see pages 7 and 8.

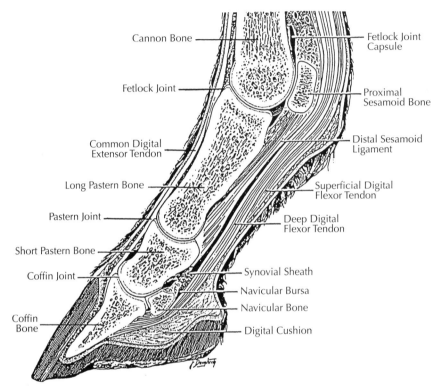

Cutaway view of the fetlock and foot.

The Laminae

The inner sensitive lamina of the hoof is called the corium. The corium is a highly vascular layer of specialized tissue modified from the *dermis* of the skin. It attaches to the coffin bone and the lower edges of the lateral cartilages. The corium manufactures the insensitive (or epidermal) lamina, which becomes the horny tissue of the hoof wall and sole.

Each part of the corium is named for one of the five insensitive laminae that it produces. These structures are the perioplic corium, which produces the periople (a waxlike waterproof covering that minimizes moisture evaporation from the hoof); the coronary corium, which produces the wall of the hoof and supplies its nutrition; the laminar corium, which lines the inside hoof wall from the coronary band to the sole; the solar corium, which produces the

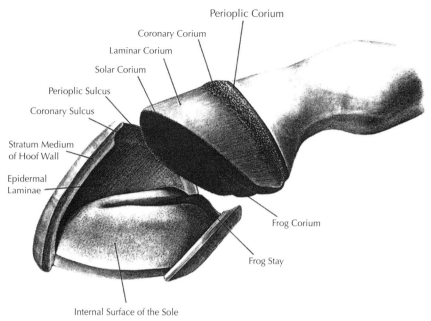

Perioplic Corium

Coronary Corium

Laminar Corium

Solar Corium

Perioplic Sulcus

Coronary Sulcus

Stratum Medium
of Hoof Wall

Epidermal
Laminae

Frog Corium

Frog Stay

Internal Surface of the Sole

Dissected view of the hoof, showing the relationship of the corium to the laminae of the hoof wall.

horn of the sole; and the frog corium, which produces the horn of the frog. The dissected view of the hoof above shows the relationship of these five inner sensitive laminae to the insensitive laminae they produce.

The Elastic Tissues

The digital cushion, hoof wall, sole, frog, and bulbs of the heel are elastic tissues, which means they are capable of changing shape in response to foot impact. The digital cushion is the main shock absorber of the hoof. It is a wedge-shaped elastic structure bounded by the lateral cartilages at the sides, the deep digital flexor tendon above, and the horny frog below. The back of the cushion forms the bulbs of the heel.

The hoof wall is composed of three layers. The outer layer consists of horn cells that give the hoof its gloss and protect it from excessive drying. Located at the hairline along the top of the hoof wall is the coronary band (also called the coronet). This is the primary source of growth and nutrition for the hoof wall. Injuries to the coronary band usually leave a permanent defect that extends the length of the hoof.

The middle layer is the stratum medium. It is thickest at the toe and gradually becomes less thick at the heels, although it is slightly reinforced at the angles where the bars are formed. (The angle of the wall and the bar is called

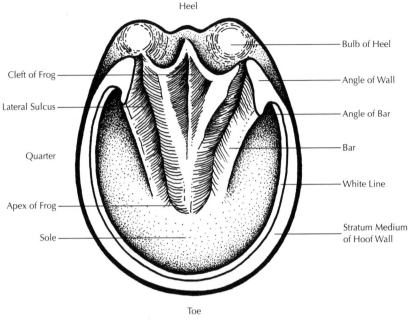

Heel

Bulb of Heel

Cleft of Frog

Angle of Wall

Lateral Sulcus

Angle of Bar

Bar

Quarter

White Line

Apex of Frog

Sole

Stratum Medium
of Hoof Wall

Toe

The ground (solar) surface of the hoof.

the buttress.) The middle layer incorporates pigment cells which, if present, give the hoof its color. An unpigmented hoof will not be any weaker than one with pigment.

The inner layer of the hoof wall fuses with the corium, which attaches to the coffin bone. This relationship is important because it means the weight of the horse is transferred to the bearing edge of the hoof wall and not to the cupped sole of the foot, as one might expect.

The ground surface of the hoof is composed of the sole, frog, bulbs, and bearing edge of the hoof wall. The ground surface has four quarters, called the toe, the heel, and the two side quarters.

The sole is a thick plate of flaky horn that covers most of the ground surface and is rounded in such a way that when viewed from the bottom, it is hollowed out or concave. This is important, because if the sole made contact with the ground, lameness would result from sole bruising.

The frog is an elastic, wedge-shaped mass of horn that fills a triangular space at the back of the foot. The triangular space is created by two ridges or bars that separate the frog from the sole. The bars converge and run forward to end just short of the apex of the frog. At the back, the bars terminate in the bulbs of the heels. Just inside the bars are two grooves called the lateral sulcii, which spread slightly when weight is placed on the frog.

In the center of the frog is a deep *depression* called the central sulcus or cleft. If you could view it from the inside of the hoof, this cleft would present as a ridge called the frog-stay. The frog-stay acts as a wedge pressing into the digital cushion.

Around the perimeter of the ground surface of the hoof is the white line, which represents the inside edge of the hoof wall at its junction with the sole. The white line marks the border between the sensitive and the insensitive sole. It serves as a guide to show where nails should be driven when shoeing the horse.

In an unshod horse, weight is carried on the bearing surface of the hoof wall, and on the bars and frog. The bearing surface of the hoof wall should be level with the frog to distribute the weight evenly.

The foot receives an excellent blood supply from the two digital arteries. Blood goes back to the heart through a network of veins called the coronary plexus. This plexus is located between the lateral cartilages and the surrounding hoof wall. In this location, the coronary plexus acts like a hydraulic cushion. Since these veins do not contain valves, blood can flow out of the coronary plexus when the foot expands and back into the plexus when the foot contracts.

The Hoof as a Shock Absorber

The shock of concussion is dissipated laterally against the hoof wall. It is not transferred vertically to the ground, which would greatly increase the force of the concussion and the number of musculoskeletal injuries. A number of shock-absorbing mechanisms aid in dissipating this force.

As the foot strikes the ground, downward pressure flattens out the concave surface of the sole. This distributes weight laterally against the hoof wall, which expands about a quarter of an inch (6 mm). Now the reason for the bars becomes clear. If the hoof wall formed a continuous ring, uninterrupted by the bars, the hoof could not expand.

With heel pressure the horny frog, aided by the frog-stay, compresses the digital cushion, which then flattens and pushes the lateral cartilages outward in opposite directions. To make room, venous blood is squeezed out of the coronary plexus.

As weight is removed from the leg, all these structures spring back to their original positions. This is called contraction and aids in propelling the horse forward.

The conformation of the knee and hock joints also helps reduce the shock of impact. These semi-flexed joints are composed of a number of bones arranged in layers and capable of yielding in three planes.

One other shock-absorbing structure is the navicular bone, which is supported by the deep digital flexor tendon and its ligaments. During concussion, the navicular bone shuttles the load from the digital cushion through to the short pastern bone, thereby bypassing the coffin bone and relieving some of its load.

All of these mechanical aids are of great importance in preventing musculoskeletal and foot injuries and maintaining the health and fitness of the horse.

Hoof Care

Horses living outdoors on varied terrain wear and grow their hooves in a natural fashion. In contrast, domestic horses living in paddocks and stables, with infrequent exercise and limited opportunity to toughen their feet, are susceptible to a number of hoof problems. A program of daily inspections and hoof cleaning, routine hoof trimming, and horseshoes for those horses who require them, will prevent many of these problems.

Good stall and paddock sanitation is essential to good foot care. Corrals, paddocks, and stalls that contain a buildup of urine and wet manure predispose the horse to thrush and canker.

It is important to clean a horse's hooves before and after each workout, daily if the horse is stabled, and at least once a week if she is on pasture. Remove all debris from the sole and frog, using the hoof pick as shown in the illustration below. Give special attention to the central cleft and both lateral sulcii of the frog.

Lack of environmental moisture has been implicated as a cause of hoof drying and cracking. Recommendations for improving hoof moisture content have included applying mud packs or commercial hoof dressings, and allowing the water tank to overflow, creating mud for the horse to stand in several times a day.

However, excess moisture, especially frequent wet-to-dry episodes that expand and contract the hoof, may do more harm than good. For example, hoof dressings and mud packs can remove the periople, a waxlike moisture

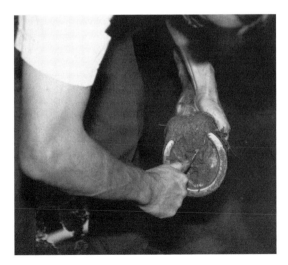

Cleaning the hoof. Start at the frog and work toward the toe. Strokes are made away from the handler.

barrier that protects the hoof wall from absorbing too much water. A hoof that absorbs too much water, or contains a persistently high moisture content, becomes less elastic. The soft, crumbly horn tends to peel and separate, and does not hold horseshoe nails well.

The health of the outer hoof is related to the health of the inner sensitive structures of the foot. Regular exercise stimulates circulation, maintains the health of the corium and elastic tissues, and balances moisture content internally. If the external moisture can be kept at a constant, relatively dry level and frequent wet-to-dry episodes can be avoided, most hoof problems related to drying and cracking will be eliminated.

Many farriers recommend that hoof dressings be used sparingly. Hoof dressings containing turpentine are particularly harmful. When hoof dressings are used for a therapeutic purpose, such as cracking of the bulbs of the heels, an animal grease product such as lanolin or fish oil is preferable. A commercial hoof sealer, which penetrates the outer hoof better than a dressing, may be of benefit as a moisture barrier when a horse must be kept in unusually wet or dry conditions.

An appropriately balanced diet is essential for normal growth and a healthy appearance of the hoof. Overfeeding and underfeeding are the chief causes of poor hoof growth in *foals*. A balanced ration should provide adequate amounts of calcium, biotin (from the vitamin B complex), and the essential amino acid DL-methionine. Supplementing a diet with gelatin, amino acids, and other dietary additives will not produce a better hoof if the foal is eating an appropriate creep or weanling ration. Inadvertently adding selenium to a diet that already meets selenium requirements can have serious and harmful consequences, including hoof wall degeneration or even loss of the foot.

HOOF TRIMMING

In a mature horse, the hoof grows about a third of an inch (8 mm) each month. In the foal, the rate is half an inch (13 mm) each month. Growth is most rapid in the spring and slowest in hot and cold weather.

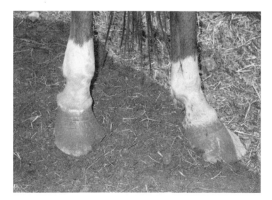

These chipped and elongated hooves are badly in need of trimming.

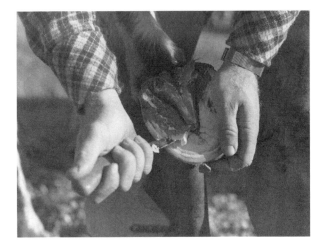

Trimming the hoof. Pare away excess sole and frog with the hoof knife.

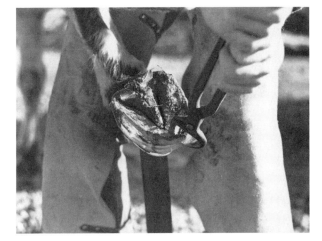

Using hoof nippers, trim the walls until they are even with the frog.

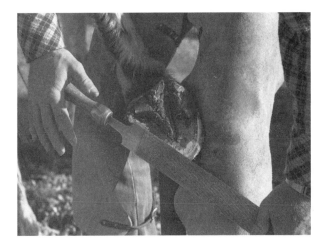

Rasp both sides of the hoof wall at the same time until they are level and smooth.

Few horses are given the amount of exercise needed to keep their hooves worn down naturally. Shod horses, in particular, require frequent trimming because the horseshoe, which is interposed between the ground and the hoof, prevents hoof wear. Accordingly, if the horse is shod, her hooves should be trimmed about every five to eight weeks. If the horse is not shod, the frequency of trimming will depend on hoof wear.

Because a horse's toe grows faster than her heel, the foot becomes unbalanced if the hoof is not trimmed frequently enough. After seven to nine weeks, the excessively long toe alters the horse's gait, which may result in injury and poor performance. The long toe also contributes to the development of sole bruises, corns, and contracted heels.

Although many horse owners employ the services of a farrier, some may decide to trim the feet themselves. The tools required for trimming are a hoof paring knife, hoof nippers, and a rasp.

First clean out the feet thoroughly. Using a hoof knife, pare away excess sole and frog. Use hoof nippers to trim the hoof walls. The object is to trim the walls evenly and to trim just enough of the walls to make the bearing edges level with the surface of the frog. This distributes weight evenly between the frog and the walls. Complete the leveling process by rasping both sides of the hoof wall at the same time, from side to side across the bearing edges.

There is a strong temptation to trim the hoof so that it corresponds to an ideal hoof and pastern axis. If the horse does not have this angle naturally, abnormal stresses will be placed on the supporting ligaments of the pastern and foot. Accordingly, the best job of trimming preserves whatever angle is normal for the individual horse.

Some errors to be avoided:

- Trimming and rasping the bearing surfaces unevenly, so that the foot is not level

- Overtrimming the heels; dropping the heels puts strain on the sesamoids and may cause lameness

- Opening the heels; only loose or torn pieces of frog should be removed, because removing the wide part of the frog, or more of the frog than is normal for the horse, weakens the heels and may lead to contracted heels

Putting on Horseshoes

Horses living outdoors on varied terrain do not require horseshoes. Horseshoes have been described as a necessary evil and a product of domestication, stabling, and circumstances that limit the availability of exercise.

However, there are situations in which horseshoeing is almost a necessity. One is to prevent excessive hoof wear when the horse is being worked or ridden on difficult terrain. Performance horses need shoes for traction. For stabled horses, shoes should be put on to prevent sole injuries from lack of foot toughness. Corrective and therapeutic shoes are indicated for orthopedic problems.

Horseshoes should be reset whenever the foot is trimmed, which is usually every five to eight weeks. The shoes of racehorses are usually reset every two to four weeks.

Most horseshoes are composed of flat plates without raised edges or appendages. However, shoes with calks, studs, ice nails, borium spots, and other traction devices can be fitted when the horse needs added traction on ice, snow, or mud. A solid raised bar on the toe of the shoe is called a grab. Calks and grabs should be of the same height on all shoes to prevent an uneven step or unnatural gait. Reining horses frequently are fitted with sliders, which are solid plates on the rear feet only to help them slide to a stop.

All traction devices have the potential to stop the shoe suddenly while the horse is moving forward. Severe sprains or fractures are possible, especially at high speeds and during performance activities. To prevent such accidents, it is important to build up the traction devices in stages. This requires the close monitoring of an experienced farrier.

Horseshoes can be applied hot or cold. Hot-shoeing is the application of a fire-heated shoe to the trimmed level hoof. The shoe can be made by the farrier from scratch or modified from a premade shoe using a forge. The hot shoe shows the edges of the hoof that may need more rasping. This ensures an optimal fit between the hoof and the shoe.

Cold-shoeing is the application of an unheated shoe to the trimmed level hoof. Most farriers can apply cold shoes that are both level and fit the horse well. Many farriers use a combination of hot- and cold-shoeing techniques.

Most horseshoes have holes for eight nails, but four to six nails will hold the average shoe. The shoe is sized and fitted to the surface of the hoof. It is then nailed into position. Horseshoe nails are made with a built-in curve. When they are driven into the white line, which marks the border between the sensitive and insensitive laminae, they curve away from the sensitive laminae and exit through the hoof wall about a half to three-quarters of an inch (13 to 19 mm) above the bearing edge. The end of each nail is twisted off and, when all nails are in, their tips are bent over or clinched. The clinches are then filed smooth, and wax or another substance is used to fill all nail holes. This prevents urine, water, and mud from entering the hoof and causing *infection*. Finally, any overhang of the hoof wall beyond the shoe should be rasped to bring it into alignment with the edge of the shoe.

Quicking, also called hot nailing or nail prick, occurs if the nail is accidentally driven into the sensitive laminae. When this happens, the horse immediately jumps or flinches. The offending nail should be taken out. As the nail is removed, blood can frequently be seen on the nail and in the nail hole. The nail hole should be flushed with 7 percent tincture of iodine. Administer a tetanus toxoid booster. If the horse's tetanus immunization history is unknown, see the table on page 100.

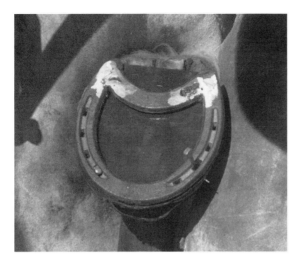

The nail exits about half an inch (13 mm) above the bearing edge. This is a pad and complete bar shoe, used in corrective shoeing.

A close nail is one that puts pressure on the sensitive lamina of the foot without actually piercing it. It may cause the horse immediate discomfort, but frequently goes unnoticed for several days or until the horse is exercised and comes up lame. The nail causing the problem can be located with a hoof tester or by tapping each nail with a hammer. Removing the offending nail usually resolves the problem.

One other cause of immediate lameness is clinching the nails too tightly. If this happens, the nails should be loosened or reset at once.

To remove a horseshoe, open the clinches at the side of the hoof using the chisel end of a clinch cutter. Holding the horse's foot between your knees, use a shoe puller starting at the outside of one heel. Pry the shoe away from the hoof wall while pulling in toward the frog. Switch to the opposite side and repeat the process. Work down the sides toward the toe. Once the shoe is loose, it should come off easily. Avoid prying excessively at any one spot, as this might bruise the sole. Check the hoof wall for nail fragments and remove any.

LOST SHOES

Eighty percent of lost horseshoes involve the front feet. The loss of a horseshoe is a cause of concern not only because of the potential for hoof wall damage associated with the shoe pulling free, but also because the unprotected hoof is at risk for bruising and cracking.

The majority of horses do not lose shoes. It has been estimated that 20 percent of horses lose 80 percent of shoes. If a horse loses a shoe more than once or twice a year, there will be a specific reason. A bad job of shoeing is seldom the cause, as long as the shoes were applied by an experienced individual.

There are a number of possible causes for repeated shoe loss. A wet, muddy environment predisposes the horse to soft hooves that do not hold nails securely. A conformation problem, such as underrun heels, may require setting shoes farther back on the hoof, where they project at the heels and can be stepped off by another horse. A horse who toes out can step off a front shoe with either foot. Horses who overreach can clip off a front shoe with a back foot.

Leaving shoes on too long is the most common cause of lost shoes. As the hoof wall overgrows the shoe, the shoe becomes embedded in the sole. The nail clinches are then too long and are pushed away from the hoof wall, resulting in the shoe working free.

Treatment: When a shoe is lost, the hoof must be protected as soon as possible. Clean the hoof and wrap it with a protective bandage or apply a commercially available protective rubber boot. Duct tape is an effective hoof protector, is easy to apply until the shoe is replaced, and will prevent chipping of the hoof wall. The horse should be kept in a clean, dry enclosure until the shoe is replaced.

All shod horses should have their shoes reset on a regular schedule to prevent hoof wall overgrowth, lost shoes, and conformational foot imbalances.

CORRECTIVE TRIMMING AND SHOEING

The purposes of remedial hoof care are to correct (or compensate for) an abnormal hoof-pastern axis, to relieve stresses associated with painful tendon and bone diseases, and to prepare the horse for conventional horseshoes.

Corrective trimming and shoeing should be part of a specific treatment program involving the cooperative efforts of both farrier and veterinarian, as each has specific skills and expertise to contribute.

Corrective trimming and shoeing forms an integral part of the treatment for most orthopedic diseases. Laminitis, sand cracks, flat feet, corns and sole bruises, navicular disease, and contracted heels are among the most common conditions for which remedial hoof care is used. Other conditions include contracted flexor tendons, tendonitis, ligament injuries, ringbone, sidebones, bone spavin, dropped sole, and cunean tendon bursitis.

Natural Hoof Care

Natural hoof care is the practice of allowing the horse to go barefoot and trimming in a nontraditional manner. Horses are shod partly because that's what has been done for hundreds of years, even though improper shoeing can lead to lameness. There is a growing body of research with wild and feral horses that examines how they remain sound and maintain "good" feet while living on rough, rocky ground. Native Americans, for example, rode their horses without shoes, and, because the horse was their sole mode of transportation and was an integral part of the success of the buffalo hunt, it was imperative that their horses remain sound.

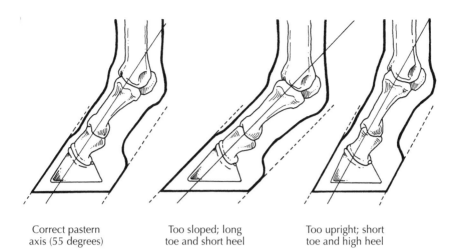

| Correct pastern axis (55 degrees) | Too sloped; long toe and short heel | Too upright; short toe and high heel |

Hoof pastern axis of the front foot.

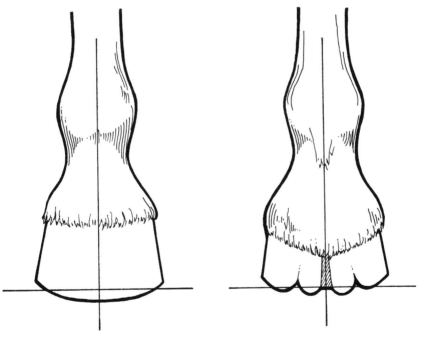

Front view   Rear view

A balanced hoof. The weight of the horse is evenly distributed and the sole makes level contact with the ground.

The biomechanics of the foot dictate that with movement more blood is pumped into the foot, increasing circulation and enhancing growth. In wild and unshod horses, usage wears away the foot and calluses the sole; this layer of callus acts as a protective barrier.

The modern horse lives under conditions quite different from the wild horse, though. We limit movement through stalling and pasturing, and most horses live and compete on very soft footing. Natural hoof care involves trimming the horse's hooves to simulate wild conditions by trimming off the parts of the hoof that would be worn off naturally. The transition to this healthier, tougher hoof takes about three to six months and requires a farrier who is educated in the art of natural hoof care, so that more problems are not created for the horse. Most important, the horse must be used so her feet will become callused. There will be times during this transition period when the horse needs help protecting her feet until they are callused. Protective boots are commercially available and come in many styles.

Horse owners in all riding disciplines are using this natural method with good success, including endurance riders (although reiners are still using sliders on the horse's rear feet). The result is that their horses are developing stronger, healthier hooves.

Foot Wounds and Injuries

Wounds of the feet are common in horses. All such wounds become contaminated and are frequently complicated by infections and abscesses.

Lacerations of the coronet are caused by barbed wire, sheet metal, and rusty nails. The coronet is quite vascular and bleeds profusely. Since the hoof wall grows from the coronet, an injury involving the coronet can leave a horny ridge or defect in the hoof wall.

Puncture wounds of the sole and frog are a common cause of lameness. In all cases of lameness, it is essential to carefully inspect the ground surface of the hoof for a puncture wound. In many cases, the object causing the puncture will be visible as a foreign body in the wound, making the diagnosis relatively easy. However, when the object is not visible, the puncture wound can be extremely difficult to detect, especially when it is located in the frog. A hoof tester, an instrument that your veterinarian may use that looks like giant tongs, is of considerable help in locating the site of tenderness.

Puncture wounds of the sole are among the most serious foot wounds because there is no effective drainage to the outside. An abscess beneath the sole may force drainage at the coronary band, but when this does not happen, serious complications arise. They may include bacterial laminitis, tetanus, septic arthritis of the coffin joint, *septic* tenosynovitis of the flexor tendon sheath, pedal osteitis, septic bursitis of the navicular, fracture of the navicular, destruction of the digital cushion, and blood poisoning (*septicemia*).

TREATING FOOT WOUNDS

All horses with a foot wound should receive a tetanus toxoid booster if the state of immunity is unknown; see the table on page 100.

Lacerations of the skin of the coronet and fetlock should be cleansed, dressed, and bandaged as described in *Wounds* (page 35). Change the dressing daily and confine the horse to a stall. Usually it is not advisable to attempt to close wounds of the coronet band with sutures because there is not enough connective tissue and because of problems with contamination. Wounds of the fetlock can be successfully sutured.

With puncture wounds on the bottom of the foot, the entire sole and frog should be cleaned and washed. It is important to establish drainage at the point the foreign body entered. This is done by cutting down into the puncture wound with a narrow hoof knife and following the tract to its deepest point, or until you reach the sensitive tissues. The external opening should be at least a quarter of an inch (6 mm) wide. Soaking the foot in an Epsom salt solution twice a day is useful therapy. The tract should be irrigated with a dilute Betadine solution (1 to 2 ml added to 1,000 ml sterile saline) or tincture of iodine, and packed with Betadine or iodine-saturated gauze. The foot should then be bandaged as described in *Wounds* (page 39).

Repeat the irrigation daily until healing is well established. The horse should be closely confined in a clean, dry stall. Antibiotics are not necessary for simple wounds, but are often prescribed for heavily contaminated wounds where you don't know when the horse was first wounded. Your veterinarian may wish to x-ray the foot to determine the depth of the wound and which, if any, internal structures of the hoof are involved.

Sole wounds that drain at the coronary band already have a tract to the outside. The ground surface of the foot should be treated as described previously, and the through-and-through tract thus created should be flushed once a day for several days. Deep and complicated wounds require veterinary management.

After the infection has been cleared and the wound is clean, apply shoes over full pads to prevent dirt and manure from getting into the cavity and reinfecting the foot.

PUNCTURE WOUNDS OF THE WHITE LINE (GRAVEL)

Gravel is a specific foot infection caused by a puncture wound or a crack in the white line that allows infection to invade the deep structures of the foot. Because these infections usually cannot drain through the site of injury, *pus* will follow the path of least resistance and travel up the white line to drain at the coronary band.

At one time, it was thought that a piece of gravel entered the sole of the foot at the white line and worked its way upward—hence the name of the condition. However, while this may occasionally happen by coincidence, it is not the cause.

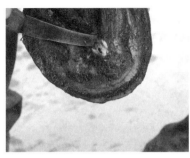

The hoof of a horse demonstrating lameness is cleaned and a puncture wound is identified.

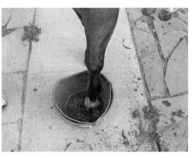

Soaking the puncture wound in an Epsom salt solution.

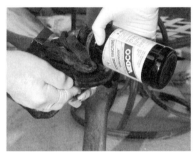

Apply tincture of iodine to the puncture. Be sure to wear gloves to protect your skin when handling this product.

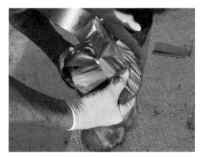

Applying a temporary bandage with duct tape keeps contaminants out and the puncture clean.

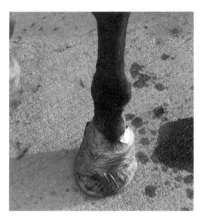

With the foot completely bandaged, this hoof will stay clean and dry, which helps the wound heal.

When you examine the white line in a horse with gravel, you will see black spots. On probing, one of these will be found to penetrate into the sensitive laminae. Pus will often exude from this wound. The sensitive area will be very painful when the foot is examined with a hoof tester.

Treatment: An abscessed pocket under the white line and sole should be drained by cutting down and paring out the tract with a hoof knife. If the tract is already draining at the coronet, this opening should be enlarged as well. In a horse with a long-standing infection, an additional drainage hole may need to be made in the hoof wall midway between the wounds of entrance and exit. Proceed as described in *Treating Foot Wounds* (page 211).

HOOF WALL CRACKS

A crack is a separation or break in the hoof wall. Cracks are identified according to their location as toe, quarter, or heel. Vertical cracks are classified as grass cracks or sand cracks. Grass cracks start at the ground surface and extend upward; sand cracks begin at the coronet and extend down.

Grass cracks often occur in unshod hooves where the bearing surface of the hoof wall is not trimmed and becomes too long, cracking with percussion. A common cause of hoof cracking and peeling is exposure of the hoof to too much moisture (rather than not enough). Especially deleterious are repeated wet-to-dry episodes, which cause expansion and contraction of the hoof wall. A vitamin or essential amino acid deficiency may be a contributing factor in some cases of cracked hooves.

Sand cracks occur as a result of cuts and injuries to the coronet. Gravel can lead to a vertical sand crack.

Horizontal cracks in the hoof wall are called blowouts. They are caused by injuries to the coronary band and hoof wall. A blowout is inconsequential unless it weakens the hoof wall and sets the stage for a vertical crack.

A horse with a hoof wall crack may or may not be lame. This depends on the location and depth of the crack. If the crack bleeds after exercise, it is deep and extends into the sensitive laminae. Deep cracks are susceptible to infection. If infection does set in, you will see a discharge of blood and pus and feel increased heat in the hoof wall.

Hoof cracks do not unite from side to side, as skin wounds do. Instead, the crack is replaced by new horn that starts at the coronary band and grows down (like a fingernail growing out from its base).

Treatment: This depends on the location and depth of the crack. The immediate goal is to prevent the crack from becoming longer and deeper. For grass cracks, this can often be done with a skillful hoof trimming. Sand cracks usually respond to a combination of professional trimming and application of corrective horseshoes. The shoes must be worn for as long as it takes the crack to grow out. For cracks at the coronet, this can be 9 to 12 months.

Large, deep cracks must be stabilized to prevent the hoof from splitting. Before a crack can be stabilized, however, it must be thoroughly cleaned to remove dirt, debris, and loose horn, which serve as reservoirs for bacterial infection. If the crack is moist or bleeding, it should be treated as described in *Treating Foot Wounds* (page 211), and should not be closed until dry.

One technique for closing a vertical crack is to drill holes in the hoof wall on either side of the split and then lace the two sides together with stainless steel wire or heavy nylon. Alternately, the crack can be patched by fastening a metal plate across it. A variety of prosthetic materials can be used to fill cracks completely or patch across them. These materials resemble the consistency of the hoof wall so closely that once applied, they can be nailed into, trimmed, and even rasped along the hoof wall as it grows down.

Another therapy that aids in supporting the hoof wall is the hoof plate. A steel shield is applied to the hoof wall using a horseshoe nail and/or screws. This stabilizes the hoof wall and allows the cracks to heal from the coronet down.

As a sequel to treatment, protect the hoof from repeated episodes of wetness and dryness, which can make the hoof brittle and less pliable. A hoof sealer, an acrylic material, is beneficial in stabilizing hoof moisture content if the horse cannot be quartered under ideal conditions.

The feed should provide adequate amounts of the amino acid DL-methionine, calcium, and biotin (a component of the vitamin B complex). To meet these needs, a nutritional supplement may be indicated.

The *prognosis* is good for both superficial and deep cracks, although reoccurrence is common; investigate the cause to improve success.

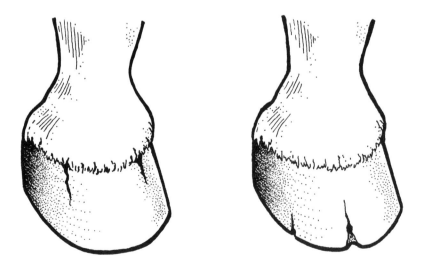

Sand Crack   Grass Crack

Hoof wall cracks can begin at the coronet or the bearing edges.

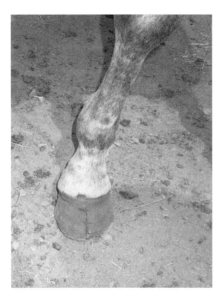

This vertical crack was laced together with wire.

CORNS AND BRUISED SOLES

Rocks and other hard objects can bruise the sole and produce lameness. The injury actually involves the underlying sensitive laminae, not the horny sole or the frog. Horses with thin soles are most often affected, as are horses with flat feet. Both of these conditions are inherited traits. Another cause of thin soles is removing too much sole or frog when trimming the foot.

Corns are bruises of the sole that occur at the buttress, the angle formed by the wall and the bar. They occur most frequently on the inside buttresses of the front feet. Improper foot care is the most common cause of corns. When shoes are left on too long, the growing hoof wall can force the heel of the horseshoe to apply pressure to the sole. Putting on shoes that are too small, bending the shoe in at the heel, and trimming the heels too low all result in excessive sole pressure over the buttress.

A dry corn is characterized by red staining in the horn. This is the result of bruising (bleeding) in the sensitive tissue beneath the horn. In a moist corn, *serum* is present beneath the involved horn. This indicates a more severe injury. In a suppurating corn, the corn has become infected, resulting in a draining abscess beneath the horn, which causes death of the adjacent sensitive lamina and digital cushion. Bruised soles are identical to corns, except that they occur at the toe or quarter instead of the heel.

Lameness is the most common sign of corns and bruises. A horse with a corn tends to favor that heel. Cleaning the flaky material from the sole with a hoof knife may reveal characteristic findings. A hoof tester helps locate the injury.

If a sole abscess becomes chronic, it can lead to a complication called pedal osteitis. This is a thinning and demineralization of the coffin bone. The result is a chronic and persistent lameness that is most difficult to reverse.

Treatment: For dry corns caused by improper shoeing, remove the offending shoe, trim the hoof wall, and rest the horse. Do not reapply shoes until the horse is free of symptoms.

Sole bruises are best treated by resting the horse. When limited use is required, the sole can be covered with a suitable hoof packing and a full pad applied beneath the shoe. Using an *NSAID* can provide some relief.

Inflamed corns and bruises that ooze pus are treated by removing all diseased horn over the bruise, down to the sensitive lamina. Soak the hoof daily in a solution of magnesium sulfate (Epsom salt) and bandage the foot (as described in *Wounds*, page 39) to prevent contamination. A tetanus vaccination may be indicated. Rest the horse until she is healed. If the horse must be used, the wall and bar in the area of the corn can be removed and a special shoe applied to protect the injured area.

The feet of a horse with thin soles can be toughened by taking the shoes off and turning the horse out to pasture on rough ground for six months. Alternately, the soles can be toughened using a topical solution containing equal parts of phenol, formalin, and iodine. This requires veterinary supervision. Corrective shoeing helps some horses with flat feet, but there is no cure for the problem.

SHEARED HEELS AND QUARTERS

The heel of the horse's foot has two bulbs, one on each side. In a balanced foot, both bulbs contact the ground simultaneously. In a horse with sheared heels, one bulb (and often its associated quarter) strikes the ground first, causing the horse to bear weight on the inside or outside of her heel. This causes an upward displacement of that heel bulb in relation to the other. An important finding on examination is that the heel bulbs can be manipulated back and forth independently and/or displaced in opposite directions.

After a period of selective weight-bearing on one side of the foot, the heel and quarter on that side become painful. The resulting lameness is like that seen with navicular disease, which may actually be brought on by sheared heels. Sheared heels also predispose the horse to hoof wall injuries and thrush.

The most common cause of sheared heels is improper hoof trimming in which one heel bulb and/or quarter is trimmed shorter than the other. In some cases, this is intentional, the belief being that changing the balance of the hoof will increase her speed at the racetrack or compensate for some fault in the horse's conformation—although this has not been proven.

Treatment: It involves bringing the foot back into balance through corrective trimming. In chronic cases, an egg bar or full bar shoe may be required.

Foot and Hoof Diseases
WHITE LINE DISEASE (SEEDY TOE)

In a horse with this disease, the white line disintegrates as the result of infection caused by bacteria, yeast, or fungus. The infection starts at ground level and works its way up the white line to the coronary band. The toe, back to the quarter, is most commonly affected. The loss of horn creates a hollow space between the hoof wall and the sole that becomes mealy or "seedy." Eventually, a deep recess, filled with cheesy material and debris, develops between the sole and the hoof wall. The loss of supporting horn, coupled with the pull of the deep digital flexor tendon, can cause rotation of the coffin bone like that seen with chronic laminitis.

White line disease seldom occurs in barefoot horses on pasture. Like many other hoof conditions, it is a disease of domestic horse management. The typical horse with white line disease is shod, given limited daily exercise, bedded in damp wood shavings, kept in a wet stall, exposed to frequent wet-to-dry episodes such as daily wash-downs, walks in wet grass or muddy paddocks, and is not trimmed regularly.

Treatment: All diseased horn and unsound tissue must be pared out and removed, down to solid, healthy horn. In some cases, the cavity should be packed with Betadine dressings and treated as a hoof infection until healthy horn is seen. The deep recesses are then filled with prosthetic hoof repair material, such as those made by Equilox. Egg bar or full support shoes are fitted. With advanced disease, special shoeing techniques are required. All predisposing conditions should be corrected.

KERATOMA

Keratoma is a rare tumor or growth arising in the horn-producing cells of the hoof wall, usually in the toe region and less commonly in the sole. There is usually a history of prior injury or hoof disease, but some cases of keratoma will arise spontaneously. Lameness results from pressure on the coffin bone or sensitive laminae.

Keratomas are typically circular and approximately 0.5 to 2.0 cm across. They may or may not produce an abnormal contour or bulge in the hoof wall. Keratomas of the sole are most commonly found during hoof trimming and paring of the sole. A deviation of the white line toward the center of the sole is suggestive of keratoma.

Treatment: If the horse is not lame, no therapy is needed. For keratomas that cause symptoms, surgical removal is the only effective treatment. Some keratomas recur after surgery and require removal again. The outlook is good when the keratoma can be removed completely without damaging surrounding structures.

DISEASES OF THE FROG

Thrush

Thrush is a painful bacterial infection involving the central cleft and the collateral sulcii of the frog. It is characterized by a putrid black discharge along with poor growth and degeneration of the horn. When the frog is cleaned with a hoof pick, a soft, puttylike material will fall away, revealing sulcii deeper than normal. The infection may extend into the sensitive laminae and infect the digital cushion. A number of bacterial species may be involved, but the *anaerobic* organism *Fusobacterium necrophorum* appears to be the most common.

Thrush is caused by the lack of proper foot care, resulting in a buildup of mud and manure that prevents air from getting to the frog. During routine hoof trimming, the clefts of the frog should be pared back to make them self-cleaning. When this is not done, flaps of frog tissue can seal in debris and make it impossible to clean out the frog with a hoof pick.

Treatment: Remove the horse from mud and manure and stable her in a clean, dry stall. Remove the shoe and thoroughly clean out the frog. Expose the clefts by removing degenerating frog with a hoof knife. Apply a drying agent such as 10 percent formalin, Kopertox, methylene blue, 10 percent bleach solution, or 7 percent tincture of iodine to the cleft and sulcii, and then follow with a topical antibiotic solution such as 10 percent sodium sulfapyridine. Bandage the foot to prevent contamination.

Repeat the treatment daily for several days, then once or twice a week until the foot is healed. Your veterinarian may suggest a bar shoe to promote frog regeneration. The prognosis is good when the sensitive structures are not involved.

Canker

Canker is a chronic infection of the horn tissues of the foot. It begins at the frog and progresses slowly to involve the sole and sometimes the wall. The disease is rare and is found almost exclusively in tropical climates.

Canker develops in horses who stand in mud or in bedding soaked with urine and feces, and who do not receive regular foot care.

The cankerous horn tissue of the frog loosens readily, and when removed discloses a foul-smelling, bleeding corium covered with a curdled white discharge. The appearance is quite similar to thrush, but can be distinguished by the characteristics of the discharge, the severity of infection, and the involvement of the sole as well as the frog.

Treatment: Move the horse to a clean, dry stable or preferably a dry, rocky pasture. Treat the foot as described for *Thrush* (above). Penicillin, both intramuscularly and topically, is an effective antibiotic. Because canker regularly involves the corium, treatment is often prolonged.

Contracted Heels

This is a disorder in which the foot is abnormally narrow or is actually contracted, especially at the heels. One or both front feet may be affected. In severe cases the bars may actually touch while the hoof wall, from the coronet down, may slope inward toward the bearing surface instead of outward.

One cause of heel contracture is too little pressure on the frog. This can happen when a horse with a painful foot stands for long periods with her heel off the ground to relieve pressure on the sole. Another cause of heel contracture is an excessively long, unbalanced foot resulting from improper trimming. It is a common practice for racing Thoroughbreds to be trimmed and shod for a long toe and underrun heel, which theoretically increases the speed of the horse. This is a foot conformation likely to predispose the horse to contracted heels.

Treatment: Therapy is directed at restoring a balanced foot by corrective trimming and shoeing. If the contracted heel is the result of a painful foot, the cause must be identified and treated.

LATERAL CARTILAGE DISEASES
Quittor

Quittor is a chronic, deep-seated infection of the lateral cartilages of the coffin bone. Destruction of the inflamed part of the cartilage results in the discharge of infected material via a sinus tract that opens at or above the coronet.

Injuries near the lateral cartilages, such as being struck by another foot, often precede the appearance of quittor, as do penetrating injuries of the sole.

During an acute attack, the horse will be lame. You can see swelling and feel heat over the lateral cartilage near the involved quarter. In the chronic stage,

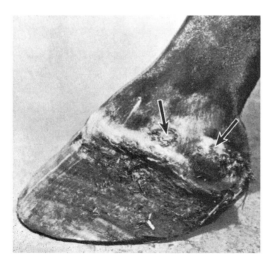

Quittor is an infection of the lateral cartilage of the coffin bone. Note the draining sinus tracts.

one or more sinus tracts are apparent. Periodically, these tracts open and drain pus. In long-standing cases, some degree of sidebones will be present.

Treatment: The most effective treatment is to remove the destroyed cartilage. Many horses recover completely. In long-standing cases, there may be enough damage to surrounding structures to cause permanent lameness.

Sidebones

This is ossification of the lateral cartilages of the coffin bone (in other words, calcium builds up in the cartilage until it is converted to bone). It can occur in all four feet but is most common in the front feet. Excessive concussion (often combined with incorrect shoeing) is believed to be the primary factor in converting the cartilage to bone. Faulty conformation is a definite predisposing factor.

Sidebones usually do not produce lameness, except perhaps in the acute ossifying stage, when pain, heat, and swelling are found over the quarters. If a horse with sidebones is lame, it is quite likely that some other condition, such as navicular disease, is responsible for the lameness.

Treatment: This is needed only for relief of lameness. NSAIDs and rest for several weeks is beneficial. The quarters can be grooved or thinned to permit the hoof to expand, which helps to eliminate pain. Full roller motion shoes diminish action in the region of the coffin joint. If lameness persists, a palmar digital neurectomy can be performed, as described in *Navicular Disease* (page 222).

Navicular Disease

Navicular disease is perhaps the most common cause of intermittent front leg lameness in horses. Quarter Horses, jumpers, cutters, racers, calf ropers, and barrel racers are especially prone to the problem. These horses are subject to unusual foot stresses with hard stops, twists at speed, abrupt changes in direction, and forceful landings on overextended fetlocks. Usually both front feet are affected, but a predominant lameness on one side may lead to the impression that the lameness is *unilateral*.

The navicular bone is located at the heel of the foot beneath the central one-third of the frog. It is suspended by three ligaments, articulates with the coffin joint, and serves as a support to the coffin and short pastern bones. Behind the navicular is the deep digital flexor tendon, which curves around and attaches to the back of the coffin. Between the navicular and the tendon is a bursa (A fluid-filled sac) that enables the deep flexor tendon to glide over the bone. All these structures make up the navicular complex.

The exact mechanism of injury and pain in navicular disease is not known, but a number of factors are predisposing. They include poor foot conformation (upright pasterns), infrequent or inadequate hoof trimming that results in a long toe and a low heel, sheared heels, contracted heels, and improper shoeing. All these abnormalities adversely affect the smooth and efficient transfer of weight through the navicular bone to the ground (see *The Hoof as a Shock Absorber*, page 201).

Among horses with navicular disease, it is believed that tissue stresses are multiplied beyond the capacity of the bone and surrounding supportive structures to adapt. Degenerate changes appear in the bone. They consist of cartilage *erosion*, bone erosion, and adhesions between the bone and the deep digital flexor tendon. These changes may be accompanied by periostitis (inflammation of the outside of the bone, also called shin splints), bursitis (inflammation of the bursae), and tendonitis (inflammation of the tendon) in the surrounding structures that make up the navicular complex.

Initially, the lameness is mild. The horse goes lame for short periods and then appears to be sound. Later, the lameness becomes more frequent. Pain in navicular disease is located in the heel. As a consequence, the horse puts her toe down first, sometimes actually stabbing it into the ground, which may cause the horse to stumble on the toe. A stiff, shuffling gait with a shortened, choppy stride is characteristic.

A standard diagnostic test is to apply a hoof tester over the center of the frog. Pain is elicited here because the bone is located beneath the frog. In contrast, a horse with laminitis reacts painfully to hoof testing over the toes. Blocking both palmar-digital nerves in the foot helps determine whether the heel is the site of pain. After an effective block, the horse with navicular disease no longer feels pain and moves out freely, unless the condition is *bilateral*, in which case the lameness shifts to the other leg. Blocking the second leg then eliminates the lameness.

X-rays may reveal changes in the bone or surrounding tissue but are not always diagnostic. A diagnosis of navicular disease usually must take into consideration all factors, including the history, the horse's characteristic gait, and the results of hoof testing, nerve blocks, and x-rays.

Treatment: Any abnormalities in hoof balance and conformation that can be to corrected should be. This will require the services of a farrier who is skilled in therapeutic hoof trimming and shoeing. Results may not be apparent for several months Corrective shoeing helps many horses with navicular disease.

Medical treatment involves the periodic use of phenylbutazone (Butazolidin) and other anti-inflammatory drugs to relieve pain. Analgesics should not be given continuously because of potential side effects, including stomach ulcers.

Isoxsuprine hydrochloride appears to offer significant relief for horses with navicular disease. Its mechanism of action is unknown, but horses receiving the drug have shown substantial improvement that can last up to a year after the drug is discontinued. Some veterinarians recommend year-round use of the drug at lower doses. Isoxsuprine hydrochloride is given by mouth. It has few known side effects and can be used along with Butazolidin.

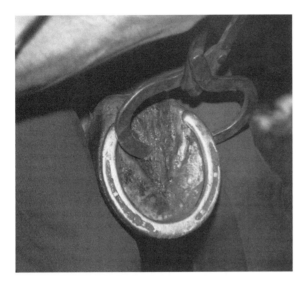

A hoof tester over the central third of the frog elicits pain in a horse with navicular disease.

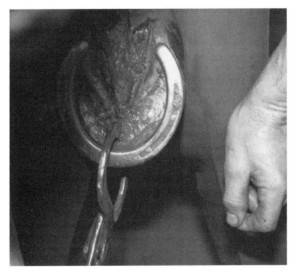

A horse with laminitis reacts painfully to hoof testing over the toe.

Some horses do not respond to conservative treatment and/or have more advanced disease. For these horses, surgery is indicated. The most common operation, palmar digital neurectomy, involves removing both digital nerves and all accessory branches that supply the back half of the foot. When successful, the horse will be free of symptoms and can be used safely for all activities, including racing and jumping. Digital neurectomy is not legal in all states on racehorses. In some states, the racing commission regulates the sites of incision.

Approximately 20 percent of horses do not respond completely after digital neurectomy. This may be because of tendon disease, adhesions, periostitis, traumatic arthritis of the fetlock joint, or complications resulting from the effects of the surgery.

A second operation is navicular suspensory desmotomy. In this procedure, the suspensory ligament of the navicular is divided close to its attachment on the long pastern bone. The operation is difficult and is not often performed.

Laminitis (Founder)

Laminitis is a metabolic and vascular disease that involves the inner sensitive structures of the feet. There are many causes of laminitis. One way the disease can begin is when bacterial *endotoxins* are released into the bloodstream and directly affect blood flow into the hoof, causing inflammation of the sensitive laminae. This may occur secondary to illness or gastrointestinal tract disease.

Endotoxins dilate the large arteries leading to the feet, increasing blood flow while at the same time causing intense constriction of the small capillary vessels that nourish the laminae. The result is a large volume of blood going down to the feet but being shunted around the laminae. Thus deprived of blood and oxygen, the laminae swell. Because the hoof is rigid, the swelling compresses the laminae and causes further tissue compromise. If the situation is not relieved, the sensitive inner structures of the feet will die.

Endotoxins may be the result of carbohydrate overload from grain or fresh green pasture. Endotoxins may also result from colic or infections in the intestines. Bacterial *sepsis* has been known to produce endotoxins.

Another cause of laminitis is mechanical overload. This occurs when one hoof or leg is injured and the horse must bear the bulk of her weight on the opposite limb. This may cause decreased blood flow to the weight-bearing limb, which causes a form of laminitis. This happened to the racehorse Barbaro following his leg injury.

Obesity in horses creates conditions that can lead to laminitis. Research is ongoing to explain the exact mechanism that is involved in this process. Obese horses with insulin resistance are associated with equine metabolic syndrome (see page 228). Current research suggests insulin resistance may cause laminitis by a combination of any or all of the following: The fat tissues may be overloaded and the stress releases inflammatory chemicals; there is a lack of insulin entering hoof cells, depriving them of nutrition; there is a decreased blood flow to the hoof, which also starves hoof cells of adequate nutrition for normal function. Equine metabolic syndrome is identified by obesity, insulin resistance, and the resulting laminitis.

ACUTE LAMINITIS

Acute laminitis may begin suddenly with high fever and chills, sweating, diarrhea, fast pulse, and rapid, heavy breathing. The digital artery at the fetlock has a pounding pulse. The feet are hot and painful. The horse alternately lifts one foot after another and gives evidence of severe pain when the sole of the foot is tapped.

There is a characteristic stance in a horse with acute laminitis in which the two front feet are placed out front to take weight off the toes. When all four feet are involved, the horse draws her feet up underneath her belly or lies down. Death in acute laminitis is uncommon but can occur. A horse with severe laminitis may slough the hard hoof wall.

Acute laminitis can result from any *systemic* disturbance, including gastrointestinal diseases, especially diarrhea, and equine Cushing's disease.

Once signs of laminitis occur, it can be difficult or impossible to prevent permanent foot damage. Accordingly, if you know or even suspect that your horse has consumed an unknown quantity of a carbohydrate such as grain, *consult your veterinarian without delay*. Treatment must be initiated *before* the signs of laminitis or colic develop.

Postpartum laminitis is a complication of a severe, often fatal bacterial infection of the *mare's* uterus that develops during or shortly after *foaling*. Retained placental tissue contributes to the infection and subsequent *endotoxemia*. Respiratory and other systemic infections are rare causes of acute laminitis.

High doses of corticosteroids, used in treating a variety of severe illnesses in horses, have been shown to increase the sensitivity of the laminar capillaries to circulating toxins and other vasoconstrictive substances—thus increasing the risk and occurrence of acute laminitis. Approximately 5 percent of horses treated with corticosteroids are affected.

Treatment: *Acute laminitis is a medical emergency.* Notify your veterinarian immediately. Do not wait for clinical signs to develop. Signs of acute laminitis, as described by the American Association of Equine Practitioners, are:

- Lameness, especially when a horse is turning in circles; shifting lameness when standing
- Heat in the feet
- Increased digital pulse in the feet
- Pain in the toe region when pressure is applied with a hoof tester
- Reluctant or hesitant gait, as if the horse is walking on eggshells
- A "sawhorse stance" with the front feet stretched out in front to alleviate pressure on the toes and the hind feet "camped out" or positioned farther back than normal to bear more weight

Remove all feed from the horse's stall; if the horse is on pasture, move her to a paddock or stall.

The object of emergency treatment is to reduce the severity of the attack and prevent rotation of the coffin bone (see *Chronic Laminitis*, page 226). If this can be prevented or minimized, the horse usually will not suffer permanent disability.

In a horse with grain laminitis, treatment is directed at eliminating the grain from the horse's intestinal tract before it reaches the colon and undergoes

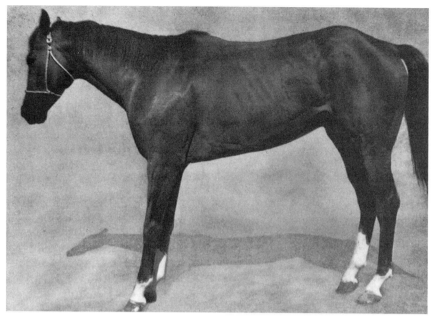

The typical stance of a horse with acute laminitis.

fermentation. Pass a stomach tube and coat the intestinal tract with a large volume of mineral oil (3 to 4 quarts, 2.8 to 3.7 l, per 1,000 pounds, 453 kg, of body weight). Mineral oil is a laxative and also prevents the absorption of endotoxins. Repeat this dose every six hours until all grain has passed through the horse's intestine.

Once symptoms of acute laminitis develop, your veterinarian may recommend gently removing the horse's shoes and applying cold packs to the feet. Keeping the hooves in cold water (colder than 40°F, 4.4°C) for 24 hours is quite beneficial. Stall rest is essential, as is providing a soft footing (6 inches, 15 cm, of sand is ideal) that is comfortable to stand on and reduces tension on the deep digital flexor tendon. One way of reducing the pull of the tendon, and thus minimizing coffin bone rotation, is to apply 18- to 20-degree wedge pads beneath the heels. A similar effect can be obtained by wrapping a roll of elastic gauze beneath the frog. Exercise contributes to coffin bone rotation and should be avoided.

Veterinary management of acute laminitis includes the administration of flunixin meglumine for its anti-endotoxic properties. Butazolidin is given for its anti-inflammatory properties. When given in combination with acepromazine (a tranquilizer), it has been shown to reduce capillary constriction and hypertension. For best results, both drugs should be given together intravenously. After 24 hours, phenylbutazone (Butazolidin) can be given orally. During the next two weeks, x-rays are taken at regular intervals to monitor the position of the coffin bone.

Dietary management involves eliminating grain from the diet and replacing it with good-quality grass hay. Begin by offering a few pounds of hay two or three times a day while watching for signs of relapse. Later, grain can be introduced at about half a pound (227 g) per day. Water should be available at all times. Overweight horses should be put on a reducing diet, as described in *Obesity* (page 420).

A horse who has foundered once is likely to do so again. Such horses should be watched carefully and not given unrestricted access to lush green pastures. They should never be fed large amounts of grain or fresh hay.

CHRONIC LAMINITIS

Laminitis becomes chronic when pain and lameness persist for more than two days or when there is permanent damage to the foot.

A serious complication of laminitis is rotation of the coffin bone. This can happen as early as 48 hours after the acute episode, but may not occur until much later. Rotation occurs when the coffin bone becomes detached from the hoof wall and, aided by the pull of the digital flexor tendon, rotates away and drops down. All degrees of rotation from mild to severe are possible. With a severe rotation, the tip of the coffin bone may penetrate the sole of the foot. This is a serious complication and is most difficult to treat.

Other complications of chronic laminitis include white line disease, thrush, separation of the hoof at the coronary band or sole, and complete loss

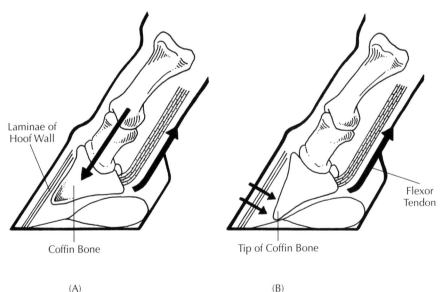

Laminae of
Hoof Wall

Flexor
Tendon

Coffin Bone

Tip of Coffin Bone

(A)   (B)

Rotation of the coffin bone. (A) Normal position within hoof. (B) Detached from the hoof wall and rotated, with the tip pointing down.

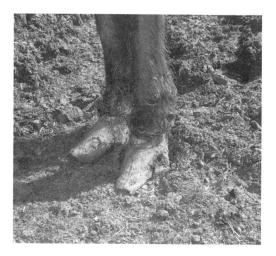

Slipper foot is caused by permanent damage to the sole corium.

of the hoof. Over time, damage to the sole corium often produces a long toe that curls up at the end (known as slipper foot).

After an attack of acute laminitis, damage to the inner sensitive laminae causes characteristic changes in the hoof wall. You may see a series of heavy founder rings on the hoof wall. These rings are caused by injury to the coronary band corium. The rings are present for life.

Signs of chronic laminitis, as described by the American Association of Equine Practitioners, may include:

- Rings in the hoof wall that become wider from toe to heel
- Bruised soles or stone bruises
- Widened white line, commonly called seedy toe, with occurrence of blood pockets and/or abscesses
- Dropped soles or flat feet
- Thick, crested neck
- Dished hooves, which are the result of unequal rates of hoof growth

Treatment: Foot care is important in the management of chronic laminitis. The goal is to prevent further rotation of the coffin bone and to realign the bone with the hoof wall and the sole. This involves corrective hoof trimming and shoeing, and the cooperative efforts of farrier, veterinarian, and horse owner.

Best results occur when symptoms resolve within the first 110 days. Any degree of rotation of the coffin bone is undesirable, but when rotation is greater than 12 degrees, it is most likely that the horse will remain lame regardless of treatment. Cracks and separations of the sole and hoof wall predispose the horse to infection of the inner sensitive laminae. These present major treatment challenges.

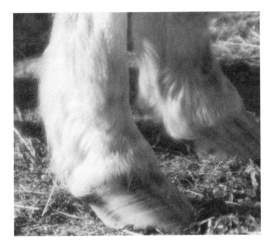

Founder rings can be seen on the hoof wall.

Equine Metabolic Syndrome

Equine metabolic syndrome (EMS) is an endrocrine disorder characterized by abnormal fat deposits (most often found on the crest of neck, tail head, and the sheath of geldings), a history of laminitis, and insulin resistance. Although it is sometimes mistaken for Cushing's disease because they share some characteristics, EMS is its own unique disorder.

Affected horses tend to be middle-age rather than geriatric, between 8 and 18 years old. Nearly all breeds have been affected, although Morgans, Peruvian Pasos, Paso Finos, domesticated Spanish Mustangs, and warmbloods seem to be predisposed. Ponies as a group tend to be overweight and often suffer from laminitis. Affected broodmares show unusual estrous cycling, which makes it difficult to impregnate these mares.

Many horses today are fed diets with high-calorie concentrates and are not worked at a level high enough to work off their excessive feeds. Obesity appears to be related to the onset of metabolic syndrome. There are many theories as to how this leads to insulin resistance, but the end result is a horse with high insulin levels that appear to be ineffective at lowering the blood glucose levels.

The most obvious sign of equine metabolic syndrome is laminitis, but in the EMS horse, the laminitis tends to be mild and therefore is frequently overlooked. Excessive insulin and vascular spasms in the laminae (the interconnected layers of tissue that ensure the integrity of the hoof) are believed to cause the chronic laminitis. The signs of chronic laminitis include abnormal hoof growth, dropped soles, unusual growth lines, and separation of the hoof at the white line.

The diagnosis of equine metabolic syndrome is based on physical characteristics, the results of glucose-tolerance testing, and eliminating similar conditions such as Cushing's disease and hypothyroidism.

A horse (or pony) must have abnormal fat distribution, which will include the crest of the neck, over the shoulders, the tail head and the rump, and the sheath of geldings. A glucose tolerance test involves administration of glucose and measuring the insulin and glucose levels in response. A horse with EMS will have high glucose and insulin levels. Cushing's disease can be ruled out with a dexamethasone suppression test (it will be normal in horses with EMS). The pituitary glands on the EMS horse will be normal, and hirsuitism does not occur in affected horses. Thyroid tests will be in normal ranges, ruling out hypothyroidism.

Treatment: The most effective treatments involve diet and exercise. To limit the amount of calories in relation to the amount of work, affected horses should be fed no more than good quality grass hay (1 to 1.5 percent of body weight) with a complete vitamin and mineral supplement. This ration is low in starch. Sources of soluble carbohydrates include grain, sweet feed, carrots, apples, and fresh pasture, and these should be avoided. There are some commercial feeds that are low in carbohydrates and starch, such as LiteBalance by Nutrena.

An exercise regimen cannot be implemented until the laminitis is under control. Once the horse is exercising and the obesity is resolving, grass hay may be supplemented with soaked beet pulp and/or fat (vegetable oil or rice bran) rather than grain. Exercise seems to be the most effective method of decreasing insulin resistance.

There is no medication suitable for treating EMS; the medications used to manage Cushing's disease are not effective.

THE
MUSCULOSKELETAL
SYSTEM

The horse's skeleton is made up of an average of 216 individual bones, connected by ligaments and surrounded by muscles. This is about 12 more bones than humans have, but most of this difference is made up of the bones in the tail.

Over the surface of each bone is a layer of dense connective tissue called the periosteum. Injuries to the periosteum result in the formation of new bone, which often leads to degenerative *arthritis*.

The union of two bones is called an articulation, or joint. Joint position is maintained by ligaments (which connect bone to bone), tendons (which connect muscle to bone), and a tough fibrous capsule, all of which combine to provide stability and strength to the joint. A layer of connective tissue cells called the synovial membrane lines the inside surface of the joint. This membrane secretes a fluid that allows for smooth movement and friction-free gliding.

Interposed between tendons and bony projections elsewhere in the body are fluid-filled sacs called bursae. These sacs enable the parts to move freely without wear and tear.

Because the horse is such an athletic animal, injuries to all these structures are common.

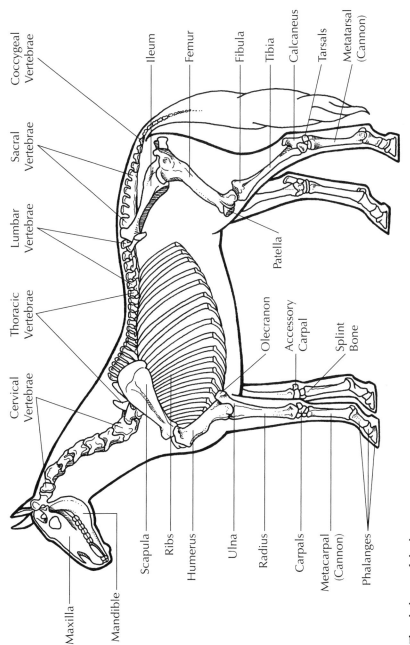

The skeleton of the horse.

Conformation and Soundness

Horse breeders, veterinarians, and horse show judges have specific terms they use to describe a horse's overall structure and composition. *Conformation* is how the various angles, shapes, and parts of the horse's body conform to the breed standard. Standards for registered horses describe the ideal conformation for each breed. These standards are based, to a certain extent, on aesthetic considerations, but they also take into account the breed's original purpose as a working animal.

Most breed standards provide some information about the desired angle or slope to the bones of the shoulder, pelvis, and limbs. These angles are determined by comparison with imaginary lines drawn horizontally and vertically through the plane of the standing horse.

Another term used to judge the physical attributes of a horse is *soundness*. When applied to the musculoskeletal system, it means that in a sound horse, all the bones and joints are in correct alignment to function as intended. In particular, good skeletal conformation is one in which the alignment of the legs is such that there is equal distribution of weight, equal bone pressure, and equal strain on the supporting ligaments when the horse is standing naturally. A horse is considered unsound when, by virtue of an old injury or a conformation defect, he is unable to perform at the level for which he was intended.

Good conformation is of great importance. Horses who do not possess it are much more susceptible to injuries and bone and joint diseases.

A blemish is a defect that usually involves the skin, connective tissue, or bone, which more or less diminishes the value of the horse by its unsightly appearance but does not interfere with or diminish his ability to function.

Judgment must be used in deciding whether a defect is a blemish or an indication of unsoundness. For example, thoroughpin and wind puffs could be the result of an old sprain. In that case, you must consider whether the sprain or injury was produced by poor conformation. If so, the horse would be considered unsound. On the other hand, the horse might have good conformation, in which case the defect is considered a blemish.

Lameness

The forelegs carry 60 percent of the weight of the horse and are subject to a higher incidence of lameness. As a general rule, 95 percent of front leg lameness occurs from the knee down, with the foot being the most frequent site of the problem. This is different in the hindquarters. Only 20 percent of lameness occurs in the foot, with 80 percent occurring in the hock and stifle joints. For information on lameness cased by foot problems, see chapter 8, "The Feet."

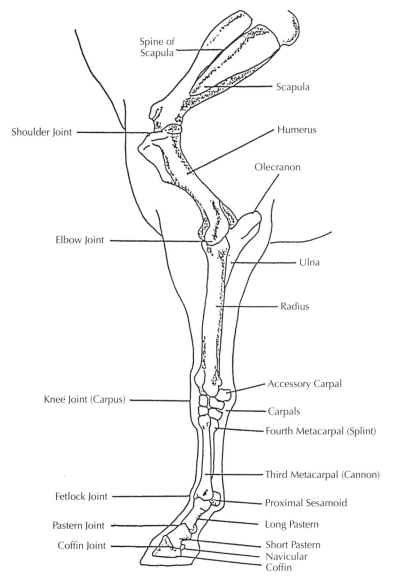

The bones and joints of the front leg.

Note that gait disturbances can be caused by neurological diseases (pain along the nerves) as well as musculoskeletal diseases. If you see bizarre behavior such as *head-pressing*, staggering, swaying, lack of coordination, head-bobbing, or paralysis, see *The Neurological Examination* (page 342).

The terms "supporting-leg lameness" and "swinging-leg lameness" are used to describe the type of lameness observed. Supporting-leg lameness is the kind that is made worse when the horse shifts his weight or support onto the sore

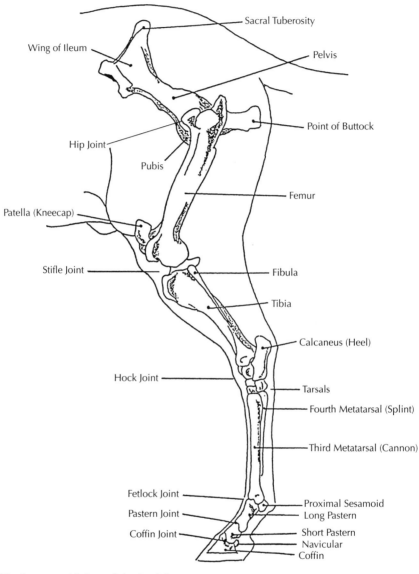

The bones and joints of the back leg.

limb. The horse will attempt to rest the painful leg by taking weight off it, and will often stand with the sore leg pointed well forward of the sound leg. Laminitis and foot wounds are examples of supporting-leg lameness, as are ringbone and navicular disease. All are discussed in chapter 8.

Swinging-leg lameness refers to the fact that the pain is caused by the swing or movement of the limb. A horse with swinging-leg lameness tries to protect the painful leg by shortening the reach of the leg. This makes for a stilted stride. Muscle strain and joint injuries are examples of swinging-leg lameness.

DETERMINING THE CAUSE

Without a systematic approach to the problem of lameness, it can be very difficult to make a diagnosis. You must consider the history and circumstances surrounding the onset of the lameness. Which limb is involved and exactly where is the problem located? Once the site of pain has been identified, you can begin to make a differential diagnosis. If the diagnosis is not apparent after inspection and examination, x-rays and special tests may clarify the problem. Finally, remember this rule: When the site of lameness is difficult to determine, think of the foot in front and the hock behind.

History

Sudden onset lameness suggests laminitis or an acute injury. What happened to the horse just before you noticed the lameness? Were his shoes changed or his hooves trimmed? Was he ridden over uneven ground or for a long distance? Could he have been kicked by another horse or have stepped in a hole? Does he have conformation faults that predispose him to injuries?

The condition of the horse is an important factor. When a horse is out of condition, even moderate work or training may sprain a muscle or pull a tendon.

Inspection

Observe the horse while he is standing still, moving, and then being ridden. Normally, a horse stands with his weight evenly distributed on all four legs and the feet more or less next to one another. If you see a horse standing with one leg flexed, you can be sure there is a reason why he is favoring that leg. A horse with a bruised sole or a painful foot usually points that foot or stands with it partly off the ground. A horse with shoulder lameness frequently stands with the heel raised and the toe resting on the ground. If the horse stands with a bend in his knee, suspect an injury to the elbow. If the heel is raised and the knee or stifle is held forward, the horse may have sustained an injury to the heel or the fetlock. With a stifle joint injury, the horse often stands and travels with the stifle turned out.

Bone fractures and joint injuries often (but not always) produce some degree of limb deformity. X-rays should be taken. Foot fractures, in particular, are difficult to diagnose without x-rays.

Standing directly in front of the horse, watch his head to see if it bobs up and down with each step. In a horse with front leg lameness, the head bobs down as weight comes down on the sound leg. In the rear leg, the head bobs down as weight comes down on the injured leg. Note that head-bobbing does not occur with mild lameness.

Next, standing directly behind the horse, see if one side of the rump appears to dip as the horse moves away. This indicates a sore hind limb on the side opposite the dipping.

With a sore stifle, the horse often travels with the stifle pointing out. In addition, he may hesitate before bringing the sore leg forward, which results in dragging the leg.

Very subtle lameness may not cause visible signs. However, when riding the horse, you may notice that he appears unwilling to step out or seems stiff in one leg. Occasionally, you can detect a hind limb lameness by changing diagonals at the trot. The horse's gait feels different on the new diagonal because now you are rising and sitting in time with the sore leg. As you listen at the walk or trot, you should hear equal beats of the hooves. If there is an irregular beat, the horse may be favoring one foot and not putting it down as hard as the others.

A supporting-leg lameness is often made worse by riding the horse in a circle or working him on a longe line, which forces the horse to put more weight on the inside leg. A left-sided lameness, for example, will show up on a counterclockwise circle to the left. A horse with a supporting-leg lameness is apt to shuffle and stumble, especially on rough surfaces such as gravel. This is particularly characteristic of navicular disease.

A swinging-leg lameness can be brought out by riding the horse down a slope. This requires the legs to move through a greater arc, which increases pain in the sore leg. The horse may compensate by swinging the sore leg out wide or dragging that toe.

Physical Examination

Starting at the feet, perform a systematic examination, working up the legs to the hips and shoulders. First, pick up each foot and examine the sole for a puncture wound and a bruised sole or corn. It will usually be necessary to clean the hoof thoroughly and possibly remove flaky horn to see the needed detail. A hot or close horseshoe nail is a frequent cause of sole lameness. A hoof tester is indispensable in examining for this and for foot wounds, laminitis, gravel, quittor, and navicular disease. Hot, painful front feet should alert you to the possibility of laminitis. (For more information on lameness caused by foot and hoof problems, see chapter 8 "The Feet.")

Run your fingers and thumb along the flexor tendons at the back of the fetlocks, looking for swelling, pain, and increased warmth (see *Tendonitis*, page 239). Swelling of the foot above the coronet is usually caused by ringbone.

Run both hands slowly up the legs. A swollen, painful joint indicates inflammation, usually from a recent injury (see *Joint and Ligament Injuries*, page 249). Swelling without pain suggests tenosynovitis or bursitis. In the front legs, a painful swelling along the inside front of the cannon bone indicates bucked shins or splints. On the hind limbs, a bony enlargement on the inside of the leg below the point of the hock is typical of bone spavin. If thickening and swelling is found at the back of the hock, consider curb.

Diagnostic Tests

Veterinarians use certain tests to diagnose lameness and to monitor the course of treatment.

- **Flexion tests.** Flexion tests are most commonly performed on the knees, pasterns, fetlocks, and hock-stifle-hip of a horse. These tests require no special equipment. The veterinarian observes the movement of the horse prior to any joint manipulation, and will then hold the joint in a flexed position for a minute or two. The handler trots the horse off on a loose lead rope as soon as the joint is released. The horse is observed for lameness, stiffness, irregularities in stride, and head bobbing. Although flexion tests can demonstrate degenerative joint disease, it is not unusual for a normal horse to limp a few steps after a flexion test. As each limb is handled, the vet is also checking for range of motion, lateral (sideways) movement, rotation, and pressure on the joint. Two sets of flexion tests may be performed, one cold and one "warm" after the horse is exercised. The horse's responses often improve after exercise.

- **Conventional x-rays.** X-rays make it possible to differentiate between soft tissue swellings and bone growths. They are absolutely necessary for diagnosing bone fractures. They do not always provide a definitive diagnosis for lameness, however, because changes seen on an x-ray may not be associated with lameness, and not all causes of lameness produce x-ray findings.

- **Digital x-rays or digital radiography (DR).** This imaging method is currently quite expensive but offers high-quality results instantly. DR can be used to *radiograph* regions that were previously difficult to image in the field, such as the neck or stifle. DR also allows for computer enhancement where there is a large quantity of soft tissue to penetrate.

- **Computed tomography (CT scan).** Previously know as a CAT scan or computer-assisted tomography, this is another variation on x-ray technology. In a *CT scan* a rotating, focused x-ray beam takes "sliced" images of the anesthetized horse. A major advantage of CT over other types of diagnostic imaging is its superior resolution. It offers three-dimensional images with magnification, often achieved using contrast dye. CT scans are useful in examining fractures. CT scanners can image equine limbs up to the knees and hocks, or the head and the first 4 to 5 inches (101 to 127 mm) of the neck. Scans are expensive.

- *Ultrasonography.* This technology uses ultrasound waves through soft tissues to create pictures that can be displayed on a television monitor. Ligaments and tendons that cannot be seen on x-rays can be seen through ultrasound. This is an excellent way to follow the progress of ligament and tendon healing. It enables the trainer to determine when the horse is ready to return to work.

- **Magnetic resonance imaging (MRI).** *MRI* is a noninvasive, usually painless imaging technique. It uses a powerful magnetic field, radio waves, and a computer to produce detailed images of internal structures. This is the only diagnostic test that can assess both soft tissue and bone, although it is best in evaluating soft tissue. MRIs are expensive, and the horse must be anesthetized and sound enough to stand still for two to three hours for the scan. Because of a horse's body mass, only the head, upper neck, and lower limbs can be examined in the adult horse. Full body scans can be performed on *foals*. This test can be used to diagnose and evaluate lameness or orthopedic injuries of the lower limbs.

- **Nuclear scintigraphy.** This method of imaging uses intravenous radioactive isotopes and scintigraphy equipment (which detects the radiation) to form a picture of the bone and surrounding tissue. Because of cost and restrictions governing the use of radioactive materials, bone scans are performed primarily at equine medical centers and schools of veterinary medicine. This imaging method is an excellent diagnostic tool for differentiating hoof problems.

- **Nerve block.** Local anesthetics are often injected around specific nerves to localize pain and lameness. Anesthesia and pain relief occur in the area supplied by the blocked nerves. Thus, if the lameness disappears after the nerve block, the site (if not the cause) of lameness has been identified. Nerve blocks do not always establish a specific diagnosis because many causes of pain may exist in the same general location.

- *Synovial fluid analysis.* Synovial fluid is a viscous lubricating liquid containing hyaluronic acid. It is found in joint, bursal, and tendon sheath swellings. The fluid can be removed using a sterile needle and a syringe. Normal synovial fluid is clear and pale yellow. The presence of blood indicates that bleeding has occurred into the synovial space. Usually this is because of an acute injury. Pus indicates an *infection* in the joint or bursa. Laboratory analysis of synovial fluid provides further information.

- **Arthroscopy.** This diagnostic procedure allows direct inspection of the interior of a joint to determine the cause of swelling. A fiber-optic scope is passed through a small incision that can be closed with a single suture. The scope works like a tiny video camera. Arthroscopic joint surgery involves removing bone fragments, cartilage, and debris using tiny instruments that fit into the fiber-optic scope. Reconstruction of ligaments is also possible. Because there is less trauma due to small surgical wounds, this procedure has become more common. It may be used for a simple examination or for surgery involving deep joints with few complications. It is limited to accessible areas within the joint, and not all bone fragments can be removed or treated.

Tendon Injuries

A tendon is a tough, inelastic band of fibers that connects muscle to bone. Tendons are classified as flexors or extensors, depending on whether they bend the limb (flexors) or straighten it out (extensors). Most tendon injuries in horses are in the lower half of the leg.

The large tendon running down the front of the horse's leg is the common digital extensor. This tendon straightens the leg and extends the fetlock, pastern, and coffin joints. In the hind limbs it also flexes the hock joint.

Running down the back of each leg are the two digital flexor tendons. The superficial digital flexor tendon forms the rear outline of the leg. The deep digital flexor tendon lies beneath the superficial tendon. The combined action of these tendons is to flex the knee and all the joints below it. In the hind limbs, the flexors also straighten the hock. Each tendon has special "check" ligaments that restrain the tendon and keep it from overstretching (see *Joint and Ligament Injuries*, page 249).

STRAIN

A strain is an injury to a tendon caused by overuse or exercise beyond the fitness level of the horse. In a horse with a severe strain, the tendon first overstretches and then tears. The area is painful and swollen. Ultrasound can be used to visualize the degree of tendon damage and monitor the healing process.

Treatment: Applying ice is beneficial in stopping inflammation. *NSAIDs* are effective in relieving pain and inflammation. Some veterinarians may inject corticosteroids around the inflamed tendon. DMSO is also useful. Your veterinarian will select the best drugs for your horse.

TENDONITIS (FLEXOR TENDONITIS, BOWED TENDONS)

Tendonitis in the horse refers to strains of the superficial digital flexor tendons of the forelegs. These injuries often occur at the end of a long race or a lengthy workout, when muscles are fatigued and the horse no longer has the muscle tone to compensate for rapid loading and overstretching of the tendon. Thus, the injury occurs most commonly in racehorses, Quarter Horses, hunters, and jumpers, but can occur in any horse as a result of a direct blow to the tendon area. Tendonitis of the hind limb is less common but does occur to some extent in harness racers.

The signs of tendonitis are generalized swelling throughout the area of injury, with warmth and pain to the touch. The horse may pull up lame or experience severe lameness shortly after the accident, and stand with his heel off the ground. If the tendon is partially disrupted, you may see "dropping" of the fetlock (the fetlock joint sinks toward the ground).

Within the injured tendon there is bleeding and leakage of inflammatory fluids. Released muscle enzymes cause further damage. A pocket of accumulated *serum* and debris can develop within the tendon itself. The blood supply to the tendon is often disrupted, along with its fibers.

In the healing stages, acute inflammatory tissue is replaced by fibrous connective tissue and scar. The tendon becomes thick and bowed out from the leg when viewed from the side. A mild to moderate degree of lameness may be present, which is exacerbated by hard work.

The bow in the tendon is described by its location. A high bow covers the upper third of the cannon just below the knee or hock. A middle bow (the most common) is found at the mid-cannon at bone level. A low bow is found at the lower cannon level in the annular ligament area. A low-low bow, indicative of deep digital flexor tendon injury, is found in back of and below the fetlock joint.

Treatment: Treatment of acute tendonitis involves reducing the swelling with ice, pressure, and anti-inflammatory medications. During the first 48 hours, it is most important to prevent further damage by resting the horse completely. Your veterinarian will perform an ultrasound of the injury so that progress can be monitored. The horse should not return to work before he has healed. Begin cold therapy with the application of ice packs for 30 minutes three to four times a day for two days. There is a commercially available machine (Game Ready) that can apply circulated ice water and compression. The wraps are simple to apply and remove and can target the cold therapy to the afflicted area. Wraps are available for the front legs, the hocks, and the back over the withers. The unit is available for rent or purchase. Cold therapy slows bleeding, reduces inflammation, and helps to relieve pain.

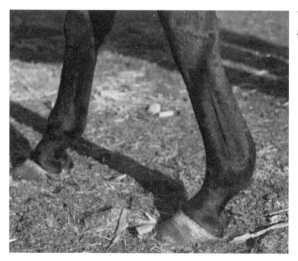

The typical appearance of a bowed tendon.

Between applications, immobilize the area and provide counterpressure by wrapping the leg as described in *Bandaging* (page 39).

After the first 48 hours, alternate the cold packs with warm packs. The warm packs should be applied for about 90 minutes (continue at 30 minutes for the cold packs). Continue alternating warm and cold packs three or four times a day for four to six days. After six days, warm packs alone are recommended to promote circulation and healing.

Flunixin meglumine (Banamine) is a strong analgesic with a rapid onset of action. Consider beginning treatment with Banamine and switching to phenylbutazone (Butazolidin) as pain and swelling begin to diminish. For more information on analgesics, see *Anti-Inflammatory Drugs and Pain Relievers* (page 590). DMSO gel has anti-inflammatory and antioxidant properties, which are beneficial in eliminating harmful inflammatory by-products at the site of injury. DMSO can be applied topically once a day beneath the bandage or two to three times a day on uncovered skin. Hyaluronic acid injections into the tendon sheath have yielded good results. Corticosteroid injections are no longer recommended for the treatment of tendonitis, because they delay healing.

At the beginning of the third week after the injury, remove the supportive bandages and begin passive exercises by gently moving the joints back and forth several times a day. Proceed to light exercise in four to six weeks.

Early surgical treatment may be indicated in selected individuals, especially those in whom ultrasound shows signs of delayed healing. Various surgical procedures have been used successfully. They include splitting the flexor tendon, cutting of the radial check ligament, and dividing the annular ligament.

Although expensive, the use of stem cells collected from the horse and injected into the injured tendon is showing promise in the healing of torn or injured tendons. Shock wave therapy is currently popular, but clinical trials showing benefits to its use are ongoing. At this time, shock wave therapy does not appear to be more beneficial than enforced long-term rest.

CONSTRICTION OF THE ANNULAR LIGAMENT

The annular ligament of the fetlock is a tough, unyielding thickening of the sheath that encircles the superficial and deep flexor tendons and forms a canal through which they pass. Constriction of these ligaments squeezes and damages the tendon and prevents it from gliding. The constricting effect is made worse when the tendon swells after an injury. Accordingly, the majority of cases of annular ligament constriction are associated with preexisting tendonitis. Direct injury to the ligament accounts for the remainder.

The typical history is that of pain and lameness associated with tendonitis that fails to improve after several months (as it should with an uncomplicated bow of the tendon) and gets worse with exercise. In many cases, swelling of the tendon sheath above the annular ligament can be seen and felt. Ultrasound examination is a useful diagnostic test for annular ligament constriction. All cases of low bow tendonitis should be examined for the possibility of a coexisting annular ligament constriction.

Treatment: An operation to divide the annular ligament and release the constricted flexor tendons is usually successful.

LACERATED OR RUPTURED TENDONS

Tendons can be severed by a deep cut through the leg. They can also be torn or ruptured during athletic competition as a result of sudden overextension or overflexion of a fatigued joint. Struggling to free a trapped leg is another cause of injury.

Damage to a tendon can weaken it to the extent that spontaneous rupture can occur even with normal stress. This can happen in a horse with a prior tendon sheath infection, with prior tendon repair, or with advanced navicular disease.

The common sites for tendon injuries are:

- **Flexor tendons of the feet.** All degrees of tear and disruption can occur in the feet. If just the superficial flexor tendon is involved, the fetlock will drop but not touch the ground. When both tendons are cut, the fetlock will drop further, bringing the toe up into the air as the horse bears weight. An infected wound increases the amount of scarring and decreases the chance for full recovery. Rupture of the deep flexor tendon usually occurs near its junction with bone at the back of the fetlock joint. Rupture is often preceded by an infection of the sole of the foot, which extends upward to involve the tendon. Navicular disease is another precursor to rupture of the deep flexor.

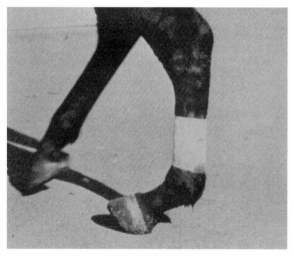

Laceration of both flexor tendons with dropping of the fetlock.

- **Extensor tendon of the knee (carpus).** This tendon assists in straightening out the knee joint. This condition may occur in foals with club feet or other angular limb deformities. Rupture occurs just above the knee, usually as a result of being kicked by another horse or by striking the knee against a wall or post. Signs of rupture are difficult to detect. Careful observation will show that the injured knee flexes more than the normal knee, especially at the trot. *Palpation* of the tendon will reveal loss of substance when compared to the normal knee.

- **Peroneus tertius.** This tendon is an integral part of the reciprocal apparatus, which mechanically bends the hock when the stifle joint is flexed. Because rupture occurs above the hock joint, the diagnosis can be made if the hock can be straightened while the stifle is bent.

- **Achilles (common calcaneal) and gastrocnemius tendons.** The Achilles tendon is easily visible as a ridge beneath the skin at the back of the hock and leg. The Achilles is made up of the tendons of the gastrocnemius muscle and the superficial digital flexor of the hind limb. It is rare for the Achilles tendon to rupture, but when it does, the hock is dropped very nearly to the ground and the limb cannot support weight. More commonly, the gastrocnemius tendon ruptures before the superficial digital flexor. Although the hock is dropped, the horse can still bear some weight. These injuries are caused by falls with the back legs flexed beneath the body, by being stopped suddenly and pulled back on the hocks, and by making strenuous efforts to keep from slipping while going downhill.

Treatment: Lacerated and ruptured tendons must be surgically repaired. If the wound is clean, this can be done at the time of injury. If the wound is dirty, it is best to treat the wound and repair the tendon at a later date. In either case, antibiotics are indicated. Stem cell therapy is expensive but may be beneficial.

In the lower leg, a partially ruptured tendon in which most of the fibers remain intact is usually treated by immobilizing the joints above and below the injured tendon. (The same immobilization is used following surgical repair.) The cast can be changed, but should be left for six weeks. Afterward, special shoes may be necessary for several months to protect the tendon from undue strain.

Rupture of the peroneus tertius requires only stall rest for eight weeks. Most cases heal and the horse can return to normal activity.

The results of tendon treatment cannot be fully evaluated for one year. They are best for extensor tendons and less satisfactory for flexor tendons. Ruptured gastrocnemius tendons are difficult to treat and usually require casting the limb from the hoof to the stifle for two to three months and placing the horse in a sling. When the Achilles tendon is ruptured, the *prognosis* is guarded.

TENOSYNOVITIS

A tendon is surrounded by a sheath of specialized tissue called the synovial membrane, which secretes fluid that lubricates the tendon and reduces friction when the tendon glides. Inflammation of this sheath is called tenosynovitis. The hallmark of tenosynovitis is fluid accumulation in the sheath, which causes obvious swelling. There are several types of tenosynovitis.

Acute Tenosynovitis

This condition is distinguished by a sudden buildup of fluid within the sheath, accompanied by pain, heat, and lameness. There may be a history of trauma. Symptoms are like those of tendonitis and, in fact, both conditions may exist at the same time. Diagnostic ultrasound is useful to distinguish between them.

Acute tenosynovitis can progress to chronic tenosynovitis, with persistent thickening and swelling of the tendon sheath and the development of fibrous bands and adhesions between the tendon and the sheath. Chronic tenosynovitis restricts tendon movement and athletic performance.

Treatment: Treatment of acute tenosynovitis is like that described for tendonitis (see page 240), except that injections of corticosteroids into the tendon sheath are recommended for tenosynovitis as long as there is no injury to the tendon. Repeated corticosteroid injections may have negative side effects, such as mineral deposits in the tendon and/or sheath.

Septic (Infectious) Tenosynovitis

In a horse with bacterial infection, the synovial fluid contains pus and inflammatory enzymes that can digest the tendon. Pain and lameness are severe. Diagnosis is confirmed by ultrasound and by analysis of fluid drawn from the infected sheath.

Treatment: Treatment involves immediate surgical drainage of the abscessed sheath, along with appropriate antibiotics. The outlook is guarded because of the potential for tendon degeneration and rupture and the presence of dense fibrous adhesions that encase the tendon.

Idiopathic Tenosynovitis

There are a number of mild conditions that produce tendon sheath swelling but do not produce pain or lameness. In some cases, chronic stress appears to be a causative factor; in others, there is a history of repeated minor trauma to the tendon sheath. Foals can be born with idiopathic tenosynovitis.

The common types of idiopathic tenosynovitis are:

- **Thoroughpin.** This is a swelling of the deep digital flexor tendon of the hind limb. The distended sheath appears as a soft, boggy prominence on the outside of the hock at or below the joint. It rarely causes problems and is considered a blemish.

- **Bog spavin.** This is a swelling of the joint capsule of the hock joint, considered here because of its similarity to thoroughpin. A stress or strain of the hock joint may be the initiating factor, but once the joint capsule becomes distended, the swelling persists. Bog spavin can be distinguished from thoroughpin by the fact that there are not one but three swellings of the hock joint. Two are present on either side of the back of the hock, the third on the inside front of the hock. Bog spavin tends to occur in young horses and disappear as the individual matures. In some *colts* with *congenital* conformation abnormalities, bog spavin may be an early symptom of osteochondritis dissecans.

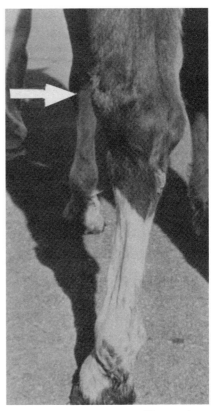

Thoroughpin is a boggy swelling on the outside of the hock at or below the joint.

- **Wind puffs (wind galls).** Generically, the term refers to synovial swellings of various joints and tendons that do not cause lameness. However, the term is usually used to describe the firm swellings in the area of the fetlock. A horse in full training who abruptly stops working frequently shows wind puffs on the front and/or back legs. Long, straight pasterns, incorrect trimming of the hoof, and heavy training on hard surfaces predisposes a horse to wind puffs, especially young horses.

Treatment: Swellings caused by idiopathic tenosynovitis can be drained and injected with a corticosteroid for cosmetic reasons. However, they have a strong tendency to recur. Those caused by hard training may respond to modification of the exercise program.

STRINGHALT

This is a peculiar condition in which there is a sudden upward jerking of the hind leg, accompanied by an involuntary flexion of the hock as the horse steps forward. In a horse with severe stringhalt, the fetlock may actually shoot forward and strike the undersurface of the abdomen.

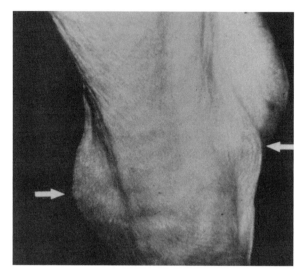

Bog spavin is recognized by swellings on either side and at the back of the hock.

Although the cause is unknown, the condition appears to involve the tendon of the lateral digital extensor muscle at the hock. Some cases follow trauma to this tendon, and adhesions may form as it crosses the outside surface of the hock joint. Although most cases are isolated occurrences, outbreaks of a stringhaltlike syndrome among horses on pasture have been reported and may be related to fungal toxins (*mycotoxins*).

Treatment: Surgery to free adhesions and divide the tendon usually affords immediate improvement, although recovery may be incomplete in some cases. Horses with the stringhaltlike syndrome usually recover spontaneously when removed from pasture.

Bursitis

A bursa is a closed sac lined by a membrane that secretes a lubricating fluid. These sacs are located at strategic points between moving parts and act as cushions to prevent friction and chafing. Trauma to a bursa—either a direct blow or the mechanical stress of racing—produces a painful swelling called *acute* bursitis.

Acute bursitis causes lameness. With rest and anti-inflammatory drugs, the acute bursitis usually resolves. However, with the stresses of repetitive motion at high speeds or heavy loads, the bursa becomes thickened and scarred, and the swelling persists. This is called *chronic* bursitis. It may or may not cause lameness.

Septic bursitis occurs when the bursa becomes infected with bacteria or, rarely, fungi. A good example is septic navicular bursitis, which follows a nail penetration injury of the frog of the foot. As the infection works its way up through the laminae of the foot, it rapidly involves the bursa behind the navicular bone. Urgent treatment is required to prevent further complications.

Treatment of septic bursitis involves wide surgical drainage of all infected pockets and appropriate antibiotics.

Common locations affected by acute bursitis are described in this section.

Bicipital (Shoulder Joint) Bursitis

Shoulder joint bursitis follows a kick or a blow to the point of the shoulder. Signs are swelling and a noticeable limp. X-rays are advisable to rule out an associated fracture. With shoulder joint lameness, a horse in motion will often swing his leg out wide in a half-circle.

Treatment: Rest the horse until signs of lameness are gone. Anti-inflammatory drugs such as flunixin meglumine (Banamine) or phenylbutazone (Butazolidin) help relieve pain and swelling. Injections of cortisone into the bursa are often beneficial.

Trochanteric Bursitis (Whorlbone Lameness)

This is a painful hip lameness caused by inflammation of a bursa beneath the tendon that crosses the head of the femur. It is the result of tendon overuse that occurs during racing or hard training. It is seen most often in Standardbred racehorses. A horse with trochanteric bursitis carries the foot inward and puts most of his weight on the inside edge of the foot.

Treatment: Injecting the bursa with corticosteroids is often effective. As an alternative, the bursa can be injected with an obliterating agent such as Lugol's iodine solution. Phenylbutazone (Butazolidin) is given to relieve pain and swelling. Rest the horse until lameness disappears.

Cunean Tendon Bursitis (Jacks)

This is a painful inflammation of the bursa beneath the cunean tendon at the inside of the hock joint. The condition is common among harness racers. In fact, it is said that most Standardbreds will be affected at some point in their racing careers.

Acute bursitis results from a shearing stress produced as the foot impacts and pushes off during extended fast pacing or trotting. Improper shoeing and incorrect conformation are believed to contribute. In the majority of cases, there is an associated bursitis of the small tarsal bones within the hock joint, causing some experts to refer to the condition as a cunean tendon bursitis-tarsitis.

Characteristically, the horse exhibits a "cold" lameness—that is, the lameness diminishes or disappears as the horse warms up. With continued abuse the lameness becomes constant, with the horse putting as little weight as possible on the affected leg and moving in shorter steps while carrying the leg to the inside.

Cunean bursitis is often *bilateral*, although usually one side is more severely affected than the other. Blocking the cunean bursa with a local anesthetic brings temporary relief and helps to make the diagnosis.

Treatment: Lameness is reversible. Treatment involves corrective shoeing, slower workouts at longer distances, phenylbutazone (Butazolidin), and a corticosteroid and/or hyaluronic acid injection into the tarsal joints.

Surgery, which involves removal of the cunean tendon, also affords relief. However, this further exposes the horse to shearing stresses and should be reserved for individuals who do not respond to other types of treatment.

Calcaneal Bursitis (Capped Hock)

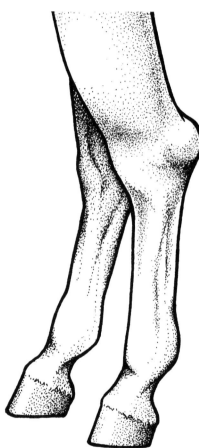

Capped hock is a soft swelling caused by repeated trauma.

This is a boggy swelling over the point of the hock caused by single or repeated trauma, such as kicking a wall or trailer gate. By itself, it is not a cause of lameness.

Treatment: Treatment is like that for olecranon bursitis (below).

Olecranon Bursitis (Capped Elbow)

This is a soft, boggy swelling of the bursa that overlies the point of the elbow. It occurs in horses who bang the elbow when getting up and down on hard surfaces. It can also be caused by a shoe hitting the elbow when the horse is recumbent. It usually does not cause lameness.

Treatment: The bursa is drained and injected with a corticosteroid or an iodine solution. This may have to be done several times. Alternately, the bursa can be opened and packed with gauze containing Lugol's iodine solution, or a drain can be left in place until the cavity obliterates. If these procedures are not successful, the bursa can be surgically removed. Prevent further injury by providing softer bedding.

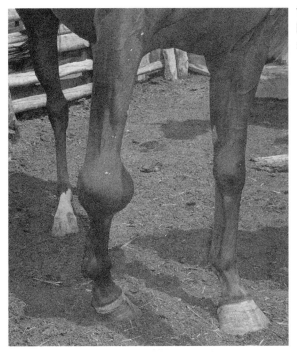

This long-standing hygroma of the knee requires surgery.

HYGROMA OF THE KNEE (CAPPED KNEE)

Hygroma is a swelling over the front of the knee caused by pawing and hitting the knee against a wall or getting up and down on hard surfaces. The swelling, which can become quite prominent, takes various shapes.

Treatment: Treatment involves needle aspiration of the fluid sac and injection of a corticosteroid. In chronic cases, permanent swelling is treated by opening and draining the hygroma or removing it surgically.

Joint and Ligament Injuries

In the horse, there is an apparatus composed of muscles, ligaments, tendons, and connective tissue. Its function is to support the horse as he stands, to diminish compression during locomotion, and to protect the horse from injuries that might occur from overextension of the fetlock, pastern, and coffin joints. This apparatus is called the stay apparatus. The stay apparatus is further subdivided as follows:

- **The check-or-stay apparatus.** This refers to ligaments that restrain the knee and hock joints, and also to the superficial and deep flexor tendons in all four legs. The check apparatus enables a horse to sleep on his feet by locking or "checking" his lower legs in an extended position with little muscular effort.

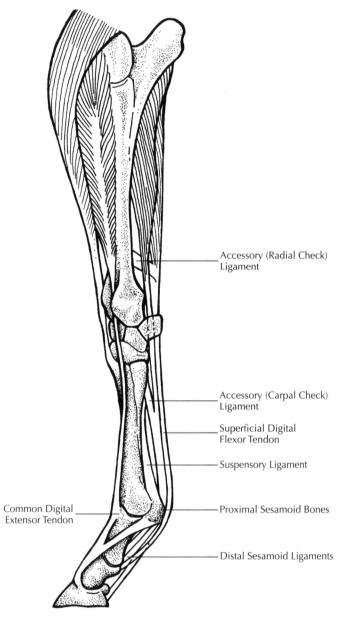

Accessory (Radial Check) Ligament

Accessory (Carpal Check) Ligament

Superficial Digital Flexor Tendon

Suspensory Ligament

Common Digital Extensor Tendon

Proximal Sesamoid Bones

Distal Sesamoid Ligaments

The stay apparatus of the front leg.

- **The reciprocal apparatus of the hind limb.** This ensures that there will be reciprocal flexing of the hock joint when the stifle joint is flexed, and that the hock will extend when the stifle extends. The reciprocal apparatus also aids in preventing fatigue when the horse is standing.

Structures in the reciprocal apparatus include the peroneus tertius muscle, the superficial digital flexor tendon, and the gastrocnemius tendon.

- **The suspensory apparatus of the fetlock.** This is of prime importance in absorbing the shock of concussion and in supporting the fetlock. The fetlock is the joint that is subject to the greatest stress. The suspensory apparatus includes the suspensory ligament, the paired sesamoid bones and their ligaments, and the superficial and deep flexor tendons. The suspensory ligament is a wide, thick, elastic, tendonlike band that arises from the back of the cannon bone above and attaches to the back of the upper third of the long pastern bone below. In its course from top to bottom, the ligament divides into two branches that surround and partly encase the two proximal sesamoid bones. Where the two branches attach to the long pastern bone, they also join the common digital extensor tendon. All these attachments serve to cushion impact and prevent extreme overextension of the fetlock joint.

A joint injury involves stretching or tearing of the joint capsule and its supporting ligaments by forced movement of the joint beyond its normal range. An injury to a ligament is called a sprain.

A mild sprain is one in which a few fibers of the ligament are torn, resulting in swelling, stiffness, and often a limp. The integrity of the ligament is not lost, so a mild sprain responds to rest and a support bandage.

A moderate sprain is one in which there is a tear of the ligament but the ends do not separate. The signs are pain over the joint, bleeding into the joint or soft tissues, swelling, and restriction of motion, causing lameness. There may be some degree of looseness in the joint. This type of injury requires casting and prolonged rest.

A severe sprain is one in which the ligament and/or joint capsule is completely disrupted. Loss of integrity may result in dislocation (*luxation*) of the joint.

INJURIES OF THE SUSPENSORY APPARATUS OF THE FETLOCK

This serious injury is a common cause of fetlock breakdown in Thoroughbreds. It occurs when the horse's weight comes down on the overextended fetlock under the extreme stress of racing. All degrees of tear of the ligament are possible, from mild sprains to complete ruptures of the suspensory ligament and its two branches.

Signs are sudden lameness and extensive swelling at the fetlock joint. The horse often stands with his entire weight on the uninjured leg. When weight is transferred to the injured leg, the fetlock may sink to the ground. Severe fetlock sprains are difficult to tell apart from fractures of the sesamoid bones, which occur because of stress and fatigue during a long race (referred to as

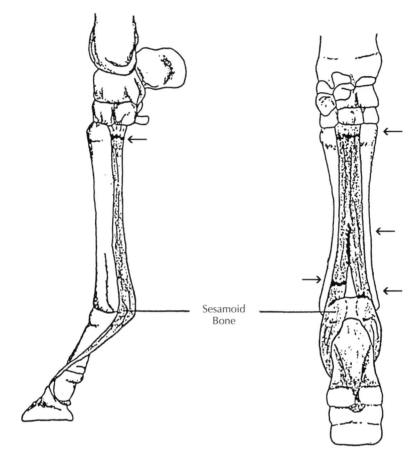

Sesamoid
Bone

Sprains of the suspensory ligament of the fetlock, showing where tears are most common.

"breaking down on the racetrack"), from sprains of the distal sesamoid ligaments, and from fractures of the fetlock joint and the long pastern bone. In fact, massive injuries can be associated with all of these, as well as injuries to the digital arteries and tendons.

Treatment: Veterinary examination and x-rays are important with all fetlock injuries. A variety of measures are used to treat fetlock sprains. They include stall rest, splints, casts, special shoes to raise the heel, and, in difficult cases, surgical fusion of the joint. With massive injuries, treatment is difficult or impossible.

SPRAINS OF THE DISTAL SESAMOID LIGAMENTS

The three distal sesamoid ligaments run between the proximal sesamoid bones and the back of the short pastern and coffin bones. Injuries occur when the horse's weight comes down on the overextended fetlock under the extreme stress of racing. The onset of lameness is sudden. Swelling is present over the course of the ligaments and pressure over the ligaments causes pain. An exact diagnosis is made with ultrasound, which is also used to monitor the progress of healing.

When trauma is sufficient to disrupt the ligaments, it may also cause fracture of the fetlock. One problem with severe injuries of this ligament is late calcification (see *Sesamoiditis*, page 259).

Treatment: Confine the horse for six weeks and support the leg with bandages. For severe strains, the leg should be put in a cast. Phenylbutazone (Butazolidin) helps to reduce pain and swelling. Return the horse to work slowly, as this area is prone to reinjury.

CARPITIS (SPRAINED KNEE)

Carpitis is an exercise-induced sprain of the ligaments that stabilize the interior of the knee joint. These sprains tend to occur in racehorses, hunters, and jumpers. Poor conformation with incorrect alignment of the knees is a major contributing factor.

Carpitis is common in young horses who have just started to train. Signs include varying degrees of heat, swelling, pain, lameness, and reluctance to bend the knee. The swelling is noted over the front of the joint.

Carpal lameness can be confirmed by a joint block. The knee should be x-rayed to exclude a fracture (see *Knee Joint (Carpal) Fractures*, page 274).

Treatment: Rest the horse for two to three weeks. Failure to do so may result in fractures of the small bones within the joint. Phenylbutazone

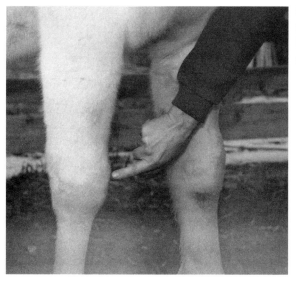

Swelling of the front of the knee, accompanied by lameness, indicates a sprained knee.

(Butazolidin) relieves pain and swelling. Joint injections with hyaluronic acid have been recommended. Most horses can return to competition with adequate rest, but poor knee conformation increases the likelihood of reinjury.

Sprain of the Accessory Ligament of the Superficial Digital Flexor Tendon

The accessory ligament (the radial or superior check ligament) of the knee is a strong, fibrous band that arises from the back of the radius and joins the superficial digital flexor tendon. The accessory ligament can be sprained during sudden overextension of the fetlock and knee joints, which forcefully elongates the flexor tendon and rips the attached ligament. This occurs primarily in racehorses.

A horse with a sprained accessory ligament walks gingerly and puts his toe and heel on the ground at the same time, as if he is walking downhill. Swelling will be seen at the back of the knee joint.

Treatment: Anti-inflammatory agents relieve pain and swelling. Confine the horse to a stall for six weeks. Apply support bandages to the knee. During the next two months the horse can be put in a short run. Ultrasound examination at 6 and 12 weeks after the injury is used to monitor healing.

Sacroiliac Strain

The sacroiliac joints are stabilized by strong ligaments that join the iliac bones to the sacrum and thus to the backbone. Ligament injuries occur after slips and falls, which may also fracture the ileum or pelvis. There is also a type of chronic sacroiliac strain associated with certain gaits, such as trotting and pacing. This is a problem among harness racers. The overall result may be a site-specific intervertebral osteoarthritis.

The signs of sprain are stiffness and pain in the hindquarters, occasionally associated with lameness in one or both hind limbs. A common complaint in hunters and jumpers is that the horse refuses to jump. When there is looseness (*subluxation*) of the sacroiliac joints, the sacral tuberosity (the wings of the pelvis) on one or both sides will become prominent over the high point of the rump (known as hunter's bump).

Treatment: Rest the horse in a box stall for one to two months. Anti-inflammatory drugs can reduce pain and swelling. The outlook for returning to previous levels of performance is guarded. In difficult cases, local irritants can be injected about the ligaments to cause scar tissue, which may help stabilize the pelvis.

DISLOCATION OF THE HIP

Dislocation of the hip is unusual because the round ligament, one of the strongest ligaments in the body, holds the head of the femur tightly in the hip socket. In fact, the ileum usually fractures before the hip will dislocate.

Signs of dislocation are shortening of the affected limb and swelling over the joint.

Treatment: A complete dislocation is a veterinary emergency. The hip must be put back in place under general anesthesia without delay. If this cannot be accomplished by traction on the limb, the joint can be opened and the hip replaced surgically. The prognosis is guarded, and many horses may never be able to return to work.

GONITIS (STIFLE LAMENESS)

The stifle joint, which includes the kneecap and its ligaments, is the largest and most complex joint in the horse. Swelling of the stifle joint, when accompanied by lameness, is called gonitis. Gonitis is a descriptive term that does not denote a specific diagnosis. Joint blocks and arthroscopy can assist in determining the cause of stifle joint swelling. A complete set of x-rays is essential in all cases. Severe stifle joint injuries are often complicated by bone fractures (see *Stifle Joint Fractures*, page 278).

As a sequel to stifle joint injury, many horses develop degenerative arthritis. These horses will not return to sound condition.

Gonitis can include any of the following conditions.

Upward Fixation of the Patella (Locked Kneecap)

In horses with this condition, one of the ligaments of the kneecap catches over the inner ridge of the femur and causes the hind limb to be locked in extension. When the horse is required to move forward, he is unable to advance the leg normally and drags the toe. There is a variation of locked kneecap in which the kneecap intermittently catches and suddenly releases, jerking the leg forward in a manner somewhat resembling stringhalt. The stifle normally locks to keep the horse standing while asleep.

A maneuver for releasing a locked kneecap is to back the horse while at the same time pushing inward and downward on the kneecap. This often causes it to release. The horse can then move forward with ease.

Horses and ponies with straight stifle joints, very young horses, and unfit horses are predisposed to upward fixation of the patella. The condition is often bilateral.

Treatment: In some horses, increased physical conditioning may be beneficial in improving muscle strength and tone, which will keep the patella from locking up. In other horses, irritants may be used to alter the pull of the

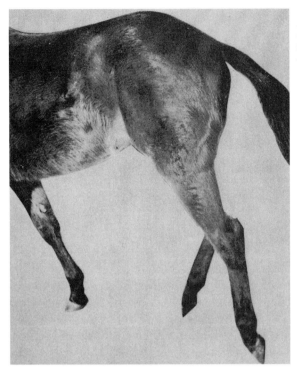

Locked kneecap: The stifle joint is locked in extension as the horse attempts to pull the leg forward.

patella and aid in preventing upward locking. For some horses, the best results may result from surgically cutting the patellar ligament on the inside of the leg so that the ligament cannot lock the patella at all. Your veterinarian will work with you and your horse to determine the best course of therapy. He or she may try the increased muscle conditioning first, and, if that is not successful, may eventually recommend the surgical approach.

Rupture of the Collateral Ligaments

The inside (medial) collateral is the ligament that is usually ruptured. The injury is caused by a sudden force applied to the outside of the joint. With rupture of either ligament, the joint becomes unstable and is subject to degenerative joint disease.

Treatment: There is no effective treatment. Chronic lameness results.

Rupture of the Cruciate Ligaments

Two cruciate ligaments are found inside the joint. They join the femur above to the tibia below. A severe wrenching or twisting injury can tear the cruciates. Often a tear of the *meniscus* or cushion inside the stifle is also involved.

Treatment: There is no effective treatment. Chronic lameness results.

Sprain of the Joint Capsule

If a joint capsule is stretched but does not rupture, recovery to performance level is possible. Unfortunately, joint capsule injuries are often accompanied by tears of the cruciates, collaterals, and meniscus.

Treatment: Treatment involves absolute stall rest for two to three months, followed by a gradual return to full activity. Irritants are sometimes injected into the sprain site to promote scarring in an effort to stabilize the joint.

SPRAIN OF THE PLANTAR LIGAMENT (CURB)

Curb is a thickening and enlargement of the plantar ligament and may also involve other soft tissue structures. It is often preceded by an injury to the ligament. The plantar ligament is located at the outside of and just below the point of the hock. Conformation defects such as cow hocks and sickle ("curby") hocks predispose a horse to curb. Occasionally a foal with faulty hock conformation is born with a curblike condition.

Sprains serious enough to cause curb occur when a horse is pulled up sharply on his haunches. Kicking walls and going too strongly over a jump are other causes.

Signs of acute sprain include lameness with pain and swelling over the ligament. The horse often stands with his heel off the ground. A horse with chronic curb may not be lame, but the tissues are thickened and swollen scar tissue is visible at the characteristic site. It is important to use ultrasound to differentiate which soft tissue structures are involved.

Treatment: The most important treatment is to rest the horse. The length of rest is determined by which structure is affected, and varies from four weeks to four months Apply ice packs for 30 minutes, three to four times a day, for two days and wrap between treatments to reduce swelling. Alternatively, a commercially available machine called Game Ready is available that includes both cooling and compression directed at the site of injury. Continue with alternating temperature therapy, as described for *Tendonitis* (see page 240). Oral and topical anti-inflammatory drugs, and hyaluronic acid injected around the ligament, reduce pain and swelling. For horses with good conformation the outlook is favorable.

Periostitis

Bones are covered by a thick layer of connective tissue called the periosteum. Inflammation of this layer is called periostitis. Injuries that result in stretching or tearing the periosteum initiate a series of events that begin with bleeding and inflammation beneath the periosteum. The mixture of blood clot, serum, and inflammatory enzymes then converts to fibrous scar tissue that contracts, calcifies, and becomes incorporated into the bone at the site of injury. This is called new bone formation. It is the distinguishing feature of periostitis.

Since ligaments attach to the periosteum, forces that stretch ligaments can stretch and tear the periosteum. One example is the chronic stretching of ligaments that occurs with prolonged training on hard surfaces. This stress is amplified when the horse lacks good conformation. Another cause of periosteal injury is a direct blow to the periosteum and bone.

Specific types of periostitis are discussed in this section.

BUCKED SHINS AND STRESS FRACTURES OF THE CANNON BONE

Bucked shin is a periostitis of the front surface of the cannon bone. It is common in the foreleg but rare in the hind legs.

Bucked shins occur frequently in young Thoroughbreds during the first weeks of training. Horses who run on turf rarely develop this problem, but horses who run on hard surfaces are likely to do so. As the foot strikes the ground, the front surface of the cannon experiences greater compression than the back. The causes the periosteum on the front surface of the cannon to buckle and tear. At the same time, the bone can develop cracks and fissures called stress fractures. The bone then responds to the percussion injury by periosteal remodeling, while new bone is deposited at fracture sites to maintain strength and durability.

Signs of acute periostitis are a warm, painful, firm swelling over the front of the cannon bone. Lameness increases with exercise. The gait is choppy. When only one leg is involved, the horse tends to rest that leg. When both legs are involved, which is the usual situation, the horse shifts his weight from side to side.

Treatment: X-rays should be taken to identify the injury and look for stress fractures. Relieve acute inflammation and swelling with ice packs, pressure bandages, and phenylbutazone (Butazolidin), as described for *Tendonitis* (page 240). Apply support bandages and rest the horse for at least one month to prevent recurrence. Cortisone injections help reduce periosteal inflammation. Stress fractures may require surgical intervention.

If the injury becomes calcified, a permanent blemish results. However, this does not interfere with performance.

SPLINTS

Splints is a strain or tear of the interosseous ligaments that bind the splint bones to the cannon bone. This is a lameness of young horses. A heavy training schedule, benched knees, improper shoeing, and developmental orthopedic diseases are predisposing causes.

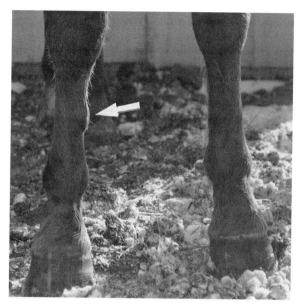

Splints in a young horse.

The periosteal swelling is typically found on the inside of the front leg about 3 inches below the knee. Pain, warmth, and a hard swelling will be noted in this area.

A splint bone can be cracked or fractured by direct trauma. This also produces a type of periostitis, but it is technically not the same as true splints because the interosseous ligament is not involved. X-rays should be taken to rule out the possibility of a bone fracture.

Treatment: Treatment of splints is similar to that described for bucked shins (see page 258), but rest is the most reliable treatment. The length of rest varies from 2 to 12 weeks. If the interosseous ligament becomes calcified, it may interfere with the suspensory ligament of the knee. This can require surgical correction.

SESAMOIDITIS

Sesamoiditis is a periostitis of the paired distal sesamoid bones. It follows sprains of the distal sesamoid ligaments (see page 252). The periostitis and new bone formation occur at points where the suspensory ligament attaches to the bone above and the two distal sesamoid ligaments attach to the bone below.

Sesamoiditis tends to occur among hunters, jumpers, and racing horses 2 to 5 years of age. Long, sloping pasterns make the horse more susceptible.

Signs include varying degrees of lameness along with pain and swelling, which is visible over the sesamoid bones at the back of the fetlock. Both front feet may be affected. X-rays are needed to confirm the diagnosis.

Treatment: Apply ice packs followed by compression dressings, as described for *Tendonitis* (page 240). Phenylbutazone (Butazolidin) relieves pain and swelling. If the lameness is severe, immobilize the fetlock joint for two to three weeks with a cast up to the knee. Corrective shoeing can relieve tension on the ligaments.

These bones have a poor blood supply and must be protected from additional trauma during the slow process of healing. This requires a prolonged period of rest (several months), followed by a gradual return to training or activity.

RINGBONE

Ringbone is the name given to all forms of periostitis and new bone formation that occur below the fetlock joint. The low ringbone disease process is also known as arthritis of the coffin bone. Most cases involve the forelegs. High ringbone involves the pastern joint area, while low ringbone affects the coffin joint area. Although new bone develops around these joints, it does not always involve the joint spaces. High and low ringbone can coexist in the same foot. When present, this leads to fusion of the pastern and coffin joints.

The initiating factor is chronic pulling and tearing of tendons and ligaments related to the stress of concussion on hard surfaces or making quick stops, sharp turns, and twisting movements at high speeds. Straight pasterns and high heels increase stress in the pastern and coffin joints and make the horse more susceptible. Occasionally, there is a history of a direct blow to the pastern, causing periosteal reaction and bone injury.

Heat, swelling, and pain are evident in characteristic locations. With high ringbone, the swelling is most pronounced over the pastern joint. In low ringbone it is found just above the coronary band. The horse may show pain when the site is squeezed. Lameness is present at all gaits and upon turning. With extensive new bone formation, the hair on the coronary band stands erect.

Buttress foot, also called pyramidal disease, is a specific type of ringbone caused by excessive strain on the common digital extensor tendon where it attaches to the front of the coffin bone. The new bone that forms in this location gives a bulky, pyramidlike look to the foot. Horses with buttress foot will always be lame and experience pain.

Rachitic ringbone is a fibrous tissue enlargement of the pastern in horses under 2 years of age. Because there is no bone involvement, it is not true ringbone. It is caused by a deficiency of calcium, phosphorus, or vitamins A, D, and C, either singly or in combination. Dietary correction is the appropriate treatment.

Treatment: X-rays are needed to diagnose ringbone and to determine the extent of involvement. Treatment undertaken during the acute phase before

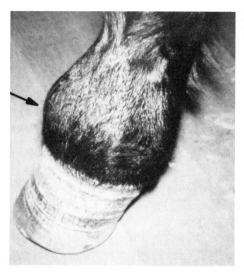

Bone enlargement above the coronet is typical of ringbone.

new bone develops involves immobilizing the leg in a plaster cast from the hoof to just below the knee. The cast should remain for four weeks.

Phenylbutazone (Butazolidin) helps relieve pain and swelling. Steroids injected into the soft tissues may be of value before the cast is applied, but injections into the joint can lead to further damage and should be avoided. Rest the horse for several months. Full roller motion shoes are of value because they shorten the horse's stride and reduce stress on the pastern and coffin joints.

Once there is new bone growth, treatment is less successful. Involvement of joint surfaces almost always leads to osteoarthritis and permanent disability. If the coffin joint is affected, there is little likelihood that the horse can return to riding condition. Digital neurectomy relieves pain.

When the pastern joint is affected, surgical fusion of the joint with screws or plates, followed by casting and a rehabilitation program, can produce a good result, especially for the hind limb.

Developmental Orthopedic Diseases

This is a group of related conditions linked by a common pathological process: a breakdown in the mechanism by which cartilage is converted to bone. Among these diseases are osteochondrosis, osteochondritis dissecans, physeal dysplasia, angular limb deformities, flexural limb deformities, and wobbler syndrome.

The mechanism by which cartilage is converted to bone is called endochondral ossification. Ossification occurs at three sites in the bone. The first, in the shaft of the bone, is called the diaphysis. The second site is the physis, or growth plate, located at the junction of the shaft and the head of the bone. The third is the epiphysis, which is the surface of the head of the bone that articulates with the joint.

The process of ossification is complex. Any mistakes along the way can either delay the ossification process or leave damaged cartilage, which fails to mature into healthy bone. Abnormal cartilage is prone to fracture, fissure, and breaks into small fragments that enter the joint and become joint mice. Cystic spaces can develop within mineralized bone. Cystic spaces are nonmineralized areas of phalangeal and carpal bones. There is a failure of mineralization of juvenile cartilage due to physical stresses; the horse develops translucent areas (holes or spaces) that fail to mineralize into normal bone. Delayed ossification or uneven bone growth can result in angular limb deformities.

Overfeeding and mineral imbalances were once thought to be the major causes of these problems, and they were known as nutritional bone diseases. Now that other influences are recognized as important contributing factors, the name of this group has been changed to developmental orthopedic diseases (DOD).

Some horses appear to have a genetic potential for developing DOD, but whether the horse develops the disease or not depends on external factors and the degree to which they influence the endochondral ossification process. Some of these external factors are either too much or too little energy in the diet; a deficiency of calcium, phosphorus, or microminerals in the diet; heavy exercise or hard training during rapid growth; bone and joint injury; hormonal diseases; and events that occurred in utero before the foal was born.

High-energy diets have long been recognized as precursors to DOD. A growing foal needs adequate amounts of dietary energy, protein, calcium, phosphorus, and the minerals copper, zinc, and manganese. Accelerating the rate of growth from 1 pound (453 g) to 2.5 pounds (1,134 g) a day increases energy and other nutrient requirements by 65 to 70 percent, and calcium and phosphorus requirements by 95 percent. If extra energy is supplied but there is insufficient calcium or phosphorus in the diet, growth still proceeds rapidly but without adequate mineralization of bone. This results in an increased risk of diseases associated with defective cartilage and immature bone. A deficiency of the minerals copper and zinc also results in defective cartilage formation. (For more information, see *Minerals*, page 400.)

The most common feeding practices responsible for nutritional imbalances in growing horses are feeding too much grain, feeding alfalfa hay without adding phosphorus to the ration, and feeding a grass hay and grain mix that does not have enough calcium, phosphorus, and protein. Adding excessive amounts of vitamins and minerals to the ration is another cause of bone disease. How to feed the growing horse is discussed in chapter 15, "Nutrition and Feeding." In some areas, copper deficiency can be a primary cause of DOD; too little copper in the native soil can lead to feedstuffs that are deficient.

To treat developmental orthopedic diseases related to overfeeding, remove alfalfa and grain from the horse's diet and provide as much good-quality grass or cereal grain hay as the horse will eat. This feeding regimen decreases the protein and energy portions in the ration and slows the rate of growth, allowing time for recovery.

Specific DODs are discussed in this section.

OSTEOCHONDROSIS AND OSTEOCHONDRITIS DISSECANS

Osteochondrosis is an extremely common disease in growing horses. One study reported osteochondrosis in more than two-thirds of all racehorses in the northeastern United States. Osteochondrosis results from a primary defect in the process by which cartilage is converted to bone. In one manifestation of osteochondrosis, thickened cartilage within the joint fragments breaks into loose pieces of cartilage called joint mice. This form of the disease, in which joint mice are present, is called osteochondritis dissecans.

Another characteristic disturbance in osteochondrosis is the subchondral bone cyst, found beneath the outer shell of the bone. Some of these cysts become quite large and are prominent x-ray findings.

The common joints affected by osteochondrosis, in order of decreasing frequency, are the stifle, hock, shoulder, fetlock, cervical spine, knee, elbow, and hip.

Symptoms commonly appear in young horses 1 to 2 years of age who have just started performance training. A typical history is that of a swollen joint accompanied by mild or no lameness. X-rays are usually diagnostic.

Treatment: The goal is to restore the horse to athletic fitness and prevent damage to the joint. Conservative treatment involves stall rest for up to six months, along with correction of dietary imbalances. Joint surgery is a widely accepted alternative and can often be done in young horses using the fiberoptic arthroscope. Most joints affected by osteochondrosis are amenable to arthroscopy. Devitalized cartilage and loose fragments can be removed through the instrument. Results depend on the location, type, and severity of the disease. Return to racing is possible.

Prevention: The frequency or severity of osteochondrosis can be reduced by good management practices, beginning with care and feeding of the pregnant *mare* as described in chapter 17, "Pregnancy and Foaling." It is important to maintain steady growth of foals from the neonatal period to 2 years of age, in particular avoiding growth spurts associated with feeding high dietary carbohydrates and energy. The daily ration should provide concentrations of copper and zinc as described in chapter 15. It is important to do a dietary analysis that compares feed quality to the nutritional requirements of the horse. In addition, the growing foal needs moderate exercise, but hard, prolonged, and stressful exercise can damage growing cartilage.

Physeal Dysplasia

Physeal dysplasia, also called physitis (and formerly—and inaccurately—called epiphysitis), is a generalized bone disease that causes lameness in young horses. The disease is characterized by enlargement of the growth plates located at the junction of the shaft with the head of the bone. This creates a flaring at the end of the bone, causing the bone to assume the shape of an hourglass (this is visible on x-rays). The bones commonly affected are the radius, tibia, and cannon bones.

Physeal dysplasia occurs in rapidly growing foals up to 2 years of age, with a peak incidence between 6 and 12 months. The disease may appear as an isolated event or affect several horses on a breeding farm. Signs include intermittent lameness and joint stiffness of varying severity. Pain, heat, and swelling are detectable at sites of bone involvement.

A combination of several factors appears to contribute to the development of physeal dysplasia. They include genetic predisposition, rapid growth, obesity, trace mineral deficiency, calcium-phosphorus imbalances, and excessive and strenuous exercise.

Physeal dysplasia is most likely to occur in overweight, active foals on high grain rations that are low in calcium and high in phosphorus. The frequency of the disease is increasing, perhaps because more breeders are selectively feeding for rapid growth and maximum mature size.

Physeal dysplasia is also known to occur in association with other developmental bone diseases, including wobbler syndrome, angular limb deformities, osteochondrosis, and flexural limb deformities.

Treatment: Perform a comprehensive analysis of the feeding program, including a ration analysis. It will often be found that dietary energy and/or protein is in excess of recommendations for growing horses (see chapter 15, "Nutrition and Feeding"). A calcium-phosphorus imbalance or deficiency may be identified. Adjust the ration accordingly.

Phenylbutazone (Butazolidin) diminishes pain and stiffness. Use it for short periods only. Rest is essential and exercise should be restricted but not eliminated, because stall confinement can cause flexural limb deformities. Many horses outgrow physeal dysplasia, especially if nutritional problems are corrected and strenuous exercise is curtailed until the bone disease becomes inactive. Some horses, however, develop cystlike areas in bones, angular limb deformities, or flexural limb deformities that ultimately impair their utility.

Angular Limb Deformities

Angular limb deformities refer to knock-knees and bowlegs. Other knee joint deformities are considered here as well.

Congenital angular limb deformities are apparent at birth. Congenital limb deformities are caused by abnormal limb positions in the uterus, nutritional

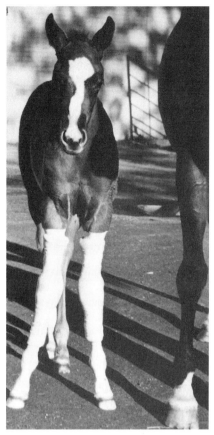

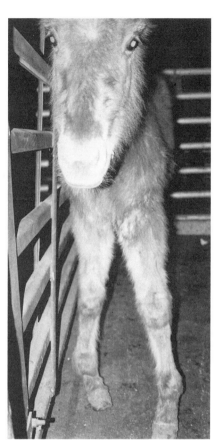

This foal with knock-knees is being treated with tube casts.

In this horse, bowlegs were caused by severe nutritional deficiencies.

imbalances in the mare, neonatal hypothyroidism, and unequal growth between the two sides of a long bone.

Developmental deformities appear days to months after birth. Developmental deformities can be secondary to incomplete ossification (or collapse) of the small cuboidal bones in the knee or hock joint. Some cases are caused by joint injury during the first few weeks of life. Premature foals are at greatest risk and should be monitored closely.

Note that many normal foals have some degree of limb crookedness, which may not straighten out until they are yearlings. On visual inspection as seen from the front, if the knock-kneed or bowlegged limb is greater than 15 degrees off vertical, the deformity is significant and a veterinarian should be consulted.

Knock-knees (carpus valgus) means the knees are deviated toward one another when viewed from the front. When the cause is congenital, the knees often straighten in a short time. Foals who acquire deformities after birth often need veterinary treatment.

Bowlegs (carpus varus) is the reverse of knock-knees; the limbs bow out. The outlook is like that for knock-knees.

Calf knees (backward deviation) is the reverse of buck knees. The knees are shallow at the front and rounded at the back. Because of abnormal stresses imposed by this conformation, chip fractures of the carpal bones are common.

Benched (popped) knees are also known as "offset knees." This is a conformation in which the cannon bones are set too far to the outside, with the result that most of the weight is carried on the inside splint bones. The majority of cases are congenital. Young horses with benched knees are prone to injuries of the knees and lower legs, particularly to splints and sprains of the fetlock joint.

Bucked or sprung knees (anterior deviation) are when one or both knees are flexed forward so that the joints appear rounded over at the front, when viewed from the side. This conformation restricts movement and causes a shortened stride. The fetlock may become knuckled. The involvement of both knees indicates the cause is congenital. When one knee is involved, a limb injury should be considered.

Treatment: Early recognition and treatment are vital. The longer a foal walks on deformed legs, the greater the likelihood of permanent damage. Treatment decisions are based on x-rays and physical findings. The simplest therapy is stall rest with five minutes of controlled exercise several times a day. A second option is splints, tube casts, or braces. Surgery is recommended when the deformity is severe or has failed to improve with conservative management. Results for surgery are best when it is performed before 3 months of age.

FLEXURAL LIMB DEFORMITIES

Flexural limb deformities, also called contracted digital flexor tendons, are seen most commonly in the fetlock joint, coffin joint, and knee joint. Young horses from birth to 18 months of age are affected. The basic condition involves a shortening of the deep, the superficial, or both digital flexor tendons in the forelegs, and occasionally in the hind limbs. Most deformities are bilateral.

The exact mechanism by which these deformities occur is unknown. One theory is that rapid growth of the long bones exceeds the ability of the flexor tendons and check ligaments to lengthen accordingly, thus pulling the fetlock joint or coffin joint into flexion. Another theory is that a painful condition causes temporary muscle contracture, which prevents elongation of tendons and ligaments. Trauma, or a developmental orthopedic disease such as osteochondrosis, may be the cause of the limb pain. Most studies have found that nutritional excesses and imbalances are common in horses with flexural deformities.

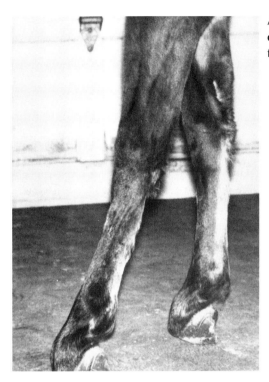

A foal with severely contracted digital flexor tendons in both front feet.

Flexural deformity of the coffin joint produces a raised heel and a club foot. With mild deformity, the pastern is straightened and the foal appears to walk on his toe. In horses with severe contracture, the foot knuckles over and the foal bears weight on the front of the fetlock.

Involvement of the fetlock joint (fetlock flexor deformity) causes knuckling at the fetlock, with the foot remaining flat on the ground. A third common contracture involves the knee joint (carpal deformity).

Treatment: In a newborn foal with mild deformity involving the coffin, fetlock, or knee joint, the tendon will usually stretch in a few days with corrective treatment. This involves walking the foal for ten minutes two or three times a day. Physical therapy includes joint extension exercises and the application of support wraps.

Deformities that appear after the first few weeks of life may also respond to conservative treatment. Reduce energy intake and balance the horse's ration. Trimming the heel helps stretch and lengthen the tendon.

When the deformity is severe or progressing in spite of conservative treatment, surgery is advised. The most frequently used operation involves dividing the inferior check ligament, which allows the flexor tendon to lengthen. The superior check ligament, and even the suspensory ligament, can be cut in advanced cases.

The prognosis for complete recovery depends on the location and severity of the flexural deformity, the age of onset, and the response to treatment. For mild congenital flexural deformities, the outlook is excellent.

Arthritis

Arthritis actually describes a number of joint ailments characterized by inflammation, degeneration, and new bone formation in and around joints.

When there is a history of an injury to a joint, or to the ligaments supporting a joint, the resulting arthritis is called post-traumatic arthritis or degenerative joint disease.

DEGENERATIVE JOINT DISEASE (OSTEOARTHRITIS)

Degenerative joint disease is the most common arthritic problem in adult horses. It is the end result of various injurious processes, many of which are discussed in this section. The lameness associated with arthritis is caused by stiffness and diminished range of motion. With an arthritic flare-up, there is joint swelling, pain, and tenderness over the joint.

Bone and joint x-rays are important in the diagnosis and treatment of all types of arthritis. Arthroscopic examination with an *endoscope* can be very useful in determining the type and severity of joint damage. It also aids in finding and eliminating fractures of surrounding bones and bone chips in the joint.

Treating Degenerative Joint Disease

Many beneficial drugs are available to ease the pain, swelling, and discomfort and slow the inflammation associated with degenerative joint disease. The use of these drugs may allow healing and repair of the affected joint. After a thorough work-up of your horse's condition, your veterinarian can determine which drugs may be the most beneficial for your horse.

- **Steroids** are actually a class of drugs called corticosteroids or glucosteroids that have a basic chemical structure similar to the cholesterol molecule. Examples are dexamethasone, methylprednisolone, and triamcinolone acetate. The short-term use of corticosteroids may stop the inflammation and degeneration associated with arthritis, but the side effects can cause laminitis and may even further damage the joint. These drugs are very powerful anti-inflammatory agents but may stop or delay healing by obstructing cartilage metabolism. Injecting corticosteroids into joints may therefore cause further joint degeneration.

- **Nonsteroidal anti-inflammatory drugs** (NSAIDs) are very useful at relieving the pain associated with arthritis, and at higher doses these drugs can stop inflammation. NSAIDs can make the arthritis patient comfortable and allow healing to begin if used in appropriate dosages. The side effects of prolonged use include stomach ulcers, bleeding, and slowing of the healing process. Examples are aspirin, phenylbutazone (Butazolidin), naproxen, and flunixin meglumine. There is one topical cream in use, Surpass, which contains diclofenac. This is an NSAID and its use is indicated to control pain and inflammation associated with osteoarthritis in the hock, knee, fetlock, and pastern joints in horses.

- **Dimethyl sulfoxide** (DMSO) is a solvent derived as a product of paper manufacturing that is useful in controlling inflammation and swelling. It also has the ability to carry other drugs, such as corticosteroids, through the skin. DMSO is known to cause cataracts in dogs, so you should wear rubber or Latex gloves when applying this drug.

- **Glucosamine sulfate** is a chemical found in the body as a precursor in building connective tissue, joint surfaces, and joint fluid. The sulfate form is the easiest to absorb from the horse's intestines and the sulfur in this form is essential for the production of connective tissues. The hydrochloride forms of glucosamine are poorly absorbed from the gut and do not appear to be as effective in joint repair.

- **Sodium hyaluronate** is most useful in treating joint capsule inflammation and increasing the quality of the joint fluid. It has poor to no effect when used in degenerative joint conditions.

In addition to drug therapies, there are alternative treatments for arthritis. The most useful and the modality that has been proven to alter the pain response in horses with degenerative joint disease is acupuncture. This and other holistic therapies are discussed in chapter 21, "Alternative Therapies."

Another emerging therapy for the treatment of degenerative joint disease, arthritis, and tendonitis is extracorporeal shock wave therapy (ESWT). ESWT has been shown to increase the growth of new blood vessels into the area of application, as well as stimulating the horse's body to produce growth factors in the treated areas. At this time, there are many research projects that are trying to validate the effectiveness of ESWT. So far, the research results have been controversial and inconclusive.

ACUTE SEROUS ARTHRITIS

Acute serous arthritis is characterized by a swollen, tender, fluid-filled joint along with a tendency to favor the limb. It is the result of either a joint stress or injury. This condition is also called acute synovitis. It does not necessarily progress to degenerative joint disease.

Treatment: Acute serous arthritis is treated like a sprain (see page 253). Rest the horse. Apply cold and alternating temperature therapy as described for *Tendonitis* (see page 240). Topical application of DMSO, with or without steroids, can reduce joint inflammation. Phenylbutazone (Butazolidin) helps to relieve pain and swelling. The joint can be aspirated or injected with corticosteroids, hyaluronic acid, DMSO, or polysulfated glycosaminoglycan (PSGAG). PSGAG occurs naturally in joint fluid and is said to promote cartilage healing. For more information, see *Anti-inflammatory Drugs and Pain Relievers* (page 590).

After a flare-up, the horse should be returned to activity slowly. Proper shoeing of a horse with faulty conformation helps relieve abnormal stresses on joints. In advanced stages, a surgical procedure may be indicated to relieve pain and improve serviceability.

SEPTIC ARTHRITIS

Infectious (septic) arthritis occurs when bacteria from the bloodstream invade joints. If the infection destroys cartilage, there will be irreversible damage. A form of septic arthritis called joint ill occurs in young foals. It is discussed on page 553.

Treatment: Septic arthritis requires high-dose broad-spectrum antibiotics while awaiting *culture* and sensitivity reports based on fluid withdrawn from the joint. Antibiotics should be given for several weeks. The joint may be drained and flushed via arthroscopy and antibiotics injected into the joint. Phenylbutazone (Butazolidin) relieves pain and swelling. This facilitates joint movement and prevents adhesions. Early and appropriate care of wounds, as described on page 35, will prevent many cases of septic arthritis and bone infection.

BONE SPAVIN (JACK SPAVIN)

This is arthritis of the hock joint. The hock is composed of an improbable column of bones that are subject to compression, rotation, and stretching of the ligaments that unite them. Hard use damages cartilage and also produces periostitis, the end result of which is degenerative arthritis. Sickle hocks, cow hocks, and very straight hocks can predispose a horse to joint injuries.

Bone spavin is seen in horses ridden hard at a gallop. It is an occupational hazard among racehorses, hunters, jumpers, and Western horses used for barrel racing, roping, and cutting.

When bone spavin has been present for some time, you will see a bony enlargement on the inside of the leg below the point of the hock. This protuberance is called a "jack." In the early stages before bony enlargement, x-rays or bone scans will show signs of bone *erosion*. This is called a "blind" spavin.

Spavin typically begins as a "cold" lameness. A cold lameness is present before exercise, disappears as the horse warms up, and returns when the horse cools down. Because of pain on the inside of the hock, the horse tries to carry most of his weight on the outside of the foot. The hoof or shoe may show wear on the outer edge.

To test for spavin, the hock is flexed by holding the foot up close to the lower abdomen for two minutes. The foot is then released and the horse immediately trotted. With a positive test, the horse shows lameness on the first few steps.

Treatment: All stressful activity contributing to the lameness must be discontinued. Intermittent use of low-dose nonsteroidal anti-inflammatory drugs, and hyaluronic acid injections into the joint, sometimes with added corticosteroids, are beneficial. Corrective shoeing is helpful. In advanced cases, dividing the cunean tendon and/or fusing the hock joint relieves pain and makes the horse serviceable.

OSSELETS

Osselets is an arthritis of the fetlock joint that begins as a chronic stress injury to the joint capsule from the repeated concussions of hard training and racing. Upright pasterns predispose the horse to this condition. One or both front feet may be affected.

In the initial stages, there is stretching or tearing of the fetlock joint capsule with signs of acute serous arthritis. This stage is referred to as "green" osselets. "True" osselets represents a more advanced stage and refers to the visual presence of swelling and new bone growth on the outside front of the fetlock joint.

The stride in a horse with osselets is short and choppy. The horse tends to plant his weight on the outside edge of the hoof.

Treatment: The outlook for "green" osselets is favorable if the horse is rested until all signs of inflammation are gone. When new bone growth involves the joint surfaces, treatment is difficult. This is especially true if the horse has upright pasterns.

OMARTHRITIS (SHOULDER JOINT ARTHRITIS)

Shoulder joint arthritis usually occurs as a complication of a joint fracture. In most cases there is a history of being kicked by another horse or running into a solid post or door. Osteochondrosis of the shoulder joint in growing horses may cause sufficient joint injury to lead to a degenerative arthritis.

A horse with shoulder joint lameness lifts his head when stepping down on the painful leg, swings the bad leg out wide instead of carrying it straight ahead, and stands with his good leg ahead of the painful leg. Swelling and tenderness about the shoulder joint may be evident.

A nerve block can help locate the site of lameness. X-rays showing arthritic bone changes within the joint are diagnostic. Arthroscopic examination is useful and can aid in treatment.

Treatment: When a chip fracture or joint mouse is identified, it should be removed. Steroid injections into the joint, followed by hyaluronic acid (HA), afford temporary relief. With new bone formation, the outlook for recovery is poor.

Broken Bones

Broken bones are caused by accidents such as being kicked by another horse, taking a hard fall, stepping into a hole, running into a fence or post, or being hit by a car. In addition, horses are prone to high-torque and compression injuries of the legs and feet.

Bone fractures are classified as open or closed. A closed fracture does not break through the skin. With an open or compound fracture, the bone makes contact with the outside, either because of a wound that exposes it or because the point of the bone punches through the skin from the inside. Open fractures are considered dirty, because they are automatically contaminated with dirt, debris, and bacteria. *Osteomyelitis*, or bone infection, is a potential hazard with all open fractures. Long-standing bone infection is called chronic osteomyelitis. It is characterized by fever, lameness, pain, and swelling, and a discharge through a sinus tract connecting the infected bone with the skin.

Comminuted fractures are multiple breaks in the bone, like a shattered car windshield. A large force is necessary to cause multiple breaks. This results in marked instability and is a most difficult problem to treat.

Bone fractures are recognized by limb deformity, shortening of the leg, swelling at the site of injury, and inability to put weight on the leg. Stress fractures of the cannon bone and chip fractures involving the joints below the elbow and stifle are not obvious on visual inspection. X-rays are needed to make the diagnosis.

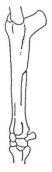 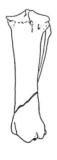 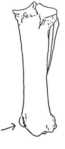 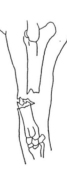 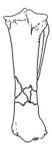

| Incomplete Fracture | Simple Fracture | Chip or Avulsion Fracture | Open Displaced Fracture | Comminuted Fracture |

TREATING BROKEN BONES

This depends on a number of factors, including the location and type of break, whether the affected bone is involved in direct weight-bearing, the age and weight of the horse, and the resources available to the veterinarian. In general, treatment falls into one of three categories.

The first is complete rest. The horse must be confined to a box stall for several weeks or months. For weight-bearing fractures, the horse may need to be placed in a sling. However, many horses will not tolerate slinging.

The second is to apply splints, braces, and casts. Lightweight polyvinyl chloride pipe splints are effective. They can be removed easily to inspect the skin for pressure sores and to administer physical therapy to the joints. Ideally, splints and casts should be applied to immobilize the joints above and below the fracture site.

The third approach is repair the fracture surgically. There are several ways to do this.

Arthroscopy is an excellent approach for chip fractures that enter the joint. The small surgical incisions heal with minimal scarring and restriction. However, arthroscopy is not suitable for all joints.

Open reduction, internal fixation involves making an incision over the joint or fracture, bringing the ends into alignment, and then maintaining the desired position with various devices, including screws, pins, plates, and wires, or rods inserted down the center of the shaft. Compression plating is a procedure in which a metal plate is laid across the fracture site and secured above and below by bone screws.

Arthrodesis (joint fusion) is a surgical procedure in which bone grafts are placed in and around the joint to fuse it. Fractures involving joints often lead to painful post-traumatic arthritis. Fusion of the joint will relieve pain and make the horse more serviceable, although some degree of permanent lameness will result. Bone grafts can also be used to heal certain types of fractures, such as those of the proximal sesamoid bones.

The prognosis for a successful outcome after any fracture is guarded if the horse will have a residual lameness or a handicap and thus cannot return to the activity for which he was intended. There is a poor prognosis for horses with multiple fractures, comminuted fractures, open fractures (often complicated by bone infection), fractures involving the weight-bearing surfaces of joints, unstable fractures, and fractures that cannot unite because of poor blood supply. In some cases, treatment is most unlikely to be successful and may even be impossible.

FRACTURES OF THE SHOULDER

These fractures are uncommon. A large force is necessary to fracture the scapula or humerus. Such a force could occur with a hard fall on the shoulder, being kicked by another horse, or running into a solid object.

The humerus usually breaks in mid-shaft, causing either a spiral or oblique fracture. The horse is unable to bear weight on the limb. The radial nerve may also be injured, producing a "dropped elbow." Treatment is complicated by rotation of the bone fragments, angular deformities, persistent radial nerve paralysis, and technical problems associated with attempts at surgical reduction and stabilization. The prognosis is guarded.

Treatment: Simple fractures of the scapular spine heal with stall rest. Comminuted fractures are more difficult to treat successfully. If the horse recovers, permanent lameness and shoulder joint arthritis are to be expected.

FRACTURES OF THE FOREARM

The radius and ulna are fused to form a single bone in which the olecranon is the remnant of the ulna. All types of fractures can occur in the forearm, usually as a result of hard falls, direct blows, and stepping into holes.

A horse with a broken forearm is unable to bear weight and exhibits obvious swelling and deformity. These fractures are difficult to immobilize.

Treatment: The prognosis is guarded to poor. However, results are good for young horses with nondisplaced stress fractures treated with stall rest for two to four months.

KNEE JOINT (CARPAL) FRACTURES

The knee is composed of three movable joints made up of eight bones arranged like blocks in two layers. One or any combination of the eight bones can fracture. Chip and slab fractures are most common. A slab fracture is a vertical fracture through one of the blocks.

Knee joint fractures tend to occur in racehorses who tire at the end of a hard race and come down heavily on an overextended knee. The direction in which the horse is raced influences which front leg is affected. Horses who race in a counterclockwise direction (as in the United States) have more chip fractures in the right leg, while those who race in a clockwise direction (as in Europe) have more chip fractures in the left leg.

The large accessory bone at the back of the knee joint also can break. This produces a characteristic swelling on the outside of the knee joint.

Treatment: Chips in the joint can be removed surgically using an arthroscope. Many horses can return to racing. Slab fractures are fixed in place with screws. The prognosis for racing is guarded. Accessory bone fractures tend to pull apart after repair; however, if left alone, they eventually form a fibrous union.

CANNON BONE FRACTURES

Breaks can occur anywhere along the lengths of these bones and can enter the joints above and below. Fractures entirely across the long axis, comminuted fractures, and those that enter joints require extended therapy and often cannot be treated successfully.

Small fissure fractures may develop in association with ligament stress and concussion (see *Bucked Shins and Stress Fractures of the Cannon Bone*, page 258). These fractures are incomplete.

Treatment: Treatment is like that for bucked shins, and usually has a good outcome.

SPLINT BONE FRACTURES

The second and fourth metacarpal and metatarsal bones are also known as the splint bones. These splint bones lie on either side of the long bone below the knee joints and the hock joints. They have been considered to be bony remnants of additional toes from many millennia ago.

Fractures of these splint bones usually occur in mature horses, possibly as a result of a loss of flexibility of the ligaments that hold the second and fourth metacarpal bones to the long third metacarpal bone. As horses mature past 2 years of age, training programs increase in intensity, which may lead to more stress on these bones. Injuries caused by blows or kicks to these bones also result in fractures.

Treatment: Treatment is usually successful if the horse is given enough time to rest—usually one to two months. A slow return to athletic activities is advised. Occasionally, the healing affects the suspensory ligament and the splint bone may be removed surgically to allow better motion of the limb.

Prevention: If the injury was caused by the horse "interfering" or his own hoof striking the splint bone, use of splint or shin guards may prevent recurrence. Slowly increasing training may aid in preventing splint bone fractures.

FETLOCK JOINT AND LONG PASTERN BONE FRACTURES

Chip fractures involving the fetlock joint are common in racehorses. These are stress fractures related to overextension of the pastern joint at racing speeds. They are often bilateral. The chip most often comes off the long pastern bone at the joint lip. The diagnosis cannot be made without x-rays.

A small chip can be treated with adequate rest for four months. Large chip fractures, and those displaced into the joint, require surgery. Arthroscopic removal is preferred. The prognosis is good if treatment has been uncomplicated.

Longitudinal and comminuted fractures of the first phalanx tend to occur in Western performance horses in whose events sudden turns, slides, and twists are combined with axial compression.

Treatment: Surgical treatment offers the best results. The prognosis is guarded.

FRACTURES OF THE SESAMOID BONES

Sitting side by side at the back of the fetlock are the two proximal sesamoid bones. Fracture of these bones is almost an occupational disease of racehorses. The forelimbs are most frequently affected in Thoroughbreds and Quarter Horses, and the hind limbs are most frequently affected in Standardbreds. When the fractures involve both sesamoid bones, the horse may actually break down on the racetrack and need to be removed by ambulance. In this situation the suspensory apparatus is lost. This becomes a most difficult problem to treat.

Treatment: Broken sesamoids heal slowly. In young horses, casting the leg for four months has been successful. In performance horses and those with displaced fractures, surgical fixation and bone grafting offer the best results. The prognosis for a return to racing is guarded.

PASTERN AND COFFIN JOINT FRACTURES

Fractures of the short pastern bone occur most often in the hind limbs of Western performance horses, especially those wearing heel calks, which prevent foot rotation when the horse changes direction. A "pop" may be heard at the time of injury. Chip fractures can be treated with stall rest or arthroscopic surgery. More extensive fractures require special casts or internal fixation with plates or screws. The prognosis for athletic performance is guarded.

Fractures of the coffin bone are stress-related. They tend to occur in the front feet of racehorses exercised on hard surfaces. The foot should be immobilized in a full bar shoe with quarter clips, and the horse should not be worked for at least eight months. The prognosis for racing is guarded.

There is a characteristic fracture that occurs at the site where the common digital extensor tendon attaches to the coffin bone. Sudden traction on the tendon can crack the bone and pull the extensor process free of the coffin bone. Unlike most fractures in the lower leg, this fracture usually does not produce acute lameness. With lack of treatment, the foot assumes a triangular shape and eventually takes on the typical appearance of buttress foot. Treatment involves applying a cast and administering anti-inflammatory drugs. The prognosis is guarded. Arthroscopic removal of small fragments and rest can return some horses to work. Larger bone fragments may also be treated surgically, but the prognosis for a return to athletic function is guarded.

NAVICULAR BONE FRACTURES

Navicular fractures are rare. Most are associated with navicular disease (see page 220). Hind limb fractures can occur from kicking walls and posts. Navicular fractures are difficult to diagnose. X-rays are required.

Treatment: The navicular bone heals poorly. These fractures often do not unite. Surgical fixation may be useful in selected cases. Treatment is similar to that described for navicular disease.

BROKEN RIBS

Broken ribs are caused by kicks and blows to the chest wall. In the newborn, they occur during the birthing process. Signs are pain and swelling over the ribs, frequent coughing, and reluctance to move. Fracture of the first rib may cause dropped elbow if the radial nerve is involved.

The end of a broken rib may enter the chest cavity and puncture the lung. If the lung collapses, the chest cavity fills with air. This is called a *pneumothorax*. In most horses, the right and left chest cavities are incompletely separated. This enables air to pass from one side to the other, in which case the pneumothorax occurs on both sides. This causes extreme difficulty in breathing and often death.

Treatment: Uncomplicated rib fractures heal spontaneously in several weeks. Complete rest is important.

PELVIC BONE FRACTURES

Horses who slip and fall on their side or struggle during casting while their hind limbs are tied may sustain a fractured pelvis. (Casting is a procedure in which ropes and lines are used to throw a horse down on his side.) The ileum can be broken in many places, but the most common sites are the wing, shaft, and sacral tuberosity.

When the tuberosity is fractured, the horse appears to have a flattened or "knocked-down" hip on that side. This type of fracture also occurs when a horse runs through a narrow gate.

Rectal and vaginal (for mares) examination may reveal pelvic bone asymmetry and bone crepitus (crackling) when the horse shifts her weight. X-rays are difficult to perform, requiring general anesthesia with the horse on her back. However, a bone scan can be done with the horse standing. Hot spots will be seen at fracture sites.

Treatment: Pelvic fractures cannot be treated surgically. Confine the horse to a box stall for at least three months. Slinging the horse is of benefit, but many horses will not tolerate it. Complete healing takes at least a year. The prognosis for return to service is guarded.

FEMUR FRACTURES

Young foals occasionally break a femur during casting and halter breaking. These injuries often involve the growth plates. In an adult horse, a considerable force is required to fracture the femur. The broken bone fragments usually override or slide past each other, which makes it difficult to maintain alignment.

Treatment: Surgical treatment is the only possible course of action, but even with compression plates and rods the prognosis for horses over 1 year of age is poor.

Stifle Joint Fractures

The stifle is a complex joint that incorporates articulations between the femur and tibia and the femur and kneecap. Fractures of the kneecap can occur from any blow to the knee such as kicks to the knee or hitting a jump during a race, or a horse's leg could strike an upright post at high speed. A force sufficient to break the patella often produces soft tissue injury to the ligaments and the capsule of the joint. The damaging blow may fracture the end of the femur as well.

Other fractures at the stifle occur as a result of crushing or twisting injuries of the limb, often associated with joint dislocations. A chip fracture in the stifle joint is rare. Consider osteochondrosis.

Treatment: Simple patellar fractures heal with stall rest for three to five months. Surgical repair is indicated for complicated breaks. The outlook is guarded.

Severe stifle joint injuries are difficult to treat successfully and often heal in a bad position. This frequently leads to serious complications, such as stifle lameness.

Tibia and Fibula (Gaskin) Fractures

The gaskin is the area between the stifle and hock joints. The tibia and fibula are the bones of the gaskin. The fibula is seldom broken because it is rather small and is well protected by muscle.

All types of fractures can involve the tibia, including those into the joint. The most common cause is a kick from another horse. Incomplete fractures are often preceded by stress fractures. With a complete fracture, the horse is unable to bear weight on the leg. If obvious deformity is not apparent at the time of injury, x-rays are necessary to make the diagnosis.

Treatment: Stress fractures are best treated by strict stall confinement for up to three months. With complete fractures, internal fixation with plates and screws has been successful in some foals. In adult horses, fractures of the tibia are very difficult to treat. The outlook for recovery is poor.

Hock Joint Fractures

The hock is a complex structure composed of ten individual bones, which make up several movable joints. Fractures generally occur because of a direct blow, such as a kick from another horse. Twisting injuries also can produce fractures. These tend to occur among barrel racers, Thoroughbreds, and horses shod with heel calks. X-rays and bone scans are used in making a diagnosis.

In young horses, hock injuries frequently involve growth cartilage, in which case healing often produces a false joint and permanent lameness.

Treatment: Broken bones in the weight-bearing axis heal poorly. Surgery has been used successfully in a few cases. It is unlikely that many horses with such fractures can return to full performance. Degenerative joint disease with permanent lameness can be expected.

Other fractures, such as those of the calcaneus, can be treated successfully in some cases by removing chips or stabilizing the fragments with screws. Badly comminuted fractures of the calcaneus cannot be treated.

SKULL FRACTURES

Fractures of the skull are usually the result of an injury with trauma to the head. For example, the horse may run into a fixed object such as a tree, fence, or post, or pulling back when tied may injure the head and neck. The two most common types of head injury are when a horse or foal is kicked by another horse or when the horse goes over backward and strikes the top of his head on the ground. Some injuries may also result from hitting the head in low stalls or horse trailers. The jaw bone may be fractured if the horse is kicked or if the side of his head hits the ground suddenly.

The bones of the skull are fixed in place, so a traumatic injury to the head may cause a fracture of the head bones in more than one location. Multiple skull fractures are found when the horse flips over backward or from direct frontal trauma to the forehead.

Signs vary according to the location and force of the injury, and whether there is injury to the brain. Sometimes a swelling may be seen on the forehead, blood from the nose or ear may be observed, or symptoms of brain injury may be the only sign if the cause of the injury is not observed. The symptoms of brain injury may include *depression*, lack of response to stimuli, fear, and even coma. (For more information see *Head Injuries*, page 348.) Occasionally, respiratory distress may be noted. A fractured jaw bone may present with obvious swelling and reluctance to eat or open the mouth.

Treatment: Some injuries to the forehead may heal with little or no residual swelling. The horse may continue to exercise and eat without problems. Usually though, there will be a hard lump on the head that can be seen and felt.

More serious injury resulting in injury to the brain or spinal cord may require immediate treatment by your veterinarian. NSAIDs such as flunixin may be given, and sometimes there will be a need for massive doses of steroids such as dexamethasone or methylprednisolone to reduce inflammation.

Intravenous salt and mannitol solutions may be given to relieve an increase in intracranial pressure. Barbiturates may be given if seizures occur.

Most skull fractures will heal after a long convalescent period, if the brain injuries can be controlled.

Fractures of the mandible or jawbone may heal on their own if balanced nutrition can be maintained. Offer water-softened feed or complete grain supplements. In more severe cases, surgery may be required to plate or pin the jaws in proper anatomical alignment. Stainless steel or titanium metal plates, pins, and/or wires are surgically implanted to achieve alignment and facilitate healing. Small bone fragments may be removed. Fracture repair is slow but possible.

VERTEBRAL FRACTURES

Fractures to the vertebral column of the foal or horse are invariably caused by some form of trauma. Foals who pull hard against a lead rope, a horse of any age who runs into fixed objects, jumping horses, or horses who rear and fall may sustain vertebral injuries.

The symptoms may include loss of balance, inability to walk in a straight line, not being able to stand, sitting like a dog, or inability to stand at all. The symptoms may help pinpoint the site of the *lesions*. Paralysis with lack of ability to lift the head off the ground indicates a neck injury. Sitting like a dog indicates a fracture of the vertebrae around the withers.

Fractures of the rump are vertebral and signs may include restlessness, reluctance to stand, or cauda equina syndrome (see page 353).

Treatment: The prognosis is guarded in all cases. Even if immediate treatment of anti-inflammatory agents is successful, new bone growth at the fracture site may impinge on the spinal cord and produce chronic symptoms. Surgery may stabilize some fractures and produce satisfactory life-sustaining results in a limited number of cases.

Muscle Injuries and Diseases
MUSCLE STRAIN

A muscle strain is an injury caused by overuse or overstretching of muscle fibers. The signs are a painful swelling accompanied by lameness. In a mild strain, only a few fibers of the muscle are stretched, swollen, or torn. In a severe strain, the entire muscle may be torn free from its attachments, or the muscle itself may tear.

The muscles most commonly involved in athletic performance injuries are those of the croup and the backs of the thighs.

Injuries severe enough to cause muscle strain may also strain ligaments and tendons. Diagnostic ultrasound helps distinguish between these conditions and monitor the healing process.

Treatment: Muscle strains respond to massage by hand, ultrasound therapy, or even rest. Anti-inflammatory medications, administered both orally and topically, are of considerable value. Naproxen (twice daily) appears to be the most beneficial drug for muscle pain. The horse should be rested until the injury is healed.

Sore Back and Loin Syndrome

The longissimus dorsi muscle runs down the back from the neck to the sacrum. This muscle, as well as the two psoas muscles that lie beneath it, are strained when the horse is racing or jumping. Ill-fitting tack is a contributing factor.

A horse with a strain of this muscle group will be stiff and drag his hind toes. Pain and spasm cause a shortened stride and gait alterations suggestive of hindquarter lameness. The horse may twist himself over the jumps instead of going over strong. With pressure over the loins, the horse may groan and drop his back. The involved muscles will be firm, warm, and painful. The abdomen is tucked-up and tense.

Treatment: Rest the horse. Anti-inflammatory drugs help relieve pain and swelling. Hot packs and ultrasound promote blood flow and relieve spasms. Vitamin E and selenium have been used in treating and preventing certain muscle disorders, and may be of benefit. Muscle relaxants may provide some relief.

Check to see if the saddle and tack are too tight by placing a string down the horse's back between the saddle and the pad. When you're in the saddle, you should be able to draw the string out easily if the tack is properly adjusted.

Overlapping of the Spinous Processes

The ridge down the center of the horse's back is composed of the spines of 18 thoracic and 6 lumbar vertebrae. Normally, these vertebral spinous processes are separated by interposed muscle. In a horse with this disease, the spines impinge on one another or overlap. This causes pain and muscle spasms. An overlap involving two or more spines can occur anywhere along the back, but most often affects the saddle area. Friction caused by the spines rubbing together results in a periostitis with new bone formation. This often leads to arthritis of the vertebral column.

In some horses with overlapping spinous processes, there is a history of falling or going over backward. This would suggest that a back injury caused the condition. However, not all affected horses have a history of back injury. Undoubtedly, many cases are caused by activities that produce maximum flexion and extension of the spine. The problem is most prevalent in hunters and jumpers. Horses with a weak or swaybacked conformation are most commonly affected.

Signs are like those described for sore back and loin (page 281). Downward pressure on the back is painful. The horse often resents being saddled and gives

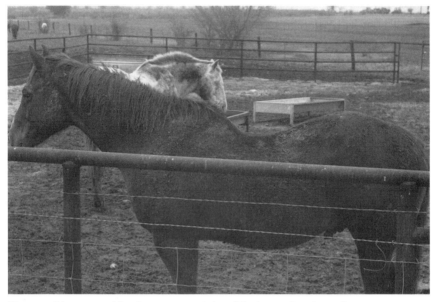

Horses with a swayed back are more susceptible to overlapping spinous processes and back pain.

evidence of pain when the cinch is tightened. Diagnosis is based on physical examination and x-rays that show narrowing of the spaces between the spines and, occasionally, an overlap. *Ultrasonography* is useful in diagnosing lesions involving the ligaments and spines of the back. Nuclear scintography may help in selected cases.

Treatment: Response to treatment varies and is not necessarily related to the severity of the lesions found during diagnostic procedures. Nonsteroidal anti-inflammatory drugs (NSAIDs) may not alleviate any of the symptoms. Local injections of corticosteroids and muscle relaxants are sometimes useful.

Alternative treatments using acupuncture and chiropractic management have been useful in cases of equine back pain. Massage therapy is useful in relieving the muscle damage caused by spinous process disease. Training may proceed during treatment but strict protocols are recommended to prevent muscle *atrophy* while allowing stability of the affected bones.

Severely affected horses may require surgery. This involves removing the tops of the spinous processes. Two months of stall rest and one month of light exercise are required before the horse can be ridden.

FIBROTIC MYOPATHY

Following a tearing injury to a muscle, healing can be complicated by the development of excessive fibrous connective tissue and, later, calcification in the muscle. This is called fibrotic *myopathy*. Characteristically, the injury occurs in the semimembranosus and semitendinosus muscles at the back of the thigh at the level of the stifle joint. In this location, these muscles are especially prone to sprains and tears.

The presence of scar and bone severely restricts the action of the muscles. There is a characteristic gait in which the back foot, just before touching the ground, is suddenly jerked back several inches. This is the opposite direction from stringhalt. The back of the thigh at the site of ossification is hard to the touch.

Treatment: The most satisfactory treatment is surgical, which involves removing the ossified muscle or dividing the tendon of the semitendinosus. Improvement usually is apparent shortly after the surgery. Not all horses remain free of symptoms, however, because new fibrous adhesions can form.

MYOPATHY OF PROLONGED RECUMBENCY

Horses who are under a general anesthetic for more than two to three hours, and horses who become recumbent for long periods in the lateral position, are subject to a myopathy caused by the weight of the horse pressing on the dependent muscles. This causes a decrease in the arterial blood flow to the compressed muscles, with oxygen deficit in the local tissue. For reasons not well understood, in one form of this disease the myopathy becomes generalized. This condition may also occur in horses with laminitis or certain neurological conditions.

The typical history is that of a long anesthesia. The horse generally stands after the operation and at first seems normal. In a short time, the horse develops signs of muscular weakness, becomes wobbly and unstable, may exhibit a dropped elbow or stifle, or knuckles over at the fetlock. The affected muscles become hard, swollen, and painful.

If the myopathy is severe or generalized, it is unlikely the horse will be able to regain or keep his feet. *Myoglobin* produced by dying muscle may appear in the urine and turn it a dark brown. Death can occur from shock or kidney failure.

Treatment: Treatment is like that described for *Exertional Myopathy* (see page 18). *NSAIDs* relieve pain and swelling. Intravenous fluids are important to aid recovery. Wrap the opposite limb with a support bandage. Attempts to minimize post-anesthetic myopathy include expeditious surgery, positioning the patient on a well-padded surface, and avoiding certain anesthetic agents that may predispose to generalized myopathy.

Prevention: When a horse goes down for any reason and requires good nursing care, it is important to maintain the *sternal position* if possible. If this is not possible, turn the horse from side to side every two hours and provide soft padding. Foam rubber eggshell padding is good bedding and also helps prevent pressure sores.

Exertional myopathy is discussed on page 18 and nutritional myopathy and myotonia are discussed on pages 567 and 568.

Hyperkalemic Periodic Paralysis Disease

Hyperkalemic periodic paralysis disease (HYPP) is an inherited muscular disease that can be traced back to a single male American Quarter Horse named Impressive. Up to 4 percent of all American Quarter Horses develop the syndrome. American Quarter Horse Crossbreds, American Paint Horses, and Appaloosas may also be affected.

Horses with HYPP have a defect in a protein that regulates the passage of potassium and sodium in and out of muscle cells. Potassium therefore leaks from inside the muscle cell into the bloodstream, raising the blood potassium level. Symptoms may include muscle twitching and weakness, increased respiratory sounds, and unpredictable episodes of paralysis that can lead to sudden death. Horses with an episode of HYPP are aware of their surroundings and do not seem to be in any pain.

HYPP is not associated with exercise but can occur following any stressful event. Episodes of HYPP can be confused with other conditions because of the muscle tremors and weakness; for example, it can resemble exertional rhabdomyolysis (tying-up syndrome). A horse will appear normal after an attack of HYPP, while horses with tying-up syndrome will have a stiff gait and painful, firm muscles. It may also be confused with colic, since a horse may go down and be reluctant or unable to stand, and the tremors may be confused with seizures. The paralysis of the respiratory muscles cause some horses to make loud breathing noises during an attack; these to can be confused with other conditions, such as choking or a respiratory condition.

Treatment: Emergency treatment from your veterinarian is required if the attack of HYPP is severe. Your veterinarian will give an IV solution of calcium and/or dextrose with added sodium bicarbonate. Karo syrup may be squirted into the horse's mouth until the veterinarian can arrive, if this is a reoccurring event and you know the cause. For long-term therapy, this condition can be managed with a carefully controlled program of exercise and diet. The diet should be grass hay with no alfalfa, and any grain supplements should not contain molasses. Do not confine the horse in a stall, but allow him to move freely in a paddock or pasture. Avoid rapid changes in diet and decrease the amount of potassium in the feed. If managing the diet does not prevent attacks, treatment with a diuretic such as acetazolamide may be useful, as recommended by your veterinarian.

Prevention: Genetic testing has been developed to help breeders and veterinarians identify carriers of this disease. Hydrochlorothiazide or acetazolamide may be used over the long term to control recurrence of symptoms in some horses.

10

THE RESPIRATORY SYSTEM

A horse's nasopharynx is made up of the nostrils (nares), nasal cavity, and pharynx. The nasal cavity is divided by a midline septum into two passages, one for each nostril. At the back, these passages open into the throat behind the soft palate. The two nasolacrimal ducts, which drain tears from the eyes, open onto the floor of the nasal cavity close to each nostril. Because of this arrangement, eye ailments with excessive tearing cause a watery discharge from the nose.

The entire respiratory tract is lined by a delicate membrane. On the surface of this membrane is a layer of *mucus* that is moved by tiny hairlike *cilia* toward the front of the nose. This *mucociliary blanket* traps bacteria and foreign irritants and acts as a first line of defense against *infection*. Exposure to cold and dehydration stops the motion of the cilia and thickens the mucus. This reduces the effectiveness of the mucociliary blanket.

The turbinates are prominent ridges of bone inside each nasal cavity. They produce air turbulence as the horse breathes in. This helps to warm and humidify the air and also traps foreign particles and irritants at the back of the pharynx, where they can be removed by the action of the cilia.

Because horses breathe through their noses, the nasal passages must be both large and expandable. During maximal exercise, air flow increases ten-fold and the nostrils flare to provide a bigger opening. Because of the large size of the horse's nasal passages, foreign bodies in the nose are easily sneezed out and rarely cause problems.

A horse's nose is normally cool and moist. There are no sweat glands in the nose. Moisture is secreted by mucous glands in the nasal cavity.

A warm nose suggests that a horse has a fever and may be somewhat dehydrated. However, this is not always the case. Occasionally, a sick horse has a runny nose that is cool because of evaporation. If you suspect your horse has a fever, confirm it with a rectal temperature.

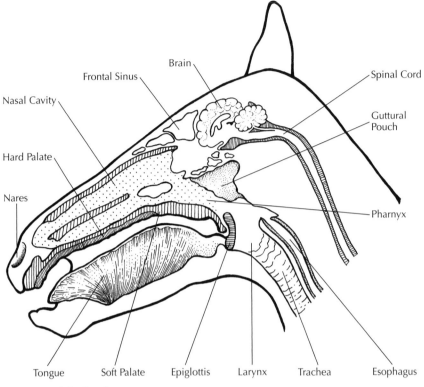

Anatomy of the head.

Six pairs of paranasal sinuses connect directly or indirectly with the nasal cavity. The frontal and maxillary sinuses are the most important because they are the most susceptible to sinus infection. In the upper jaw, the roots of the cheek teeth are imbedded in the floor of the maxillary sinuses. In young horses these roots occupy most of the space in the sinus, but as the horse matures, the roots recede and the sinuses become correspondingly larger.

At the back of the pharynx are the paired eustachian or auditory tubes that connect with the middle ear and equalize air pressure across the eardrum. Each auditory tube has a specialized out-pocket or sac called the guttural pouch. These pouches are unique to horses. Ordinarily they are not visible in the neck, but when filled with fluid or air, they can be seen as distinct bulges on each side of the neck just behind the angles of the jaws. The purpose of the guttural pouches is unknown.

Nasopharyngeal Endoscopy

Nasopharyngeal *endoscopy* has greatly simplified the diagnosis of upper respiratory diseases. In this procedure, a fiber-optic *endoscope* is passed into the nasal cavity to view the turbinates, the openings of the sinuses and the gutural pouches, the palate, the back of the throat, and the larynx. *Cultures* and biopsies can be taken with precision through the instrument. The endoscope can also be used to accurately place catheters into a sinus or guttural pouch to irrigate and infuse medications.

Bronchoscopy is an endoscopic procedure in which a long scope is passed into the trachea and down into the larger breathing passages. Bleeding may be detected in the trachea of horses with exercise-induced pulmonary hemorrhage.

Bronchoalveolar lavage (BAL) is a procedure in which sterile saline is flushed through the scope into the lower respiratory tract, and then the fluid is recovered by suctioning it through a channel in the scope.

Transtracheal aspiration involves inserting a needle through the skin of the neck into the trachea. A sterile catheter is passed through the needle into the trachea. Secretions are withdrawn through the catheter.

The secretions obtained using these methods are cultured and examined under a microscope. This assists in making an exact diagnosis and in guiding treatment. Cultures taken from the nostrils of horses are unreliable because of the many types of bacteria that normally inhabit this area. Accurate samples can only be taken during endoscopy, or your veterinarian can pass a swab or catheter into the nasal cavity to take cultures.

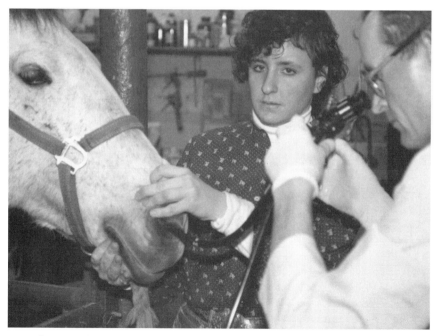

Nasopharyngeal endoscopy has greatly assisted the diagnosis and treatment of upper respiratory diseases.

Signs of Nasal Irritation

Horses don't catch colds the way people do. Human cold viruses do not affect the horse, and vice versa. However, young horses are afflicted by a number of viruses of the adenovirus/rhinovirus species that produce mild symptoms much like the human cold. Usually, they are accompanied by a cough, runny eyes, and a sore throat. Signs of a sore throat would be discomfort or reluctance to eat or drink. For more information, see *Equine Viral Respiratory Diseases*, page 84.

Nasal Discharge (Runny Nose)

A discharge that persists for more than a day indicates a disease in the nasal passages, sinuses, or guttural pouches.

Often you can tell whether a discharge is significant by observing its appearance. A watery discharge with sneezing can be due to irritants such as dust or vegetable matter trapped on the mucous membranes. Environmental allergies may occasionally produce a clear nasal discharge, but allergic reactions in horses primarily involve the skin and the gastrointestinal tract.

A mucoid discharge from both nostrils is characteristic of an equine viral respiratory disease. A thick yellow *mucopurulent* discharge from both nostrils indicates a bacterial or fungal infection. In the upper airway, the most likely sites of infection are the nasal passages, sinuses, guttural pouches, and pharynx. In the lower airway, consider pneumonia and lung *abscess*.

When you see a puslike discharge from one nostril, suspect sinusitis, guttural pouch mycosis, or a nasal foreign body, polyp, or tumor. Pharyngitis and rhinitis may produce a discharge from just one nostril. Note that in a horse with a guttural pouch infection, you can occasionally see a *purulent* discharge from both nostrils, even though only one pouch is affected.

The nasal cavity drains best when the head is down. That is why many nasal discharges, particularly those from the sinuses and guttural pouches, are most apparent after a horse has been grazing.

A horse with eye discharge often has nasal discharge. This is because the nasolacrimal ducts drain into the nose.

Sneezing

Sneezing is a reflex resulting from stimulation of the lining of the nose. When a horse sneezes off and on for a few hours but shows no other signs of illness, the sneezing may be due to minor nasal irritation. Sneezing that persists all day suggests a nasopharyngeal or respiratory tract infection.

Foreign bodies in the nose cause bouts of violent sneezing. The foreign body is almost always expelled, but the irritation caused by it may continue to cause sneezing.

If one nostril appears to be obstructed, a persistent sneezing problem may be due to a foreign body, polyp, or tumor. Check to see if there is less air coming from the nostril by holding a mirror up to the nose and checking for vapor condensation.

EPISTAXIS (NOSEBLEEDS)

Nosebleeds do not occur spontaneously in horses. The majority bleeds are due to trauma. Most other nosebleeds are related to guttural pouch mycosis and ulcerations in the nasopharynx caused by infections, polyps, tumors, and ethmoid *hematomas* (see *Nasopharyngeal Tumors*, page 292). Bleeding tends to occur intermittently, often when the horse is at rest. The blood may be mixed with a mucopurulent discharge.

Bleeding from guttural pouch mycosis can be massive and life-threatening. Major bleeds are often preceded by intermittent minor bleeds from one nostril.

Trauma to the face, especially when accompanied by a fracture of the nasal bones, is another cause of nosebleeds.

A nosebleed may be a manifestation of a clotting disorder such as hemophilia, liver disease, warfarin poisoning, or dicumarol (moldy sweet clover) poisoning. These are rare causes of nosebleed.

Exercised-induced pulmonary hemorrhage occurs commonly in racehorses. Infrequently, blood will be seen at the nostrils—suggesting a nosebleed—but the bleeding is actually in the lungs. See *Exercise-Induced Pulmonary Hemorrhage*, page 307, for more information.

The Nasopharynx
PROBLEMS WITH THE NOSTRILS

Lacerations of the nostrils sometimes result in unsupported flaps of skin that can block the airway as the horse breathes in. Failure to repair the injury often results in an obstructing flap of skin or narrowing of the nostril due to scarring. The laceration is best managed by careful suture repair at the time of injury.

Alar fold stenosis (narrowing of the opening of the nostrils) occurs occasionally in young horses. *Stenosis* can result in a fluttering noise when the horse exhales or it can cause a respiratory obstruction. It may be apparent only during exercise. When the narrowing in the nasal openings causes breathing difficulties, the folds can be removed.

Congenitally narrowed nasal passages are another uncommon condition. Horses with this disorder usually have a narrow face and exhibit noisy breathing. These horses will always have exercise intolerance.

Deviation of the nasal septum occasionally occurs as a *congenital* deformity, but most often it is caused by facial trauma or a growth in a nasal passage. The deviated part of the septum can be surgically removed. The operation is difficult and in most cases must be performed at a center that has the equipment to provide the necessary support.

RHINITIS (NASAL CAVITY INFECTION)

Rhinitis is characterized by nasal discharge with sneezing, sniffling, and noisy breathing. Most cases are associated with an equine viral respiratory disease, such as equine influenza. The nasal discharge is watery at first but soon becomes mucoid, yellow, and thick. Other signs include fever, tearing, blobs of mucus in the eyes, coughing, and lethargy.

Another cause of nasal cavity infection is strangles. Strangles is accompanied by high fever, loss of appetite, a dry and throaty cough, and swelling of lymph nodes at the angle of the jaw and the back of the throat. The discharge may be profuse and is always purulent.

A bacterial infection can become established when the nasopharynx has been weakened by a previous viral respiratory disease. Bacterial infections also spread to the nasal cavity from the paranasal sinuses and the guttural pouches. A bloody discharge indicates deep involvement with ulceration of the mucosa.

Fungus infections can invade the nasal cavity. The most common is *rhinosporidiosis*. This noncontagious disease produces flat-based or polyplike growths, usually on one side of the nose only. These growths bleed easily and occasionally grow large enough to obstruct the flow of air. They should be removed.

A foreign body in the nasal cavity produces a malodorous discharge and occasionally bleeding (or blood-tinged mucus) from one nostril. Most foreign bodies can be removed using forceps.

Treatment: The objective of treatment is to restore normal breathing, prevent or treat infection, and make the horse as comfortable as possible. Gently wipe the nostrils with moist cotton balls to remove dried crusts. Vaporizers help humidify and restore the integrity of the mucociliary blanket. They are most effective in stalls and closed areas. A purulent discharge suggests a bacterial infection and indicates the need for antibiotics.

When the discharge persists, diagnostic studies are needed to determine the cause. Fiber-optic endoscopy is the best way to examine the nasal passages, sinuses, and guttural pouches.

SINUSITIS

The paranasal sinuses connect with the nasal cavity and are lined by a mucous membrane similar to that of the nose. Therefore, nasal cavity infections, particularly those caused by *Streptococcus* bacteria, can extend to involve the sinuses. Other causes of sinusitis include abscessed teeth, tumors, and fungal infections of the sinus.

Signs of sinusitis include a purulent discharge from one side of the nose, an eye discharge, and painful swelling or deformity involving the face. Tapping over the sinus produces a dull rather than a hollow sound.

A common cause of secondary sinusitis is dental disease, found most often in middle-age horses. The roots of the upper cheek teeth are embedded in the floor of the maxillary sinuses. When one or more of these teeth become infected, the infection can invade the maxillary sinus. A particularly severe form of purulent sinusitis then ensues. In addition to a copious purulent discharge from the nose, you may notice difficulty breathing, blood in the discharge, a fetid odor, and painful chewing. An opening between the oral cavity and maxillary sinus can develop. This is called a sinus fistula. If present, you may see food or plant particles in the nasal discharge.

The diagnosis of sinusitis is made by physical examination and occasionally by sinus x-rays and fiber-optic endoscopy.

Treatment: Bacterial sinusitis following a respiratory infection is best treated by instilling a catheter into the sinus through a small hole in the bone. The sinus is flushed and irrigated at regular intervals for several days. For severe sinusitis, more than one opening may have to be made into the sinus

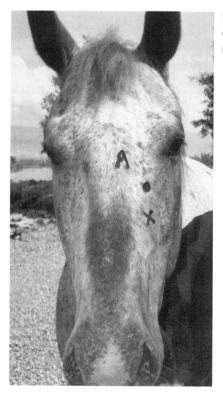

Sites used to bore through the bone to drain the frontal, frontomaxillary, and maxillary sinuses.

cavity through the face. Large volumes of fluid are flushed into and out of the sinus, which helps dilute bacteria and debris. Continuous *lavage* is carried out for two to three days. Antibiotics can be used along with flushing and drainage, but are not effective when used alone.

Abscessed teeth should be removed, as described on page 196.

Exercise and grazing help to promote drainage. Turn the horse out to pasture as soon as possible.

Paranasal Sinus Cysts

These are congenital defects resulting from abnormal development of a tooth bud. They occur most often in young, growing horses. As the cyst enlarges, it often produces a yellow nasal discharge, swelling of the face, and deviation of the nasal septum.

Treatment: Successful treatment involves removing the entire cyst.

NASOPHARYNGEAL TUMORS

Tumors of the nasopharynx interfere with airflow in the nasal passage, producing noise when the horse inhales, nasal discharge, intermittent nosebleeds, and swelling or deformity of the face. The nasal discharge may be mucoid or mucopurulent and blood-tinged.

The most common malignant tumor is squamous cell carcinoma of the nasal turbinates. The most common benign tumor is the nasal polyp. *Sarcomas* and carcinomas can arise in the paranasal sinuses and guttural pouches. Tumors of dental origin are found in the maxillary sinuses.

A condition called progressive ethmoid hematoma affects the nasal turbinates. This nonmalignant tumor is actually a growth of fibrous connective tissue and blood vessels. It usually first presents with mild nosebleeds. The tumor mass can become quite large, fill the entire nasal cavity, and become visible at the nostrils. The cause is unknown.

Treatment: Benign tumors such as polyps can be cured by simple removal. Malignant tumors, especially those that deform the face, are extensively invasive and often metastatic. Treatment usually is not effective. Ethmoid hematomas have been successfully treated with *chemotherapy*, laser treatment, and surgical removal.

The Guttural Pouches

The guttural pouches are a pair of sacs, each with just one opening. There is one on each side of the neck just in back of the angle of the jawbone. They develop as out-pockets of the eustachian or auditory tubes. Guttural pouch disease produces nasal discharge and swelling in the neck on the affected side.

The swelling may involve the area of the parotid salivary gland, which overlies the guttural pouch and extends up toward the base of the ear. Pressing on this area produces pain and the horse will often resist.

Guttural Pouch Empyema

A pouch infection with an accumulation of pus is called *empyema*. There is usually a history of exposure to an infectious respiratory illness, such as strangles. Young horses are most often affected. The principal sign is a chronic, intermittent, nonresponsive, *unilateral* nasal discharge. The discharge is purulent, often bloodstained, and may contain food particles.

A swollen guttural pouch can press on the pharynx, causing difficulty in swallowing and, in very severe cases, respiratory obstruction.

A long-standing empyema is associated with drying and hardening of pus. Over a period of time, the pus becomes molded into calcified nodules called chondroids. A pouch may contain 30 or more chondroids, some of them quite large and others the size of a small bean.

Nasopharyngeal endoscopy helps make the diagnosis and obtain pus for culture. X-rays may show fluid in the distended pouch, which is not normal.

Treatment: Pus in the guttural pouches is best drained by placing a catheter into the pouch through the nose and then irrigating the pouch at regular intervals for several days using a nonirritating saline-antibiotic solution or 1 percent Betadine. The horse's head should be lowered to facilitate drainage and prevent aspiration. For thick pus and chondroids, drainage must be done through a surgical incision in the neck, or with an endoscope. A catheter is left in place for flushing and the neck wound is left open for drainage. Horses with respiratory obstruction require an emergency tracheotomy.

Guttural Pouch Mycosis

This is a fungal infection. *Aspergillus* species are the most common fungi found in guttural pouches. Horses may acquire the fungus from eating damp, moldy hay. In addition, the guttural pouches are dark, warm, humid, and poorly ventilated. These factors favor the growth of fungus.

The most common sign of guttural pouch mycosis is a nosebleed on the affected side. It usually begins as a mild, intermittent *epistaxis*, followed in two to three weeks by a sudden, massive hemorrhage. Fungal plaques adhere to the carotid artery and its branches. These arteries pass close to or through the guttural pouches. Weakening of the arterial walls causes bleeding. When the artery finally ruptures, the horse bleeds massively through the nose. This type of hemorrhage can be fatal.

Involvement of a major nerve plexus adjacent to the guttural pouch produces a number of cranial nerve palsies (see *Cranial Nerve Paralysis*, page 343).

The most common is a paralysis of the nerves that initiate swallowing. Horses with this problem often regurgitate food and water through the nose. Horner's syndrome (drooping of the upper eyelid), paralysis of the larynx (roaring), paralysis of the facial nerve (drooping of the ear, muzzle, and lower lip), and muscle wasting (*atrophy*) of the tongue can occur. Cranial nerve palsies are associated with advanced guttural pouch disease.

Signs of middle ear involvement include head-tilt, staggering, head-shaking, and rapid eye movements.

Treatment: When the diagnosis is made before a fatal hemorrhage, tying off the offending artery in the neck can be attempted to stop the bleeding. Nasopharyngeal endoscopy is the only way to effectively examine the guttural pouch and determine which artery is causing the bleeding.

Guttural pouch mycosis is treated much like empyema (see page 293), except that drugs effective against fungi are used in the irrigating solution. Surgical drainage usually produces better results than medical management, although the outlook for cure is guarded with all forms of treatment. Occasionally, a horse with mycosis improves spontaneously.

TYMPANY OF THE GUTTURAL POUCH

Guttural pouch tympany, or "bullfrog" disease, is a condition in which the pouches become distended with air. It occurs in *foals* from birth to 18 months of age. An abnormal flap of mucosa over the pharyngeal opening of the eustachian tube causes a build-up of pressure as the one-way valve traps air in the pouch. The result is a soft, balloonlike swelling in the neck extending from the base of the ear to the angle of the jaw.

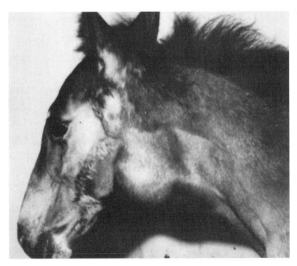

This horse shows the ballooned-out guttural pouch of tympany.

This does not seem to bother most foals, but the guttural pouch may progressively enlarge to the extent that it narrows the pharynx. This can interfere with swallowing and even cause respiratory distress.

Treatment: The pouch can be deflated by passing a catheter into the auditory tube or using a needle inserted through the neck. These measures are temporary; the pouch rapidly refills. They are necessary to relieve an acute pharyngeal obstruction.

Tympany may temporarily correct spontaneously, but it is usually necessary to surgically remove the obstructing flap and drain the pouch externally through the neck.

The Soft Palate and Epiglottis

The soft palate is a flap of tissue at the back of the pharynx. In its normal position the soft palate is down, which seals off the oral airway and opens up the nasal airway. Because horses are obligate nose-breathers, the soft palate is always down except when the horse swallows. As the horse swallows, the epiglottis flips over the trachea like a lid, preventing food from entering the lungs.

The relationship between the positions of the soft palate and the epiglottis is important. In the normal relationship, the epiglottis is dorsal to (behind) the palate, as shown in the illustration *Anatomy of the Head* (page 286).

There are certain disorders in which the soft palate and the epiglottis produce respiratory symptoms that interfere with athletic performance. These include swelling of the palate from pharyngeal lymphoid hyperplasia, dorsal displacement of the soft palate, paralysis of the nerves to the palate, epiglottic entrapment, and pharyngeal cysts.

DORSAL DISPLACEMENT OF THE SOFT PALATE

In a horse with this problem, the normal relationship between the soft palate and the epiglottis is reversed: the epiglottis is in front of, rather than behind, the soft palate. This displacement causes a narrowing in the diameter of the nasopharyngeal airway. The displacement is intermittent and usually occurs with forced breathing. There are a number of muscular, developmental, and neurological causes of dorsal displacement. In some horses, the cause is unknown.

Symptoms of displacement usually occur during exercise as the horse reaches high speeds. The horse has sudden difficulty breathing, drops his speed, and produces a gurgling noise referred to as "choking down." The diagnosis is confirmed by nasopharyngeal endoscopy and lateral x-rays of the head.

Treatment: There are various surgical options; all involve removing a part of the palate and dividing the muscles that raise the larynx during strenuous exercise. The choice depends on what is thought to be the cause of the displacement. When the appropriate surgery is done, the outlook for athletic performance is good.

Epiglottic Entrapment

In a horse with this condition, mucosal folds surrounding the epiglottis become excessively large, creating a mass that envelops the epiglottis and narrows the airway. Some cases are associated with a hypoplastic epiglottis (an epiglottis that is smaller or less well developed than normal). Although not common, epiglottic entrapment occurs most often in Standardbred and Thoroughbred horses.

As a consequence of the narrowed airway, affected horses are exercise-intolerant, breathe noisily, and cough during exercise or after eating. Nasopharyngeal endoscopy reveals redundant folds, often swollen and ulcerated, obscuring the view of the epiglottis.

Treatment: Treatment involves surgically removing the redundant mucosal folds. Complications include recurrent entrapment (when too little tissue is removed) and dorsal displacement (when too much tissue is removed). A horse with a hypoplastic epiglottis presents a special problem and has a poor *prognosis* for athletic performance.

Pharyngeal Cysts

These noncancerous growths arise from the back of the pharynx. They are relatively uncommon and are seen most often in 2- to 3-year-old racehorses. Signs are similar to those of a soft palate disorder. Diagnosis is by nasopharyngeal endoscopy.

Treatment: Pharyngeal cysts can be removed surgically.

The Throat

Horses do not have tonsils. However, they do have aggregates of lymphoid tissues scattered over the back of the pharynx. These lymphoid *follicles* are well developed and prominent in young horses, but usually regress and disappear at 3 to 4 years of age.

Pharyngitis (Sore Throat)
Acute Pharyngitis

Sore throats are associated with respiratory infections such as strangles, rhinopneumonitis, and equine influenza. The throat appears red and inflamed. A purulent discharge coats the back of the pharynx. Other symptoms include fever, noisy respirations, coughing, gagging, pain in the throat on swallowing, and loss of appetite. Enlarged lymph nodes may be felt beneath the angles of the jaws.

Treatment: Anti-inflammatory drugs relieve pain and encourage the horse to eat. Provide a soft diet, or better yet, turn the horse out onto fresh green pasture. Antibiotics, alone or in combination with corticosteroids, are often sprayed three times a day on the back of the throat through a nasopharyngeal catheter. The effectiveness of this treatment should be evaluated by the response of the individual horse.

Frequent vaccination with respiratory virus vaccines (every four to six months) may prevent some episodes of pharyngitis.

Pharyngeal Lymphoid Hyperplasia

In a horse with this condition, the lymphatic tissue at the back of the pharynx becomes quite large and diminishes the size of the nasopharyngeal airway. This can cause varying degrees of airway obstruction. Signs include decreased exercise tolerance, a blowing sound when the horse becomes slightly winded, and a chronic cough—especially at the start or finish of a workout.

One complication of chronic lymphoid hyperplasia is guttural pouch tympany (see page 294). The tympany may be caused by a blockage of the auditory tube from enlarged follicles.

Lymphoid hyperplasia tends to affect racehorses 2 to 3 years of age. Exposure to one of the equine respiratory viruses often precedes the hyperplasia. Exposure to air pollutants found around racetracks is another predisposing factor.

If the diagnosis is uncertain and there is a question of lymphoma, nasopharyngeal endoscopy with biopsy of a follicle will clarify the diagnosis. Chronic lymphoid hyperplasia usually resolves spontaneously by 3 years of age.

Treatment: Ideally, the horse should be rested for at least two months to allow swollen follicles to get smaller. If rest is not feasible, the horse can be placed on a broad-spectrum antibiotic and treated with nonsteroidal anti-inflammatory medications and topical steroids. If the horse is still unable to return to training and competition, the obstructing lymphoid tissue can be removed by cryosurgery, laser surgery, or electrocautery. General anesthesia is required.

Early recognition of pharyngeal hyperplasia, combined with frequent vaccination with influenza and rhinopneumonitis vaccines (every four to six months), may alter the course of the disease for the better and even prevent recurrences.

The Larynx

The larynx, sometimes called the voice box, is an oblong box situated between the nasopharynx and trachea. It is composed of a number of cartilages, including the paired arytenoids. Within the larynx are the two vocal cords that open and close the airway. The vocal cords and the muscles of the larynx are supplied by the two recurrent laryngeal nerves.

At the top of the larynx is the epiglottis, a leaflike flap that covers it during swallowing, thus preventing food from going down the trachea. The larynx is the most sensitive cough area in the respiratory system.

Laryngitis

Laryngitis is inflammation of the larynx. It frequently follows respiratory infections that are complicated by a chronic or persistent cough. Other causes include smoke inhalation and foreign bodies in the larynx.

Signs of laryngitis include a persistent, harsh cough that is initially dry but later becomes soft and moist. There may be a nasal discharge. Swallowing can be difficult and painful.

Laryngeal *edema* is a condition in which the vocal cords and laryngeal cartilages become fluid-filled and swollen. The resultant narrowing of the airway produces a croupy sound, or *stridor*, as the horse breathes in. In its most severe form, laryngeal edema results in complete airway obstruction and death from asphyxiation.

Treatment: The cough is best treated by confining the horse in a warm, dry enclosure and humidifying the atmosphere. Offer a soft or liquid diet. Laryngeal edema requires urgent treatment, including intravenous corticosteroids. The airway must be kept open. This may require the veterinarian to insert an endotracheal tube or perform an emergency tracheotomy.

Laryngeal Hemiplegia (Vocal Cord Paralysis, Roaring)

Roaring is a common laryngeal problem. It is due to paralysis of one of the recurrent laryngeal nerves (nearly always the left one). When one nerve is inoperative, the vocal cord on that side becomes paralyzed and does not retract to open the larynx as the horse breathes in or out. The resultant narrowing of the air passage is responsible for the characteristic roaring or whistling sound that begins as the horse is exercised. In addition, the horse performs poorly and seems unfit. The degree of nerve paralysis may vary, producing a range of disability.

Evidence suggests that some cases of vocal cord paralysis are due to a degenerative process affecting the recurrent laryngeal nerves. This paralysis is most likely an inherited trait. Less common causes include direct trauma to the laryngeal nerve, accidental injection of irritating substances (such as a phenylbutazone shot) around a blood vessel, and plant and chemical intoxications. All breeds may be affected, but there is a higher prevalence among males and among long-necked and larger breeds. The principle clinical signs of laryngeal hemiplegia are noise upon inhalation during exercise and exercise intolerance. The horse will have an unusual whinny due to the paralyzed larynx, but will be asymptomatic at rest.

Fiber-optic endoscopy will reveal a cord that does not open as the horse breathes in. In addition, endoscopy helps to exclude other causes of roaring, such as laryngitis, arytenoid chondritis, and dorsal displacement of the soft palate.

Treatment: If the condition interferes with the horse's utility, larynx surgery can be considered. There are different procedures. Results vary and complications can occur. Athletic performance will improve, but the horse is unlikely to fulfill her potential.

ARYTENOID CHONDRITIS

Inflammation of one of the paired arytenoid cartilages (chondritis) results in progressive enlargement and distortion of the cartilage, eventually leading to partial obstruction of the larynx and symptoms of roaring (see page 298).

Arytenoid chondritis usually occurs in young racehorses, but it has been observed in other horses. It usually involves only one side. The cause is unknown.

Treatment: Medical treatment has not been successful. However, many horses with mild disease are able to perform satisfactorily if strenuous exercise is not required. Surgical removal of the affected cartilage can be considered for horses in whom obstruction interferes with athletic fitness. The postoperative complication rate is high. About 50 percent of such horses can return to full athletic performance.

The Lower Respiratory System

The lower respiratory system is made up of the trachea or windpipe and the lungs, which contain the bronchi (large airways), the bronchioles (small airways), and the alveoli. As the airways branch, they become progressively smaller until they open into the air sacs. It is here that air exchanges with the blood. The ribs and muscles of the chest, along with the diaphragm, function as a bellows, moving air into and out of the lungs.

A horse at rest takes about 10 to 30 breaths per minute. Determine the breathing rate by observing and counting the movements of the nostrils or flanks. The respiratory motion should be smooth, even, and unrestricted. Abnormal breathing patterns are discussed in this section.

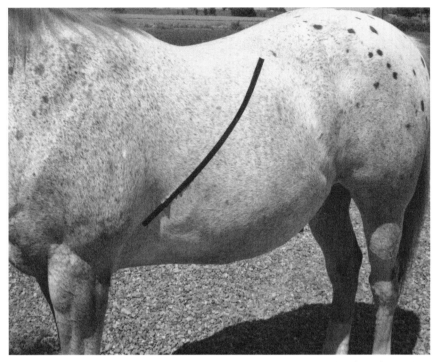

The tape shows the position of the diaphragm, which separates the chest from the abdomen.

Dyspnea

Dyspnea is rapid, labored breathing. It can be caused by fear, pain, fever, shock, or dehydration. A horse who is winded after exercise may be unfit and out of condition. In the absence of exercise, a rate of 30 breaths per minute or greater indicates a serious problem.

A horse with severe dyspnea stands with her feet spread apart, neck stretched out, and head extended. You may see flaring of the nostrils and an anxious expression, with protruding eyeballs. Movement of the chest wall is exaggerated and the flanks heave.

Dyspnea is associated with shock and *sepsis*, heart failure, pneumonia, fluid in the lungs, overexertion, and recurrent airway obstruction (RAO). Cyanosis is the condition in which the blood turns blue because of inadequate oxygen. The bluish discoloration can be seen in the mucous membranes of the mouth, lips, and conjunctiva. This is a grave sign in horses.

Broken wind occurs in horses with RAO and long-standing airway disease affecting the bronchioles. You will observe a prolonged phase of expiration, followed by a second effort to exhale in which the horse contracts her abdominal muscles to squeeze the remaining air out of the lungs. This is often accompanied by wheezing.

NOISY BREATHING

Abnormal breathing sounds are most apparent when the horse inhales, but may also be heard when she exhales.

Whistling and roaring are produced by air flowing through an abnormally narrow passage in the nasopharynx. Whistling is a high-pitched sound. Roaring is a deep sound and indicates a greater degree of obstruction. The most common causes of both are vocal cord paralysis and displacements of the soft palate.

Blowing occurs on both inhalation and exhalation. It can be caused by pulling back too forcefully on the bit, which arches the horse's neck and narrows the cross-sectional diameter of the pharynx. A persistent blowing noise at rest, or at the beginning of exercise, suggests a growth or some other partial blockage in the nasopharynx, larynx, or trachea.

Thick wind is a temporary form of blowing that occurs in out-of-condition horses. It disappears as the horse's fitness improves.

Trumpeting or high blowing is an expiratory noise that occurs in fresh, high-spirited horses at the outset of exercise. It is caused by flapping of the nasal folds and is of no consequence.

Wheezing is a whistling, sometimes musical sound heard over the trachea and lungs. It indicates narrowing of the airways from spasm or bronchoconstriction. Wheezes are characteristic of acute bronchitis and recurrent airway obstruction.

Crackling and bubbling are heard with a stethoscope over the lungs. These sounds are usually present in a horse with pneumonia or congestive heart failure.

SPLINTING (SHALLOW BREATHING)

Splinting is a guarded effort to avoid the pain of a deep breath. To compensate, the horse breathes more rapidly but less deeply. The pain of pleurisy and rib fracture causes splinting. Fluid in the chest (blood, pus, serum) will produce shallow breathing, but without pain.

COUGHING

A cough is a reflex produced by an irritation of the airways. Coughs are caused by infectious diseases, smoke and other inhaled irritants, grass seeds, and foreign objects in the airway. Upper airway coughs include those caused by acute respiratory infections, pharyngitis, guttural pouch infections, sinusitis, and soft palate disorders. Lower airway coughs include those caused by acute bronchitis, RAO, pneumonia, pleuritis, and pleural effusion. Lungworms and the larvae of ascarids also produce bouts of lower airway coughing.

A cough accompanied by fever, sneezing, noisy breathing, and nasal or eye discharge is a sign of a infectious respiratory disease.

The circumstances surrounding a cough may suggest its cause. A cough that occurs when the horse is stabled is most likely caused by dust or some other inhaled atmospheric irritant. When it occurs after drinking, it may be due to sinusitis, guttural pouch disease, or leakage of fluid into the trachea from faulty closure of the epiglottis.

Coughs can be strong and forceful or weak and soft. Loud, harsh, nonproductive coughs are indicative of upper airway disease and are commonly caused by acute respiratory illnesses such as equine influenza, sore throat, guttural pouch disease, and laryngitis. Moist, weak coughs are heard in horses with advanced RAO. Soft, painful coughs are heard in horses with pleuritis, rib fractures, and acute pleuropneumonia.

Moist coughs suggest active infection in the lower respiratory system, particularly pneumonia. They occur whenever mucus accumulates in the airways. The mucus or phlegm coughed up may contain blood. If the blood appears in streaks, it probably originates somewhere in the upper respiratory tract. The phlegm of a horse with pneumonia is homogeneous in color and red or reddish-brown.

Coughs are self-perpetuating. Coughing, by itself, irritates the airways, dries out the mucous lining, and lowers resistance to infection. This leads to further coughing.

Treatment: Minor coughs of brief duration are best treated by removing the horse from the source of the irritant. Smoke, aerosol insecticides, stable dust, and mold should be eliminated from stables and barns, as discussed in the treatment of RAO (see page 304). Barns and stables should be open and well ventilated. Closing a stable to keep the horse warm is not a good practice, because it invariably increases atmospheric pollutants.

Except in unusual circumstances, cough suppressants should not be given to horses because the cough is important in eliminating infected secretions from the airways. Mucous thinners (mucolytics) and expectorants can be of value if the mucus is thick and difficult to cough up. Your veterinarian can suggest an appropriate medication. Bronchodilators such as clenbuterol may aid in eliminating mucus.

If a cough persists for more than two days, something is wrong in the respiratory tract. Consult your veterinarian. It is important to diagnose and treat the cause of a persistent cough. Fiber-optic bronchoscopy is the best and most productive test for investigating airway disease. It is indicated for a horse with a persistent cough for which the cause is not apparent on physical examination or chest x-ray.

Bronchitis

Inflammation of the bronchi is called *bronchitis*. It is characterized by repeated coughing, often precipitated by cold air and vigorous exercise. The coughing further irritates the lining of the trachea. For this reason, the term *tracheo-bronchitis* may be more accurate.

Acute bronchitis occurs with equine viral respiratory infections and strangles. After the acute infection, the cough may persist for two to three weeks and then should disappear. However, if the problem is complicated by a secondary bacterial infection, the cough persists much longer. In time, the inflammation may involve the bronchioles, at which point it becomes recurrent airway obstruction (below).

Other causes of acute bronchitis include inhaling smoke, irritant fumes, and industrial pollutants. Using an artificial airway during general anesthesia may irritate the air passages and produce postoperative bronchitis.

Chronic bronchitis is not a specific diagnosis in equine practice. A chronic cough is considered part of the RAO syndrome.

Treatment: Treat the cough as described in *Coughing* (page 301). It is important to restrict exercise in horses with bronchitis.

RECURRENT AIRWAY OBSTRUCTION (HEAVES)

Recurrent airway obstruction (RAO), commonly known as heaves, sometimes erroneously referred to as emphysema, is a common but easily preventable respiratory ailment in horses. The main feature of RAO is obstruction of the bronchioles, leading to chronic cough, shortness of breath, and exercise intolerance. The obstruction is reversible until scarring in the airways results in permanent damage. The obstruction can be caused by plugs of mucus and debris in the lower airway, or it may take the form of bronchospasm (constriction of the muscles controlling the bronchi) and wheezing. Inflammation and spasm of the bronchioles is called bronchiolitis.

A common cause of RAO is repeated exposure to molds and fungus spores in hay and straw present in barns and stables, and particularly in the horse's bedding. Dust, ammonia, smoke, and other environmental irritants are contributory factors. Exposure to these airborne irritants triggers attacks of coughing, often asthmaticlike and accompanied by wheezing. These attacks are believed to be an allergic or hypersensitivity reaction to the inhaled substance. RAO often follows an acute respiratory illness that impairs the horse's ability to clear airborne pollutants from the respiratory system.

A seasonal allergy appears to be caused by airborne pollens.

Horses mildly affected with RAO breathe normally at rest but become short of breath with exercise. Coughing is intermittent, usually when the horse is exposed to dust or cold. The cough is dry and unproductive. With continued exposure to the respiratory irritant, the horse coughs more frequently, especially after exercise and feeding. The cough becomes productive and may be accompanied by nasal discharge. Exercise tolerance becomes limited.

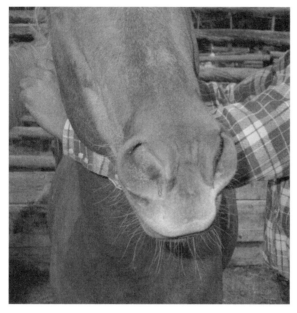

The flared nostrils, shortness of breath, and clear nasal discharge of a horse with heaves (advanced RAO).

In the late stages (known as heaves), there is chronic infection and scarring in the lower airways. The cough is soft and moist and accompanied by wheezing, increased respiratory rate at rest, weight loss, flared nostrils, and a prolonged double phase of exhalation. The abdominal wall muscles are used to assist in exhalation, since the lung tissue has lost much of its elasticity. As the abdominal muscles become strongly developed, you will see a "heave line," which is a ridge of muscle running obliquely down the middle of the flank over the rib cage toward the back of the elbow. Horses with heaves are severely restricted in their ability to exercise and may become short of breath just walking across a paddock.

Early diagnosis is essential to prevent the disease from reaching an irreversible state. Transtracheal aspiration will show inflammatory cells typical of RAO. Bacterial infection is usually absent. When present, it indicates secondary bacterial involvement or pneumonia. Fiber-optic endoscopy is useful in distinguishing upper airway diseases from RAO.

Lungworm infection may mimic RAO and should be excluded as the cause of a chronic cough.

Treatment: Bronchospasm is a major problem. A bronchodilator drug can be administered during an acute attack; if the wheezing clears and breathing is easier, continued use may be indicated. Bronchodilators are usually given for short periods while adjustments are made in the horse's environment. This is the most important treatment in helping prevent future occurrences and making sure the condition does not become chronic.

A mask inhaler system, or *nebulizer*, has been developed for horses that enables metered-dose bronchodilators and other drugs to be delivered quickly and effectively directly to the airways. Sodium cromoglycate, administered by nebulizer, is effective when environmental control is genuinely impossible. Corticosteroids are used to reduce the inflammatory response in a particularly severe attack, and are often the most common treatment. These drugs should be prescribed by your veterinarian. Clenbuterol (a decongestant and bronchodilator) is effective when given orally twice a day.

Mucolytics and expectorants loosen secretions and clear the airways. A vaporizer also serves this purpose. Antibiotics selected based on culture and sensitivity tests are indicated for acute infectious relapses. A full course should be given to prevent the emergence of resistant bacteria.

The vast majority of horses with mild to moderate RAO can be managed with proper treatment and remain asymptomatic. The most important step in treating (and preventing) RAO is to provide fresh air and a dust-free environment.

- Keep horses on pasture or in open paddocks and out of barns and stables whenever possible.
- Use peat, shredded paper, or wood shavings for bedding; avoid hay and straw.
- Remove dust, cobwebs, and loose feed from indoor enclosures. Barns and stables should be kept open and well-ventilated. Stalls should be cleaned and the bedding changed every day. A heated stable that will not be open to cross-ventilation should have a ventilating fan with a capacity of 100 cubic feet (2.83 cubic meters) per adult horse. In cold weather, only a quarter of the capacity of the fan is required. Closing a barn to keep horses warm is not a good practice.
- Horses should be stalled in well-ventilated boxes with the top door open.
- The concentration of fine particles in the air is highest when a stall is being cleaned and bedded. At such times, move the horse outside.
- Feed hay flakes in hay nets; soak the flakes for a few minutes until wet to reduce dust. It should be noted that large, round bales of hay are more likely to contain high levels of mold spores due to the method of storage. A round bale will not pose a hazard if it is stored in a dry place and you only feed as much as your horse will eat in one feeding.
- Fungal spores can be present even in the best-quality hay. Consider switching a horse with RAO to pelleted feeds, hay cubes, or wafers.
- Harvesting hay at higher than usual moisture content and preserving the hay with organic materials, such as a mixture of propionic and acetic acids, will reduce dust in the hay.
- Cold, dry weather and hot, humid weather may trigger flare-ups.

Pneumonia

Pneumonia is an infection of the lungs. Usually it is classified according to its cause: viral, bacterial, fungal, parasitic, or aspiration.

Bacterial pneumonia usually occurs after one of the equine viral respiratory infections. The most common causative bacteria is *Streptococcus zooepidemicus*, but numerous species can cause pneumonia. Individuals most likely to be affected are stressed horses (such as horses who are transported long distances), old horses, horses who are malnourished and debilitated, and very young foals. Foal pneumonia is discussed on page 554.

The general signs of pneumonia are a *productive cough*, high fever, purulent nasal discharge, loss of appetite and weight, and shortness of breath. On listening to the chest with a stethoscope, one can often hear moist, crackling breath sounds or rattling and bubbling noises. The absence of lung sounds is also abnormal. Transtracheal aspiration is used to obtain infected secretions for culture and sensitivity testing. An ultrasound of the chest confirms the diagnosis and may be needed to look for lung abscesses and pleural effusion (below).

Treatment: Veterinary attention is required. Move the horse to warm, dry quarters. Humidify the air. Provide plenty of fresh water. Maintain hydration, since this is critical in liquefying secretions so the horse can clear them from the respiratory tract. Do not use cough suppressants, because coughing helps to clear the airways. Bronchodilators and plain expectorants may be beneficial if the horse has labored breathing.

Intravenous or intramuscular antibiotics are used to treat bacterial pneumonia, and are often used *prophylactically* in cases of viral pneumonia to prevent secondary bacterial infection. An antibiotic may be started while awaiting the results of antibiotic sensitivity tests. Your veterinarian will prescribe the most effective antibiotic treatment for the bacteria present. The chosen antibiotic is usually continued for at least one to two months to prevent the secondary complications of lung abscess and pleural effusion.

Immune stimulants such as EqStim are available as an adjunctive treatment and may decrease recovery time and protect against relapses. After recovering from pneumonia, a horse should be rested for at least three weeks.

Pleuritis and Pleural Effusion

Pleuritis is a painful inflammation of the *pleura*—the membrane that lines the inside of the chest cavity. Infection of this membrane results in fluid accumulation in the space between the lungs and the ribs. This is called *pleural effusion*.

Pleuritis and pleural effusion develop as a complication of pneumonia or lung abscess, or as a result of congestive heart failure. Rapid, shallow breathing and splinting in a horse with a cough suggests pleuritis. A characteristic grunting sound may be heard with each breath, and the horse may stand with her elbows turned away from her body. As fluid accumulates in the pleural space, breath sounds heard with a stethoscope will become diminished or absent over the lower part of the chest. Ultrasound examination of the chest is of great assistance in determining the amount of fluid accumulation, as well as its composition and exact location.

Acute pleuropneumonia is a particularly severe form of pleuritis, accompanied by pneumonia. A primary form occurs in racehorses and horses undergoing the stress of shipping. When a horse is carried in a trailer, she cannot lower her head to clear mucus from the nasopharynx. Horses with nasopharyngeal and/or guttural pouch infections are quite likely to aspirate fluid, food or water under these circumstances and infect both pleural spaces.

Signs are like those of pleuritis, except that the respiratory distress is usually more severe and you may also see colic, tying-up syndrome, and swelling of the limbs or lower chest. The pleural fluid may be brown and foul-smelling, which indicates an *anaerobic* bacterial infection. In this situation the outlook is guarded.

Treatment: It is like that described for pneumonia (see page 306). Long-term antibiotics are administered, selected based on culture and sensitivity reports. An antibiotic effective against anaerobic bacteria is often required. Furosemide may be prescribed for a horse with pleural effusion due to heart failure (see *Heart Failure*, page 319, for more information).

A large pleural effusion should be removed by your veterinarian using thoracentesis. In this procedure, a catheter is placed into the pleural space through a large-bore needle inserted between the ribs. The needle is removed, leaving the catheter in place for drainage. A horse will exhibit marked improvement in breathing after the removal of a large pleural effusion. Fluid is submitted to the laboratory for diagnostic tests.

For prolonged drainage, the catheter is exchanged for a large-bore chest tube or a one-way flutter valve. These devices can be left in place for weeks. On occasion, a window must be made in the ribcage to remove thick, tenacious pus.

Maintain nutrition and rest the horse until she is fully recovered and back to a normal weight. Pain control is very important.

EXERCISE-INDUCED PULMONARY HEMORRHAGE (BLEEDERS)

Exercise-induced pulmonary hemorrhage (EIPH) is defined as bleeding from the lungs during intense exercise. It is common among all equine athletes, historically associated with racing Thoroughbreds. The importance of EIPH is related to its possible *etiology* as a cause for poor athletic performance. Today's equine athletes face the challenge of staying sound: lameness is the most significant problem, followed by exercise-induced pulmonary hemorrhage.

An example of bleeders would be the horse who performs well in the first three-fourths of the race but falls off markedly toward the end. The horse coughs and repeatedly swallows (blood is being swallowed), cools out slowly, and exhibits respiratory difficulty with rapid, labored breathing. Bleeding through the nostrils (epistaxis) is observed in 5 percent of racehorses either immediately after the race or when the horse returns to her stall and lowers her head.

Studies of the airways of racehorses shortly after maximal exercise using endoscopy reveal blood in the trachea in the majority of horses. The amount of bleeding varies a great deal. In some horses, the amount of blood in the airways is extensive and may actually cause the horse to choke. In the majority of horses, bleeding is relatively mild but is serious enough to affect performance.

As horses are expected to perform competitively at higher and higher levels, EIPH is being recognized with greater frequency. Event horses are being diagnosed more frequently with EIPH, but any equine athlete performing at an intense level is susceptible to pulmonary hemorrhage.

The exact mechanism by which bleeding occurs in EIPH is a matter of debate. A great deal of research is ongoing, due to the significance of this debilitating condition. There doesn't seem to be one single cause, but multiple factors contribute. Any lung disease that causes inflammation, such as infection, allergy, or RAO, will increase the blood flow with a decrease in airway size. Lung tissue is irritated and small blood vessels may then rupture during exercise. A horse's fitness level may also contribute to the development of EIPH: overexertion may lead to circulatory stress with elevated blood pressure. Some research suggests EIPH results from failure of the pulmonary system to accommodate a massive increase in cardiac output to meet the demands of high-intensity exercise. Eventually, research may also show that there is a genetic link, contributing to weaker pulmonary blood vessels.

The diagnosis of EIPH is made by fiber-optic bronchoscopy for observation of blood in the airways 30 to 90 minutes after exercise. The presence of blood in the upper airway may be due to other conditions, especially gutteral pouch mycosis (see page 293) and ethmoid hematoma (see *Nasopharyngeal Tumors*, page 292), which present similar symptoms. If the horse cannot be examined after exercise, a cytologic examination of bronchoalveolar lavage fluid (a cellular examination of lung washings) can be stained for diagnosis. A chest x-ray is not useful in the diagnosis or management of EIPH.

Treatment: Pulmonary hemorrhage cannot be prevented by the diuretic furosemide, but it has been proven to reduce the severity by 70 percent and improve race performance. Horses with and without EIPH demonstrate improvements in race performance with furosemide, indicating that the drug may enhance performance due to mechanisms unrelated to EIPH. It is important to note that while furosemide is legal for horses racing in the United States and Canada, it is illegal in most other countries. There is a withdrawal period prior to other sanctioned athletic events.

Nasal dilator bands have been studied on horses running on a treadmill and show a 33 percent reduction of blood in the bronchoalveolar fluid. Alternative treatments, including procoagulant agents (such as vitamin K and conjugated estrogens,), antihypertensive drugs, bronchodilators, prolonged rest, dietary supplements, and anti-inflammatory drugs, have not been shown to have any therapeutic benefit for exercise-induced pulmonary hemorrhage.

Inhalation therapy with a nebulizer may help manage the disease.

Prevention: There is no proven way to prevent EIPH, but you can help your horse by maintaining healthy lungs and keeping her free from infection and any allergic inflammatory disease. Proper conditioning and preparation for any athletic endeavor will also improve her chances of not developing EIPH. Some researchers have suggested boosting the immune system with products such as Equistim and Equimune to help the lungs fight off any *subclinical* infections before they can cause damage.

AMMONIA TOXICITY

Ammonia gas, released from urine and manure in bedding, can be a problem in poorly ventilated barns and stalls. Ammonia is an irritant that destroys the natural defense mechanisms of the mucus that protect the respiratory tract and thereby, decreases the immune response.

Neonatal and young foals are more susceptible to ammonia toxicity than older horses because of their immature respiratory tracts, and because they are closer to the source of gas. However, chronically exposed individuals, whether young or old, run the risk of developing pneumonia.

Treatment: Once you are able to smell ammonia in the stall, the gas is already present in harmful concentrations. Move the horse to a well-ventilated area. If the horse exhibits symptoms such as eye, nose, and throat irritation, coughing, bronchospasm, or, with severe cases, *pulmonary edema*, treat for cough (see page 302) or pneumonia (see page 306). Ammonia is also corrosive to the skin, eyes, and gastrointestinal tract.

Prevention: Ammonia cannot be completely eliminated from the barn, but you can limit your horse's exposure with good management practices.

- Do not overfeed protein. Consult an equine nutritionist to eliminate unnecessary protein, which leads to excess urine production.
- Limit stall time. The fresh air limits ammonia exposure and free movement enhances your horse's quality of life.
- Provide ample ventilation.
- Bedding should be changed daily, especially in winter months when stables and barns are often closed.
- Choose absorbent bedding and an ammonia-neutralizing agent. However, be aware that some neutralizers, such as lime, carry their own risks.

11

THE CARDIOVASCULAR SYSTEM

The cardiovascular system of the horse is made up of the heart (a blood pump); the blood vessels, which consist of arteries (blood distribution), the capillary beds (oxygen exchange), and the veins (to return blood to the heart); and of course, blood (to carry oxygen to the tissues). An adult horse weighing 1,000 pounds (454 kg) has about 3,500 cc (35 cc per pound) of blood within his circulatory system, or about 9 gallons (34 l).

The heart is a pump made up of four chambers: the left and right atriums act as receiving chambers, and the left and right ventricles pump the blood. The heart is divided left from right by a wall of muscle called the septum, and has four valves that keep the blood flowing in one direction. A horse's heart is about the size of a large melon and weighs approximately 10 pounds (4.5 kg).

Blood enters the heart through two large veins, the anterior and posterior vena cava, emptying oxygen-poor blood from the body into the right atrium. It then flows through the open tricuspid valve into the right ventricle. When the right ventricle is full, the tricuspid valve shuts, preventing blood from flowing backward into the atrium while the right ventricle contracts.

Blood leaves the right ventricle through the pulmonic valve, and flows into the pulmonary artery. The pulmonary artery branches into smaller vessels and finally into capillaries around the air sacs or alveoli in the lungs. Oxygen passes through the walls of the capillaries and into the blood. At the same time, carbon dioxide, a waste product of metabolism, passes from the blood into the alveoli, and leaves the body when the horse exhales.

The oxygenated blood flows through the pulmonary veins to the left atrium. It then is pumped through the open mitral valve into the left ventricle.

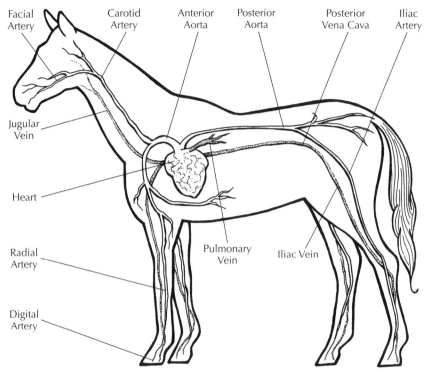

The cardiovascular system.

When the left ventricle is full, the mitral valve shuts, preventing blood from flowing backward into the atrium while the left ventricle contracts.

Blood then leaves the left ventricle through the aortic valve, flowing into the aorta. It passes through progressively smaller arteries until it reaches the capillary beds of the skin, muscle, brain, and internal organs. At these end locations, oxygen and nutrients are released and carbon dioxide and other waste products are collected. Blood is carried back to the heart through progressively larger veins, thus completing the cycle.

The arteries and veins are under the control of the nervous system and of the hormones. They can expand or contract to maintain a stable blood pressure.

The heart has its own internal electrical system that controls the rate and force of contraction. This system is responsive to outside influences, so the heart speeds up when the horse exercises, becomes excited or frightened, overheats, goes into shock, runs a fever, or requires greater blood flow to tissues. Heart rhythms follow a fixed pattern that can be seen on an electrocardiogram (EKG or ECG). Whether the beat is fast or slow, the sequence in which the various muscle fibers contract remains the same. This sequence causes a synchronized beat, allowing both ventricles to empty at the same time.

If the heart rate is very slow, this is called bradycardia. If the heart rate is too fast, this is called tachycardia. When the rate is so fast that the normal sequence of contraction is disturbed, the condition is called fibrillation. *Arrhythmia*, an absence of a regular rhythm, upsets the normal pattern of the heart muscle contraction, causing inefficient pump action.

Horses rarely have heart attacks. Common human conditions such as degenerative heart disease and cardiac *myopathies* almost never occur in horses. If they do, they are usually secondary to a preventable problem such as parasites. That being said, there are certain conditions and diseases of the heart that are seen in horses and that are important for horse owners to understand.

Evaluating the Circulation

There are certain physical signs that help to determine whether a horse's heart and circulation are working properly. Among the most useful exams that you can do yourself are taking the pulse, checking the capillary refill time, and looking for edema. Familiarize yourself with normal findings so you can recognize abnormal signs if they appear. Loss of condition, increased fatigue during exertion, shortness of breath, and increased rate of effort in breathing are other signs of heart problems in the horse that you should be aware of.

PULSE

The pulse, which is a reflection of the heart rate, can be taken at any spot in the horse's body where a large artery is located just beneath the skin. A convenient place to take the pulse is where the external maxillary artery crosses the lower border of the jawbone. To locate this pulse, press lightly with the balls of your fingers as shown in the photo on page 313. The pulse is easiest to locate after the horse has exercised.

The radial pulse is taken at the inside back of the knee. The knee of the horse corresponds to the wrist in people. Thus, taking the pulse here is like taking the wrist pulse in a person.

The digital pulse is taken just below the fetlock at the inside of the ankle. Feel for the pulse by firmly pressing with your thumb and fingers in the grooves between the pastern bones and the flexor tendons. Normally, the digital pulse is barely detectable; however, it will be strong and pounding in a horse with acute laminitis.

Another way to count the pulse is to feel the beat of the heart itself. Place your hand on the left side of the horse's chest just above the point of the elbow. If the horse is not fat, you should be able to feel the impact of the heart with each contraction.

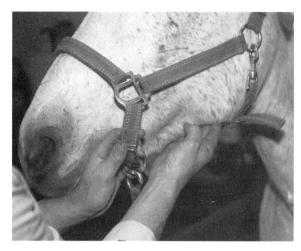

Taking the jaw pulse. With the first two fingers, feel along the inside of the jawbone just below the heavy muscles of the cheek.

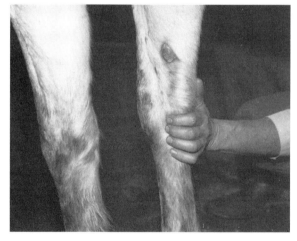

The radial pulse can be taken at the inside back of the knee.

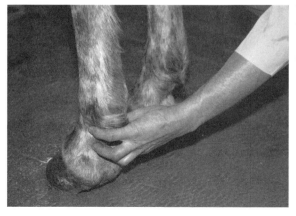

The digital pulse can be felt on the inside, just below the fetlock. The digital pulse is pounding in a horse with acute laminitis.

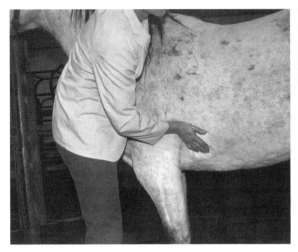

The pulse can also be taken by feeling the heartbeat over the chest just above the point of the elbow.

The pulse rate is determined by counting the number of beats per minute. Mature horses have a heart rate of 35 to 45 beats per minute at rest. In 2-year-olds, it is slightly faster. In foals 2 to 4 weeks of age, the pulse is 70 to 90 beats per minute.

The pulse should be strong, steady, and regular. A slight alteration in the pulse occurs as the horse breathes in and out. A very fast pulse (over 80 beats per minute in the adult horse at rest) is seen with severe dehydration, blood loss, shock, infection, heat stroke, advanced heart and lung disease, and *septicemia*. A very slow pulse (under 20 beats per minute) suggests low body temperature, heart disease, pressure on the brain, or a preterminal state with collapse of the circulation. It is important to note that a very physically fit horse may have a rate of 24 to 30 beats a minute.

Jugular Venous Pulse

Changes in the diameter of the jugular veins in the neck are associated with filling and emptying. During inspiration, the veins empty rapidly and the walls collapse. During expiration, the veins fill rapidly from above. Normally, these pulsations are scarcely visible. An exaggerated or very obvious jugular pulse is seen in horses with chronic obstructive lung disease, valvular heart disease, congenital heart disease, and right-sided congestive heart failure—all of which are associated with increased pressure in the venous circulation.

If the jugular veins do not collapse, the veins remain visibly enlarged throughout the entire respiratory cycle. Vein distension, especially when it extends more than halfway up the neck, has the same significance as an exaggerated jugular pulse.

MURMURS

The normal heartbeat is divided into two separate sounds. The first is a LUB, followed by a slight pause, and then a DUB. Together, the sound is LUB-DUB, evenly spaced and steady. Veterinarians use a stethoscope to listen to the heart. Its amplification enables them to hear any abnormal heart sounds, such as murmurs.

Murmurs are caused by turbulent blood flow. Most murmurs are not serious and are called functional—that is, there is no disease, just a degree of turbulence. It is estimated that as many as 40 percent of foals have a functional heart murmur up until 3 months of age.

One cause of turbulent blood flow is anemia. The turbulence heard is caused by the low viscosity of the blood.

Murmurs of a more serious nature are caused by valvular heart disease and constrictions in major blood vessels. These murmurs are called organic.

The character, sound, location, and amplitude of a heart murmur indicate to the experienced clinician whether the murmur is organic or functional, and it often suggests the diagnosis. Further evaluation can be done using an *echocardiogram*, which provides detailed images of the inside of the heart and can detect abnormal blood flow patterns.

CAPILLARY REFILL TIME

By examining the color of the horse's gums, you can obtain important information about the state of the circulation. A pink color is a sign of adequate circulation. A pale color indicates anemia. A gray or bluish tinge indicates a deficiency of oxygen (*cyanosis*). This grave sign can be seen in horses with heart disease, lung failure, and severe *colic*.

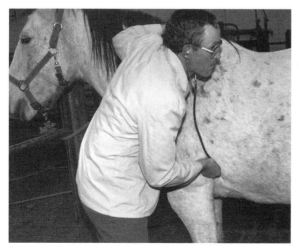

Murmurs, arrhythmias, and abnormal heart sounds can be heard with a stethoscope.

Noting the time it takes for the gums to pink up after being firmly pressed can test the quality of the circulation. This interval is called the *capillary refill time*. With normal circulation, a pink color should return to the blanched area within two seconds. If the finger impression remains pale for three seconds or longer, the horse may be severely dehydrated or in shock.

EDEMA

This is the abnormal accumulation of fluid in the tissues beneath the skin. *Edema* may occur in the underside of the abdomen (ventral edema), the *prepuce* in males, over the sternum or breastbone, and in all four legs (especially the hind limbs). Edema is characteristic of right-sided congestive heart failure. However, it also occurs in horses with liver disease and in cases of severe diarrhea associated with large protein losses. Malnutrition (a low-protein diet) is another cause. Severe edema can be recognized by the fact that it "pits"—when you press the area, an indentation remains.

Swelling in the legs that is not accompanied by edema in other locations may not be an indicator of heart disease or nutritional deficiency.

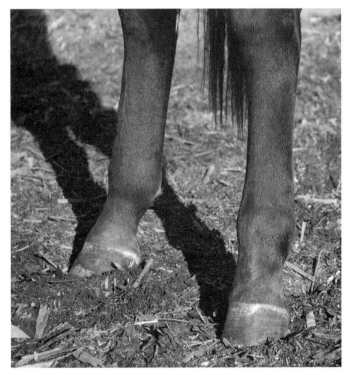

Note the round, symmetrical swelling of the lower legs and fetlocks in this case of stocking up.

There is a condition called stocking up that occurs in unconditioned or inactive horses who are abruptly put to strenuous physical exercise. After exercise, the lower half of the horse's legs may swell. Turning the horse out in a paddock or providing regular exercise each day improves conditioning and prevents stocking up.

DIAGNOSTIC TESTS

The electrocardiogram (EKG or ECG) is used principally in diagnosing cardiac arrhythmias and determining if there is evidence of heart disease. Since arrhythmias can appear or disappear with exercise, placing the horse on a treadmill while performing the EKG helps determine if the arrhythmia is significant and is likely to have an impact on athletic performance.

The echocardiogram, which is an ultrasound of the heart, is the method of choice for diagnosing the cause of heart disease. A two-dimensional echocardiogram is a cross-section of the heart. This shows the chambers, partitions, valves, and any abnormal structures within the heart. M-mode or real-time echocardiography shows the size of the chambers and major vessels, and reveals any abnormal motion of the valves. Color-flow Doppler

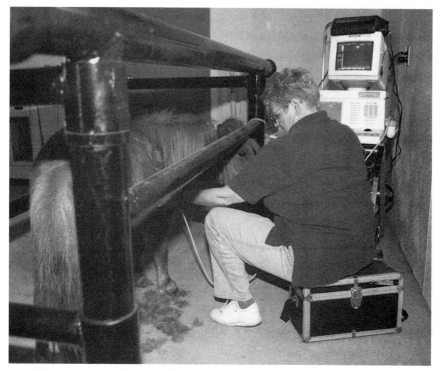

This Miniature Horse's heart defect has been diagnosed by echocardiogram.

studies map normal and abnormal blood flows. With all this information, the diagnosis, as well as the degree of cardiac impairment, can usually be determined.

Arrhythmias

Heart rhythms follow a fixed pattern that can be seen on an EKG. Whether the beat is fast or slow, the sequence in which the heart muscle contracts remains the same. This sequence is synchronized so the heart chambers can fill and empty efficiently. Various electrical disturbances in the heart's conduction system, called cardiac arrhythmias, can upset this pattern.

Not all arrhythmias are significant. Physiologic (not harmful) arrhythmias of various types are common in horses. Such arrhythmias occur at slow to normal heart rates and disappear with exercise.

Other arrhythmias, most notably atrial fibrillation, are likely to appear with sustained or maximal exercise and can cause a sudden drop in blood pressure (see *Cardiovascular Collapse*, page 12). Arrhythmias producing collapse can occur in horses with apparently normal hearts; however, in many cases, there is underlying (and often unsuspected) heart muscle disease, either myocarditis or cardiomyopathy.

ATRIAL FIBRILLATION

Atrial fibrillation is the most common clinically significant arrhythmia in horses. Episodes of atrial fibrillation can occur in horses with healthy hearts. In these cases, signs of cardiac insufficiency are not recognized when the horse is at rest or during light work, but they are more obvious with strenuous activity. As the episode begins, the heartbeat converts from a normal rhythm to one in which random electrical impulses are sent from the atrium to the ventricles. When the heart rate is fast, the ventricles do not fill and empty effectively. The blood pressure drops during exercise and causes the horse to collapse.

Treatment: A number of cardiac drugs used to control arrhythmias and heart failure in humans are used for the same purpose in horses. These drugs require close monitoring and usually are used for short-term therapy. Quinidine is used to convert persistent atrial fibrillation to a normal rhythm. However, it is complicated to administer and requires frequent stomach tube placement or an indwelling tube. Side effects, including *depression* and colic, are significant. There is ongoing research into alternative drug therapy, including flecainide, which can be administered orally.

When treating arrhythmias, it is equally important to search for and correct any underlying *electrolyte* or metabolic problem that may be responsible for the problem.

Congestive Heart Failure

Congestive heart failure is the inability of the heart to provide adequate circulation to meet the body's needs. It is the end result of a weakened heart muscle. The liver, kidneys, lungs, and other organs are affected by the circulatory insufficiency, causing a multiple organ-system problems.

A diseased heart can compensate for many months or years without signs of failure. Then, heart failure can appear quite suddenly and unexpectedly—often immediately after strenuous exercise.

When a diseased heart begins to weaken, signs of right- or left-sided congestive heart failure will appear. Symptoms are described in the next two sections.

RIGHT-SIDED HEART FAILURE

Signs of right-sided heart failure are more common than those of left-sided heart failure, even though in many cases both sides of the heart fail at the same time.

In right-sided failure, blood pressure increases in the venous circulation, causing dilated neck veins, an exaggerated jugular pulse, edema, and shortness of breath. Edema is visible in the chest area (brisket), abdomen, prepuce, and lower legs. As fluid accumulates inside the abdomen (*ascites*), the horse develops a potbellied appearance.

The slowed circulation causes less oxygen to be delivered to body tissues. The horse appears lethargic and loses appetite, weight, and condition. Even slight exertion causes muscular weakness and rapid heavy breathing. Murmurs, abnormal heart sounds, and arrhythmias may be present.

LEFT-SIDED HEART FAILURE

In left-sided heart failure, fluid backs up into the lungs. Early signs are diminished exercise tolerance, coughing, and shortness of breath. They may go unnoticed in a sedentary horse.

As blood pressure increases in the pulmonary circulation, the lungs become congested and fluid accumulates around the air sacs. This is called *pulmonary edema*. An accumulation of fluid in the chest cavity (*pleural effusion*) further reduces the ability of the lungs to expand. Respiration becomes noisy and is often accompanied by wheezing.

In the advanced stages, breathing is labored and the horse assumes a characteristic stance with his feet spread apart and his head extended to take in as much air as possible. The pulse is rapid, weak, and often irregular. Murmurs can be heard over the chest. Any sudden stress or exertion may be followed by collapse.

Treating Heart Failure

An accurate diagnosis regarding the type of heart disease is essential in planning therapy. This is established through chest x-ray, EKG, and echocardiography.

The two most commonly used drugs are furosemide and digoxin. Furosemide is a diuretic used to relieve a fluid buildup. Digoxin increases the force of heart contractions and thus slows the heart rate. When using this drug, horses should be monitored carefully for signs of drug toxicity and evidence that they are responding to the drug. Little information is available on the long-term use of digoxin, since most horses are treated only for an acute attack. Many other cardiac drugs are not used in horses, because the cost is prohibitive. Restrict activities to those well within the horse's exercise tolerance. This is of prime importance. Sudden death can occur in horses who are exercised too vigorously. The treatment of cardiac arrhythmias is discussed on page 318.

Cardiovascular Disease

The chief causes of cardiovascular disease in horses are valvular heart disease, myocarditis, cardiomyopathy, pericarditis, bacterial endocarditis, and congenital heart defects. All of these conditions can produce heart failure. Heart attacks from coronary artery disease do not occur in horses as they do in humans. However, horses with chronic heart disease do suffer collapse in association with arrhythmias and congestive heart failure.

Valvular Heart Disease

The exact cause of valvular heart disease in horses is unclear. It has been suggested that degenerative changes in heart valves associated with aging are responsible. Diseased valves are commonly found postmortem, but in most cases the heart compensates and performance is not affected. When heart failure does occur, it is because the damaged valves don't close securely. This causes reversed blood flow through the leaky valve, creating extra work for the heart, which in time begins to fail. Echocardiography is the most accurate and least invasive way to diagnose valvular heart disease.

Treatment: There is no treatment for valvular insufficiency. With mild to moderate disease, the horse may be used at mild to moderate physical activity. If the condition is more severe and is accompanied by other cardiac symptoms, such as atrial fibrillation or enlargement of the heart, the prognosis is poor and there is a strong recommendation against riding or forced physical activity.

CARDIOMYOPATHY

Cardiomyopathy is any acute or chronic disorder of the heart muscle, (the myocardium) from an unknown or *idiopathic* cause. Myocarditis is an inflammation of the heart muscle where the cause of the inflammation can be determined.

MYOCARDITIS

Myocarditis is any inflammation of the muscle of the heart. The damaged muscle loses strength and contracts less forcefully. A variety of infections and toxins can damage the heart. The chief cause of myocarditis is the bacteria *Streptococcus equi* subspecies *equi*, which causes strangles and other strep infections. Salmonella, *Clostridium tetani, Borrelia burgdorferi*, and strongylosis have also been shown to cause myocarditis. Numerous viruses also attack the heart, including equine influenza, equine viral arteritis, and equine infectious anemia. The long-term use of anabolic steroids has been associated with severe heart damage.

Myocardial degeneration occurs in foals with white muscle disease (see page 567), as well as with mineral deficiencies such as iron, selenium, and copper. Deficiencies of vitamin E and selenium may cause myocardial *necrosis*. Cardiac toxins include antibiotics such as monensin (an additive to cattle and poultry feed) and salinomycin, cantharidin (blister beetle poisoning), *Cryptostegia grandiflora* (rubber vine), and *Eupatorium rugosum* (white snakeroot).

Typically, the horse will exhibit signs of congestive heart failure (see page 319), heart murmurs, irregular pulse, and an abnormal EKG. An echocardiogram will show dilation of the heart chambers and poor muscle contractility. Lab results may show an increased white blood cell count, a high fibrinogen level, and increased cardiac isoenzymes.

Treatment: Treatment is directed at improving the ability of the heart to contract, relieving congestion, and reducing constriction of the blood vessels. Digoxin and dobutamine, along with the diuretic furosemide to relieve the edema, are commonly prescribed. Corticosteroids have been used to reduce heart muscle inflammation, except in cases of viral myocarditis, because steroids are known to lower the body's immune response to viral infections. With minimal heart muscle damage, the outlook is good. Stall rest is of great importance, since physical activity makes the heart more susceptible to injury.

PERICARDITIS

The pericardium is the thin membrane that surrounds the heart and the roots of the great blood vessels. Pericarditis is inflammation of the pericardium. The pericardium has an inner layer and an outer layer with a small amount of lubricating fluid between them. When the pericardium becomes inflamed, the amount of fluid between the two layers increases. This buildup of fluid in the pericardial sac is called a pericardial effusion.

The pericardial sac is not elastic. Accordingly, fluid in the sac presses directly on the heart and interferes with filling of the chambers. The volume of blood entering the heart is severely restricted. Signs of right-sided congestive heart failure can appear slowly or suddenly, depending on the rate of fluid production.

A characteristic sign of pericarditis is the friction rub, a scratchy or leathery sound heard with a stethoscope with each beat of the heart.

A second effect of pericarditis is to cause fibrous scarring and contracture of the pericardium, a condition called constrictive pericarditis. The effect on cardiac performance is the same as that of pericardial effusion.

Viral pericarditis can occur as a consequence of a viral respiratory infection. However, most cases are of bacterial origin. The infection first involves the lungs and the *pleura*, and then extends to involve the pericardium. In some cases, the origin of the pericarditis is unknown.

Treatment: Bacterial pericarditis is treated with antibiotics for two months or longer. Pericardial effusion can be relieved by pericardiocentesis. In this procedure, a long needle is inserted through the chest wall into the pericardial sac to draw off fluid. This immediately improves cardiac output. If fluid recurs, surgery to remove the pericardium can be considered. However, such surgery is difficult to perform in horses and has been associated with serious complications and death. In general, the long-term outlook for recovery is poor.

Congestive heart failure and cardiac arrhythmias resulting from pericarditis are treated as discussed earlier in this chapter.

Congenital Heart Disease

Congenital heart defects are present at birth. A horse may be born with more than one congenital heart defect. The most common congenital heart defect in horses is ventricular septal defect. Another defect, patent ductus arteriosus, is rare in horses beyond 1 to 2 weeks of age. These defects are usually discovered within the first week or two of life, when a heart murmur is heard with the stethoscope.

Ventricular septal defect is a hole in the septum, which separates the two ventricles. Because of the opening, blood can flow from the right to the left side of the heart without going through the pulmonary circulation and receiving oxygen.

Patent ductus arteriosus (PDA) is a defect of the ductus arteriosus. The ductus arteriosus is a large vessel connecting the pulmonary artery of the fetus to the aorta, enabling blood from the right ventricle to bypass the nonfunctioning lungs. The ductus constricts at or shortly after birth, eliminating the fetal connection and allowing normal development of the blood vessels of the lungs. This defect occurs when the ductus arteriosus fails to close. A coarse "machinery" murmur as a result of a still-patent ductus is normal for the first week of life. If the ductus does not close by then, it is considered persistent or patent ductus arteriosus. Aortic blood shunting through the pulmonary circulation leads to the development of severe pulmonary hypertension (high blood pressure), heart failure, and death.

The extent and severity of symptoms in horses with congenital heart defects depends on the type and location of the defect. A small septal defect often does not interfere with the utility and performance of the average pleasure horse, and is compatible with a normal life. Defects that cause exercise intolerance early in life tend to be the most serious and are the least likely to have a good prognosis.

Treatment: With the exception of patent ductus arteriosus, there is no surgical treatment for congenital heart disease in horses. To be successful, a patent ductus must be closed early in life, before the development of pulmonary hypertension.

Most congenital heart defects have a genetic basis. In the interest of breed soundness, horses with all types of congenital heart defects should not be bred.

Vascular Diseases

Vascular disease can be any disorder that affects primarily the blood vessels. Atherosclerosis, vascular disease associated with increased blood pressure, and high cholesterol, although common in humans, are exceptionally rare in horses. Therefore, heart attacks and strokes are also quite rare.

JUGULAR VEIN THROMBOPHLEBITIS

The jugular vein is the usual site for intravenous injections in the horse. Various drugs and irritating solutions injected either into the vein or inadvertently around the vein can lead to inflammation and clotting of the vein (thrombophlebitis). Indwelling catheters can introduce bacteria into the vein. When this happens, an infected clot develops, a condition called septic thrombophlebitis.

The signs of thrombophlebitis are a tender, swollen cord in the neck (the clotted jugular vein), sometimes accompanied by heat, redness, and swelling of the surrounding tissues. With a severe infection, devitalization or death of surrounding skin can occur. Rarely, there can be damage to the nerve plexus in the neck, which results in signs of cranial nerve paralysis (see page 343). An infected clot can give rise to blood poisoning.

Treatment: Apply hot packs and topical DMSO to the neck three times a day until the swelling subsides. Ultrasound examination of the neck is helpful in visualizing a clotted vein and documenting its progress or resolution. Anticoagulants (such as aspirin or low-dose heparin) are considered in special circumstances.

An infected indwelling catheter should be promptly removed and, if necessary, replaced in another vein. Your veterinarian will culture the tip of the catheter to discover the source of the infection, so appropriate antibiotics can be administered.

When drugs are accidently deposited outside the vein, injecting large volumes of saline around the vein can dilute the irritant. This may prevent tissue injury. In uncomplicated cases, the clot dissolves and the vein returns to normal.

Arterial Vascular Disease

There are two major diseases that cause arterial damage in horses: aorto-iliac thrombosis and arterial *thromboembolism*.

Thrombosis is clot formation within an artery. An embolus is a blood clot or thrombus that forms in the heart or a large artery, breaks loose, and travels downstream to a smaller artery, where it lodges. The blockage interferes with the blood supply to the organ or tissue affected.

Aorto-iliac Thrombosis

There is a characteristic disease involving thrombosis of the abdominal aorta and its major branches that occurs almost exclusively in heavily exercised horses. The mechanism of arterial injury and thrombosis is unknown. One theory holds that these horses are subjected to a routine of training that requires high cardiac output and maximum blood flow to the muscles of locomotion. The pressure of the blood in the aorta and the iliac arteries (which supply blood to the lower trunk and the hind legs), along with the forceful expansion and rapid contraction of these vessels, causes small tears to develop in the walls of the arteries. As these injuries heal, scars and areas of contracture form. Eventually, the passageway narrows and the rate of blood flow through the channel declines to the point that clotting occurs. In a sense, this is a disease of usage that would not occur in the wild.

The onset of symptoms can be sudden but more often is gradual. The horse is not able to perform as well. Unexplained lameness develops and there is a peculiarity of gait affecting the hindquarters. These gait disturbances become worse with strenuous exercise. The horse may go rigid in the rear, stumble, or collapse. After a lengthy period of rest, the horse does not get better.

On examination, the hind limbs are cool and sweating may be absent over the hindquarters. The digital pulses are often weak or absent. The horse sometimes inexplicably treads up and down or kicks out with his back feet. Rectal examination may disclose a large aorta without a pulse.

Treatment: The horse must be retired from training and competition. This does not improve the vascular disease, which is irreversible by the time the diagnosis is made. Degenerative changes in the walls of the large arteries may weaken them and predispose the affected vessels to rupture and bleeding. The most common sites are the root of the aorta in the *stallion* and the uterine artery in the mare.

Parasitic Arteritis

This common condition is due to vascular migration of the larval forms of the intestinal parasite *Strongylus vulgaris*. It causes a dilation of the artery, and can cause an aneurysm or rupture of the artery wall, and thrombosis with potential obstruction, usually at the origin of the large arteries to the intestine.

Treatment: This condition can usually be treated or prevented with an appropriate anti-parasite program (see chapter 2, "Parasites").

Anemia

Anemia can be defined as a deficiency of red blood cells (*erythrocytes*) in the circulation. The purpose of red blood cells is to carry oxygen to the tissues and remove carbon dioxide from the tissues.

The number of red blood cells in horses is relatively small. Breedwise, Thoroughbreds in training tend to have the highest number of circulating red blood cells. Unconditioned horses have somewhat fewer, and "cold-blooded" and draft breeds have the fewest of all. When there are fewer than 6 million erythrocytes per cubic millimeter of blood, the horse is anemic.

A horse's spleen stores about one-third of all the red blood cells in the body. During any crisis in which additional red cells are needed, including intense exercise, these cells are pumped from the spleen into the circulation. Unlike in most animals, erythrocytes remain in the bone marrow of the horse until they are fully mature—even though the horse may have lost a consider-able amount of blood. Thus, once the spleen's reserve is used up, there could be a lapse of several days before red blood cell volume is restored by the release of new erythrocytes from the bone marrow. Accordingly, the actual number of red blood cells in circulation after a bleeding episode can vary con-siderably. A series of blood counts done over different time intervals can determine if the red cell count is increasing or continuing to decrease. Once anemia is identified, its cause can be determined by other blood tests. Causes of anemia include bleeding, *hemolysis*, infection, and inadequate red blood cell production. Bone marrow *biopsy* helps determine whether erythrocyte production is normal.

Inadequate Red Blood Cell Production

Most anemias in horses are due to inadequate red blood cell production. As the erythrocytes become old, they are replaced by new red blood cells that are manufactured by the horse's bone marrow. If the metabolic activity of the bone marrow is depressed for any reason, new red blood cells are not manufactured as fast as the old ones are destroyed. Anemia is the result.

Chronic illnesses are the most frequent cause of depressed erythrocyte production in the horse. This includes equine viral arteritis, chronic pneumonia, abdominal abscesses, liver and kidney failure, lymphomas, and other types of cancer.

Iron, trace minerals, vitamins, and fatty acids are all incorporated into red blood cells. Thus, a deficiency in one or more of these nutrients could slow down or stop erythrocyte production. However, this is not a common cause of anemia because these nutrients are found in almost all horse feeds in more than adequate amounts to meet daily requirements.

Iron deficiency anemia is the one exception. Iron deficiency occurs when iron is lost from the body faster than it is being replaced through the diet. The two situations in which this can happen are chronic gastrointestinal bleeding and a heavy infestation of bloodsucking insects. Intestinal parasites and stomach ulcers are the usual causes of unsuspected chronic gastrointestinal bleeding. Gastrointestinal bleeding can be diagnosed by checking the manure for *occult* (microscopic) blood.

When the bone marrow fails to produce red blood cells, the condition is called aplastic anemia. Aplastic anemias are associated with heavy metal poisoning and exposure to insecticides, organic solvents, and hydrocarbons. Bone marrow depression has been found after prolonged use of phenylbutazone (Butazolidin), an anti-inflammatory and analgesic drug.

Idiopathic aplastic anemia, in which the cause is undetermined, can occur in horses.

Treatment: The primary cause of the anemia must be treated first. If this is a chronic, on-going anemia, the horse may tolerate low levels of red blood cells without clinical signs of anemia. If the primary cause is not corrected, a blood transfusion may be necessary to ensure adequate oxygenation.

Hemolysis and Hemolytic Anemias

Red blood cells survive in the circulation for about 150 days, after which they are broken down and destroyed. The iron is recycled by the bone marrow to make new erythrocytes. An unusual acceleration of the breakdown process is called hemolysis.

Red blood cells break down into bilirubin and hemoglobin. When hemolysis is sudden and acute, these breakdown products overload the plasma.

Accordingly, in a horse with an acute hemolytic breakdown, expect to see *jaundice* (a yellow cast to the eyes and mucous membranes) and *hemoglobinuria* (the passage of dark-brown urine that contains hemoglobin). Common causes of hemolysis include toxins and infections.

Oxidizing agents that act on the surface of the red blood cell and cause hemolysis are found in wild and cultivated onions (onion poisoning) and the leaves of the red maple tree (red maple leaf poisoning). The venom of rattlesnakes and pit vipers causes red blood cell hemolysis.

Infectious diseases associated with hemolysis include equine infectious anemia, equine ehrlichiosis, and equine piroplasmosis. Bacteria of the *Clostridia* and *Staphylococcus* species produce toxins that cause hemolysis.

Neonatal isoerythrolysis, a hemolytic disease of newborn foals, is discussed on page 562.

Treatment: It is imperative to treat the cause of the hemolysis; for example, treat the infection or remove the horse from the pasture with maple trees. Shock may accompany severe hemolysis, and the horse will need supportive care, as well as transfusion therapy. Kidney failure may develop as a result of severe hemolysis.

BLOOD LOSS

Blood loss may be due to wounds or other physical trauma. Spontaneous bleeding beneath the skin and from the nose, in the absence of trauma, suggests a clotting deficiency. The most common clotting deficiency in horses is disseminated intravascular coagulation (DIC), a condition triggered by overwhelming infection, shock, and acute colitis. DIC is characterized by clotting throughout the entire capillary circulation, followed by spontaneous bleeding when all clotting factors have been consumed. Horses with DIC are extremely ill and often die.

Other causes of spontaneous bleeding include hemophilia, dicumarol and warfarin poisoning (these follow exposure to moldy sweet clover or rat poisons), and drug-induced immune reactions. Massive bleeding from the nose occurs in horses with guttural pouch mycosis. Special laboratory studies are required to identify and diagnose these problems.

A more insidious loss of blood takes place from the gastrointestinal tract as a result of intestinal parasites (especially strongyle infection), stomach and duodenal ulcers, and cancer of the stomach.

Bloodsucking external parasites (lice, ticks, or biting flies) can produce surprising amounts of blood loss in a horse with a heavy parasite load.

Treatment: Stopping blood loss is discussed in *Wounds* (page 33). Severe loss may require blood transfusions and plasma transfusions to provide extra clotting factors. Horses normally have an extended bleeding time, so they can lose what appears to be a large volume of blood without consequence. Your veterinarian will determine by clinical signs if the horse requires a transfusion. Wounds involving arterial bleeding may result in significant blood loss quickly, as can guttural pouch mycosis.

Equine Blood Types

Red blood cells (also called erythrocytes) circulate throughout the body in blood vessels, picking up oxygen in the lungs and transporting it to all the cells within the body. Hemoglobin is the protein within the red blood cell that actually carries the oxygen molecule.

The surface of each red blood cell is covered with a number of structures called *antigens*. These antigens enable the body to recognize the cell. The antigens on the red cells are inherited from both parents. These antigens are given specific names (usually letters) depending on their structure, and are then placed in various groups. This is the basis for blood typing.

Horses have eight blood systems: A, C, D, K, P, Q, U, and T. The first seven systems are internationally recognized, and T is important in research. There are more than 30 known antigens (also called factors) on the surface of the red blood cells, and anywhere from one to eight different types of antigens within a given blood system. Equine blood groups are designated with an uppercase letter for the system and a lowercase letter for the antigen.

When an animal is exposed to a blood type that is different from his own, problems can arise. If this new blood has antigens on it that the body does not recognize, antibodies will be produced in an effort to destroy the new red blood cells, which are perceived as invading organisms. There are two kinds of antibodies horses can have to blood group antigens: those that occur naturally and those that develop after an exposure to blood. Acquired antibodies are most often produced after a blood transfusion of incompatible blood or, in the *mare*, during pregnancy with an incompatible *stallion*. With either type, the antibodies cause red blood cells to clump or be destroyed.

When red blood cells are destroyed, hemoglobin and other substances within the cell are released into the bloodstream and the cell can no longer function properly. The lack of oxygen-carrying ability and the resulting presence of hemoglobin in the blood can lead to serious health problems.

All horses also lack a unique red cell factor that donkeys possess, and therefore produce antibodies when exposed to *donkey* blood (such as in *mule* pregnancies).

Blood typing is useful in selecting blood donor horses for transfusions and to determine mare-stallion compatibility before breeding to predict the potential for neonatal isoerythrolysis (see page 562). Some of the most common indications for whole blood transfusion include trauma with acute blood loss, ruptured uterine artery, maxillosinus complications, guttural pouch infection, and neonatal isoerythrolysis. The recipient should have a blood type and antibody screen.

The most clinically significant blood systems are Aa and Qa, because when a horse who is positive for these factors is exposed to blood from a horse who is negative for these factors, serious hemolytic reactions (destruction of red blood cells) can result. However, other blood groups can also cause neonatal isoerythrolysis. The incidence of Aa and Qa blood factors varies by breed. The table below shows the percentage of horses in several breeds who are negative for these two factors, which might lead to a blood incompatibility.

Percentage of Horses Who Are Negative for Aa and Qa Blood Factors, by Breed					
	Thoroughbred	Arabian	Standardbred	Quarter Horse	Morgan
Aa	15%	18%	44%	51%	43%
Qa	39%	79%	100%	83%	99%

Source: Comparative Coagulation Laboratory at Cornell University

Your veterinarian can do a simple *hemagglutination crossmatch* and will be able to identify a large percentage of incompatibilities. A few specialized veterinary diagnostic laboratories offer blood typing for the most common blood groups, including the Animal Health Diagnostic Center at Cornell University, the Equine Parentage Testing and Research Lab at the University of Kentucky, and the Veterinary Genetics Laboratory at the University of California-Davis.

COLD-BLOODED, HOT-BLOODED, WARM-BLOODED

None of these terms refers to a horse's blood at all. These are terms used to describe breed types. Hot-blooded breeds include the Thoroughbred horse, the Arabian, Barb, Turk, Syrian, or a mixture. The heavy draft breeds and the majority of cross-bred horses are often referred to as being cold-blooded. Breeds such as the Hanoverian, Trakehner, and Dutch Warmblood are considered warm-bloods and can trace their roots to the draft breeds with refinement from breeds such as the Thoroughbred and Arabians.

THE URINARY SYSTEM

The urinary system is composed of the kidneys, ureters, bladder, and urethra. The kidneys are a pair of organs located on either side of the spine near the eighteenth ribs. Occasionally, the left kidney may be felt by rectal palpation. The urinary system aids the respiratory and digestive systems in eliminating metabolic waste products. The kidneys filter the blood and remove nitrogen products that are produced by the body's metabolism. They also maintain the *electrolyte* and acid-base balance of the body, as well as the water balance—all under the active influence of the hormone system.

Each kidney has a *renal pelvis*, or funnel, that siphons the urine into a ureter. The ureters transport urine down to the pelvic brim and empty into the bladder. The bladder empties into the urethra. The opening of the urethra is found at the tip of the penis in the male and between the folds of the vulva in the female. The decision to void or urinate is under the conscious control of the brain. Once the horse decides to urinate, the actual mechanism of emptying the bladder is carried out by a complicated spinal cord reflex.

Equine urine normally is cloudy, strong smelling, alkaline, and often rather mucoid. After standing for some time, it frequently takes on a dark coffee color, the result of oxidation of pigments.

Fresh urine that is dark and coffee-colored suggests the presence of *myoglobin*, as seen in azoturia (tying-up syndrome), hemoglobin (as seen in hemolytic anemia), or bile (as seen in *jaundice*). Certain drugs may cause the urine to turn red when exposed to light.

A urinalysis performed at the veterinarian's office will distinguish between natural pigments and those present from other causes. Blood in urine cannot be distinguished from pigment unless clots are seen.

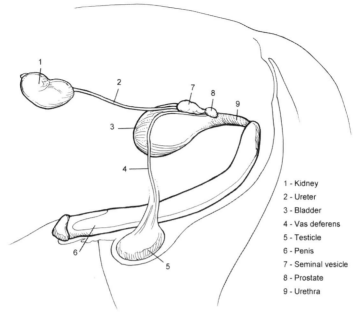

1 - Kidney
2 - Ureter
3 - Bladder
4 - Vas deferens
5 - Testicle
6 - Penis
7 - Seminal vesicle
8 - Prostate
9 - Urethra

The urogenital system of the male horse.

Signs of Urinary Tract Disease

Most urinary tract disorders cause some disturbance in the normal pattern of voiding. There are a number of signs to look for.

- **Dysuria (painful urination).** Dysuria and straining to urinate are the two most important signs of lower urinary tract infection. *Cystitis*, urethritis, and bladder stones are the usual causes. Azoturia should be considered, since passing myoglobin can produce pain on urination. Blister beetle poisoning is an unusual cause of dysuria. A horse with dysuria assumes a stretched-out posture for voiding but does not immediately void. Groaning and contracting the abdominal wall muscles are signs of straining. In males, the penis is often relaxed and protruded. A horse with dysuria often voids frequently in small amounts. Mares may have urine scalds of the *perineum*.

- **Hematuria (blood in the urine).** Microscopic *hematuria* is blood visible under a microscope. Microscopic hematuria can also be identified using a urine dip stick. When clots are visible to the eye, the problem is either cystitis or urinary tract stones.

- **Myoglobin in the urine.** Myoglobin is a protein in heart and skeletal muscles. When muscle is damaged, myoglobin is released into the bloodstream. It is filtered out of the bloodstream by the kidneys and eliminated in urine, often imparting a brown or "coffee" color. In large quantities, myoglobin can damage the kidneys and break down into toxic compounds, causing kidney failure.

- **Polyuria (excessive urination).** The bladder capacity of the adult horse is about 1 gallon (3.8 l). Horses normally void several times a day. The normal adult horse who is fed alfalfa hay and has access to water will produce about 4 gallons (15 l) of urine per day. Much larger volumes are seen in horses who consume large amounts of salt. *Polyuria*, if not otherwise explained, suggests chronic kidney failure. A horse with polyuria exhibits extreme thirst and drinks a lot more than usual to compensate for urine losses. In fact, extreme thirst and continual drinking (polydypsia) are more likely to call attention to the problem than is the large urine output.
- **Incontinence or dribbling.** If the horse is dribbling urine, it could be a sign of urinary tract disease. Neurological causes must be ruled out.

Diagnosing Urinary Tract Diseases

Because of overlapping symptoms and the fact that more than one organ may be involved, it is difficult to make an exact diagnosis based on the symptoms alone. Laboratory tests can be of considerable help. Routine tests are *urinalysis*, which may show a urinary tract infection, and blood chemistries, which provide information about kidney function. By taking a blood and urine sample at the same time, your veterinarian can compare levels of creatinine (a muscle-energy waste product), electrolytes, and enzymes. An excessive amount of waste products in the blood or nutrients in the urine may point to irregular kidney function. Elevated creatinine does not occur until 70 percent of the *nephrons* in both kidneys are severely damaged. Excess calcium may also appear in the blood if the kidneys are unable to excrete this mineral. Because there is heavy bacterial contamination in voided specimens from horses, urine is best obtained by inserting a catheter or obtaining a midstream specimen. The urethra in mares is short and wide. It can be catheterized easily using a rigid catheter. In the male, the urethra is long and narrow. To facilitate handling the penis and passing a catheter, the horse should be tranquilized. This also paralyzes the muscle that retracts the penis, so the penis will protrude.

Sterile techniques should be used when inserting a catheter to avoid introducing bacteria into the lower urinary tract and causing infection. This should be done by a veterinarian.

Rectal palpation is a useful examination. It often indicates the condition of the bladder and the presence of stones in the lower urinary tract. An enlarged kidney, ureters, or bladder may be detected by palpation.

Transrectal or abdominal *ultrasonography* is useful in visualizing the size and appearance of structures in the urinary tract. Small, shrunken kidneys, stones, and abnormalities not apparent on palpation are often revealed on ultrasound. Ultrasound visualization is also helpful in placing a needle in the correct position for a kidney *biopsy*.

Fiber-optic cystoscopy or transurethral endoscopy provides the opportunity to visualize and biopsy the interior of the bladder.

X-rays using injected dye to outline the urinary collecting system (which includes the kidneys, ureters, and bladder) are difficult to perform in adult horses and generally are useful only in foals. Ordinary x-rays of the pelvis may show urinary tract stones, but will require general anesthesia.

Urinary Tract Infections

Infection in the urethra (*urethritis*) is associated with diseases of the male reproductive system. It is discussed on page 494.

CYSTITIS (BLADDER INFECTION)

Inflammation of the lining of the bladder is called cystitis. Infections of the urethra in both males and females usually precede the development of cystitis.

The bladder of horses is relatively resistant to infection. Accordingly, cystitis usually does not occur unless there is an additional problem that prevents the bladder from emptying or lowers the body's natural defenses. Such predisposing conditions include late pregnancy, prolonged labor, bladder stones, and paralyzed bladder.

Signs of bladder infection are frequent, painful voiding, hematuria, and straining. A male horse may stand with his penis dropped and a mare may have a vaginal discharge with scalding of the skin. A catheterized urine specimen reveals *pus*, blood, and bacteria. Fever and loss of appetite do not occur unless the upper urinary tract is also infected (*pyelonephritis*), which is more serious than cystitis. It is important to exclude the presence of bladder stones.

Treatment: Early diagnosis and treatment will decrease the risk and occurrence of chronic cystitis and/or pyelonephritis.

A urine culture and sensitivity test should be done to screen for the antibiotic most effective against the bacteria in question. A first attack should be treated with antibiotics for 14 days, and a second or recurrent attack for one month. Repeat the urine culture one week after starting treatment. Change to a new antibiotic, as prescribed by your veterinarian, if the sensitivity studies show that the first antibiotic was not effective or if bacteria are still present in the urine.

PYELONEPHRITIS

Pyelonephritis is a bacterial infection of the upper urinary tract (kidneys and ureter). It may affect one or both kidneys. Cystitis often precedes pyelonephritis. Most cases occur in *postpartum* mares, presumably as a result of infections created by placental membranes wicking bacteria from a dirty environment during foaling.

Signs of pyelonephritis include fever, *colic*, weight loss, loss of appetite, and *depression*. These signs are not specific and do not necessarily point to the urinary tract. However, when cystitis is also present, urinary symptoms will be noted.

The urine contains pus, bacteria, blood, protein, and epithelial cells. Rectal palpation and ultrasound studies show enlargement of the kidneys or ureters. When infection has been present for several weeks, laboratory tests and *ultrasonography* are apt to reveal reduced kidney function and small, shrunken kidneys.

Treatment: The treatment is like that described for *Cystitis* (see page 333). Antibiotics, selected after *bacterial sensitivity* tests, should be continued for four to six weeks. Reculture in two weeks and change the antibiotics as circumstances warrant. Culture again at the end of treatment to be sure the infection has been eliminated. If bacteria are still present, continue treatment.

Pyelonephritis is insidious and chronic in horses. Recurrent episodes ultimately lead to kidney failure. The longer the horse is impaired, the worse the prognosis. Many cases are not discovered until there is extensive loss of kidney function and localized pockets of pus that are difficult to eradicate with antibiotics. If only one kidney is badly damaged and the other kidney is normal, the damaged kidney may be surgically removed to eradicate the source of infection.

Paralyzed Bladder

Paralysis of the bladder accompanies spinal cord injuries, cauda equina syndrome, and equine herpes *encephalomyelitis*. These diseases are described in chapter 13, "The Nervous System."

Sorghum cystitis ataxia is a type of bladder paralysis that occurs in horses who graze pastures containing Sudan grass, Johnson grass, Columbus grass, and sorghums. These types of pastures are found in the southwestern United States. Sorghum cystitis ataxia causes degenerative changes in the sacral spinal cord that causes bladder paralysis and failure of the bladder to empty. Regardless of the cause, a paralyzed bladder empties only when it overflows. The characteristic sign is dribbling urine. When the horse coughs or strains, urine spurts from the urethra. In males, the penis is often relaxed and extended. In mares, the vulva and skin of the buttocks may be scalded. Rectal palpation reveals a large, flaccid bladder, often containing stones. There is a pool of static urine and sediment that serves as a culture medium for bacteria of many species.

In addition to the bladder problem, horses with spinal cord disease show varying degrees of hindquarter unsteadiness, with a weaving gait and a tendency for the legs to buckle. There is loss of anal sphincter control, leaving an open or gaping anus.

Treatment: Horses with sorghum cystitis ataxia may improve after the toxic grass has been removed from the diet. Complete recovery is rare.

Management of a paralyzed bladder involves intermittent drainage by urinary catheter, as determined by the horse's level of comfort, ability to tolerate the full bladder, and status of infection. Drugs are available that can stimulate bladder emptying and relax the uretheral muscles. Success is uncertain.

Attacks of acute cystitis or pyelonephritis occur in conjunction with bladder paralysis, and require continuous catheter drainage and antibiotics. *Prophylactic* use of antibiotics may reduce the frequency of such episodes. Applying petroleum jelly will help to prevent urine scalds. Manual evacuation of stool from the rectum is often necessary to prevent impaction.

Uroliths (Urinary Tract Stones)

Uroliths are not common in horses. The majority occur in the bladder or urethra. Kidney and urethral stones, although common in people, are rare in horses. They are usually bilateral and produce chronic renal failure before they are diagnosed. These uroliths in the horse can vary in size from ¼ inch (5 mm) up to 8 inches (20.5 mm) and weigh up to 14 pounds (6.5 kg) Bladder and urethral stones rarely affect young horses, but are seen more frequently in middle-age and older horses, and are more common in males.

Most stones are composed of calcium carbonate, with struvite (magnesium-ammonium-phosphate) uroliths seen occasionally. The mechanism of urolith formation in horses is not known, although the alkaline pH and high mineral content of normal equine urine may favor crystal formation and precipitation. Normal equine urine also contains large amounts of mucoproteins, which may serve as a cementing substance for crystals. *Forages* that contain large amounts of calcium, ammonia, and magnesium predispose the horse to stone formation, as do grains with high phosphorus content.

The irritation of the stones, along with pooled urine, creates an ideal environment for infections. Diagnosis is tentatively based on history and clinical signs, and confirmed by rectal palpation of a firm oval mass at or near the neck of the bladder. Transrectal ultrasonography allows visualization of the urolith. Urinalysis reveals red blood cells, white blood cells, calcium carbonate crystals, and proteinuria.

Clinical signs of urinary tract stones depend on their location. Most are located in the bladder and cause painful urination, frequent urination at short intervals, and hematuria. Hematuria is most evident after exercise and toward the end of a voided urine stream. Affected horses frequently stretch out to urinate and may maintain this posture even after urinating. Geldings and stallions may protrude the penis flaccidly for prolonged periods while intermittently dribbling urine.

Stones in mares usually pass easily and cause few signs. This is because the urethra of the mare is short and wide. In stallions and geldings, the long, narrow urethra prevents the passage of most bladder and urethral stones, which can cause obstruction. Signs of incomplete obstruction are straining, painful urination, and passing blood clots—often noted at the end of urination. Complete, unrelieved urethral obstruction is characterized by severe colic with groaning and rolling. It is likely to progress to rupture of the bladder and subsequent *peritonitis*.

The diagnosis of bladder and urethral stones can be made by rectal palpation and/or transrectal ultrasound. Fiber-optic cystoscopy is useful in determining the size, number, and location of the stones. This information is useful in planning treatment.

Treatment: Passing a catheter to decompress the bladder may dislodge an impacted stone. Several surgical procedures are available for urolith removal, including laser lithotripsy. In this minimally invasive procedure, the veterinarian inserts a cystoscope into the horse's urethra and proceeds up the urinary tract to locate the stone. A fiber-optic line is run up the endoscope, with a laser that disintegrates the stone. Prophylactic antibiotics and urinary acidifiers (such as ammonium chloride) after treatment may help prevent the formation of new stones.

Management of a ruptured bladder depends on the size of the tear and whether the horse is voiding after removal of the blockage. The two alternatives are antibiotics alone or antibiotics plus surgical repair of the bladder. Rupture of the bladder in newborn foals is discussed in *Ruptured Bladder* (see page 564).

Kidney Failure

The chief functions of the kidneys are to regulate fluid, electrolyte, and acid-base balance and to excrete the wastes of metabolism. This is accomplished by millions of nephrons, the basic working units of the kidneys. A nephron is composed of a globe of blood vessels (called the *glomerulus*) that filters waste from the blood plasma and passes it through a system of renal tubules that reabsorb water and electrolytes. This concentrates the liquid waste, which becomes urine. Damage to nephrons or tubules leads to kidney failure.

Kidney failure is the inability of the kidneys to remove nitrogen and other wastes from the blood, resulting in a buildup of toxic chemicals called uremic poisoning. The most common diseases that can cause kidney failure are discussed in *Kidney Diseases* (see page 339).

ACUTE RENAL FAILURE

Acute renal failure comes on suddenly. The predominant signs are severe depression with marked loss of appetite. In horses with early acute renal failure, the urine output is decreased or absent. In the acute phase, the horse fails to drink and thus is dehydrated. However, as the horse begins to recover, she will drink more, but her kidneys are not concentrating the urine, so urine volume is much greater than normal.

Blood work shows elevated serum creatinine and blood urea nitrogen (BUN). Urinalysis may show increased protein and numerous white cells. The presence of pathogenic bacteria indicates an infection. Large amounts of hemoglobin or myoglobin pigment in the urine indicate tubular disease secondary to azoturia or hemolytic anemia. Abdominal or transrectal ultrasound may reveal uroliths or pyelonephritis.

Causes of acute renal failure include:

- Shock, when due to sudden blood loss, rapid dehydration, or endotoxemia
- Complete blockage of the urethra by a urolith
- Blockage of both ureters by uroliths
- Rupture of the bladder with urine peritonitis (peritonitis caused by urine in the *peritoneal cavity*)
- Myoglobinuria, caused by azoturia or prolonged recumbency
- Hemoglobinuria, caused by a hemolytic anemia
- Exposure to drugs that are toxic to the kidneys
- Exposure to plants that are toxic to the kidneys, especially cultivated and wild onions, certain oak species, withered red maple leaves, wild jasmine, locoweed, certain fungal toxins in cereal grains, and blister beetles in alfalfa
- Exposure to heavy metal poisons (mercury, arsenic, selenium, and copper)

Treatment: Treating acute renal failure is directed at correcting shock and dehydration, eliminating urinary tract infections and obstructions, stopping exposure to drugs and poisons that are toxic to the kidneys, and supporting the horse during the acute phase of the illness.

CHRONIC RENAL FAILURE

Horses with chronic renal failure do not begin to show signs of failure until 70 percent of the kidney's nephrons are destroyed. At this point, the causative illness often is no longer present, making its identification difficult or impossible. Causes of chronic renal failure include:

- Acute kidney failure that has progressed to a chronic stage
- Glomerulonephritis
- Interstitial *nephritis*
- Chronic pyelonephritis
- Vitamin D toxicity
- Exposure to substances that are toxic to the kidneys
- Kidney tumors

The most important sign of chronic renal failure is unexplained weight loss. Unfortunately, this is not specific for kidney disease. Failing kidneys lose the ability to retain protein, concentrate urine, and conserve water. Accordingly, horses with chronic renal failure have dilute urine and must drink a large volume of water to compensate. You may notice that the horse seems to be extremely thirsty, or that her stall is a lot more wet than usual. Urinalysis will reveal that the specific gravity of the urine is low (indicating dilute urine) and the protein level is high.

Because damaged kidneys do not retain protein, the serum protein is low on blood work, which favors fluid accumulation in the subcutaneous tissues of the abdomen (ventral edema) and marked swelling of the lower extremities. Edema is particularly characteristic of chronic glomerulonephritis.

As kidney function deteriorates further, the horse retains ammonia, nitrogen, potassium, acids, and other wastes in the blood and tissues, a syndrome called uremic poisoning or uremia. Signs of uremia include depression, refusal to eat, weight loss, anemia, ammonialike odor to the breath, mouth ulcerations, and excessive buildup of tartar on the teeth. At the end, the horse falls into a coma.

Treatment: Your veterinarian may wish to make an exact diagnosis via a kidney *biopsy*. This helps to plan treatment and determine prognosis.

It is important to provide unlimited access to fresh water. A salt block should be available as long as the horse does not develop edema or hypertension, in which case salt should be restricted. It is important to restrict calcium in the diet, since uremic horses retain calcium.

To reduce stress on the kidneys, it is important to supply an easily digested diet with low protein and low carbohydrates. Replace grain with a soluble fiber such as bran, beet pulp, or low-protein corn. Good-quality timothy or grass hay are desirable, because they are low in calcium. Avoid alfalfa and feeds that are high in protein, which will increase nitrogen consumption and thus contribute to uremia. The horse's serum electrolytes (sodium, potassium, and bicarbonate), phosphorus, calcium levels, and kidney function indicators should be monitored at frequent intervals. This may anticipate and prevent *acidosis* (acid blood pH), mineral and electrolyte imbalances, and other complications. Some exercise is good for a uremic horse, but stressful activity should be avoided.

Kidney Diseases

Diseases of the kidney attack either the glomerulus or the tubules. Untreated, they lead to kidney failure.

GLOMERULONEPHRITIS

Glomerulonephritis is an inflammatory disease that targets the glomerulus. It is the most common cause of chronic renal failure in horses.

This disease appears to be related to a malfunction of the horse's immune system. The virus of equine infectious anemia has been identified as a specific cause. Certain strains of *Streptococcus* bacteria have also been shown to cause acute glomerulonephritis in horses. In many cases the cause is unknown.

The diagnosis is established by needle biopsy of the kidney.

Treatment: Corticosteroids may suppress the immune reaction and slow the progress of the disease. However, glomerulonephritis eventually leads to chronic renal failure.

INTERSTITIAL NEPHRITIS

Interstitial nephritis is an inflammation of the tubules and the spaces between the tubules and the glomeruli. It is a common cause of acute and chronic renal failure.

A number of drugs that are toxic to the kidneys can cause interstitial nephritis. Among the most common are the antibiotics gentamicin and neomycin; butazolidin and other *NSAIDs*; sulfonamide antibiotics; dewormers containing carbon tetrachloride and tetrachloroethylene; and insecticides containing toxaphene. Problems with the antibiotics and NSAIDs occur when the recommended dosage is exceeded or when the drug is administered over a long period or when the NSAIDs are given to a dehydrated animal.

Pyelonephritis and stones that block the ureters are other causes of interstitial nephritis.

Treatment: Treatment is directed at the primary disease. Drug-induced kidney failure is reversible if the drug is withdrawn before permanent damage is done. Most (but not all) horses recover within a few weeks. Those who do not recover develop chronic renal failure.

ACUTE TUBULAR NEPHROSIS

Acute tubular nephrosis is kidney damage that occurs with an infection of rapid onset, accompanied by *endotoxemia* (a condition in which *endotoxins*, toxic substances associated with certain bacteria, get into the bloodstream), dehydration, and circulatory collapse. Most cases occur in horses with intestinal clostridiosis (high intestinal counts of *Clostridium perfringens* type A) and other forms of infectious colitis.

Myoglobin is a pigment released from oxygen-starved muscle. Hemoglobin is released from destroyed red cells. Diseases that cause the sudden release of large amounts of these pigments (such as azoturia and hemolytic anemias) will result in the formation of pigment casts, made of a proteinaceous accumulation, in the nephrons that obstruct the flow of urine and impair circulation to the kidneys. The kidney failure is usually reversible if the horse recovers from the causative illness.

Treatment: Treatment is directed at the primary disease. Early and aggressive treatment of the endotoxemia and circulatory failure offers the best prospect for kidney recovery.

THE NERVOUS SYSTEM

The central nervous system of the horse is composed of the cerebrum, cerebellum, midbrain (which includes the cranial nerves and the brain stem), and the spinal cord.

The cerebrum has two hemispheres and is the largest part of the brain. It controls learning, memory, reasoning, behavior, and voluntary motor control. A horse's voluntary actions are initiated here. Diseases affecting the cerebrum are characterized by seizures, mild to marked *depression*, and alterations in personality and behavior. A well-socialized horse may exhibit signs of aggression or hyperexcitability; wander aimlessly or turn in circles; toss his head or press his head against objects; exhibit varying degrees of blindness; yawn continually or make strange noises; have muscle tremors and facial and muzzle twitching, and head-tossing. Foals may exhibit ineffective nursing behavior, wander away from the mare, appear dumb, and vocalize in a peculiar fashion.

The cerebellum is relatively large and well developed in the horse. It also has two lobes. Its main function is integrating the motor pathways of the brain to maintain the horse's coordination and balance. Injuries or diseases of the cerebellum result in incoordination, staggering gait (*ataxia*), and muscle tremors. Uncoordinated body movements include awkward jerking of the limbs and head bobbing. Gait disturbances can be distinguished from paralysis in that there is no loss of muscle strength in the quarters.

In the midbrain and brain stem are the centers that control levels of consciousness, respiration, heartbeat, blood pressure, and other activities essential to life. At the base of the brain and closely connected to the midbrain and brain stem are the hypothalamus and pituitary gland. These structures are vitally important in regulating the horse's body temperature and hormone systems. They are also the centers for primitive responses such as hunger, thirst, anger, and fright. Diseases affecting this part of the brain cause paralysis of many of the cranial nerves, the effects of which are discussed on page 343. A

341

set of 12 nerve pairs called the cranial nerves pass directly out from the mid-brain into the head and neck through special holes in the skull.

The spinal cord passes down a bony canal formed by the arches of the vertebrae. The cord sends out nerve roots that combine with one another to form the peripheral nerves, which carry motor impulses to the muscles and also receive sensory input from the skin and deeper structures. Diseases of the spinal cord produce various degrees of weakness, stiffness, muscle incoordination, and paralysis of the limbs.

The cauda equina is the termination of the spinal cord and contains the nerve branches to the sacrum and coccyx. Diseases of the cauda equina produce loss of sensation over the rump, paralysis of the tail, loss of bladder and bowel control, and paralysis of the anal sphincter.

There are multiple causes for central nervous system disease. Trauma to the nervous system is the most common cause. Although group outbreaks are rare, if multiple cases of central nervous system disease occur at one location it suggests an infectious or toxic cause. Bacterial infections typically are not as common as viral infections, and even less common causes are liver and electrolyte disturbances.

The Neurological Examination

In assessing brain and nerve diseases, the horse's history is of great importance. Your veterinarian will ask whether your horse has a recent history of head or neck trauma. Could the horse have been exposed to poisonous vegetation? Is there a history of a recent respiratory infection or *abortion*? Could a skin laceration or recent surgical incision be the focus of an infection? What is the vaccination and deworming history? Has the horse spent time on another farm, or been turned out with a new horse? Has he been exposed to other horses who are ill? Is the horse taking any drugs? When did you first notice the symptoms? Have the symptoms progressed? If so, has the progression been rapid or gradual? These are all important points to consider.

Age, sex, breed, and color of the horse are important, as well, because certain neurological disorders are genetically determined.

Next, the veterinarian will evaluate the horse's general behavior, mental status, head carriage, coordination, and cranial nerve function, looking for abnormal signs. Finally, there will be a complete examination of the horse's general body posture and gait, looking for signs of cerebellar, spinal cord, or peripheral nerve involvement.

To further evaluate a neurological disorder, special tests may be needed. These may include a complete blood panel, including a CBC, chemistry analysis of the serum, and even *titers* for infectious diseases, x-rays of the skull and vertebral column, diagnostic nerve blocks with local anesthetics, muscle and nerve conduction studies, and nerve and muscle *biopsies*. A *spinal tap* (a procedure in which fluid is removed from the spinal canal and submitted for laboratory analysis) may be necessary. A *myelogram* is a spinal tap in which dye is introduced into the spinal canal so signs of spinal cord compression can be seen on x-ray studies. Myelograms in the horse are performed under general anesthesia.

ASSESSING POSTURE AND GAIT PROBLEMS

- **Ataxia** is an inability to coordinate voluntary muscle movements that is symptomatic of some central nervous system disorders and injuries. The horse should be walked and, if possible, trotted in a straight line. Other maneuvers include walking him on the side of a hill in a circle, walking him over a curb, and making him walk backward. Signs of ataxia include swaying of the trunk and pelvis, stumbling, dragging the toes, wide circling, crossing the legs, and awkward foot placement such as stepping on the opposite foot. At rest, the horse will often assume a wide stance. When you pick up a foot and cross his legs, the horse may leave them crossed. Signs of ataxia are caused by diseases of the cerebellum, vestibular system, or spinal cord. Cerebellar ataxia is usually accompanied by head-bobbing and fine muscle tremors. Blindfolding the horse makes cerebellar ataxia worse but has little effect on spinal cord ataxia, in which the stumbling and swaying are caused by a lack of limb strength. Vestibular ataxia is discussed on pages 173 and 344.

- **Spasticity** is stiffness or rigidity of the limbs, and is seen in horses with spinal cord and cerebellar diseases. There is a shorter than normal stride in a spastic leg, while a longer than normal stride is seen in a weak leg. The difference in stride length is best detected by walking next to or behind the horse, matching him stride for stride.

- **Weakness** is an indication of partial paralysis. It is present in diseases of the spinal cord, musculoskeletal system, or peripheral nerves. A peripheral nerve paralysis is localized to one limb, is not accompanied by ataxia, and is often associated with localized loss of muscle volume (*atrophy*). Hind leg weakness can be confirmed by walking behind the horse and pulling on his tail. A normal horse can resist this, but a weak horse is easily pulled to the side. Dragging a foot, lacking the ability to extend a joint, and being unable to bear weight on a leg are all signs of a peripheral nerve paralysis.

Cranial Nerve Paralysis

The 12 pairs of cranial nerves arise from the midbrain and brain stem and pass directly out into the head and neck through openings in the skull. Damage to any of them can cause very specific symptoms. The most frequently encountered cranial nerve palsies in the horse are:

- **Optic nerve (II).** Damage to the optic nerve, or the optic center in the brain, produces varying degrees of blindness. The usual causes are trauma, brain abscess, and encephalitis.

- **Oculomotor nerve (III).** This nerve controls the size of the pupil. Shining a light into the eyes should cause the pupils to constrict and get smaller. When there is damage to the paired oculomotor nerves close to the brain stem, both pupils become dilated and unresponsive to light. Head trauma and brain abscesses are the most common causes of oculomotor paralysis.

- **Facial nerve (VII).** This nerve controls the muscles of facial expression. Paralysis causes drooping of the ear, inability to shut the eye (resulting in corneal ulcers and occasional loss of the eye), inability to flare the nostrils, loss of skin wrinkles around the nostrils and muzzle, and drooling from the corner of the lip. All these occur on the side of the face that is paralyzed. The most common causes of facial paralysis are guttural pouch infections, jugular vein thrombophlebitis, and trauma to the side of the face. Pressure on the nerve from failure to pad the side of the face during general anesthesia is another cause.

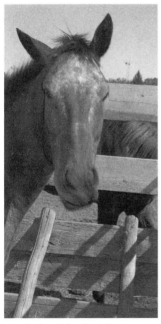

Paralysis of the facial nerve causes this horse's right ear, nostril, and lip to droop.

- **Vestibulocochlear nerve (VIII).** The nerves to the inner ear are important for balance and coordination. Horses with eighth nerve paralysis often exhibit a wide stance and a staggering gait. There is a tendency to lean, circle, and fall toward the side of involvement. Vestibular disorders are discussed in *Labyrinthitis* (page 173).

- **Glossopharyngeal, vagus, and spinal accessory nerves (IX, X, XI).** The primary functions of these nerves are to control swallowing and to produce sounds. Accordingly, signs of involvement include difficulty in swallowing, and a characteristic roaring or whistling sound as the horse is exercised. The most common causes of paralysis of one or all of these nerves are guttural pouch mycosis and jugular vein thrombophlebitis. Also consider the possibility of lead poisoning, botulism, or rabies.

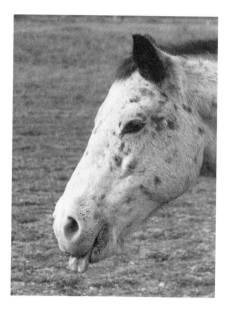

Paralysis of the tongue is associated with hypoglossal nerve injury.

- **Hypoglossal nerve (XII).** The 12th cranial nerve controls the muscles of the tongue. When one side is paralyzed, there is muscle wasting on that side of the tongue but little difficulty in grazing and swallowing. When both nerves are affected, the tongue is paralyzed and the horse is unable to eat or drink. Consider rabies, encephalitis, botulism, and poisoning from ergot, *forage*, lead, yellow star thistle, and Russian knapweed poisoning.

Peripheral Nerve Injuries

Peripheral nerve injuries result from trauma, infection, and toxicity. When a major nerve is injured, there is loss of sensation and muscle weakness or paralysis in the area served by that nerve. Most nerve injuries are associated with major limb trauma. Occasionally, a horse will have an isolated nerve injury. Such injuries are caused by bruises, stretches, tears, and lacerations.

One cause of nerve paralysis is injecting an irritating medication into or around a nerve. This problem is infrequent but can be a source of concern. The correct locations for giving injections are described in *Injections*, page 599.

Diagnostic studies that can be helpful in evaluating nerve function include nerve blocks with local anesthesia, muscle and nerve conduction studies, and nerve and muscle biopsies.

Common nerve injuries are discussed in this section. All cause lameness in one limb.

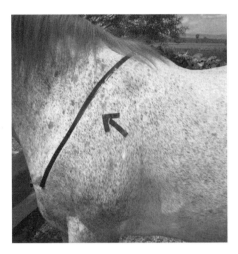

The location of sweeny, a wasting away of the muscles on either side of the scapula.

SUPRASCAPULAR NERVE (SWEENY)

A sweeny is caused by damage to the nerves that supply the supraspinatus and infraspinatus muscles. These muscles lie on either side of the shoulder blade. Denervation of these muscles causes atrophy. Loss of muscle volume and shrinkage of tissue result in a characteristic prominence of a ridgelike spine of the shoulders.

Nerve damage can occur from continuous pressure on the nerve, from a direct blow to the area, or from a stretch caused by a sudden backward thrust of the foreleg as the horse slips. Sweeny used to be common in draft horses when yokes were used to pull plows.

A horse with sweeny swings his front leg to the side because the shoulder is forced in an outward motion away from the body, a condition called lateral slippage of the shoulder. Slippage may be accompanied by an audible popping sound. The peculiar shoulder action may further stretch the nerve and aggravate the problem. The lateral slippage occurs before muscle atrophy, which takes several weeks to become evident.

A horse with sweeny can walk without difficulty but has a supporting leg lameness and is not able to participate in athletics. Treatment involves medical management, as described in *Treating Peripheral Nerve Injuries* (page 348). Surgery to remove a notch of bone to decompress the nerve may be beneficial. It takes six months for the full effects of treatment to become evident.

RADIAL NERVE

The radial nerve in the foreleg is responsible for advancing the leg as the horse steps forward. Injury to the radial nerve can occur with a fracture of the humerus below the shoulder blade, a fracture of the first rib, or pressure on the nerve from prolonged lateral *recumbency* (lying stretched out on the side of the body). If the radial nerve is injured high in the leg, the horse has a dropped elbow and cannot advance or bear weight on the leg. With a low paralysis, the horse stumbles and knuckles over and has a noticeable limp, but is able to bear weight.

FEMORAL NERVE

This large nerve in the hind limb straightens the stifle joint. It can be injured by a kick or a blow to the stifle area. Other causes of injury include exertional myopathy and overstretching the stifle during vigorous exercise. With femoral nerve paralysis, the horse holds the stifle in a flexed position, has difficulty advancing the leg, and will be unable to extend the stifle to put weight on the leg.

SCIATIC NERVE

The main trunk of the sciatic nerve is situated inside the pelvic canal. Most sciatic nerve injuries are associated with fractures of the pelvis and sacrum. In foals, deep injections close to the bone in the sciatic area can injure the nerve. The function of the sciatic nerve is to extend the hip and flex the stifle. Paralysis results in major gait disturbances. The limb is dragged, and there are signs affecting both major branches of the sciatic nerve (the tibial and peroneal nerves), as described in the next two sections.

Tibial Nerve

This branch of the sciatic nerve straightens the hock and flexes the ankle. The nerve is well protected and isolated injuries are not common. With paralysis, the leg is held with the hock flexed and the ankle straight. This causes the hip to drop on the affected side. The overall stride is strikingly like that of stringhalt (see page 245).

Peroneal Nerve

The peroneal branch of the sciatic nerve flexes the hock and extends the pastern. The nerve is easily injured in the upper leg near the stifle joint, where it is relatively unprotected by overlying muscle. Trauma from kicks and prolonged lateral recumbency are the usual causes.

Paralysis produces a characteristic stance in which the horse holds the leg straight out to the rear with the hoof knuckled over and the front surface of the hoof resting on the ground. As the horse advances and attempts to put weight on the back leg, the foot is dragged along the ground and then jerked to the rear.

Treating Peripheral Nerve Injuries

A nerve that has been bruised or stretched (but remains intact) may recover with time. The immediate need following injury is to suppress swelling and inflammation. This can be accomplished by applying ice packs and dimethyl sulfoxide (DMSO), or a topical *NSAID* such as diclofenac (Surpass) to the traumatized area. The horse should be rested in a stall for several weeks or months and gradually returned to full activity.

A severed nerve should be surgically repaired as soon as possible. However, the timing of repair depends on the condition of the wound. Dirty wounds are likely to become infected, which will compromise the repair. In such cases, the repair should be postponed for three to five weeks.

Healing nerves regenerate slowly—at the rate of about 1 inch (25 mm) a month. Following repair, the joint or limb must be protected while the nerve heals. This is done with splints and bandages. Physical therapy involves gentle massage and passive exercises that flex and extend the joints to maintain range of motion. Swimming is a good exercise because the water supports the paralyzed limb.

Occasionally, a traumatized nerve becomes trapped in scar tissue or forms a sensitive mass of nerve fibers at the severed ends. This mass is called a neuroma. Surgery can free up the nerve or remove the painful neuroma, but the neuroma may reoccur.

Head Trauma

The horse's brain is encased in bone, surrounded by a layer of fluid, and suspended in the skull by a system of tough ligaments, so it takes a major blow to the head to fracture the skull and injure the brain. Such injuries can be caused by kicks from other horses, running into posts, and rearing and falling over backward to land on the poll. Horses are naturally cautious animals, making them quite prone to head injuries, particularly of the poll.

Skull fractures can be linear, star-shaped, depressed, compound (open to the outside), or closed. Fractures at the base of the skull often extend into the ear, orbit, nasal cavity, or sinuses, creating pathways for brain infection. Open fracture should be suspected if there is bleeding from the ear canals or the nasal passages. Injuries serious enough to fracture the skull are often associated with bleeding into and around the brain from ruptured blood vessels. When the horse is known to have suffered head trauma, the possibility of skull fracture should be investigated.

Even head injuries without skull fracture can cause severe brain damage. Brain injuries are classified according to the severity of damage to the brain, as follows.

Contusion (bruising) is the mildest sort of injury and there is no loss of consciousness. After a blow to the head, the horse is dazed, wobbly, or disoriented. The condition then gradually clears.

Concussion means the horse was knocked out or experienced a loss of consciousness. A mild concussion is one in which there is only a brief loss of consciousness; with a severe concussion, a horse may be unconscious for minutes or even hours. After a severe concussion, a horse may exhibit a set of characteristic signs and symptoms called post-concussion syndrome. In this syndrome the horse appears depressed, lethargic, or in a stupor; he may wander in circles toward the side of the brain injury; and he often exhibits blindness or his tongue protrudes. These signs are due to brain swelling. If treatment is undertaken and the swelling does not extend to the midbrain, the outlook is favorable.

Brain swelling or a blood clot from ruptured vessels can follow severe head injury. Both produce increased intracranial pressure. Brain swelling, technically called cerebral edema, is always accompanied by a depressed level of consciousness and often coma. Since the brain is encased in a bony skull that does not expand as the brain swells, swelling of the brain leads to pressure on the brain stem. As the cerebellum is forced down through an opening near the base of the skull, the vital centers in the midbrain become squeezed and compressed. If this happens suddenly, it leads to death. Head trauma is a common cause of cerebral edema. Inflammation of the brain from encephalitis is another cause.

Death also occurs when the brain is deprived of oxygen. Complete interruption of the circulation and oxygen supply for only five minutes produces irreversible damage to the cells of the cerebral cortex. This could happen with cardiac arrest or suffocation.

Blood clots can occur between the skull and the brain, or within the brain itself. A blood clot produces localized pressure which does not, at least initially, compress the vital centers. The first indication is a depressed level of consciousness. Often one pupil is dilated and doesn't constrict when a light is shined in the eye. A paralysis or weakness may be present in one or more limbs. Progressive signs indicate the clot is expanding.

Inner ear (vestibular) syndrome is a characteristic set of signs caused by a blow to the poll with hemorrhaging around the brain stem. Typically, the horse experiences dizziness, incoordination, and loss of balance. In addition, the horse may exhibit head tilt, rapid jerking eye movements, circling, and evidence of facial nerve paralysis. Horses with vestibular injury often thrash and struggle violently in an effort to stand and therefore are quite likely to injure themselves or their handlers. Horses who recover from labyrinthitis (see page 173) may exhibit head-bobbing, or a coarse tremor of the head, that is most apparent when eating or drinking.

Signs of Brain Injury

Following a blow to the head, you should watch for signs of increased intracranial pressure caused by brain swelling or a blood clot. These signs can appear any time during the first 24 hours.

The most important thing to observe is the level of the horse's consciousness. An alert horse is in no danger. A stuporous horse is sleepy but responds to his handler. A comatose horse cannot be aroused. Any change in level of consciousness is an indication that treatment is imperative!

Checking the pupils of the eyes after any head trauma is a good way to monitor the horse's condition. Be sure to check the horse's pupils every hour. They should be equal in size and should constrict when a light is shined in the eyes. A dilated pupil that does not respond to light is a serious sign. Notify your veterinarian immediately. Also notify your veterinarian if the horse lies down or if his breathing becomes rapid and shallow. The horse may lie down during the course of the night but should respond to his handler. Once a horse becomes comatose, it is often too late to begin treatment.

Treating Brain Injuries

A severely injured horse may have other life-threatening conditions, such as a blocked airway, severe external bleeding, fractured ribs, or a punctured lung. Treatment of these takes precedence over the head injury.

Do not attempt to handle a frightened, thrashing, injured horse without professional assistance. Place the horse in a quiet, private enclosure (such as a stall), alone with nothing on which he can hurt himself. Many times the horse is not near his stall at the time of injury, so an enclosure must be improvised. The horse should be sedated first to prevent further injury and to facilitate a safe examination.

The objective of medical management is to control intracranial pressure and prevent brain swelling. This is accomplished by intravenous medications. The corticosteroid dexamethasone, with or without DMSO (dimethyl sulfoxide), is used for this purpose. Mannitol also is effective, but should be avoided if there is active bleeding into the cranial cavity. Seizures are controlled with an intravenous drug such as diazepam (Valium), pentobarbital, or xylazine. Antibiotics are indicated for open skull fractures.

Good nursing care is crucially important in a recumbent horse to prevent respiratory complications, muscle damage, and bedsores. Provide a well-padded bed for the horse to lie on and keep the area clean and dry. Roll the horse from side to side every four to six hours, or better yet, maintain a sternal position if possible to prevent pressure sores and the muscle wasting that is characteristic of prolonged recumbency. Petroleum jelly is a good water repellent and can be applied to the skin to prevent scalds. Maalox (an antacid that contains aluminum hydroxide and magnesium hydroxide) can be applied topically to help heal skin sores and abrasions.

An indwelling bladder catheter may be advisable; alternately, the horse can be catheterized several times a day.

If neurological signs develop despite treatment, it is an indication of increased intracranial pressure from cerebral edema or intracranial bleeding. Exploratory surgery should be considered. It must be done in a well-equipped equine surgery center. Further injury may result by transporting a horse in this condition, so consult with your veterinarian before moving the horse.

When coma persists for more than 36 hours, the chances for recovery are slight. However, if the horse shows steady improvement throughout the first week, the outlook for recovery is good. Horses who recover from brain injuries may continue to suffer from seizures, head tilt, head-bobbing, head tremors, and varying degrees of blindness.

Spinal Cord Problems
VERTEBRAL TRAUMA

Vertebral fractures are among the most frequent injuries sustained in athletic training and competition, particularly in racing and jumping. A horse who rears and falls over backward, or stumbles and falls in a somersault, can fracture his spine. Neck fractures may be associated with somersaults, head-on collisions, getting the head stuck between the bars of a pipe stall, or even struggling against a tied lead rope. Injuries to the lower spine are most likely to occur when a horse rears and falls over backward, or when he stumbles while backing up and slides into a sitting position.

Fractures of the vertebrae may or may not be accompanied by injuries of the spinal cord. It depends on the nature of the injury. Following a serious injury to the spinal column, if the horse is recumbent and is able to lift only his head, it is likely the horse has damaged his spinal cord high in the neck. If the horse can raise his head and neck, the injury is in the mid-to-lower cervical spine. If the horse can get up into a sitting position, the injury is at or below the second thoracic vertebra. If the horse can stand yet is ataxic and weak in the hindquarters, the injury is in the lumbar spine (toward the end of the back). Paralysis of the tail, along with urinary or fecal incontinence, indicates sacral cord involvement (the sacral spine is the large, triangular bone made up of the five fused vertebrae beyond the lumbar region).

The diagnosis and location of a spinal cord injury can be determined by testing for sensation, muscle function, and the presence of abnormal reflexes. X-rays of the neck and back are helpful in showing fractures and dislocations, but do not necessarily reveal the true extent of spinal cord injury. A myelogram (x-rays using a contrast dye) is the best way to tell to what extent the spinal cord is compressed or swollen.

Treatment: A horse with a vertebral fracture but no neurological signs of spinal cord injury requires only stall rest and observation. When neurological signs are present, treatment is directed at preventing further spinal cord injury or swelling. Medical treatment is like that described in *Treating Brain Injuries* (see page 350).

Surgery to remove bone fragments or to decompress the spinal cord is considered in all vertebral injuries in which the intact cord is in jeopardy. However, if the cord has been cut, torn, or crushed, the injury is permanent and surgery is unlikely to benefit the horse.

A paralyzed horse who is recumbent and shows no signs of improvement on medical or surgical treatment during the first two to three days can be considered to have irreversible damage to the spinal cord and should be euthanized to prevent further suffering.

Cervical Vertebral Myelopathy (Wobbler Syndrome)

Cervical vertebral myelopathy (CVM) is the most common neurological disease in horses. It is estimated that CVM affects 10 percent of Thoroughbred horses. The wobbly gait and other neurological signs are caused by narrowing of the spinal canal (stenosis) and compression of the spinal cord from malformed vertebrae. CVM occurs frequently in foals under 1 year of age, but the predominant age group is 1 to 4 years.

CVM does not have one specific cause. There are genetic predisposing factors, but CVM does not follow a simple hereditary pattern. Nutritional factors contribute to the development of disease, especially feeding a high-energy diet to foals, which stimulates rapid bone growth. Foals with CVM have a higher incidence of osteochondrosis, suggesting that CVM may be one of the developmental orthopedic diseases discussed in chapter 9, "The Musculoskeletal System." Trauma and biomechanical stresses are also important factors in some cases.

CVM is classified according to whether symptoms are made worse by movement of the spine. In horses with dynamic stenosis, the most common type, symptoms either appear or are made worse when the horse flexes his neck. In horses with static stenosis, symptoms are present but are not exacerbated by movements of the neck. This type is relatively uncommon.

Typical signs of CVM include progressive ataxia of the hindquarters (or all four limbs), characterized by clumsiness and wobbling, and a peculiar walk like that of a toy soldier. The neck is usually held stiffly. The horse frequently stumbles and scuffs his toes, or gets his legs crossed and then trips over them and falls. Backing up can be awkward.

Symptoms may be made worse when the horse goes up or down a hill. Because of weakness in the hindquarters, pulling the tail to one side as the horse walks causes the horse to stumble or sway to that side. This wouldn't happen in the normal horse.

Horses with CVM are subject to frequent falls. Owners and handlers often become aware of the horse's wobbliness and ataxia after a fall. This may give the impression that the fall was the cause of the symptoms, rather than the reverse.

The diagnosis is made by x-rays of the neck. However, x-rays may not be diagnostic for CVM and may point to some other cause for the ataxia, such as equine degenerative myeloencephalopathy or equine herpes *encephalomyelitis*. When x-rays are consistent with CVM, a myelogram may be requested for more detailed study.

Treatment: Medical therapy is directed at minimizing inflammation at the site of spinal cord compression. Anti-inflammatory drugs are used, including corticosteroids, phenylbutazone, NSAIDs, and DMSO, either singly or in combination. Stall rest for prolonged periods (six months or longer) is mandatory for most affected horses. Food and water should be provided at a height of 2 to 3 feet (60 to 90 cm) above the floor to minimize neck movement. Foals with mild x-ray changes may stabilize or improve when placed on a low-energy diet. In most cases, CVM is a progressive neurological disease and medical treatment alone is often unsuccessful. Surgery may be considered in selected individuals. Two procedures are used for surgical stabilization: the most often used is dorsal laminectomy, in which excess bone pressing on the spinal cord is removed; the other is intervertebral fusion, in which two or more adjacent vertebrae are joined together to stabilize the spine. These operations are difficult and may result in complications. The results are best when the surgery is performed on young horses with mild symptoms of short duration. A small number of horses return to athletic performance, and about a third can be used for pleasure riding.

CAUDA EQUINA SYNDROME

The cauda equina is made up of nerves that form the terminal extension of the spinal cord. Injuries to the sacrum that damage the cord can produce paralysis of the tail, anus, perineum, bladder, and rectum. This is called the cauda equina syndrome. Other conditions associated with the cauda equina syndrome include equine protozoal myeloencephalitis, sorghum grass poisoning, toxicity caused by haloxon (an organophosphate), parasite migration, and neuritis of the cauda equina.

Neuritis of the cauda equina is a disease of unknown cause that begins gradually or acutely with the horse rubbing and chewing at the tail head, and progresses over several weeks. The tail hangs limply and the anal and bladder sphincters are paralyzed. Urine drips continuously from a gaping vulva or protruded, relaxed penis, while feces may appear at the opening of the dilated anus. Hindquarter ataxia and gait disturbances can occur.

This disorder can also affect the cranial nerves, producing a head tilt or facial nerve paralysis. This suggests that an infectious or autoimmune process is at work.

Treatment: There is no cure. Manual evacuation of the rectum, catheterization of the bladder, and treatment of urinary tract infections may prolong the life of the horse.

Brain and Spinal Cord Infections

Encephalitis is inflammation of the brain and *myelitis* is inflammation of the spinal cord. Most cases of myelitis are actually less serious than an associated encephalitis. Specific infections of the brain and spinal cord are discussed in this section.

ENCEPHALITIS

Encephalitis is a common and very serious problem in horses, mainly because of the frequency of equine viral encephalomyelitis (see page 356). Signs of encephalitis include fever, depression, behavior and personality changes, head tilt, circling, decreased appetite, ataxia, incoordination, paralysis, seizures, and coma. How the horse behaves depends on which parts of the brain are most severely affected.

Bacteria also can cause encephalitis. Bacteria gain entrance to the brain via the bloodstream, after head trauma, or directly from an infection in the nasopharynx, sinuses, or guttural pouches. Fungi are rare causes of encephalitis, the principal one being *Cryptococcus*.

Treatment: Treatment of encephalitis is directed at the primary disease. It is important to prevent brain swelling and to provide good supportive nursing care, as discussed in *Treating Brain Injuries* (page 350).

EQUINE PROTOZOAL MYELOENCEPHALITIS

This disease is caused by the protozoan *Sarcocystis neurona,* which invades the brain and spinal cord. Opossums are the primary hosts of this protozoan. The organism is shed in the opossum's feces and contaminates feed and water, or may be picked up and distributed by birds. The horse is not a primary host, which helps explain the wide variation in clinical signs.

Equine protozoal myeloencephalitis (EPM) occurs most often in young horses 1 to 6 years of age, although it may also be seen in older horses. It is a disease of the western hemisphere, following the natural geographic range of opossums. Most cases are isolated. Outbreaks have not been reported.

The ingested protozoa migrate randomly through the spinal cord and brain, producing a variety of unexplained and highly variable neurological signs. The horse often stumbles or falls repeatedly and may exhibit a head tilt. Over a period of days, weeks, or months, the horse develops weakness, lameness, and muscle wasting in one or more limbs, frequently on different sides of the body. The ataxia and muscle weakness are progressive. Finally, the horse goes down and is unable to get up.

EPM mimics many neurological diseases. However, it should be a top consideration for any horse with unexplainable neurological signs that include weakness, ataxia, and muscle wasting. These signs are more severe in the hind limbs and occasionally can be asymmetrical.

The diagnosis is based on clinical suspicion, neurological findings, and antibody testing. The antibodies are detected using a cerebrospinal fluid sample and the Western blot test (usually a blood test). Using the Western blot test with blood alone is unreliable because of the high number of false positive results (because exposure is common among horses). However, a blood test can serve as a screening tool to rule out EPM. The polymerase chain reaction test (PCR) using cerebrospinal fluid is an accurate test, and its significance may be increased by concurrently performing the Western blot test on a cerebrospinal fluid sample. PCR may be positive well before a horse has an immune response, and therefore a positive Western blot test.

Treatment: The drugs diclazuril, nitazoxanide, and ponazuril are now available; they decrease the treatment time to about four weeks (it used to take several months). Your veterinarian will select the best treatment regimen for your horse. Pyrimethamine (Daraprim) and sulfa are older treatment options that are still used in some cases for economic considerations.

Prevention: Rodent-proofing feed containers, protecting *forages* from wildlife, and excluding birds may help reduce the risk of exposure. To further minimize contamination, pick up dead cats, armadillos, skunks, and raccoons, and dispose of the carcasses. This prevents opossums from eating the carcasses and excreting more of the infected cells, which are called sporocysts. A vaccine is available for use in regions where there is a high incidence of EPM. Discuss with your veterinarian whether vaccination is recommended in your area.

PARASITIC MYELOENCEPHALITIS

This disease is similar to EPM, but it is caused by the larval stages of *Strongyles vulgaris*, Habronema, Hypoderma, and other worms that migrate aimlessly through the brain and spinal cord. Parasitic myeloencephalitis, also called worm encephalopathy, is less common than EPM, but the symptoms are nearly indistinguishable.

Treatment: Ivermectin, thiabendazole in high doses, and febendazole are effective against the larval tissue stages of worms. Anti-inflammatory drugs reduce inflammation and swelling around the killed parasites. Corticosteroids may be used as directed by your veterinarian. Improvement follows treatment, but neurological deficits may persist.

Equine Degenerative Myeloencephalopathy

Equine degenerative myeloencephalopathy (EDM) is a progressive disease involving the spinal cord and brain stem. Most affected horses develop clinical signs by 1 year of age, but it can strike at any age. EDM produces symptoms like those of CVM (see page 352). EDM is found primarily in the northeastern United States, but it may occur throughout North America and in parts of Europe. It may affect one or many foals on the same farm.

Evidence suggests that EDM is related to a deficiency of vitamin E. Foals with EDM often have a history of being fed pelleted feeds and cured hay, and not being fed fresh hay or forage that contains ample amounts of vitamin E. There is also a hereditary predisposition to EDM in a number of breeds including Standardbreds, Thoroughbreds, Arabians, Appaloosas, and Morgans. Thus, it appears that both a familial predisposition and a vitamin E deficiency may play a role in the development of the disease.

EDM begins either gradually or suddenly, usually in foals 4 to 8 months of age. Initial signs are clumsiness and weakness in the legs. The gait is erratic, with the feet sometimes crossing and interfering. The hindquarters frequently are more severely affected than the forequarters, resulting in a wobbly ataxia with pelvic swaying, scuffing of the back feet, and sliding back on the rear into a sitting position.

EDM is difficult to distinguish from CVM and other forms of myeloencephalopathy, but it can be suspected when a young horse develops unexplained weakness and ataxia. X-rays of the neck are normal in a horse with EDM. In horses with CVM, neck x-rays show spinal column abnormalities.

Treatment: When a foal is diagnosed with EDM before 12 months of age, daily administration of 6,000 IU of dl-alpha tocopherol (vitamin E) mixed in grain with 2 ounces (60 ml) of corn oil has been shown to at least partially reverse the neurological signs, especially with mild disease. Improvement begins in three to four weeks. In older horses with spinal cord degeneration, the signs are irreversible and the disease is chronic and progressive.

Prevention: On farms where EDM occurs as a familial trait, giving foals 2,000 IU of vitamin E per day has been shown to offer protection. Pregnant mares near term may be given a vitamin E and selenium injection to increase vitamin E levels in the milk.

Equine Herpes Myeloencephalitis

Equine herpes myeloencephalitis virus occurs in several forms. The most common are EHV-1 and EHV-4, which are responsible for major outbreaks of paralytic disease throughout North America and the world. It also causes abortions in pregnant mares and respiratory disease in young horses. Transmission requires direct contact with secretions that contain the virus.

Neurological disease usually affects the hindquarters, although occasionally there will be a head tilt characteristic of cranial nerve paralysis. Symptoms develop rapidly, reach their worst within 48 hours, and usually do not progress thereafter. Initial signs are ataxia and alterations in gait that affect the rear. The horse is reluctant to move and often drags his toes. Tail paralysis, bladder paralysis with dribbling of urine (which may cause *cystitis*), and loss of sensation over the hindquarters are common signs. The horse may sit on his rear and crawl around in the stall.

The diagnosis can be made by recovering virus in blood or cerebral spinal fluid samples, or by serum antibody tests. A technique to identify the DNA sequence of EHV viruses from nasopharyngeal secretions can provide another means of diagnosis.

Treatment: Anti-inflammatory agents and DMSO are recommended. The anti-viral drug acyclovir has been of benefit in some horses and foals. Mildly affected horses continue to eat and drink and often recover completely in 3 to 12 weeks. The prognosis for the recumbent horse is guarded, although many horses will recover if given intensive nursing care, as described in *Treating Brain Injuries* (see page 350). Complications of recumbency are the usual causes of death.

The cystitis may be treated with sulfonamides.

Prevention: Vaccination does not prevent the neurological form of EHV-1 and EHV-4. However, maintaining a high level of immunity in the local horse population through vaccinations may serve as a barrier to the multiplication and spread of the virus. For vaccination information, see the table on page 103.

MENINGITIS

Meningitis is an infection of the membrane covering the surface of the brain. It is not common in adult horses. Most cases are caused by blood-borne bacteria from an infection elsewhere in the body. Occasionally, an infection of the nasopharynx, guttural pouch, or head and neck wound will extend into the brain.

Neonatal meningitis occurs in newborn foals who do not suckle during the first 18 hours of life and so fail to acquire protective maternal antibodies (see *Lack of Colostrum* in chapter 18, "Pediatrics"). The infection is blood-borne, originating from a septic site such as an infected umbilical stump.

Horses with meningitis have fever and behavior changes, including depression, circling, walking into walls, and falling over. These signs are followed by reluctance to move the head (stiff neck) and by indications of cranial nerve involvement, including blindness. Ataxia, weakness, epileptic-like seizures, and coma develop rapidly. The diagnosis is confirmed by finding the bacteria in the cerebrospinal fluid.

Treatment: Antibiotics in high doses are initiated on suspicion of meningitis. Drugs can be changed later in accordance with culture and sensitivity tests. Intravenous fluids are given to correct dehydration. Alcohol sponge baths reduce fever. Seizures are controlled with diazepam (Valium).

West Nile Virus

West Nile virus can cause encephalitis or meningitis. It was first encountered in the eastern United States in 1999, and has since spread throughout North America. Birds are the vector or the carrier and mosquitoes spread the infection, which can also affect humans. Horses are very susceptible to infection. For more information, see *West Nile Virus*, page 83.

Brain Abscess

Brain abscesses are not common. Most occur as complications of strangles. Bacterial infections about the head and neck can extend along the paths of the cranial nerves to involve the brain.

Signs are like those of meningitis. They include behavioral changes, head tilt, head pressing, aimlessly wandering, circling, dehydration, and starvation. In advanced stages, the horse begins to convulse. Seizures are followed by coma and death.

Treatment: Treatment is like that for meningitis (see page 357).

Seizures

A seizure is a sudden, uncontrolled burst of brain activity that begins with anxiety, followed by sweating, jaw clamping, rolling up of the eyes, collapse, spastic jerking of the legs, and loss of urine and stool. There is a brief loss of consciousness (usually up to 60 seconds) followed by a gradual return to normal. Usually the horse is able to stand within a few minutes. A post-seizure phase, ranging from mild depression to stupor and blindness, can last several hours.

Some seizures involve a small area in the brain. They are called partial seizures. Instead of the classic convulsion just described, the horse exhibits strange and inappropriate behavior such as twitching of the face or limbs, *head-pressing*, compulsive running in a circle, and self-biting.

Arrhythmias cause fainting spells that are often mistaken for seizures, as are the cataplexy spells of the fainting foal syndrome (see page 562).

Seizures commonly are associated with head trauma, brain infections, poisoning, insufficient oxygen to the brain, rabies, and liver failure. When they are due to head trauma, the seizure usually begins several weeks after the injury. Caution should always be exercised when approaching or working near a seizing horse.

Poisons that typically produce severe and sustained seizures include strychnine, antifreeze (ethylene glycol), insecticides, moldy corn poisoning, locoweed, rye grass, fiddleneck, common groundsel, yellow star thistle, and heavy metals.

Hyperkalemic periodic paralysis (HYPP) produces tremors, noisy breathing, and unpredictable paralytic episodes that may lead to death. This condition is often confused with tying-up syndrome. See pages 18 and 284 for more information.

Hypocalcemia (low blood calcium) produces seizures and ataxia, inability to chew or swallow, profuse sweating, and high fever. Most cases are associated with lactation. Others are due to blister beetle poisoning, excessive sweating, urea poisoning, and heat stroke.

Epilepsy is a recurrent seizure disorder of the brain. It is far less common in horses than it is in people. When the cause is unknown, it is said to be idiopathic. When it occurs after head trauma or brain inflammation, it is classified as acquired.

In some horses with idiopathic epilepsy, seizures appear to be brought on by specific events, such as feeding or saddling. There is a syndrome involving recurrent seizures in estrous mares that appears to be associated with circulating estrogen. It may improve if the ovaries are removed or the mare is given progesterone.

A convulsive syndrome in weanling Arabian foals is the only known form of inherited epilepsy in horses. Seizures appear abruptly and increase in frequency over days to weeks. Episodes can be mild to severe and are usually generalized. Eventually the foal is having seizures many times a day. The post-seizure state is often quite marked. Most foals appear to outgrow the problem. For more information, see *Neonatal Epilepsy* (page 574).

Treatment: If a horse begins to have a seizure, stand well aside to avoid being injured when the horse collapses and kicks out. Do not attempt to gentle or quiet the horse. After the seizure, notify your veterinarian. He or she may want to examine the horse to determine if the horse has been injured or has any findings that may suggest a cause.

Seizures lasting more than 60 seconds may be associated with chemical poisoning. Continuous seizures should be stopped to prevent injury to the brain. Diazepam (Valium) or pentobarbital can be given intravenously to stop a continuous seizure. Normally this is possible only when a trained professional is in attendance.

Seizure disorders such as those in Arabian foals or in horses with *idiopathic* epilepsy can be controlled with drugs. Phenobarbital is the most commonly used anticonvulsant. It is given once a day. The dosage can be reduced if the horse remains free of seizures for three months. Riding a horse who has a seizure disorder is not recommended.

14

THE DIGESTIVE SYSTEM

The equine digestive tract is a complex system that begins at the mouth and ends at the anus. The lips, teeth, tongue, mouth, and pharynx have been discussed in preceding chapters. The remaining organs are the esophagus, stomach, small intestine, large intestine, pancreas, and liver. (Horses do not have a gallbladder to store bile, as people do. Bile from the liver empties continuously into the small intestines.)

The esophagus is a muscular tube 5 feet (1.5 m) long that conveys food from the throat down to the stomach. This is accomplished by rhythmic contractions. The lower esophagus enters the stomach at an acute angle, which creates a one-way valve. When the stomach is distended by food or air, pressure closes the valve and prevents *reflux* into the esophagus. One disadvantage of this mechanism is that the valve also prevents the horse from vomiting to relieve an excessive buildup of gas and fluid. This increases the risk of gastric rupture.

The stomach is relatively small when compared with the size of the remaining gastrointestinal tract. Although it is capable of holding 4 gallons (15 l), it functions most efficiently when filled to about 2 gallons (7.6 l). Food in the stomach is acted upon by acid and pepsin. Pepsin breaks down proteins into chains of amino acids.

Digestion begins as soon as food enters the stomach. When the stomach is about two-thirds full, the sphincter at the outlet of the stomach relaxes and food passes in a steady stream into the *duodenum* and small intestines. Rapid ingestion of a large volume of feed causes the stomach to empty rapidly, before the stomach enzymes can act upon the entire meal. This interferes with total digestion and the proper use of feed. This is the main reason why frequent small meals are preferable to a single large one. This makes sense when you consider that the horse is naturally a grazing animal.

The small intestine is 70 feet (21.3 m) long and has a capacity of about 12 gallons (45.4 l). It is located principally in the forward part of the left abdominal

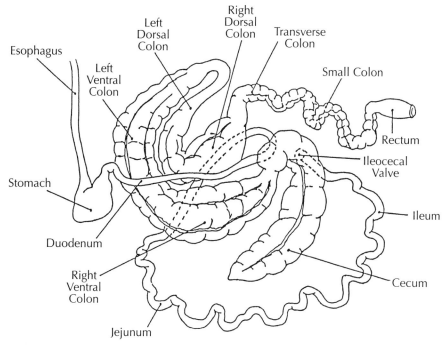

The digestive tract.

cavity and is divided into the duodenum, jejunum, and ileum. The small intestine absorbs nutrients, as does the large and small colon.

As food enters the upper small intestine, it is acted upon by bile salts from the liver, digestive enzymes from the pancreas, and a mixture of digestive enzymes secreted by the small intestine itself.

The end products of digestion are then absorbed and enter the bloodstream, flowing to the liver. The liver has numerous functions connected with metabolism. Here the materials of the horse's meal are converted into stored energy.

The remains of the meal, consisting mostly of liquid fiber and roughage, move on into the large intestine (also known as the bowel). The large intestine is approximately 25 feet (7.6 m) long. It is divided into the cecum, large colon, small colon, and rectum.

The cecum is a blind sac that is 4 feet (1.2 m) long and holds 7 to 10 gallons (26.5 to 37.8 l). This part of the digestive tract is primarily responsible for hindgut fermentation and may be one of the reasons that the equine gastrointestinal tract is sensitive to any changes. It is a comma-shaped structure located in the right flank, with its tip extending toward the diaphragm. The contents of the cecum are liquid. The cecum contains a large population of bacteria, which feed on the partially digested food from the stomach and, by the process of fermentation, break down cellulose. These bacteria also produce essential fat-soluble vitamins and acids that are absorbed by the horse and later used for energy.

The large intestine is made up of the large colon, the small colon, and the rectum. The large colon is 10 to 12 feet (3 to 3.6 m) long and holds about 20 gallons (75.7 l) of semi-liquid stool. It is subdivided into the right lower (ventral) colon, left lower (ventral) colon, left upper (dorsal) colon, right upper (dorsal) colon, and the transverse colon. All these names refer to the positions of these segments within the *peritoneal cavity*.

The small colon is also 10 to 12 feet (3 to 3.6 m) long. In the small colon, water is absorbed and the end products of digestion are formed into soft round balls.

The rectum is about 1 foot (30 cm) long. It stores the waste material until it is passed out of the horse's body during the act of defecation.

The pancreas is located behind the stomach and is connected to the duodenum. In addition to producing digestive enzymes, the pancreas manufactures insulin. A deficiency of insulin causes diabetes mellitus. This disease is extremely rare in horses.

Horses are hindgut fermenters. Hindgut refers to the part of the intestine after the small intestine—the cecum, the large and small colon, and the rectum. Fermentation is the process by which microbes break down components of feed (the structural carbohydrates of hay) into molecules that the horse can use for metabolism.

The Esophagus

A horse with esophageal disease regurgitates, swallows painfully, and drools. *Regurgitation* is the expulsion of swallowed food. It is due to a blockage or malfunction of the swallowing mechanism. When the blockage is low in the esophagus, regurgitation occurs about ten seconds after swallowing.

When the blockage is located at the back of the throat or in the upper esophagus, attempts to eat or drink produce coughing, gagging, and regurgitation of food and saliva through the nose. Food may be inhaled into the lungs, causing aspiration pneumonia. With a complete blockage, the horse cannot swallow anything—not even water.

Choking is the most common cause of sudden blockage of the esophagus. A slow progressive obstruction is characteristic of tumors and strictures. Cleft palate is the diagnosis in a newborn foal who regurgitates milk.

Central nervous system poisons include botulism, moldy corn poisoning, yellow star thistle, and Russian knapweed. These poisons produce paralysis of the tongue and throat, accompanied by regurgitation and drooling.

Dysphagia is painful swallowing. It occurs under the same circumstances as regurgitation. A horse with dysphagia is noticeably anxious and makes repeated efforts to swallow by lowering her head and stretching her neck. If the horse cannot swallow, she drools. In a horse with strangles, swollen lymph nodes at the back of the throat are a cause of painful and difficult swallowing.

When the esophagus has been blocked or paralyzed for more than 24 hours, a horse becomes apathetic, stops trying to swallow, and stands quietly beside her water trough.

CHOKING

Choking occurs when the esophagus is blocked by a large bolus of food or foreign material. It does not cause respiratory obstruction because the impaction in the esophagus is below the level of the larynx.

Choking tends to occur in horses who eat rapidly and swallow their feed without chewing it thoroughly. It also occurs in horses who do not chew their food completely because of defective teeth or who bolt their food to avoid painful chewing, usually older horses. Some horses choke because their esophagus is narrowed by inflammation, ulceration, or stricture.

A horse who chokes displays sudden, anxious behavior, backs away from her feed, salivates profusely, coughs, arches her neck and attempts to swallow repeatedly, and regurgitates food and saliva through the nostrils.

Horses can choke on dry grain, which swells when it becomes wet. Sugar beets, a large carrot, pelleted rabbit food, and even hay can cause choking. Pelleted feeds, however, do not seem to cause choking any more frequently than do sweet feeds.

Other foreign bodies that can lodge in the esophagus and cause choking include wood and wood shavings, corncobs, milk teeth, fruit pits, and large pills. Trauma to the esophagus can cause choking by creating a stricture. Usually, external signs of the trauma are visible. The esophagus can also rupture secondary to choking or trauma.

Treatment: Place the horse in an empty stall that contains no food, water or bedding and notify your veterinarian. The impaction will often soften up with saliva and pass into the stomach in a matter of hours. If not, it may do so after the horse has been tranquilized and given an analgesic that helps to relax the esophagus.

With a persistent impaction, your veterinarian may elect to pass a nasogastric tube and gently flush the upper esophagus with warm water to loosen up the wad. This may need to be repeated several times over the next 24 to 48 hours. If this is not successful, the impaction can usually be dislodged under general anesthesia, using a scope to extract the wad or push it down into the stomach. Rarely, it will be necessary to open the esophagus and remove the impaction manually. Following such surgery, there is a high incidence of esophageal stricture.

After recurring episodes of choking, the esophagus should be examined with a fiber-optic gastroscope to determine whether the esophagus has ulcerated, and also to be sure the horse does not have a stricture or tumor of the esophagus. As an alternative, the esophagus can be x-rayed using barium paste given orally. The barium serves as a contrast medium to help visualize the walls of the esophagus.

If the esophagus is normal after the impaction has been relieved, it is safe to resume feeding after 12 to 24 hours. However, if there is ulceration or an inflammatory stricture, withhold feed (but not water) for three to four days and then begin feeding a soft diet as described for *Strictures* (below). A soft diet can be made by adding warm water to pelleted feed to make a mash.

Prevention: Correct any dental problems that may be the cause of improper chewing (see *Taking Care of Your Horse's Teeth*, page 186). Feeding small amounts more often, and moistening the grain, can help prevent recurrent episodes of choking. If the horse persists in gobbling her food, spread the feed over a large surface, mix it with chopped hay, or add several large, smooth stones (too large to swallow) to the feed box and scatter the pellets so the horse will have to pick them out one at a time.

Prevent your horse from chewing wood and plastics. Remove wood shavings from stall floors.

STRICTURES

A stricture is a narrowing of the esophagus caused by inflammatory swelling or scarring. Nearly all strictures are caused by choking. Following an episode of choking, a temporary stricture caused by swelling of the mucosal layer of the esophagus may lead to repeated choking episodes for several weeks. These episodes can occur even though you are soaking the horse's feed in water and feeding it softened.

The depth of the mucosal injury determines the depth of the stricture and whether it will respond to treatment. Ulcerating injuries that involve all layers of the esophagus tend to heal with permanent scar tissue.

A squamous cell cancer of the esophagus is a rare cause of stricture.

Treatment: The stricture should be investigated by your veterinarian using barium contrast x-rays or fluoroscopy, and/or an esophageal *endoscopy*. A mucosal swelling may subside if the horse continues on a soft diet for several weeks. A soft diet consists of a slurry of pelleted feed with added roughage such as chopped alfalfa. Pelleted rations that are nutritionally complete and require no additional roughage are also available.

Tight fibrous strictures that remain fixed often respond to the passage of esophageal dilators that stretch out the scar. Multiple (and occasionally, periodic) stretchings are required to maintain an adequate passage. In these instances, a soft diet will be necessary for life. Tight, fixed strictures that do not respond to dilatation require esophageal surgery. The surgery is difficult and usually requires referral to a veterinary specialty center.

Prevention: Many strictures can be prevented by prompt treatment of the initial episode of choking.

The Stomach

Diseases of the stomach are associated with indigestion, failure to thrive, and severe colicky pain in the abdomen. Because there is a powerful sphincter mechanism at the *gastroesophageal junction*, both vomiting and the reflux of stomach fluid into the esophagus are uncommon in horses. In most cases, what is thought to be vomiting is actually choking on unswallowed food rather than stomach contents coming out through the nostrils.

GASTRIC DILATATION

Acute gastric dilatation is a sudden painful distention of the stomach due to a buildup of fluid and gas. The most common cause is grain engorgement. The grain forms a packed mass in the stomach that ferments and draws in fluid. Gases produced by fermentation cause bloat. Inflammation of the stomach lining or an obstruction of the small intestines can also cause dilatation.

A secondary type of gastric distension occurs when there is an obstruction in the small intestine or the colon. The fecal contents of the bowel back up into the stomach. The stomach progressively enlarges because the horse cannot vomit to relieve the pressure.

The pain of acute gastric dilatation is severe and violent. Signs include rolling, sweating, kicking at the abdomen, and turning the head as if to bite at the abdomen. Heart and respiratory rates are increased. The horse may exhibit shock, with cold extremities. A rectal exam will show displacement of the spleen. A peritoneal tap (as described for *Colic*, page 381) will show

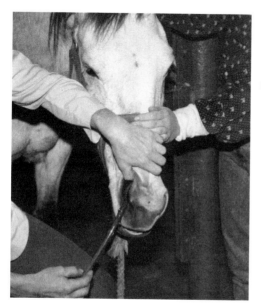

Passing a nasogastric tube is an important initial step in diagnosing acute gastric dilatation, bowel obstruction, and moderate to severe colic.

whether the stomach has ruptured. Finding ingested food in the peritoneal fluid confirms this diagnosis and is an ominous sign.

Chronic gastric dilatation is a milder condition found in horses who *crib* and swallow large amounts of air. It also occurs in horses who suffer from gastritis. The diagnosis of gastric dilatation is confirmed by passing a nasogastric tube. When the tube enters the stomach, air and fluid will rush out the end of the tube. The appearance of the gastric reflux fluid gives some indication of whether the gastric dilatation is primary or secondary to a bowel obstruction. In the latter instance, the gastric reflux is brown and fecal-like. Horses with bowel obstruction require further treatment (see *Intestinal Obstruction*, page 372).

Treatment: If the horse shows signs of abdominal distress, notify your veterinarian at once. Passing a nasogastric tube will bring immediate relief, as air and fluid are expelled. Gastric rupture is a fatal complication of acute gastric dilatation and is likely to occur if the distended stomach is not decompressed.

Irrigating and flushing the stomach will relieve a problem caused by overeating or overdrinking. Dioctyl sodium sulfosuccinate (DSS) helps to soften a grain impaction. Mineral oil, which must be given by tube, is also useful for its anti-fermentation effects.

Most horses with gastric dilatation are dehydrated and have *electrolyte* and acid-base imbalances. These should be corrected by appropriate intravenous therapy.

Note that acute laminitis may accompany or follow an episode of acute gastric dilatation.

Gastric Rupture

Rupture of the stomach follows severe untreated gastric dilatation. As the stomach tears during acute gastric dilatation, there is a brief period during which the pain of distention is relieved and the horse appears to be better. However, within 30 minutes the horse becomes bathed in sweat, develops a rapid heart rate, goes into shock, and dies within a matter of hours.

Other causes of gastric perforation are ruptured stomach and duodenal ulcers. Rarely, a perforated stomach is caused by bots or Habronema worms that invade the wall of the stomach.

The diagnosis of gastric perforation can be confirmed by an abdominal tap, which shows ingested feed in the peritoneal fluid.

Treatment: Surgical repair is not possible. The horse should be euthanized as soon as the diagnosis is confirmed.

Equine Gastric Ulcer Syndrome

Gastric ulcers in horses are now recognized as much more common in all ages of horses than had previously been thought. With the use of endoscopic examination, equine gastric ulcer syndrome (EGUS) has been found to occur in up to one half of all foals and 90 percent of horses past the age of weaning.

The causes of EGUS in horses can usually be associated with three major risk factors, occurring singly or in combination: feeding rates, stress, and the use of non-steroidal anti-inflammatory drugs (*NSAIDs)* over time. Horses evolved as grazing animals who require frequent but small amounts of food entering the stomach. Humans have altered that continuous grazing pattern by confining horses to stalls and stables. A horse in a confinement situation is usually fed once or twice a day. But the horse's stomach produces acid throughout the day; in the absence of food, this prolonged acid exposure in the empty stomach erodes the normal stomach surfaces and creates ulcers.

The mechanism by which EGUS develops is complicated by chemical imbalances, other existing clinical disorders, and stress. The bacterium *Helicobacter pylori* is a primary cause of peptic ulcers in humans, but has not been found in horses. However, recent studies suggest that another *Helicobacter* species may be involved in EGUS.

Stress-induced EGUS has many causes: strenuous training and showing for the high-performance horse, boarding the horse alone without contact with others, and feeding high-grain diets all may contribute.

The prolonged administration of NSAIDs is a well-established cause of EGUS in the horse. The length of NSAIDs treatment that will produce EGUS varies from individual to individual. Usually, more than ten days of treatment increases the risk of developing EGUS. This risk will be greatly increased if the horse is following an arduous racing or training schedule.

The diagnosis of ulcers usually cannot be made based solely on the symptoms, which include intermittent *colic*, going off feed, and restlessness characterized by repeatedly getting up and down. However, when a horse is under stress or taking anti-inflammatory drugs and exhibits these symptoms, endoscopic examination is worthwhile. A screening test is now available to detect blood that is present within the gut. This test can be useful in diagnosing ulcers.

Treatment: The first step is to remove all stressful conditions that may be causing the ulcer. Anti-inflammatory medications the horse may be taking should be discontinued, if possible.

Omeprazole (Gastrogard or Ulcergard) is effective in treating the ulcer, as is sulcralfate (a mucosal coating agent) and antacids that contain aluminum hydroxide, such as Mylanta. These drugs are best taken in combination and should be given several times a day, under the guidance of your veterinarian. Treatment is continued for at least three to four weeks. A follow-up *gastroscopy* may be advisable to ensure that healing is complete. Omeprazole at one half its therapeutic dose has also been used as a preventive.

GASTRIC OUTLET OBSTRUCTION

The scarring associated with ulcers may cause a ring constriction or deformity, which prevents the stomach from emptying. The obstruction may be partial or complete. Horses with gastric outlet obstruction experience pain immediately after eating, are reluctant to eat and drink, lose weight, become dehydrated, and experience intermittent abdominal bloating and gastric dilatation.

Squamous cell cancer and lymphoma are other causes of gastric outlet obstruction.

Treatment: Strictures caused by ulcers can be corrected surgically, with a good prognosis.

Gastritis

Gastritis is an inflammation and irritation of the lining of the stomach. Unlike a stomach ulcer, gastritis involves large areas. The mucosa throughout much of the stomach appears red and swollen, and contains many small ulcerations or areas of erosion. Gastritis occurs in both the acute and chronic form. It is less common than equine gastric ulcer syndrome.

Acute gastritis is caused by ingesting moldy or spoiled feed, sand, chemicals and toxins, or by overeating or blister beetle poisoning. The horse with acute gastritis salivates and drools excessively, refuses to eat, and exhibits colic. A severe case of acute gastritis is indistinguishable from acute gastric dilatation (see page 365). In fact, acute gastric dilatation often develops along with the acute gastritis.

Laminitis can accompany or follow an episode of acute gastritis.

Chronic gastritis is associated with the long-standing ingestion of poor-quality feeds or foreign materials such as wood shavings, sand, or stones. These indigestible materials irritate the lining of the stomach and often remain for long periods, during which they conglomerate with feed to form impacted food balls called *bezoars*. The bezoars are too large to pass into the small intestines but are small enough to intermittently obstruct the outlet of the stomach. The retention of gastric contents creates a favorable environment for the overgrowth of bacteria.

Other causes of chronic gastritis include cribbing, with swallowing large amounts of air, and infection of the lining of the stomach by bots, Habronema, hairworms, or certain bacteria such as *Helicobacter sp.*

Signs of chronic gastritis include intermittent colic, lack of appetite, weight loss, unthrifty appearance, a rank odor to the breath, and emaciation. The stool is pasty and soft. The diagnosis is made by gastroscopy performed to evaluate stomach symptoms.

Treatment: The initial treatment of acute gastritis is the same as that described for acute gastric dilatation (see page 365). A tube is passed and the stomach is thoroughly irrigated to remove the ingested irritant. Intestinal protectants (mineral oil or Kaopect, a kaolin and pectin suspension) help soothe an inflamed stomach. Anti-ulcer medications (see *Equine Gastric Ulcer Syndrome*, page 366) are often prescribed.

After an episode of acute gastritis, provide an easily digestible diet, such as one that contains bran mashes, green feeds, or fine hay fed continuously. After one to two weeks, switch to a high-quality maintenance diet as described in chapter 15, "Nutrition and Feeding."

It is important to identify and remove the source of the problem. Chronic gastritis is treated by correcting the underlying cause of the condition. This may involve treating a dental problem causing improper chewing. Gastric parasites are eliminated with appropriate anthelmintics (see chapter 2, "Parasites"). Horses who eat wood and foreign material should be turned out to pasture and provided with exercise and companionship. An obstructing bezoar requires surgical removal.

Peritonitis

Inflammation of the lining of the abdominal cavity is called *peritonitis*. Peritonitis can be acute or chronic, and localized or generalized.

ACUTE PERITONITIS

Acute peritonitis occurs when the peritoneal cavity is suddenly contaminated by foreign material and bacteria. The common causes are gastric rupture, rectal tears, strangulation of the intestines, bowel obstruction, ruptured bladder, penetrating wounds of the abdominal cavity, and the breakdown of a suture line following bowel surgery.

In *mares*, peritonitis can be caused by vaginal tears during intercourse, rupture of the large colon during labor and delivery, uterine *torsion*, or rupture of the pregnant uterus.

In *foals*, peritonitis can be caused by a ruptured bladder during delivery, navel infection, *strangulated* hernia, foal *septicemia*, foal pneumonia, or ruptured gastric ulcer.

Horses with acute spreading peritonitis exhibit intense pain in the abdomen, break out in a sweat, and usually lie down and roll on the ground. Listening with a stethoscope reveals absent bowel sounds. Pressing on the abdomen causes the horse to groan. The belly and flanks feel somewhat rigid or boardlike, because of reflex spasms of the abdominal wall muscles. Diarrhea may be noted.

When peritonitis is caused by intestinal rupture, signs of shock and dehydration will be evident in the red or muddy mucous membranes, prolonged *capillary refill time* (three seconds or longer), and rapid thready pulse (over 60 beats per minute). Death can occur in a matter of hours.

Tapping the abdomen and examining the peritoneal fluid (as described in *Diagnosing Colic*, page 381) is the quickest way to confirm the diagnosis.

Treatment: It varies with the cause of the peritonitis. In general, horses with acute peritonitis require intensive intravenous fluid therapy, broad-spectrum antibiotics, and correction of acid-base and electrolyte imbalances. Flunixin meglumine (Banamine) is given for pain relief and may help control endotoxic shock.

Inserting a nasogastric tube to decompress a distended stomach can lead to dramatic initial improvement. It is advisable to leave the tube in place or to pass it at frequent intervals.

A horse with a continuing source of contamination may be a candidate for surgical exploration. Alternately, in the absence of such a source, your veterinarian may decide to perform peritoneal *lavage*. Catheters are inserted into the peritoneal cavity and large volumes of salt solution are flushed into and out of the abdomen. This reduces the concentration of bacteria and foreign particles.

With massive contamination or advanced shock and *sepsis*, the likelihood for success is so remote that it is often advisable to euthanize the horse.

CHRONIC PERITONITIS

Peritoneal infection can localize to form an abscess, or chronic peritonitis. Abdominal abscesses also occur in horses with strangles or foal pneumonia. Migrating larvae of *Strongyles vulgaris* have been implicated in some cases of chronic peritonitis.

Signs of chronic peritonitis include gradual weight loss, poor appetite, failure to thrive, and intermittent episodes of colic. If diarrhea develops, the outlook is poor. An abdominal ultrasound may help locate an abscess, which is an uncommon cause of chronic peritonitis.

Treatment: It is directed at the underlying disease. Antibiotics and deworming agents, such as ivermectin, may be effective in some cases. Your veterinarian may suggest surgical exploration to establish a diagnosis or to drain an abscess.

The Small Intestines

Diseases of the small intestine are characterized by colic and intestinal obstruction.

Diarrhea is not a sign of small intestinal disease in adult horses. The length and size of the horse's colon compensates almost completely for disorders of the small intestines. Diarrhea originating in the small intestines only occurs when there is also disease of the colon. This does not apply to foals, in whom the capacity of the colon is not fully developed. Diarrhea in foals is discussed in *Foal Diarrhea* (see page 555).

Enteritis

Enteritis is any inflammatory disease of the small intestines. Since most cases also involve the colon, and diarrhea is a prominent feature, enterocolitis is a more accurate term. Infectious diseases are the most common cause of enterocolitis. They include enteric salmonellosis, actinobacillosis, equine viral arteritis, and rotavirus infection.

Intestinal parasites are another cause of enterocolitis. Adult worms of several species attach to the lining of the small and large intestines and produce inflammation, bleeding, anemia, loss of protein, impaired digestion, and in some cases severe diarrhea.

The migrating larvae of S. *vulgaris* may initiate recurrent episodes of severe colic caused by clotting of the blood supply to a segment of the small intestines. Diarrhea is not a feature.

Treatment: It is directed at the specific infectious disease. Protect your horse by keeping vaccinations current and by maintaining a good parasite control program (see chapter 2, "Parasites").

Duodenitis-Proximal Jejunitis

This severe and sometimes fatal enteritis begins suddenly with unexplained colic. *Clostridium difficile* and *Salmonella species* have been suggested as causes of duodenitis-proximal jejunitis (DPJ). Dehydration and toxicity develop rapidly. The small intestines cease to function and passively fill with large amounts of gas and fluid that back up into the stomach, producing secondary acute gastric dilatation. The picture closely resembles mechanical small intestine obstruction or intestinal strangulation. The findings on peritoneal tap (as described for *Colic*, page 382) help to differentiate these diseases. This is important because, unlike the other conditions, horses with DPJ do not require surgery.

Treatment: It involves inserting a nasogastric tube and removing large amounts of fluid and gas. This brings relief from colic and also eliminates the risk of gastric rupture. Large amounts of intravenous fluids are administered to correct electrolyte imbalances, along with antibiotics. Prolonged nasogastric tube decompression (up to seven days) is typical of horses with DPJ. These two steps usually restore normal intestinal function.

Granulomatous Enteritis

This disease of the small intestines and colon is occasionally associated with chronic diarrhea. However, most horses experience colic, *depression*, and weight loss. The cause is unknown. A hypersensitivity reaction to some as yet unknown *antigen* has been suggested. Rectal examination may disclose enlarged nodes in the mesentery (the ligament that holds the gastrointestinal tract together and is attached to the backbone) of the small intestine.

Treatment: Some horses respond to corticosteroids, but relapses occur when the medication is stopped.

Intestinal Obstructions

The diagnosis of intestinal obstruction is suspected based on the history and behavior of the horse. The onset is abrupt and signs are severe. The horse becomes noticeably depressed and exhibits signs of colic and pain in the abdomen. The heart rate increases (often to greater than 60 beats per minute), the pulse is weak and thready, the mucous membranes are muddy or cyanotic, *capillary refill time* is greater than three seconds, and the extremities become cool. The horse may roll repeatedly in a violent manner.

These signs are more pronounced in cases of strangulation and unrelieved obstruction. They are due to dehydration, loss of fluids into the distended bowel, and, in some cases, to toxicity from endotoxins and degenerating gut, and peritonitis.

Inserting a nasogastric tube may show reflux of partially digested food from a distended stomach. This indicates either a high intestinal obstruction or an obstruction of long standing. When the obstruction is early or low (in the colon), there is generalized bloating of the belly but little undigested food and gas in the stomach.

Rectal examination is of utmost importance in all cases of suspected bowel obstruction. An experienced observer can frequently tell the type and location of the obstruction by whether the bowel is in its usual position and by the feel of the distended loops.

A peritoneal tap (as described in *Treating Colic*, page 382) is another important diagnostic test and can be performed in the field. Fluid is withdrawn and inspected for blood, pus, protein, bacteria, and ingested plant material. This helps determine whether the bowel is becoming gangrenous or if rupture has occurred.

The common causes of intestinal obstruction are discussed in this section.

STRANGULATION

Any interference with the blood supply to the walls of the intestines is called strangulation. Strangulation is characterized by rapid deterioration in the horse's *condition*. Signs of strangulation are difficult to distinguish from those of peritonitis. The pain of both is severe and unrelenting. Sweating is pronounced. The horse rolls from side to side and often lies on her back. Dehydration and toxicity occur rapidly. Endotoxic shock occurs when bacterial toxins and toxic products of degenerating equine intestinal tissue are released into the circulation. Multiorgan system failure can result.

If blood flow to the strangulated bowel is not restored within four to six hours, the bowel becomes devitalized and dies. This is called *infarction*. It is may not always be followed immediately by rupture and peritonitis; however, if treatment is to be successful, it must be undertaken before the bowel ruptures. The only effective treatment is to operate and remove the infarcted intestine.

The most common causes of strangulation are listed here.

Volvulus

A segment of intestine can twist. If the twist is less than 360 degrees, it is called a torsion. A twist of 360 degrees is called a volvulus. A volvulus results in a sudden shutting-off of the blood supply to the twisted portion of the bowel. The bowel itself may be twisted shut at one or both ends.

Volvulus of the small intestine can be caused by adhesions, worm impactions, and motility disorders (lack of normal *peristalsis*, the normal contractions of the gut) associated with changes in diet. Migrating strongyle larvae have been known to cause motility disorders. Lipomas are a common cause of torsion and volvulus. A lipoma is a fatty tumor on a long stalk attached to the mesentery of the bowel. The lipoma may become displaced and cause strangulation and infarction. Groin and navel *hernias*, internal hernias, and diaphragmatic hernias are other causes of twists and obstructions. An internal hernia occurs when a loop of bowel becomes trapped in a pocket between internal organs. A diaphragmatic hernia is a hole in the diaphragm that allows a portion of bowel to pass into the chest. Most hernias are apparent at or shortly after birth, causing severe respiratory distress in the neonatal foal. These hernias are rare in older horses, but may be considered in cases of trauma. Volvulus of the colon is not uncommon. The colon in horses is extremely large when compared to that of other animals, and is loosely attached to surrounding structures. For these reasons it is easily displaced, twisted, and kinked. It has been suggested that a horse who rolls from side to side may incur a volvulus, torsion, or displacement of the colon.

Treatment: The treatment of volvulus is surgical unwinding of the twisted bowel. If the bowel is devitalized (the tissue has died), that segment must be surgically removed.

Intussusception

Intussusception occurs when the small intestines telescopes into an adjacent segment of bowel. It occurs frequently in young horses as a result of enteritis, heavy worm infestation, or dietary changes that result in abnormal peristalsis.

Ileocecal intussusception involves the telescoping of the terminal ileum into the cecum. This is the most common type of intussusception and produces complete obstruction. Ileal-ileal intussusception (in which the ileum folds in on itself) often results in partial obstruction. Intussusception of the colon does occur, but much less often.

Depending on the location, symptoms develop abruptly or gradually. An acute intussusception is indistinguishable from strangulation. When the obstruction is not complete at the onset, signs develop more slowly and may initially suggest spasmodic colic.

Treatment: The treatment of all types of intussusception is surgical removal of the involved bowel. The sooner this is done, the better the prognosis.

Nonstrangulating Infarction

The wall of the bowel can become devitalized as a result of arteritis and arterial *occlusions* produced by migrating strongyle larvae. This does not happen often, because the intestinal blood supply of horses contains numerous channels that provide alternate pathways for perfusion (liquid circulating through tissue). When infarction does occur, the cecum and large colon are the most common sites.

Episodes of recurrent *thromboembolism* without infarction occasionally cause colic and abdominal pain in yearlings and young adults. Bowel obstruction is not a factor, although the migrating larvae may also produce an intestinal motility disorder that predisposes the horse to or causes intussusception or volvulus.

Treatment: Surgical *resection* is the only effective treatment for an infarcted bowel. For recurrent thromboembolism, the treatment of choice is ivermectin or moxidectin to remove parasite larvae in the arteries. Of course, your veterinarian must identify and treat the underlying cause of any infarction.

Prevention: A conscientious deworming program using ivermectin every two months for life will prevent such episodes.

IMPACTIONS

Impactions are mechanical blockages that occur when inadequately digested feed or foreign material forms an obstructive mass in the cecum or the large colon. Meconium impaction in newborn foals is a special case and is discussed in *Meconium Colic* (see page 525). Impactions tend to occur in horses who consume coarse, poor-quality feed. Horses with dental disease who are unable to chew their feed are also candidates for an impaction, as are horses who simply bolt their meals. In all such cases, the feed is presented to the colon in a poorly chewed, semisolid state.

Horses recovering from surgery and anesthesia are especially prone to impactions of the cecum. Decreased water intake, most likely in winter when the water supply freezes, is a common cause of colonic impactions. Ingesting sand is another cause.

Intestinal parasites are responsible for worm impactions in the small intestines and may predispose the horse to colon impactions. Abscesses and tumors in the intestinal tract are infrequent causes.

Large Bowel Impactions

Impaction of the large colon begins with mild colic, apathy, loss of appetite, increased thirst, and the passage of small amounts of hard manure covered

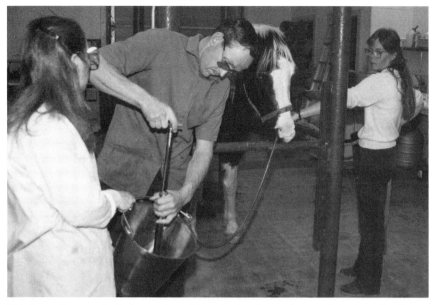

This horse has a colonic impaction. After she has been vigorously hydrated, mineral oil is given to facilitate passage of the impaction.

with thick, sticky mucus. The horse's expression is somewhat anxious. The heart rate is less than 50 beats per minute, the pulse is strong and regular, and the breathing rate and temperature are normal. The mucous membranes are pink, with a capillary refill time of less than two seconds. Listening to the abdomen with a stethoscope reveals the presence of bowel sounds. Pushing on the belly does not intensify the pain.

The early signs of an impaction may go unnoticed. However, with the passage of time, abdominal pain becomes more severe and the horse becomes notably anxious or depressed. The heart rate increases to 55 beats per minute (sometimes to more than 60). The pulse becomes weak and occasionally irregular, and the respiratory rate is increased. Pale mucous membranes indicate vasoconstriction or internal bleeding. A capillary refill time of more than three seconds indicates impending shock. Dry mucous membranes and loss of skin elasticity are signs of severe dehydration. Bowel sounds are absent if the horse has peritonitis.

Cecal impaction is a serious condition that may be secondary to an unrelated problem, such as staying at a surgical facility or extended stall rest. It is often difficult to medically manage and resolve. It begins with mild, intermittent, colicky abdominal pain and depression. These symptoms may persist for days. When untreated, complete cecal impaction leads to rupture of the cecum. In fact, some horses may be found dead as a result of sudden, overwhelming peritonitis.

Treatment: A horse with a suspected impaction must be examined by a veterinarian. The most important step is to soften the impaction and facilitate its passage by liquefying the intestinal contents. With a mild impaction, withholding feed and allowing the horse to drink water may accomplish this. As the impaction softens up and begins to pass, the pain subsides. The horse develops an appetite and appears brighter. Temporarily reduce the ration, as advised by your veterinarian, for two to three days. If grass is available, the horse may have a few nibbles. Once the horse is passing manure, discuss with your veterinarian how to increase the ration and overall feeding plans.

Severe impactions must be treated aggressively. The horse will be sedated by your veterinarian to control pain and relax the bowel. Vigorous hydration is accomplished by administering large volumes of water (6 to 8 quarts per 1,000 pounds of body weight, 5.7 to 7.5 l per 453 k) by nasogastric tube every two hours. If the water refluxes from the tube, fluids are given intravenously through large-bore needles placed in both jugular veins.

Dioctyl sodium sulfosuccinate, a laxative and stool softener, may be given at 1 ounce of 5 percent solution per 1,000 pounds body weight (per 453 k)—noting that only one dose per colic episode may be given. Mineral oil (3 to 4 quarts, 2.8 to 3.8 l, repeated every 12 hours) is another option to soften the stool. Either should be given by nasogastric tube. Note that dioctyl sodium sulfosuccinate and mineral oil should not be used together in the same treatment, although they can be used separately to treat a colic that is unresolved.

Magnesium sulfate (Epsom salts mixed with water) is also effective as a laxative, although it may cause cramping and loose stool. The magnesium sulfate draws fluid into the intestinal passage, which helps soften the impaction.

In the seriously ill horse, frequent rectal examinations and peritoneal taps are necessary to monitor progress. Failure to improve, or the advent of signs suggesting impending peritonitis, call for immediate surgery. To be effective, surgery must be performed before the colon ruptures.

Prevention: If you are able to identify and correct a predisposing cause, there is less likelihood of recurrence. Review feeding practices to be sure the ration is of high quality and digestibility, and that there are no sudden feed changes. It is important that a source of fresh water is available at all times. Perform any necessary dental procedures. Make sure the horse's deworming regimen is up-to-date.

Sand Impaction

Some horses eat sand for reasons unknown. In areas with sandy soil, unintentional ingestion is possible when grass is short-grazed or pulled out by the roots. Sand is also consumed when hay is fed on sandy ground. For both these reasons, these kinds of impactions are more prevalent in certain areas; Florida and California are among the states where they are most likely to be a problem.

Sand tends to accumulate in the cecum and large colon. However, if a significant amount is consumed at one time, a sand impaction can develop in the ileum or the ileocecal valve. A continuous low-level intake of sand leads to colic and diarrhea, a condition called sand enteropathy. The enteropathy may persist for weeks or months, often leading to an acute impaction. The weight of the sand in the large colon can cause displacement of the colon from its normal position, torsion, or volvulus.

Rectal palpation will diagnose a sand impaction if the impacted segment is within reach. When not within reach, the volume of sand in the feces can be estimated by filling a rubber glove with balls of fresh manure, adding water, mixing, and observing the amount of sand that settles out in the fingers of the glove. Greater than 2 teaspoons (10 ml) is significant.

Treatment: It is like that described for *Large Bowel Impactions* (see page 374). It is important to administer large volumes of water during the acute attack, either by nasogastric tube or intravenously. Failure to replenish fluids lost by diarrhea, dehydration, and sweating makes sand impactions drier and most difficult to pass.

The laxative of choice is a soluble fiber derived from psyllium seed husk (Sand Clear and Equine Enteric Colloid are two of several brands sold for horses). Psyllium forms a jelly in the intestinal tract that collects the sand and lubricates its passage. Administer 1 pound (453 g) of psyllium mixed in 2 gallons (7.6 l) of water by nasogastric tube. To prevent gel from forming in the nasogastric tube, mix the psyllium with water just before the solution is pumped into the stomach. Repeat as necessary, until well after the colic subsides. Usually a considerable amount of sand remains after the first treatment. This leads to recurrence if treatment is stopped too soon.

Surgical removal is necessary for difficult sand impactions and those with unrelieved signs of intestinal obstruction.

Prevention: Prevent sand impaction by feeding hay in racks or mangers. When horses graze on sandy soil that has caused impactions in the past, dry psyllium powder can be added to sweet feeds as a form of prevention. There are also prepared psyllium products, such as Sand Clear. These horses may be fed psyllium daily for five to seven days each month.

Worm Impaction

Following the use of a rapid-acting deworming agent, such as piperazine, in a heavily parasitized weanling foal or yearling, paralyzed *ascarids* can conglomerate into masses, which partially or completely obstruct the small intestines.

Signs include mild to severe colic, which begins shortly after deworming, and, in some cases, gastric distension. Worms may be present in the feces. In the most severe form, signs are those of an acute intestinal obstruction. Perforation and rupture of the stomach or small intestines is a possibility. Heavy ascarid loads may also be associated with intussusception (a problem with the intestines in which one portion of the bowel slides into the next, much like the sections of a telescope).

Treatment: Treatment is like that described in *Large Bowel Impactions* (see page 374). If that treatment is not successful, surgery may be necessary to remove worm masses.

Prevention: Deworming foals at 8 weeks of age or earlier (as discussed in chapter 2, "Parasites") and then every six to eight weeks until they are year-lings, can prevent worm impactions.

Fecal Impaction

Fecal material in the small colon and the rectum can become so dry and hard that the horse is unable to expel it despite forceful and prolonged straining. The fecal mass appears at the anal opening, which is widely dilated and often everted.

Water deprivation is a common cause of fecal impaction. It is most likely to occur in cold weather, when water sources are either frozen over or are so cold that horses will not consume enough water to prevent dehydration. Other causes of fecal impaction are described in *Constipation* (page 388).

Treatment: Restrain the horse and manually remove stool from the anus and rectum. Intravenous sedation by a veterinarian is often necessary for this. Administer a soap water enema to stimulate colonic contractions. The enema also helps lubricate the anal canal and wash out balls of hard stool.

To give a soap water enema, dissolve a piece of Ivory bar or dish soap in 2 to 3 quarts (1.9 to 2.8 l) of lukewarm water until the water becomes milky. Fill an enema bottle or bag with the solution and connect the tubing of the bag to a flexible rubber catheter. Lubricate the nozzle or catheter with mineral oil and carefully insert it 8 to 12 inches (20 to 30 cm) into the anal canal, depending on the size of the horse. Allow the fluid to run in by gravity. Repeat as necessary.

Following removal of the impaction, the horse should be given 3 to 4 quarts (2.8 to 3.8 l) of mineral oil by nasogastric tube to break up any impaction in the large colon that may have developed because of the obstruction in the small colon or rectum.

Prevention: Determine the cause of the impaction and take steps to prevent recurrence. This includes ensuring there is a constant source of fresh water that is not too cold; horses will drink more if their water is not too cold. Heated buckets, tank heaters, or automatic waterers should heat the water to at least 45 to 54°F (7 to 12°C).

ENTEROLITHS AND FOREIGN BODIES

Enteroliths are stones that form around a foreign object in the intestines of horses. They form when mineralized salts are deposited around a central nidus, such as a pebble or other foreign object. A single enterolith is usually round. When there are two or more enteroliths in the same space, the grinding effect produces multifaceted concretions.

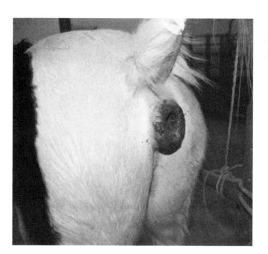

Despite forceful straining, the horse was unable to expel the impacted feces.

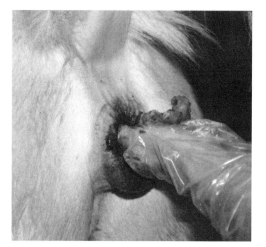

The first step in treatment is to remove the dry manure manually.

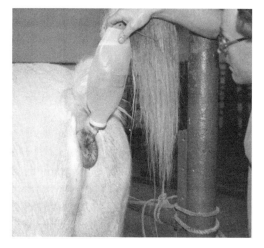

Next, a soap water enema is given to flush out remaining balls of hard stool.

Horses with enteroliths are found primarily in California and neighboring states, where high concentrations of magnesium ammonium in soil and *forage* are instrumental in the development of stones. A familial predisposition has been recognized in Arabians.

Enteroliths become symptomatic when they grow large enough to obstruct the bowel. Obstruction usually occurs in the right dorsal colon, transverse colon, or small colon, because the bowel is narrower in these locations.

The enterolith frequently acts as a ball valve before it becomes tightly wedged in the bowel. Accordingly, signs of intestinal obstruction are often preceded by bouts of severe abdominal pain and the passage of liquid feces. A horse with these symptoms will often be thought to have an impaction. However, when treatment for impaction is not successful, an enterolith may be the cause. The diagnosis can be confirmed by an x-ray showing the mass.

Foreign bodies in the intestinal tract tend to occur in young horses who eat hay nets, rubber, synthetic fibers, nylon, burlap, and other miscellaneous objects.

Treatment: Enteroliths must be removed surgically. If a swallowed foreign body fails to pass spontaneously, it will cause signs of bowel obstruction similar to those of an enterolith and will also need to be surgically removed.

Displacement of the Large Colon

The large colon moves freely within the peritoneal cavity, and when distended by gas, it can be displaced from its normal position. Large-framed horses are especially prone to displacements. In fact, the larger the horse, the greater the risk. The affected segment of colon becomes partially entrapped, twisted, or pinched off. Torsion, volvulus, or strangulation often complicates the problem.

An uncomplicated displacement usually produces intermittent bloating with mild to moderate colic. Although there is loss of appetite, there is little change in the horse's overall condition for a considerable length of time.

The displaced segment can often be felt on rectal palpation. This establishes the diagnosis as well as the type of displacement.

Treatment: There are several types of displacement. Your veterinarian can determine the best method of treatment depending on the specific type.

Fasting for one to two days, or inserting a nasogastric tube into the stomach, often relieves gas in the bowel and enables the colon to return to its normal position. On occasion, rolling the anesthetized horse as well as temporarily laying her on her back may cause the colon to flip back over. Some displacements can be reduced by rectal palpation.

Abdominal surgery is indicated for displacements that fail to resolve and those with signs of obstruction or strangulation. Approximately 50 percent of patients are euthanized during surgery due to finding devitalized colon tissue.

Prevention: A horse with a previously displaced colon is prone to recurrence. Treatment of worm parasites and/or a change in diet may prevent some of these recurrences.

Colic

Colic is the most common medical emergency encountered by the horse owner. Colic is not a specific disease; rather, it is an indicator of abdominal pain, manifested by signs of anxiety that include tail-switching, pawing, looking back, kicking at the abdomen, sweating, rolling on the ground, and urinating and defecating in small amounts.

Colic occurs in horses with indigestion, intestinal spasms, impactions, constipation, intestinal obstructions, feed toxicities, migratory worm infections, peritonitis, and dozens of other conditions, including diseases of the stomach, liver, ovaries, uterus, kidneys, and bladder.

Although the causes are many and varied, it is believed that the majority of colic cases in adult horses are caused by impactions of the cecum and large colon, and spasmodic and flatulent colic (discussed on pages 374, 388, and 384, respectively). Retained meconium and gastric ulcers are the principal causes of colic in foals (see pages 366 and 525).

A variety of management practices can be implemented to reduce the risk of colic. Horses with a history of colic frequently develop colic again. Changes in diet, the type and amount of hay fed, and feeding large amounts of whole grain concentrates increase the risk. Increased grazing time decreases the risk. Water must be easily accessible, clean, and, in the winter, warm enough to encourage drinking.

Both increases and decreases in activity can trigger colic. Increased time in a stall is a risk factor for colon impaction. Regular veterinary health management, including regular rather than infrequent parasitic treatment, prevents ascarid impactions.

The onset of colic usually is sudden. The horse may sit back on her haunches like a dog. Male horses frequently stretch out and relax the penis without urinating. A horse with colic often drops to the ground and thrashes violently while thrusting her feet up in the air. Abrasions and contusions from accidental injury are not uncommon.

DIAGNOSING COLIC

Colic is an emergency. Call your veterinarian. The first thing he or she will do is examine the horse to determine the nature and severity of the colic.

Passing a nasogastric tube and flushing out the stomach is an important diagnostic step and is indicated in all horses with moderate to severe colic. The appearance of the stomach contents may suggest the cause of the colic. In addition, decompression of a distended stomach can lead to dramatic improvement.

Rectal examination is of utmost importance in all cases of colic. It should be performed by a veterinarian, because of the risk of rectal tears in a colicky horse. Intravenous sedation is often necessary to facilitate the procedure. An experienced examiner can often tell the cause of the colic by palpating the small intestines, pelvic colon, bladder, and reproductive organs.

A peritoneal tap helps determine whether the horse has a bowel obstruction with impending or actual peritonitis. The tap is performed in the midline of the belly at its lowest or most dependent portion. A long needle is inserted through the skin and into the peritoneal cavity. Fluid is withdrawn and inspected under the microscope for blood, pus, protein, bacteria, and ingested plant material.

As a further step, your veterinarian may decide to administer an analgesic such as xylazine (Rompun). Horses with mild colic frequently respond to pain medication alone and require no further treatment.

TREATING COLIC

All forms of moderate to severe colic require intensive medical treatment. In addition to decompressing the stomach and relieving pain, fluids must be given to correct dehydration. This can often be accomplished by giving 1 to 2 gallons (3.8 to 7.6 l) of water by nasogastric tube every hour. The IV route is used if the horse exhibits signs of peritonitis or intestinal obstruction—or if there is a brown, foul-smelling reflux from the stomach tube, which indicates that the stomach is not emptying.

Further medical management is undertaken based on the presumed cause of the colic, as described in the next section.

Signs of peritonitis, strangulation, or obstruction indicate the need for rapid surgical intervention. These signs include persistent, severe pain not relieved by a stomach tube and analgesics; toxemia with a rising temperature; a heart rate greater than 60 beats per minute; a respiratory rate greater than 30 breaths per minute; finding blood, bacteria, or plant material on the peritoneal tap; or finding a bowel obstruction or displacement of the colon on rectal palpation.

Approximately 50 percent of horses recover from colic surgery. This figure drops to 25 percent if bowel resection is required; the best results are obtained when surgery is performed before the need for bowel resection.

TYPES OF COLIC

For descriptive purposes, colic has been classified into several types. The type helps determine the course of treatment. For more information on bowel sounds, see *Borborygmus* (page 622). This information will be important in diagnosing colic.

Impaction Colic

This is a common cause of colic. Most impactions are diet-related—the horse consuming poor-quality or improperly chewed feed. Water deprivation is another cause. Signs depend on the location and duration of the impaction. If the large intestine alone is involved, initially the bouts of pain are intermittent and mild. The manure is hard and dry.

Treatment: See *Impactions* (page 374).

Flatulent (Tympanic) Colic

The horse appears bloated and distended and has a great deal of gas throughout the digestive tract. Tapping on the side of the belly produces a hollow, drumlike or tympanitic sound, indicative of a large volume of air in the colon and cecum. Bowel activity is increased, which is reflected by the loud, high-pitched sounds heard with a stethoscope.

Primary tympany is a form of gaseous indigestion caused by bacterial fermentation of intestinal carbohydrates, often following the overconsumption of lush green grasses, grain, or commercial horse feeds. Occasionally, it is due to ingesting spoiled feeds. Abdominal pain is intermittent and moderate to severe. Horses with primary flatulence pass a great deal of gas via the rectum.

Secondary tympany accompanies bowel obstructions of the cecum or colon. Horses with secondary tympany are acutely ill and soon develop signs of toxicity. They pass little or no gas via the rectum.

Treatment: Passing a stomach tube helps to distinguish between primary and secondary tympany. The latter is characterized by a foul-smelling reflux from the nasogastric tube.

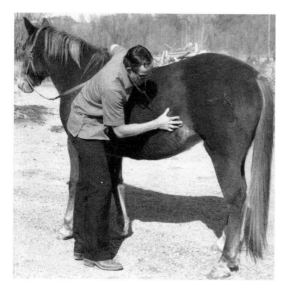

Bowel sounds are increased in cases of spasmodic and flatulent colic. They are decreased in horses with impaction colic and absent in peritonitis.

Primary tympany responds well to the administration of the antispasmodic dipyrone and the analgesics flunixin meglumine (Banamine) and xylazine. One gallon (3.8 l) of mineral oil is instilled into the stomach to prevent constipation and to treat intestinal irritation. Walking the horse promotes the passage of gas via the rectum.

Secondary tympany requires surgery to correct the blockage. When the bowel is so distended that rupture is imminent, the distension can be temporarily relieved by inserting an instrument called a trocar either through the right flank into the cecum or through the rectum into the large colon.

Spasmodic Colic

This type of colic is caused by powerful contractions of the bowel, which can be recognized by increased bowel sounds and peristaltic rushes. It is believed to be the most common cause of colic. Nervous, high-strung horses appear most susceptible to spasmodic colic, which may be triggered by fright, anxiety, or drinking cold water after a hot workout.

During spasmodic episodes, usually lasting about ten minutes, the horse rolls, paws, shakes, and kicks. The bowel sounds are loud and rushing, and are often audible without a stethoscope. Between attacks, the horse stands quietly. Patchy sweating on the neck is a characteristic finding.

Treatment: Most horses recover spontaneously in less than an hour. For those who do not, treatment is the same as that for primary tympany (see page 383).

Peritonitis Colic

The pain is severe, often unrelenting. There are signs of shock, dehydration, and toxicity. Pushing on the abdomen intensifies the pain and the horse will resist. When the cause is not obvious, consider a bowel obstruction complicated by strangulation, infarction, or perforation.

Treatment: For more information, see *Peritonitis* (page 369).

The Liver

The liver serves many vital metabolic functions. These functions include synthesizing enzymes, proteins and sugars; removing ammonia and other wastes from the bloodstream; and detoxifying drugs and poisons.

The most common signs of liver failure are *jaundice*, hepatoencephalopathy, and photosensitivity.

- **Jaundice.** The liver removes bilirubin from the blood. A buildup of bile turns the tissues yellow. This is noted in the yellowish appearance of the whites of the eyes and the mucous membranes of the mouth and tongue. Bile excreted in urine changes it from yellow to the color of tea.

- **Hepatoencephalopathy.** This is a type of encephalitis (brain inflammation) caused by high levels of ammonia and other toxins in the blood. Ammonia is a product of protein metabolism. It is removed from the circulation and metabolized by the liver. When the liver fails, ammonia accumulates to toxic levels and exerts a poisonous effect on the brain. Signs of hepatoencephalopathy include loss of appetite, mental depression, aimless wandering, circling, *head-pressing*, staggering, and frequent yawning. Affected horses often appear to be blind or oblivious to their surroundings and may injure themselves by walking into fences and stepping into ditches. Weight loss and constipation may occur. Coma is a late occurrence.

- **Photosensitivity.** This occurs in about 25 percent of horses with liver disease. For more information, see *Photosensitivity Reaction* (page 131).

Ascites (fluid in the belly) and *edema* (swelling of the abdominal wall and lower legs) are not as common in horses with liver disease as they are in cases of congestive heart failure. Major blood loss from spontaneous bleeding is rare.

LIVER FAILURE

A number of diseases, drugs, and toxins can affect the liver and cause the death of cells. Involvement of the liver is frequently just one aspect of a generalized disease.

Chronic liver disease is associated with cirrhosis; a condition in which liver cells are destroyed and the liver becomes scarred. Liver failure does not occur until at least 60 percent of cells are destroyed. When 80 percent are destroyed, recovery is impossible.

Serum hepatitis (Theiler's disease) is most often caused by a hypersensitivity reaction to a horse antiserum. Tetanus antitoxin is the antiserum implicated in nearly all cases. Because of this association, passive immunization with antiserum should be avoided in favor of active immunization whenever it is possible.

Cases of serum hepatitis that are not associated with the administration of horse antiserums usually occur in summer and autumn. Several horses may be affected at the same time. This suggests an infectious cause.

Serum hepatitis begins insidiously with malaise and loss of weight that progresses over several weeks or months and then suddenly culminates in acute liver failure and death in a matter of days. The diagnosis is confirmed by a liver biopsy. On occasion, a mildly affected horse responds to treatment and recovers.

Chronic active hepatitis is an inflammatory liver disease of unknown cause. There is no connection with the virus that produces hepatitis in humans. The encephalopathy of chronic active hepatitis is often less severe than it is in other forms of liver disease. The diagnosis is made by liver biopsy. Corticosteroids have been used successfully in some cases. In general, the prognosis for recovery is guarded.

Pyrrolizidine alkaloid toxicity is caused by ingesting plants that contain pyrrolizidine alkaloids. This is a common cause of cirrhosis and liver failure in some midwestern and western parts of North America. These plants, such as cestrum, dusty miller, fiddleneck, hound's tongue, or heliotropium, are not palatable, but accidental ingestion can occur when they are cut and baled with alfalfa or when contaminated grain is threshed and the screenings are fed to horses. See *Forage Toxicities*, page 427, for more information.

Cirrhosis caused by plant alkaloids has a poor prognosis. By the time liver failure becomes apparent, the liver is too damaged to recover.

Aflatoxin toxicity is the result of molds found in stored corn and other feeds, which produce a series of mycotoxins called aflatoxins that are highly toxic to the liver. Fortunately, horses are more resistant to these toxins than are most other domestic animals. Signs are like those of *Moldy Corn Poisoning* (see page 430).

Chemicals and drugs known to cause liver toxicity include carbon tetrachloride and tetrachloroethylene (both present in some dewormers), and toxic amounts of copper, lead, phosphorus, selenium, and iron. Drugs adversely affecting the liver include inhaled anesthetic gases, antibiotics, diuretics, sulfa preparations, anticonvulsants, arsenicals, and some steroids. Most drugs damage the liver only when the recommended dosage is exceeded or the drug is administered for an extended period.

Other rare causes of liver failure include bile duct obstruction by roundworms and bots. The horse does not have a gallbladder. However, gallstones can form in the bile ducts and produce obstruction. This is rare, but should be considered in a horse with unexplained jaundice. Cancers and liver abscesses are other causes of unexplained jaundice. Very rarely, liver flukes may cause liver disease in horses.

Liver function tests are used to diagnose liver insufficiency and to follow its progress. A liver *biopsy* is the best way to make a diagnosis when it is important to determine the exact cause of the disease.

Treatment: Treatment of acute liver failure is directed at supporting the horse until there is clear evidence of irreversible damage or the horse shows signs of recovery. Return of appetite is a good sign.

Horses with hepatoencephalopathy should be stalled and sedated to protect against self-injury. Intravenous fluids containing 10 percent glucose will maintain an adequate blood sugar level. Administering Neomycin, mineral oil, or lactulose by stomach tube can reduce serum ammonia levels. Alfalfa hay has a high protein content and should be avoided in favor of mixed-grain rations containing beet pulp, molasses, sweet feeds, and milo or other sorghums. Offer four to six small meals a day. Vitamin B, vitamin K, and folic acid supplements can be helpful. Good-quality oat hay can be introduced as the horse's appetite returns.

Protect the horse from photosensitivity by keeping her indoors from dawn to dusk.

The Rectum and Anus

Prolapse, trauma, and fecal incontinence are the most common problems of the rectum and anus. Pinworms, Culicoides-induced dermatitis, and tail mites can cause severe itching about the anus.

PROLAPSE OF THE RECTUM

Protrusion of the rectum through the anus is called prolapse. Often just the *mucous* lining prolapses, giving the appearance of a large doughnut. Rarely, the entire rectum can turn inside out through the anus and hang over the buttocks.

Heavy straining is the cause. Thus, rectal prolapse is associated with constipation, colic, diarrhea, rectal tumors, obstructed bladders, and mares who strain during difficult labor.

Treatment: Notify your veterinarian. The prolapse must be reduced before it becomes excessively swollen. In most cases, an epidural block (infusion of a local anesthetic into the spinal canal) is needed to prevent further straining and to relax the anal sphincter. Reduction is then done by the veterinarian, who will massage the swollen tissue and work it back inside the rectum. Following reduction, mineral oil or dioctyl sodium sulfosuccinate (DSS) is given to soften the stool and to prevent straining.

When the rectum has been prolapsed for several hours, the swollen and dried-out mucosa becomes devitalized. A surgical procedure to remove the dead layer and repair the mucosa is required. A rectal stricture may follow surgical repair.

Prevention: To prevent recurrent episodes of prolapse, see *Constipation* (page 388).

LACERATIONS AND TEARS

The anal canal and the lower rectum in the mare can be torn or lacerated during a difficult delivery as the result of an abnormal foal presentation. Breeding accidents and pelvic fractures are other causes.

The most common cause of a torn rectum is *iatrogenic*, meaning it is caused by treatment for another disorder. Rectal injury is a potential hazard whenever a horse is examined by rectal palpation. Some horses have a small rectum, while others have a thin, delicate rectum and narrow colon.

It is most important that horses be restrained for rectal examinations. Often this involves the use of xylazine (Rompun) to sedate the horse and to relax the rectum. In addition, rectal examinations should be done only by experienced personnel.

An injury to the wall of the rectum produces bleeding and the appearance of blood on the glove of the examiner. Shortly thereafter, the horse breaks out in a sweat and strains as if to pass feces. If the tear is deep and extends into the abdominal cavity, signs of peritonitis develop rapidly.

Treatment: Straining is prevented by first giving an epidural block, which also relaxes the rectal canal. The rectum is now carefully examined by finger palpation to determine the extent of the tear. Tears that do not involve the full thickness of the rectal wall have a favorable prognosis and usually heal on their own. Antibiotics are given to prevent infection. Dioctyl sodium sulfosuccinate or mineral oil can be given to soften the stool and prevent straining.

A laceration that involves all layers of the rectum but stops just short of entering the abdominal cavity can often be repaired. This is major abdominal surgery and must be done at a center equipped to provide the necessary support. A temporary diverting colostomy (artificial opening in the colon) is required until healing occurs. A tear that extends into the peritoneal cavity results in fecal contamination and peritonitis. The outlook for recovery is poor even with early treatment. The finding of fecal material on peritoneal tap confirms the diagnosis. For treatment, see *Peritonitis* (page 369).

FECAL INCONTINENCE

Loss of control of the rectum occurs when there has been an injury to the spinal cord. Bladder paralysis and a limp tail accompany fecal incontinence. In the male there is prolapse of the penis; in the female, gaping of the vulva. These signs also occur with cauda equina syndrome (see page 353).

A laceration of the perineum during a difficult delivery can create a passage between the rectum and vagina (rectovaginal fistula) through which stool passes via the vagina. This can give the appearance of fecal incontinence.

Treatment: Treatment is directed at the primary cause. Rectovaginal fistulas can be surgically repaired. With spinal cord paralysis, the stool should be kept soft with DSS and manually removed from the rectum as necessary. See also *Paralyzed Bladder* (page 334).

Constipation

Constipation is the infrequent passage of firm, dry manure. Usually, constipation is accompanied by some degree of straining. Constipation should be distinguished from colic, a symptom complex characterized by sudden, severe pain in the abdomen and sometimes—but not always—associated with mechanical blockages and fecal impactions.

A characteristic type of constipation occurs in newborn foals. Treatment is discussed in *Meconium Colic* (page 525). Constipation is more common in older individuals, although it may occur at any age. A constipated horse may pass only small amounts of firm, possibly mucus-covered manure. She may have a rough haircoat and fail to thrive.

One predisposing cause is dental disease, which results in improper grinding of feed and therefore improper digestion. Another cause is damage to the lining of the intestinal tract caused by worms, leading to reduced motility. Feeding too much finely ground grain can cause constipation. In some horses, the intestinal tract simply seems to slow down with age.

Treatment: The horse should have her teeth examined to see if corrective treatment is possible. Put the horse on a good parasite control program. Provide continuous access to clean, fresh water. Make sure the horse's water does not freeze and is not too cold to drink.

When the manure is persistently hard and dry, the powdered form of DSS can be added to sweet feeds. To avoid toxicity (severe diarrhea), the daily dose should not exceed 9 mg per pound (453 g) of body weight, given every other day. Do not use concurrently with mineral oil.

Milk of magnesia (magnesium hydroxide) is a safe laxative to give for mild to moderate constipation. The single individual dose for an average-size horse is 8 to 16 ounces (236 to 473 ml). Do not give a laxative to a horse who appears colicky or exhibits any signs of abdominal discomfort without veterinary approval.

Prevention: Giving a warm bran mash twice a week is a good preventive measure for older horses.

Diarrhea

Diarrhea is the passage of loose, unformed manure. In most cases, there is a large volume of stool and an increased number of bowel movements. This depends to some extent on whether the diarrhea is acute or chronic.

Because of the extraordinary size and length of the equine colon, the horse is able to compensate in large part for any inflammatory or irritative process in the small intestines and still maintain a stool of normal consistency. Accordingly, diarrhea is a factor only when there is disease in the colon.

This does not apply to foals, in which the colon is still immature. (Foal diarrhea is discussed on page 555.)

ACUTE DIARRHEA

Diarrhea of sudden onset indicates an infectious disease or acute poisoning. Poor-quality feed, spoiled feed, and ingested irritants do not cause diarrhea in horses the way they do in animals with shorter digestive tracts.

When diarrhea is profuse, watery, explosive, foul-smelling, dark green to black, blood-tinged, or bloody, the horse is suffering from infectious colitis. Salmonellosis is the most common cause.

Certain antibiotics (especially lincomycin and tetracycline) can alter the normal colonic flora and produce acute diarrhea that is indistinguishable from an infectious colitis.

Nonsteroidal anti-inflammatory drugs, when used over an extended period, can disrupt the blood supply to the mucosa of the cecum and colon and produce a severe diarrhea that is slow to respond to treatment.

Less common causes of acute diarrhea include arsenic and lead poisoning, equine viral arteritis, selenium toxicity, plant poisoning, blister beetle poisoning, and peritonitis.

Treatment: Treatment is directed at the cause of the diarrhea.

CHRONIC DIARRHEA

Diarrhea that persists for weeks or months is a frustrating problem. Horses with chronic diarrhea gradually lose weight despite having a good appetite. Stools are soft and watery and the amount is greater than normal. Large quantities of water are consumed to compensate for losses in the stool.

It is difficult to establish the cause of chronic diarrhea, even with laboratory studies and endoscopic biopsies. One of the following may be the cause of the diarrhea:

Chronic salmonellosis occurs in horses who recover from salmonellosis and become carriers and shed salmonella in their feces. The stool varies from soft and unformed ("cow pie") to profuse and watery. Treatment with antibiotics is possible, but improvement is often temporary. In addition, the carrier horse remains a danger to other animals and to humans, who are quite susceptible to salmonellosis. Care should be used in handling such horses during a bout of diarrhea.

Intestinal parasites, especially migrating larvae of strongyles, have been implicated in cases of chronic diarrhea in horses. Although most horses with chronic diarrhea do not have strongyles infection, treatment directed at killing migratory larvae is worth the effort and, if successful, is followed by cure of the diarrhea. Failure to recognize and treat protozoal diarrhea (see page 556) sometimes leads to diarrhea that continues for weeks or months. The stool is soft and has the consistency of cow manure.

Sand in the intestinal tract can be a cause of chronic diarrhea (see *Sand Impaction*, page 376).

Chronic liver disease may be accompanied by low-volume diarrhea. The stool is the consistency of cow manure.

Tumors and growths in the digestive tract can produce malabsorption and diarrhea. Lymphoma and squamous cell carcinoma are the most common intestinal tract tumors.

Malabsorption syndrome is characterized by a failure to absorb nutrients from the small intestines. These horses are malnourished and fail to thrive.

Because of protein deficiency, they frequently accumulate fluid in the dependent portion of the belly wall (ventral edema). There are changes in the consistency, color, and amount of stool, but the principal sign of malabsorption in the horse is chronic weight loss.

Most malabsorptions are caused by an episode of viral enteritis (in the neonate) or salmonella enteritis (in the neonate or adult). The infectious agent attacks and destroys the nutrient-absorbing villous cells in the lining of the small intestines.

Malabsorption has also been associated with granulomatous enteritis, cryptosporidiosis, liver disease, long-standing worm infections, congestive heart failure, heavy metal poisoning, zinc deficiency, and atrophy of unknown cause of the villous cells. The diagnosis is difficult, and treatment is usually not rewarding.

Treatment: If the cause can be determined (such as cryptosporidiosis, worm infections, or congestive heart failure), it can be treated. Absorption of nutrients returns as the bowel heals. Some causes are of unknown origin, and treatment may not stop the unrelenting diarrhea.

15

NUTRITION AND FEEDING

The quality of nutrition for the horse directly affects his health and is one facet of horse care that you have a great deal of control over. A nutritionally complete diet for a horse must supply sufficient amounts of water, energy (calories), protein, carbohydrates, fatty acids, minerals, and vitamins. A certain amount of fiber is also important for proper digestion. A number of feeds meet these requirements. The choice depends on the circumstances under which the horse is kept, the convenience of feeding, availability of hay and pasture, and relative expense. These and other considerations will be discussed in this chapter.

Nutritional Requirements
WATER

The amount of water a horse needs depends on his body temperature, the environmental temperature, his level of activity, and the amount of water present in the grass or hay he eats. In general, a mature horse will drink about 10 to 12 gallons (38 to 45 l) of water a day. Hard-working performance horses require up to twice that amount. A lactating *mare* needs 75 percent more water to replace the water lost in her milk.

When deprived of water for two days, a horse generally refuses to eat and may show signs of *colic*. With ideal weather and good health, a horse might be able to live for five or six days without water.

The best policy is to provide plenty of clean, fresh water and allow the horse unlimited access. It is safe to let a horse drink as much as he wants—except immediately after exercise. Frequent drinks during any strenuous athletic endeavor enable the horse to alleviate thirst, which is a signal of dehydration. Common sense dictates small, frequent drinks to help cool the equine athlete and prevent dehydration. Not all water sources are safe for the horse. In some parts of the country, such as western parts of the United States, the salt content of water is too high or the water may contain unacceptable levels of fluoride, selenium, arsenic, lead, or other minerals. Water with a heavy blue-green algae growth may contain a toxin that is released after the algae bloom dies and is poisonous. Stagnant water in ponds or troughs can cause diarrhea and intestinal upsets and should be avoided. The accepted criterion for sanitary water is the absence of coliform bacteria. Presence of *E. coli* correlates with other infectious organisms, including salmonella and giardia. In summary, if you are not sure of the purity of your water source, have it analyzed.

Water troughs should be emptied and cleaned frequently, especially in hot weather. An automatic water delivery system is convenient, although it is difficult to monitor water consumption with this type of system. Galvanized pipes should never be connected to copper tubing, because this results in the release of toxic amounts of zinc.

ENERGY

Energy for metabolism is supplied by dietary carbohydrates, fats, and proteins. The feeds consumed by horses are not highly digestible. Therefore, differences in digestibility must be taken into account when comparing one feed with another. One method is to compare the total energy in the feed with the residual energy in the feces. The difference between these two represents the digestible energy (DE), which is the amount of energy the horse is able to extract from the feed. Thus, if the horse required 16,500 calories per day, he would need to consume the amount of feed that would produce 16,500 calories of DE—not simply 16,500 calories of food.

The minimum daily DE requirements for various types of horse are shown in the table on page 395, but these are only guidelines. Many factors influence the amount of energy needed by each individual horse. These factors include:

- The mature weight of the horse
- His general health and whether he is in optimal condition or recovering from an illness
- The effects of cold and inclement weather
- The horse's individual metabolism

Energy requirements are highest for pregnant horses, lactating mares, and growing horses. Horses engaged in athletic activity also require additional calories. According to the National Research Council (2007), DE requirements increase by 25, 50, and 100 percent for horses engaged in light, medium, and intense work, respectively. Examples of light work include Western and English pleasure riding, and bridle path hack and equitation. Examples of medium work include range riding, roping, cutting, barrel racing, and jumping. Intense work includes race training, polo, and endurance events. The *Nutrient Requirements of Horses* (revised in 2007) is an excellent nutritional resource for horse owners. Although it is quite technical, it is also quite practical and has information on the nutritional needs of horses and other *equids*. Also available is a free computer program that is downloadable. For more information, you can go online to www.nap.edu/catalog/11653.html.

Dry Basis

Different types of foods have different amounts of water. Therefore, to make meaningful comparisons of nutrient levels between different foods types, you need to convert the nutrient content to a dry basis—how much nutrient the food has if all the water is taken out. The percentage of dry matter is 100 percent minus the percentage of moisture in the food. Therefore, if a food is 10 percent water, it's 90 percent dry matter (100 minus 10).

Most feed tags list the dry matter nutrient analysis, but if they don't, it's not difficult to figure out. The feed tag should at least list the moisture content of the food, and you can use that to figure out the rest. For example, if a particular food has 25 percent moisture, that means it has 75 percent dry matter. If it has 8 percent crude protein, divide the 8 by 75 to get .10. Multiply that by 100 to get 10 percent dry matter protein.

The newly revised *Nutrient Requirements of Horses by the National Research Council* (6th edition, 2007) has a free online program that can provide you with the nutrient content of a variety of feedstuffs. For more information, go to www.nap.edu/catalog/11653.html.

A horse's ability to digest a type of feed can be influenced by his overall health and *condition*. Dental disease and loss of teeth are common causes of impaired digestion, as are mouth ailments that interfere with the ability to chew. A heavy parasite infestation is another cause of inadequate energy. A diet deficient in calories or protein will result in a steady loss of weight. Most serious health problems are accompanied by weight loss, which may be the only indication of a chronic problem.

A chronic deficiency of energy causes loss of weight, lethargy, impaired performance, rough haircoat, and unthrifty appearance. Mares may experience delayed estrus and fail to breed. Young horses have a reduced rate of growth and a delay in the onset of sexual maturity. Despite these outward clues, many owners who see the horse every day fail to recognize weight loss until the situation is advanced. It is a good policy to weigh or score your horse at regular intervals and keep monthly records. A weight graph or body condition score is a much better indicator of body condition than is visual inspection alone. Weight tapes will help you determine weight for feed and medications; the body condition score will enable you to judge whether your feeding regimen is adequate (see *Body Condition Scoring System*, page 422). It takes practice, but once you can achieve consistency, it will be most useful.

Minimum Daily Nutrient Requirements

Type of horse	Weight*	Digestible energy (calories)	Crude protein (grams)	Lysine (grams)	Calcium (grams)	Phosphorus (grams)	Potassium (grams)
Mature horse, maintenance**	1,100 lbs (500 kg)	16,650	630	27	20	14	25
Mare, late pregnancy	1,100 lbs (500 kg)	18,490	759	33	28	20	25
Lactating mare, first 3 months	1,100 lbs (500 kg)	30,610	1,468	80	56	36	46
Nursing foal, up to 3 months old	341 lbs (155 kg)	11,770	673	29	39	22	12
Weanling, up to 6 months old	462 lbs (215 kg)	15,540	676	29	39	21	13
Yearling, up to 12 months old	715 lbs (325 kg)	18,780	846	36	38	21	17
2-year-old	990 lbs (450 kg)	18,700	770	33	37	20	22

Source: *Nutrient Requirements of Horses*, 6th ed., National Research Council (2007).

*Assumes 1,100 lb (500 kg) mature weight. For every 100 lb (45 kg) above or below, add or subtract 8 percent from the values given.

**Digestible energy, mineral, and vitamin requirements for light, medium, and intense work can be estimated by increasing the maintenance requirements by 25, 50, and 100 percent, respectively.

Determining Your Horse's Weight

When weighing by scale is not practical, the weight of the horse can be esti-mated rather accurately using a horse's weight tape (available from feed stores and tack shops). How to use the tape is illustrated in the photographs on page 397. The tape is marked in pounds (or kilograms) of body weight, as measured at the circumference of the heart girth. The heart girth is the meas-urement taken around the horse's barrel just behind the front legs. In near-term pregnant mares, the tape underestimates weight by 150 to 200 pounds (68 to 91 kg). This should be added to the result given by the tape.

If a commercial tape is not available, use an ordinary measuring tape and the information in the table below.

Determining Your Horse's Weight			
Heart girth		Weight	
Inches	Centimeters	Pounds	Kilograms
30	76	100	45.5
40	102	200	91
45.5	116	300	136.5
50.5	128	400	182
55	140	500	227
58.5	148	600	273
61.5	156	700	318
64.5	164	800	364
67.5	171	900	409
70.5	178	1,000	455
73	185	1,100	500
75.5	192	1,200	545
77.5	197	1,300	591

PROTEIN

Proteins are chains of amino acids. Protein is needed to build muscle and body tissue. It is also metabolized to provide energy.

Crude protein is the total amount of protein in a feed. Digestible protein is the amount of protein in the feed that can actually be used by the horse. Both the crude protein and the digestible protein content of a feed can be deter-mined by laboratory analysis. When protein alone is stated or given on the

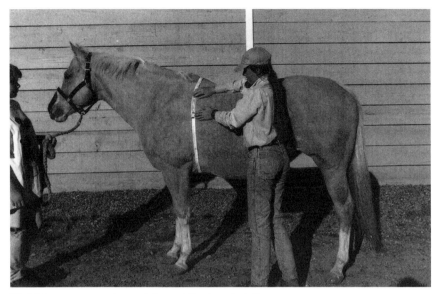

Weight measurements are taken at the heart girth.

label of a food product, crude protein is generally what is meant. Most protein in natural feeds for horses is about 75 percent digestible. Thus, if the horse is receiving 16 percent crude protein in his ration, he is getting 12 percent digestible protein.

Estimates of the minimum daily crude protein requirements for various types of horses are shown in the table on page 398. Protein requirements for working horses do not increase greatly over maintenance levels. In general, the increased feed intake needed to supply the additional energy for the performance horse will also provide adequate additional protein.

Most feedstuffs are sources of protein, but the quality and amount vary considerably. Hays, both legume and grasses, can be good protein sources. Good-quality pasture also provides protein. The online supplement to *Nutrient Requirements of Horses* by the National Research Council is an excellent resource for the nutritional analysis of a variety of feeds.

When the feed intake is inadequate to meet the horse's metabolic needs, there will be protein deficiency and energy deficiency. Horses with higher protein needs include those undergoing intense training, those at hard physical labor, growing horses, and pregnant and lactating mares. Underfeeding, relative to the horse's need, is one cause of protein deficiency. Protein deficiency may also result from prolonged grazing on pastures containing mature grasses deficient in protein or from feeding poorly digestible dietary protein that has been damaged by heat (for example, during processing).

In mature horses, protein deficiency depresses metabolic activities. The horse becomes lethargic and mentally dull, refuses to eat, loses endurance, becomes anemic, and assumes an unthrifty appearance. Protein deficiency in the pregnant mare can cause intrauterine growth retardation. In the *foal*, it causes suboptimal growth and delayed sexual maturity.

Protein Supplements

Many feeds do not contain enough protein to meet the nutritional requirements of lactating mares and growing foals. In these cases a protein supplement, such as soybean meal or a milk product, can be added to the grain or concentrate mix to make up the deficit. This is called top dressing.

Crude Protein Requirements for Horses	
Age of Horse (months)	Crude Protein (grams per day)
6	676
9	758
12	846
18	799
24	770
48	630

Most protein supplements are of plant origin. They are the by-products of extracting oil from soybeans, cottonseeds, flaxseeds (linseed meal), and other oil seeds. These supplements contain 32 to 50 percent crude protein by weight.

Protein supplements are rated according to quality. High-quality sources contain all the amino acids needed by the horse, in correct amounts. Low-quality sources are deficient either in protein or in certain amino acids.

There are at least three amino acids considered essential for growth, but only a lysine deficiency appears to be important as a growth-limiting factor. Dietary requirements for lysine can be found in the online supplement to *Nutrient Requirements of Horses*. Soybean meal, rapeseed and canola meal, fish meal, and dried milk and milk products are the protein supplements highest in lysine.

Soybean meal is the most commonly used and therefore the most important protein supplement. It is preferred for young horses because it is high in lysine. Soybean meal is rated highest in quality among all plant-source protein supplements.

Soybean meal is sometimes given for 30 days at the end of winter. This aids in the process of shedding and gives a gloss or bloom to the new spring coat.

Cottonseed meal is second in popularity. It is more palatable than soybean meal but lower in protein quality and in lysine. This may not be a disadvantage in mature horses. The major concern in feeding cottonseed meal is a substance called gossypol that interferes with digestion. Although adult horses may tolerate gossypol when fed in moderate amounts, it is undesirable for feeding foals. It should be noted that cottonseed meal is low in vitamin A. The following guidelines should be followed if you are feeding cottonseed meal.

- No more than 25 percent of the protein source should come from cottonseed meal.
- Lysine must be supplemented.

Rapeseed meal and canola meal (an extract of rapeseed) are important oil seed crops in Canada, Europe, and Asia. These high-quality protein supplements are palatable and contain adequate amounts of lysine. Like soybean meal, rapeseed and canola can be used as the sole source for protein supplementation.

Linseed meal has long been credited with giving a bloom to the coat. However, current methods of extraction remove more oil and fat, so linseed meal no longer has this advantage over other supplements. Linseed meal is palatable and quite digestible. The protein quality is somewhat lower than that of soybean meal. The lysine content is also low. Linseed meal contains a substance that softens stools. Thus, it may have a laxative effect.

Milk products, including dried milk, are somewhat more expensive but are an excellent protein source for growing horses because they are high in lysine. Since horses older than 3 years of age lack the enzyme lactase, milk products, if fed in sufficient quantity, will cause diarrhea. This is not a problem in young horses.

Peanut meal, safflower meal, sunflower meal, gluten meal, fish meals, and various brewer's pellets and grains are other protein sources that can be fed to horses.

CARBOHYDRATES AND FIBER

Carbohydrates are composed of simple sugars. They are classified as either fiber or nonfiber carbohydrates. Nonfiber carbohydrates, composed of monosaccharide and disaccharide sugars, are the major source of energy. Depending on the feed sources for the horse, hindgut fermentation of fiber may produce 30 percent to 70 percent of the horse's energy needs. This fermentation produces volatile fatty acids, which are absorbed from the intestines and converted to energy. These volatile fatty acids are highly digestible and rapidly metabolized by the body. When energy needs are low, nonfiber carbohydrates are converted to glycogen and stored in the liver and muscles.

Fiber carbohydrates are the part of the feed that is high in cellulose and lignin (a component that makes plants woody), both of which are poorly digestible and therefore low in energy. Fiber is important for lower intestinal motility and aids in the production of a bulky, well-formed stools.

Feed consisting of plants or plant parts containing more than 18 percent crude fiber is called roughage. Dietary fiber is the total fiber content of food; crude fiber represents what remains after the plant material has been removed, and is about one-fifth to one-third of the total value. A mature horse needs 12 to 16 ounces (340 to 454 g) of roughage for every 100 pounds (45 kg) of body weight per day.

Feeds containing low fiber content, such as grain, contain 50 to 60 percent more DE per pound than hay, which has a higher fiber content. The average percentage of crude fiber in several common sources of feed is about:

Grass hay: 30 to 32 percent

Alfalfa hay: 24 to 30 percent

Oats: 11 percent

Soybean meal: 7 percent

Wheat: 2 to 3 percent

Corn: 2.5 percent

ESSENTIAL FATTY ACIDS

Essential fatty acids (EFAs) are necessary fats that cannot be synthesized but are obtained only through diet. EFAs support the cardiovascular, reproductive, immune, and nervous systems. They are helpful in repairing and manufacturing cell membranes and in the production of prostaglandins, which regulate body functions such as blood pressure, blood clotting, fertility, inflammation, and fighting infection.

Although most feeds contain less than 6 percent fat, this appears to be adequate to meet the nutritional needs of horses. Fatty acid deficiency has not been described in the horse. Thus a dry, lusterless coat is unlikely to be due to fatty acid deficiency. However, experience indicates that coat conditioners and vegetable oil supplements containing fat or fatty acids may give a horse a glossier coat or help the horse shed his coat earlier in the spring. Add 1 to 2 ounces (28 to 57 g) of any polyunsaturated plant or vegetable oil to the horse's ration twice a day. (Fatty acid supplements are discussed in *Feeding the Adult Horses*, page 415.) Fats are a good way to provide extra energy without extra carbohydrates, which may make the horse excitable or "hot."

MINERALS

Minerals are needed for the formation of structural components of the body, enzymatic cofactors, and energy transfer. Some minerals play an important part in the synthesis of vitamins, amino acids, and hormones. At least 21 minerals are required in the horse's diet, but the major ones of concern in feeding horses are calcium, phosphorus, salt (sodium chloride), and, in some geographical areas, selenium. Copper and zinc are essential for growth. Although a number of mineral deficiencies and toxicities can occur in the horse, with the exception of selenium, calcium, and phosphorus, they are uncommon or rare—provided that average or better quality feeds are used, trace-mineralized salt is available, and excess mineral supplements are not added to the ration.

Plants, and the soil in which plants are grown, are the mineral sources for horses. Mineral imbalances can result from too little or too much mineral content in the soil; or factors in the soil may diminish the ability of the plants to obtain the essential elements. For example, there are large areas in which the soil is deficient in iodine and areas in which the soil contains either an excess or a deficiency of selenium. Such areas are well known and have been mapped. Information about the mineral composition of the soil where you live can be obtained from your local extension service or regional United States Department of Agriculture office.

Salt (Sodium Chloride)

Horses have a natural craving for salt. In fact, this is the only mineral for which they have a natural appetite. An adult horse at pasture will consume about half a pound (227 g) of salt per week, although this varies. Horses in training and lactating mares will consume more.

Salt provides sodium and chloride, which are necessary for cell functioning. A lack of salt causes decreased appetite and weight loss. It may be responsible for a tendency to lick at urine or to eat wood, dirt, manure, and stones. Salt toxicity can occur if water is restricted and salt is not. The symptoms include *colic*, diarrhea, paralysis, and death. This could occur if a horse drank salt brine or if a salt-starved horse obtained access to salt but not to water.

To ensure that salt needs are met, 0.5 to 1 percent salt can be added to the daily ration or, more conveniently, a salt block or loose salt mix can be made available for free-choice consumption. If salt is available, the horse will consume enough to meet its needs. There is no danger of salt intoxication provided the horse has continuous access to fresh water.

Salt can be provided in loose or block form. More salt may be consumed in the loose form, but adequate amounts will be consumed in either form. A variety of salt blocks and free salt mixes are commercially available. The least expensive is plain salt containing only sodium and chloride. For feeding horses, trace-mineralized salt containing iodine, zinc, copper, and other minerals is a better choice, because it provides trace minerals that may be absent or deficient in some *forages*, hays, and grains (see *Trace Minerals*, page 405).

Trace-mineralized salt containing higher levels of copper, zinc, and/or selenium is also available, as is salt containing high levels of iodine. Note that none of these salts contain calcium or phosphorus. When additional calcium and/or phosphorus are required, you can purchase a block or loose salt mix containing equal parts of trace minerals, calcium, and phosphorus.

Calcium and Phosphorus

Calcium and phosphorus are of great importance in the horse's diet. The mineral content of equine bone is 34 percent calcium and 17 percent phosphorus. Horses require calcium and phosphorus in relatively large amounts for bone growth and maintenance. Growing horses especially need adequate amounts of calcium and phosphorus to support active skeletal growth and development. Horses are more likely to suffer from calcium or phosphorus deficiency than from any other mineral deficiency.

Very important is the ratio of calcium to phosphorus in the horse's diet. This ratio should be about 1.2:1 (ranging from 1:1 to 3:1). That is, there should be at least as much calcium as phosphorus in the diet. So the daily intake for an adult horse would be 20 grams of calcium and 14 grams of phosphorus; a pregnant mare requires 28 grams of calcium and 20 grams of phosphorus; a weanling needs 39 grams of calcium and 21 grams of phosphorus; and a yearling needs 38 grams of calcium and 21 grams of phosphorus. Phosphorus intake that is higher than the calcium intake can result in nutritional secondary hyperparathyroidism and bone demineralization. As long as the intakes remain within an acceptable range and sufficient quantities of both minerals are provided, the horse will adjust his excretion of calcium and phosphorus to maintain the necessary ratio.

A diet deficient in calcium, phosphorus, or both will result in mineral deficiency, delayed bone mineralization, and delayed growth. Weanlings and yearlings fail to attain mature stature and may experience pain and lameness from joint and bone injuries, including fractures. Calcium deficiency in the young mature horse produces a condition called big head, also known as bran disease. The disease is characterized by a bulging of the face between the eyes and the nostrils, giving the head a deformed appearance. It used to be more common when bran was fed as a principal ration; bran is low in calcium, although it is high in phosphorus.

Many grass hays are low in calcium and/or phosphorus. Horses who eat marginal hay or forage, with or without a grain supplement, are at risk of developing a deficiency of calcium, phosphorus, or both.

Plants that contain harmful amounts of oxalate may be found in pasture grasses during summer months. Oxalate binds calcium, decreasing its absorption from the small intestine. A calcium deficiency can occur if the forage does not provide enough calcium to compensate for the losses caused by oxalate. Lactating mares and weanlings, whose calcium requirements are highest, are most likely to be affected by oxalate plants.

Cereal grains do not contain sufficient calcium to support rapid growth. If a young horse receives a high-energy diet containing cereal grains and protein supplements, but does not receive supplemental calcium, growth problems are likely.

Calcium and phosphorus requirements increase dramatically during the last three months of pregnancy and during lactation. Unless forage is excellent, mares on pasture should be supplemented (see *Care and Feeding During Pregnancy*, page 504).

Calcium and/or phosphorus deficiencies or imbalances can be prevented by ensuring that adequate amounts of both minerals are present in the horse's diet (see the tables on pages 395 and 404) and that the diet contains at least as much calcium as phosphorus. Alfalfa and other legumes are a good source of calcium. When feed sources are marginal, or when legumes are not available, provide supplemental minerals by offering a free-choice loose salt mix or salt block containing equal parts of calcium, phosphorus, and trace-mineralized salt. Remove other mineral sources to encourage consumption.

To treat a calcium or phosphorus deficiency, it is best to give the minerals directly rather than free choice. One method is to add these minerals directly to 1 pound (453 g) of sweet feed or moistened grain. Feed half in the morning and half in the evening. When calcium deficiency alone is the problem, you can give limestone (calcium carbonate) at a rate of 1 ounce (28 grams) for every 11 grams of calcium the horse requires in his diet. When both minerals or only phosphorus are deficient, you can give a dicalcium phosphate supplement, such as Dical. One ounce of Dical contains about 6 grams of calcium and 6 grams of phosphorus.

Horses who are ill and stop eating may experience low blood calcium and develop a condition called thumps. This is a diaphragmatic flutter, not in syncope with breathing, that may appear to be like hiccups. These horses usually need intravenous calcium.

Calcium excess is rarely a problem. Horses can tolerate a dietary calcium intake five times greater than what they need for maintenance for long periods without suffering adverse effects. Excess phosphorus, however, is more serious and can lead to a calcium deficiency. However, an excess of either mineral is unlikely to occur unless the horse is consuming mineral supplements in amounts well beyond daily requirements, or, in the case of phosphorus, when bran constitutes a large part of the diet.

Approximate Calcium and Phosphorus Content of Some Common Mineral Supplements*

Supplement	Calcium (%)	Phosphorus (%)	Calcium (grams per ounce, 28 g, of supplement)	Phosphorus (grams per ounce, 28 g, of supplement)
Limestone (calcium carbonate)	38	0	11	0
Dical (dicalcium phosphate)	22	19	6.5	5.7
Bone meal	30	14	9	4
Monodicalcium phosphate	16	22	4.8	6.6
Oyster shells	38	0	11	0
Pro-Phos 12 copper mineral	12	12	3.4	3.4

*These are approximate or average values. If you are using some other supplement, to find the number of grams of mineral in 1 ounce of supplement, multiply the percentage listed on the package for the mineral by 0.28.

Potassium

Potassium is important for proper cell function. Dietary potassium deficiency ordinarily is not a problem because nearly all feeds provide adequate amounts. However, diets high in grain and low in forage—most often fed to horses in training and at hard work—may be deficient in potassium. These horses also lose potassium through sweat, and therefore have a greater need.

An acute potassium deficiency can occur in horses undergoing strenuous training or endurance racing in hot, humid weather. Severe diarrhea is another cause of acute potassium loss.

Signs of potassium deficiency include muscle weakness, lethargy, and diminished intake of water and food. Treatment of loss involves correcting the cause, rehydrating the horse, and replacing *electrolytes* orally, by stomach tube, or, in severe cases, by intravenous fluids.

Potassium deficiency is most likely to occur in the high-performance or endurance horse during intense physical activity. Consider a potassium salt supplement for such horses. The most effective salt is "lite," also called low sodium salt, which is readily available at grocery stores. Lite is half sodium chloride and half potassium chloride, and contains 26 percent potassium. Add 2 to 3 ounces (57 to 85 g) to the horse's daily grain ration.

Trace Minerals

There are a number of minerals horses need in very small amounts. Generally, they are present in sufficient quantity in the horse's diet. But in some parts of the United States the soil is deficient in one or more of these minerals and therefore the feedstuffs grown in these soils are also deficient. Some trace minerals that are commonly supplemented are discussed here.

Other minerals required by horses include manganese, cobalt, molybdenum, magnesium, sulfur, and fluoride. Fluoride toxicity is discussed on page 439. In general, average or better forage and most feedstuffs provide adequate levels of these minerals. Deficiencies are rare. Problems are more likely to occur when these minerals are consumed or supplemented in excessive amounts.

Selenium and vitamin E work together to protect cells from damage caused by free radicals. Free radicals are produced when a bond is broken between two atoms that form an unstable molecule. Once free radicals are produced, they can cause a chain reaction, the final result of which is disruption of a living cell. Some free radicals are produced as a normal consequence of metabolism. The immune system may create free radicals to neutralize virus and bacteria. However, environmental factors such as pollution, radiation, herbicides, and pesticides may create free radicals. Antioxidants "neutralize" free radicals.

A deficiency of selenium has been recognized in the Great Lakes area, along the Eastern seaboard and in the Northwest of the United States. The dietary selenium requirement for all types of mature horses is estimated to be 1 mg per day. The requirements for the foal range from from 0.16 mg per day at 1 month of age to 0.86 mg per day at 2 years of age. In very young foals, selenium deficiency produces nutritional myopathy (see page 567). In older horses, selenium deficiency may be associated with a decreased immune response, lowered fertility, reduced milk production, and muscle atrophy.

Selenium deficiency is treated by giving the horse an intramuscular injection of selenium and vitamin E. In areas where selenium deficiency in foals has been a problem in the past, a prophylactic injection should be given to the pregnant mare in the last trimester and to the foal shortly after birth. Oral selenium supplementation is also available.

Trace-mineralized salt containing higher levels of selenium is commercially available and should be offered free-choice in areas where selenium deficiency is a problem. Remove other sources of salt to ensure consumption.

Selenium toxicity, a much more common problem than deficiency, is discussed on page 428.

Iodine is required to synthesize thyroid hormone. Thyroid hormone deficiency produces hypothyroidism. This is a rare condition in the adult horse, but has been described in Standardbreds and Thoroughbreds. An excess of thyroid hormone produces hyperthyroidism, which has not yet been documented in adult horses.

Iodine excess is caused by oversupplementing with iodine, usually by giving products such as seaweed that are known to contain high levels of this mineral, but occasionally by giving other horse products containing iodine.

An iodine deficiency has been noted in high mountain areas and throughout sections of the midwestern and western United States and Canada. Feeds grown in these areas may contain iodine levels below those needed to meet the horse's requirements. Pregnant mares with iodine deficiency (or excess) can give birth to foals with neonatal hypothyroidism (see page 571). This is the major concern with iodine imbalances in the horse.

Iodine deficiency can be prevented by giving the horse access to a trace-mineralized salt block. However, because there is a wide variation in salt consumption among mares during pregnancy and lactation, a mare at risk of iodine deficiency is best supplemented by adding 1 ounce (28 g) of trace-mineralized salt to her daily grain mix.

Copper and zinc are important for growing horses. The dietary concentrations of copper and zinc adequate for horses, as recommended by the National Research Council, are 100 mg per day for copper and 400 mg per day for zinc.

Increasing the concentrations of copper and zinc in the diets of nursing and weanling foals decreases the risk and occurrence of developmental orthopedic diseases. Copper and zinc play important roles in bone formation and metabolism. Concentrations in rations for rapidly growing horses 3 to 12 months of age should be somewhat lower, at 35.5 mg per day for copper and 113.5 mg per day for for zinc. These recommended concentrations have not been associated with any adverse effects.

Iron is found in hemoglobin (red blood cells) and myoglobin (muscle cells), and plays a key role in oxygen transport. The minimum daily dietary requirement for iron is 400 mg per day for adult horses and 113 mg per day for foals. Levels of consumption above 2 grams per day are toxic to mature horses. Much lower concentrations are toxic to neonatal foals.

Iron deficiency is extremely uncommon in horses. It occurs only with chronic or severe blood loss, usually related to stomach ulcers or to a heavy infestation of worms. A number of vitamin-iron-mineral supplements are available at feed stores. Their value as appetite improvers and energizers is questionable. Those that contain high concentrations of iron pose the possibility of toxicity.

VITAMINS

Vitamins are organic substances required in minute amounts for normal body metabolism. Not all vitamins are dietary essentials. Most vitamins are synthesized by bacteria in the horse's large intestines. In fact, only vitamins A and E must be supplied entirely by the diet.

Vitamin A (Retinol)

Vitamin A is the only vitamin that may be inadequate in rations routinely fed to horses. This vitamin is essential for eye health, bone growth, sperm and egg production, and growth of the cells that line the respiratory and digestive tracts and the reproductive organs. Vitamin A is important for horses who have little or no access to fresh grass, horses who are breeding, and those prone to skin disorders.

A deficiency of vitamin A makes a horse more susceptible to respiratory and reproductive tract infections, may cause *fertility* problems, and can lead to eye difficulties such as night blindness and excessive tearing. It may also cause the horse to develop a dry rough coat. An excess of vitamin A causes brittle bones, shedding of skin, and symptoms much like those of a deficiency.

Forage plants and grasses contain the vitamin A precursor carotene, which is converted to vitamin A in the horse's body. This process is not especially efficient. Therefore, carotene levels are not good indicators of vitamin A levels.

The best sources of carotene are rapidly growing spring and early summer grasses. Horses who consume such forage for four to six weeks store enough vitamin A in their liver to maintain adequate levels for three to six months. However, when a horse uses up that supply and does not have access to feeds or supplements containing adequate amounts of vitamin A, a deficiency will ensue.

Properly harvested early-cut legume hay, such as alfalfa, has adequate amounts of carotene even though much is lost during handling. However, after hay has been stored for six months, it loses about half its carotene content and may become deficient. The color of hay alone does not indicate vitamin A content.

Accordingly, to prevent vitamin A deficiency when poor-quality hay must be fed for long periods, or when pasture without a significant amount of green color is being consumed for more than three months, add 15,000 IU vitamin A to the daily diet. Feed twice this amount to broodmares during the last 90 days of pregnancy and throughout lactation. Supplements containing vitamin A are available at all feed stores. As an alternative, an intramuscular injection can be given by your veterinarian, which is good for at least three months.

Vitamin E

Vitamin E, along with selenium, enhances the body's immune system. Vitamin E is an antioxidant and is essential to muscle function. Vitamin E deficiency has been implicated as a cause of equine degenerative myeloencephalopathy. Vitamin E is present in sufficient amounts in green forages and natural feeds to more than meet daily nutritional requirements. A deficiency could occur if a horse were fed pelleted feeds and/or cured hay for an extended period, because both feeds may contain low levels of vitamin E. Pregnant and adult horses require 500 IU per day.

Wheat germ oil and alfalfa meal are excellent sources of vitamin E.

Vitamin D

Vitamin D helps the body to use calcium. Deficiency of this vitamin is rare because horses synthesize vitamin D in their skin in response to ultraviolet light, which is present in unfiltered sunlight. Remaining outdoors for two hours a day is sufficient exposure. Good quality sun-cured feeds also produce ample quantities of vitamin D.

Vitamin D intoxication is the most common vitamin toxicity in horses. Vitamin D is incorporated into most vitamin supplements but has little if any therapeutic value. However, such supplements are frequently given in the misguided belief that adding vitamin D will increase the rate of growth or improve maximum adult size. The unfortunate result is a decline in health and organ function resulting from calcium deposits in bones, soft tissue, heart, kidneys, and blood vessels. The effects of excessive vitamin D consumption are cumulative. It can take several weeks or months for signs to become evident.

One other cause of toxicity is ingesting plants that contain vitamin D glycosides. These plants are found primarily in Florida, Texas, southern California, and subtropical areas throughout the world.

Vitamin K

Vitamin K is necessary for blood coagulation and liver function. Horses synthesize vitamin K in the intestinal tract. However, if a horse ingests a vitamin K antagonist, a deficiency characterized by spontaneous bleeding will occur. For more information, see *Rodenticide Anticoagulants* (page 25). Vitamin K deficiency also can occur in horses with diseases or conditions that decrease the population of colonic bacteria that manufacture vitamin K. Some of these include prolonged antibiotic therapy, heavy infestation of worms, diarrhea disease, and colitis.

Vitamin C

Vitamin C is essential to the production of connective tissues such as tendons, ligaments, and cartilage. It also acts as an antioxidant. Vitamin C supplementation is not needed, because adequate amounts are manufactured by the horse's liver.

B-Complex Vitamins

The B-complex vitamins are especially important for horses who are not eating normally or are under stress from such things as age, heavy exercise, illness, injury, transport, surgery, or infection. B-12 aids in red cell production. All B-complex vitamins are produced by bacteria in the horse's intestinal tract and are present in natural feedstuffs in more than sufficient amounts to meet the horse's needs. A deficiency could occur if the horse were sick and not eating, or, if for the same reasons described for vitamin K, there were a decreased number of bacteria in the colon.

B-complex supplements are frequently given to hard-working and performance horses. Although benefits are difficult to quantify, many horsemen attest to their value.

Vitamin B deficiency may be marked by nervousness and irritability. When B-complex deficiency is suspected or when additional vitamins are desired, you can safely give up to 30 grams a day of a broad-spectrum commercial vitamin preparation. A similar result can be obtained by giving 12 to 16 ounces (340 to 453 g) of brewer's yeast. Brewer's yeast is high in all of the B vitamins except B-12, which is not needed in the horse's diet.

Feedstuffs

Feedstuffs for horses are generally divided into those that contain a lot of fiber—roughages such as hay—and those that do not—concentrates such as grain. There is also a wide variety of commercial horse feeds. The online supplement to *Nutrient Requirements of Horses* by the National Research Council is an excellent resource for the nutritional analysis for a wide variety of feeds. This is free and can be found at http://www.nap.edu/catalog/11653.html.

ROUGHAGES

Roughages are feeds consisting primarily of bulky, coarse plants or plant parts with high fiber content and low total digestible nutrients. By definition, a roughage contains more than 18 percent crude fiber. Hays and forage pastures provide roughage. These are the most natural and frequently the least expensive feed for horses; therefore, they should provide the basis for all horse feeding programs. If the ration for the horse is based primarily on hay, the hay must be of a high enough quality to provide the required nutrients. The starting guideline is 1 percent body weight per day should be feed as roughage. For example, a 1,000-pound (453 kg) horse should eat at least 10 pounds (4.5 kg) of hay or grass per day.

Hays

The three types of hay are legumes, grasses, and cereal grains.

Legumes are higher in protein than grasses. Legumes absorb nitrogen from bacteria that live in their roots. These plants then "fix" or convert the nitrogen to protein. The major legumes are alfalfa, clover, birdsfoot trefoil, and lespedeza.

The leaves of legumes contain much more protein than the stems. Accordingly, the amount of leafiness is a good indication of the hay's nutritional value. If the harvest is damaged by weather or excessive handling, the leaves will not be firmly attached to the stems and can be lost during feeding. Legume hay past its bloom when cut is too mature and will not make a good feed.

Grasses commonly fed to horses include timothy, bromes, orchard grass, Bermuda, bluegrass, fescue, wheatgrass, and others. Grass hay should be harvested at early maturity, when nutrient value and digestibility are best. Grass hay with heads over half an inch (13 mm) long is too mature.

Cereal grain hay, in which the grain is left on the stem and not removed during harvesting, can be cut and used for hay. This type of hay will have minimal protein content. If the heads of the grain are lost, only straw remains, resulting in a poor quality hay.

Alternate Forages

In years of drought and hay shortages, horse owners may be scrambling to find quality forage. Several acceptable alternatives to hay include beet pulp and cottonseed hulls. It is prudent before starting any new feeding regimen to consult with an equine nutrition specialist, your veterinarian or a knowledgeable county agent or local extension specialist. See *Adding to or Changing the Ration*, page 418. Commercial complete feeds may also be considered as an alternative.

Pasture

Good quality pasture is a nutritious and frequently inexpensive source of feed for horses. Grasses that provide good forage will vary in different geographic areas according to soil content, temperature, and rainfall. A county agent or local extension specialist can provide information on conditions in your area or perform a chemical analysis.

Pastures that contain a mixture of legumes and grasses, a clean water supply, and trace-mineralized salt will meet all the nutritional requirements for most horses. However, foals, hard-working horses, and pregnant and lactating mares may require more dietary energy than some pastures can provide.

Grass Clippings

Although not recommended, fresh lawn or pasture clippings can be fed with extreme care. Pockets of mold may develop quickly within the warm, moist masses. Unfavorable consequences, such as choking or the grass molding, may be prevented by spreading out the clippings and discarding whatever isn't consumed in 30 to 60 minutes. Keep in mind that grass from a lawn may have elevated nitrates if fertilizer was used, and the lawn mower may leave a residue of oil or gasoline. It may be safer to let your horse graze on the unmowed lawn.

CONCENTRATES

Concentrates include a broad class of feedstuffs that are high in energy and low in crude fiber (under 18 percent)—generally, grain. Concentrates, because they are low in crude fiber, provide a high concentration of dietary energy in a small volume.

High-energy foods have the potential to be overfed and can be associated with laminitis, acute gastric dilatation, azoturia, developmental orthopedic disease, and colic. The maximum amount of grain concentrate that is safe to feed is not more than 0.75 percent of the horse's body weight per feeding. So a 1,000-pound (453 kg) horse should receive no more than 7 pounds (3 kg) of grain at a feeding, except as part of a carefully balanced feeding program, as discussed in the section *How to Feed Your Horse* (see page 414).

Cereal Grains

Cereal grains are the principal high-energy food source for horses. Pound for pound, cereal grains contain about twice as much digestible energy as does hay. As a general rule, a mature horse may be given up to half a pound (226 g) of cereal grain per 100 pounds (45 kg) of body weight per day. Hard-working horses and lactating mares can be given up to 1 pound (453 g), depending on the energy content and nutrient quality of the roughage in the diet.

Oats have higher fiber content than most other grains and therefore are considered by many horse owners to be among the safest of grains because they are the least likely to cause laminitis. Oats are expensive, when cost is compared to energy content. One advantage of oats is that they are much less likely to be overfed, since the horse would have to eat a larger volume to extract the same amount of energy as in corn, for example. A horse will founder on oats if he eats enough.

Corn is a popular feed due to its ready availability. Many horse owners prefer not to feed corn because they feel it is too "hot" a food (that is, too high in energy). Although corn does contain twice as much energy as an equal volume of oats, when both corn and oats are fed by weight to provide equal amounts of energy, corn does not have a greater tendency to make a horse more high-spirited than do oats. Corn is palatable, consistent in quality, and is the only common grain that has significant vitamin A. Corn can be fed whole, cracked, or by the ear. It should not be ground finely, because it becomes dusty.

Wheat bran is a poorly digested cereal grain with low energy content. It does increase the volume of feces excreted and is useful in certain circumstances for this purpose. Contrary to popular belief, it is not a good laxative. In fact, if adequate water is not consumed, it may actually lead to an impaction. This is why bran is generally mixed with water to make a mash.

Wheat, barley, milo, and rye should not make up more than one-third to one-half of the total grain ration. The reason is that they contain a hard kernel or shell that makes them difficult to digest unless they are processed (crimped, rolled, cracked, coarsely ground, or steam-flaked). Wheat has a high gluten content and can produce a doughy ball in the stomach if fed in large amounts. Rye is more susceptible than other grains to a toxin called ergot. Barley is high in fat, so often this grain is added to the ration if weight gain is desirable.

Molasses

Molasses improves taste and decreases dust, which is why commercial manufacturers often combine it with processed cereal grains to make sweet feeds. Wet molasses may be added to a concentrate mix (5 percent of the weight of the mix) to increase its free-choice consumption and prevent the horse from sifting out added minerals.

Molasses is a good vehicle for giving medications. It can also be used as an added source of calories.

Grain Quality and Storage

Cereal grains containing only a few broken kernels and less than 13 percent moisture can be stored for long periods without loss of nutritional value, provided that they are kept in metal containers or dry, rodent-proof bins. Plastic containers are not suitable; rodents can rapidly eat through plastic. Grain stored in sacks can become moist and moldy. If that happens, do not feed the grain. Mold or bacterial growth and insect proliferation generally do not occur at moisture levels below 13 percent.

Galvanized garbage cans with tight-fitting lids are good storage containers. Large galvanized metal bins are good for bulk storage.

Always store grain in a room with a horse-proof latch or in some other secure location where horses cannot get to it. This will prevent overeating and its attendant dangers of gastric dilatation, colic, diarrhea, endotoxemia, and founder. Despite such precautions, if the horse gets into the grain supply and consumes an unknown quantity of grain, notify your veterinarian at once.

COMMERCIAL HORSE FEEDS

Commercial horse feed manufacturers have developed a variety of feeds that are nutritionally formulated to meet specific feeding requirements.
Complete horse feeds containing alfalfa meal, soybean meal, and other cereal grains can be fed as the *sole* source of daily nutrients. Forage is not necessary.

Complete feeds are a good choice when good-quality hay or pasture is either unavailable or more expensive than the feed. Other advantages of complete feeds are that less space is required for storage, the horse cannot sort through his food (and therefore wastes less), and they are more digestible for older horses with poor teeth.

Not all commercial feeds are "complete." Some are meant to be fed as a supplement to forage, to provide nutrients not found in the forage. Other products contain cereal grains and/or protein supplements intended to provide extra energy for recreational activities and hard work. Grain supplements are available for late pregnancy and lactation, and for the nursing and growing foal. Be sure to read the labels.

National manufacturers produce high-quality grain mixes that meet or exceed nutrient content requirements for the type of horse for which the feed is intended. The majority of these feeds also contains vitamins A and E, and trace minerals including selenium, copper, and zinc, in amounts that when fed according to recommendations, supply all the vitamins and minerals needed in the horse's diet.

State and federal laws regulate the production, labeling, distribution, and sale of animal feeds. The feed label provides useful information, including the minimum percentage of crude protein and fat, and the maximum percentage of crude fiber. Although guarantees for minerals and vitamins are not required unless the feed is advertised as either a complete feed or a specific supplement, most national name-brand manufacturers show the complete guaranteed analysis on the label. Labels on products from local feed suppliers may not show a complete analysis, but the dealer or the company should be able to provide this information. If not, consider having the feed analyzed or use a different product. In choosing among competing products, consider the relative cost, nutrient content, quality control, and services provided by the dealer. The feed should be appropriate for the use intended. For example, one formulated for mature horses would not be appropriate for growing horses. Feeds for growing horses should contain protein supplements high in lysine, derived from soybeans or milk products. Because feeds are designed to be fed with forage, failure to provide the needed roughage can lead to digestive disturbances.

Commercial feeds formulated for cattle and other animals should not be fed to horses because they do not meet the horse's specific nutrient requirements and may contain toxic ingredients. Rumensin, frequently added to cattle feed to prevent coccidiosis, is highly toxic to horses and will cause heart failure and death. Lincomycin, an antibiotic added to swine feeds to increase their growth rate, can cause diarrhea and fatal colitis in horses.

Commercial horse feeds are made up in the form of pellets, cubes, and loose mixes of grain. Loose grain mixes generally contain molasses, which increases palatability. These feeds are called textured or sweet feeds. In hot, humid weather they may spoil unless they are properly stored. Hay is often pressed into wafers or cubes about 1 to 3 inches (25 to 76 mm) in size.

Complete feeds are frequently pelleted. Pellets are made by grinding seeds and roughage and mixing them with molasses, then forcing the mixture through a sieve. Dehydrated pellets are made from fresh-cut alfalfa hay that has been processed to remove the water. Pelleting decreases waste, enables you to store the feed longer without spoilage, and provides uniform delivery of nutrients. Pellets are easier for horses to chew than grains and may result in better digestibility, especially for older horses.

Pellets vary in size, the average being about one-quarter to three-quarters of an inch (6 to 19 mm) long. While smaller pellets tend to be eaten more slowly, there is no evidence that pellet size, or pelleted feeds in general, cause choking any more often than sweet feeds. Regardless of the feed, the more rapidly it is eaten, the greater the likelihood of choking. For the horse who bolts his feed, you can make him eat more slowly by feeding smaller amounts more frequently, spreading the feed over a large surface, mixing it with chopped hay, or adding several large, smooth stones or a salt block to the feed box so the horse will have to sort through the rocks to get to the pellets or grain.

How to Feed Your Horse

Horses choose feeds according to appetite and taste appeal. If given a choice, a horse with a mineral or vitamin deficiency will not necessarily select a feed that is high in the missing ingredient. The only way to be certain each horse receives the right amount of calories and essential nutrients is to make sure the correct concentrations are present in the daily ration and that each horse receives his proper share.

It is most important to feed rations by weight and not by volume. Nutrition tables always give the horse's needs by weight of the horse and percent of each nutrient by weight in the feedstuff. This enables you to directly compare energy and nutrients from feed to feed. This kind of comparison is not possible when comparing volumes.

For example, a 3-pound (1.36 kg) coffee can holds 2 to 3 pounds (.9 to 1.4 kg) of oats. The same can holds 4 to 5 pounds (1.8 to 2.3 kg) of corn. Since corn is more energy-rich than oats, a can of corn may contain two to three times more energy than a can of oats.

Hay is frequently fed in flakes, which are sections of the compressed bale. A flake varies in weight, depending on how thick it is and how tightly the hay was compressed when baled. It is a good practice to weigh several samples to get an idea of the average weight of a bale and a flake.

How Often to Feed

Horses have a relatively small stomach when compared with cattle and other large animals. This limits the amount a horse can safely consume in a single meal. Under natural pasture conditions, a horse grazes 50 to 70 percent of the time, both day and night. Under such conditions, the stomach is never overdistended.

Overloading occurs when too much feed is given in a single meal. This causes overdistension of the horse's stomach, increases intestinal motility, produces a sudden loss of fluid from the plasma into the gut, and increases the risk of colic. These problems can be avoided, and the efficiency of digestion maximized, by feeding stabled and paddocked horses using the following guidelines.

- Provide enough hay so that the horse will always have something to eat.
- Feed the horse equal meals at least twice a day, but more often if possible. Horses fed on a consistent schedule are less likely to bolt their food or develop boredom-related vices.

- Feed as little grain as necessary. With small amounts, that is, 1 pound (453 g) or less, there is no advantage to feeding grain more than once a day.

- When horses are fed as a group, make sure a dominant or aggressive horse does not drive away a subordinate horse. Put out extra feeders at widely spaced intervals to prevent this, or feed in separate areas, if possible.

FEEDING ADULT HORSES

Care and feeding during pregnancy and feeding during lactation are discussed in chapter 17, "Pregnancy and Foaling." Feeding nursing foals and growing horses is discussed in chapter 18, "Pediatrics."

Pasturing

Depending on where you live, a horse usually can be pastured for five to six months a year. During the winter, he'll need another feed, such as hay or a commercial grain mix.

Most pastures contain more than one type of forage. A mixture containing bluegrass, tall fescue, and orchard grass, or one containing legume hay and grass, provides excellent nutrition. Keep in mind that a green field is not necessarily a pasture; pasture contains plants that are healthy and nutritious for the horse.

Horses at pasture should have access to clean, fresh water and trace-mineralized salt. To preserve pasture integrity and prevent plant injury and soil compaction, remove horses from pasture after a heavy rain and before irrigating.

A horse should be put out to pasture in a graduated manner to prevent gastric dilatation, colic, diarrhea, endotoxemia, and founder. This is especially important for fresh green pastures and pastures high in legumes. Begin by turning the horse out after a regular meal of hay, for two hours or less the first day. Increase this gradually over the next week. The regular meal helps prevent the horse from overeating. After two weeks, it should be safe for the horse to remain at pasture full time.

Feeding Hay

A horse who weighs 1,000 pounds (453 kg) needs about 10 to 15 pounds (4.5 to 6.8 kg) of good-quality hay per day. In selecting hay, the major consideration is not necessarily the kind of hay or even the cutting, but the quality of the hay and its nutritional value in relation to cost—assuming that it is readily consumed and does not contain toxic weeds and plants. To determine the exact composition and nutritional value, you need to have the hay analyzed. Local extension services can provide information on where this can be done and the cost of the service.

Hay bales should be taken apart and examined for dust and mold, which are quite likely to be present if the hay was baled while damp. The inside of a properly cured bale of hay should be green and should have a pleasant odor. Musty or offensive smells suggest mold, which makes the hay totally unsuitable for horse feed.

Ideally, hay should be fed in a hay rack or a wooden feeder. Feeding in a hay net above shoulder level is not a good practice because the horse is more likely to inhale dust and fine plant material, predisposing him to bronchitis and heaves. When hay is fed on the ground, there is considerable loss due to trampling and scattering, and also contamination of the hay by parasite eggs and the risk of ingesting sand.

Feeding Concentrates

Cereal grains are always fed in combination with a roughage. Because cereal grains are so high in energy, it is recommended that a grain or concentrate mix never make up more than half of the total amount of feed consumed each day, except for horses under 1 year of age, and for athletic horses undergoing intense physical training. In addition, grain concentrates that make up more than half the diet decrease forage intake and create problems caused by a lack of fiber.

Rations containing 75 percent hay and 25 percent grain by weight are appropriate for mares in late pregnancy, yearlings to 18 months, and adult horses doing light work.

Grain can be fed in wooden feeders, feeding buckets, or nonmetallic feed pans. Horses should be fed individually to prevent overconsumption by a dominant horse. Feed bags are a good way to ensure that each horse receives the correct amount. Remove the feed bag as soon as the horse finishes the grain.

Feeding Commercial Horse Feeds

A commercial feed should meet the requirements for protein and minerals, as determined by the National Research Council. Consult the label to be sure the product meets these specific requirements. Guarantees for minerals and vitamins are often provided but are not required unless the feed is advertised as a complete feed or a specific supplement. Feed according to the directions on the label.

If the ration is a complete feed, the horse will not need additional fiber, but you may see boredom activities, such as wood chewing. If this happens, feed some additional roughage, such as long-stemmed hay.

Rations can be calculated, or you can use the user-friendly companion to *Nutrient Requirements of Horses* by the National Research Council at www.nap.edu/catalog/11653.html. Just put in the animal specification, for example, "lactating mare-3 months," and then the forage type, the concentrates used, and any additional feeds, and the program will tell you the value of each feed stuff and any deficits in the overall ration.

Vitamin and Mineral Supplements

The majority of commercial horse feeds contain vitamin and mineral levels that meet or exceed the horse's daily needs. Green forages (pasture or hay) are good sources of vitamins A and E. These are the only vitamins that are not synthesized by the horse and therefore the only vitamins that must be provided in the diet. With the possible exception of equine degenerative *myelopathy*, vitamin E deficiency has not been described in the horse.

Vitamin A deficiency can occur if a horse does not consume green forage or some other dietary source of vitamin A for several months. Hay older than one year has lost nearly all its vitamin A and is unlikely to be suitable as a dietary source of vitamin A. Horses consuming such hay should be supplemented (see *Vitamin A*, page 407).

Additional vitamins above the daily requirements may possibly benefit the following individuals:

- Draft horses, endurance horses, and racehorses, who may have marginal intake of B vitamins (especially thiamin) relative to their needs
- Nervous, hyperactive, stressed horses, particularly when traveling or showing
- Broodmares, if there is any doubt about the adequacy of the diet to meet the vitamin needs of pregnancy and lactation

To prevent vitamin overdose, choose a supplement (preferably in solid form, which is easier to use than injectable and the horse likes it better, too) that provides additional quantities of all vitamins without excessive amounts of any specific vitamin. Administer only according to the manufacturer's directions.

There are specific situations for giving calcium and phosphorus, and the microminerals copper and zinc, as discussed earlier in this chapter.

Allowing the horse free access to trace mineralized salt will ensure that he receives adequate amounts of trace minerals, and will correct any deficiencies that may be present in feeds. In selenium-deficient areas, use trace-mineralized salt containing higher levels of selenium. Remove other sources of salt to ensure consumption.

Fat and Oil Supplements

Most horse feeds contain 2 to 4 percent fat, but horses will adapt to diets containing 10 to 20 percent fat if they are given enough time to adjust. The purpose of adding fat to the diet is to increase energy density without incurring the problems associated with high concentrations of grain. These problems include founder, colic, diarrhea, exertional myopathy, and excitability. Fat supplements can supply the added energy needs without increasing grain intake or decreasing roughage intake. For hardworking performance horses, growing horses, hard keepers (horses who have trouble keeping weight on), and senior horses who need extra calories, fat is an excellent addition. Fat also aids in the absorption of vitamins A, D, E, and K during digestion.

Plant or vegetable oils and animal fats are used for energy more efficiently than all other sources of feed. Vegetable oils provide about three times more DE than an equal weight of cereal grain. Animal fats provide slightly less.

Studies show that adding 10 percent fat to the ration of lactating mares increases the fat percentage of milk and causes the fat content to remain higher as lactation advances. Adding 12 percent fat to the diets of racing or cutting horses improves muscle glycogen storage and athletic performance. Beyond 12 percent, performance did not improve and glycogen storage began to decrease.

Among several fat supplements studied, all appeared to be equally effective. Corn, soy, and other vegetable oils were the most palatable.

Because fat supplements are rich in energy, it's necessary to adjust the ration when feeding these supplements. If the workload does not increase, too much energy will be supplied unless the daily feed intake is reduced. Vegetable oils provide about 4,000 calories DE per pound (453 g), or about 8,000 calories DE per quart (about 1 liter).

Adding 1 quart (2 pounds, 907 g) of vegetable oil to 8 pounds (3.6 kg) of grain results in a 20 percent fat supplement. If the grain and vegetable oil combination makes up half the ration by weight, the concentration of fat in the total ration is 10 percent. Using these figures, you can formulate a 10 or 12 percent fat supplement.

Horses should be started slowly on a fat supplement to prevent digestive upsets and diarrhea. Top dress the feed with half a cup (118 ml) of oil for a 1,000 pound (453 kg) horse: gradually increasing the daily amount to 1 to 2 cups (237 to 474 ml) over the course of three weeks. The oil can be added to the grain mix at each feeding. Monitor the horse's weight, eating behavior, and general well-being.

ADDING TO OR CHANGING THE RATION

Most horses prefer the feed they are accustomed to. Accordingly, when the feed is changed, the horse will usually eat less of it—unless the new feed is much more palatable than the old one.

Any change in a horse's feeding program, either in type or amount of feed, should be undertaken gradually over a period of several days. When adding a new concentrate to an established ration, begin on the first day by giving half a pound (226 g) of the new concentrate mixed in with the old concentrate. Then add half a pound a day until the desired level is reached. Be sure to cut back on the amount or hay or forage to avoid giving the horse too much dietary energy. This should prevent colic and founder.

When taking the horse off an exercise or training program, decrease the grain in the horse's diet at the same rate as you decrease the amount of exercise. An injured or ill horse may also need a decrease in grain.

When changing the type of hay or grain, replace only 25 percent every other day. It should take about one week for the new feed to completely replace the old. Most manufacturers provide guidelines for adding their products to a current feeding program. Follow these recommendations.

Finally, watch your horse closely as he eats. A sudden change in appetite indicates something is wrong with the feed or the horse.

COLD WEATHER CARE AND FEEDING

Horses adapt well to cold weather and can live outdoors in winter in most parts of the country, as long as they have adequate shelter from wind, rain, and snow. A shed open on one side is an ideal shelter for all seasons. Horses grow a long winter coat and store a layer of fat beneath their skin, both of which provide excellent insulation. However, when a horse is kept in a heated stable, he does not adapt and is more likely to suffer from chilling and pneumonia when taken outside.

Horse blankets can be used to prevent chilling. For a horse in winter with a dry coat, or one who is used to being inside, the blanket is beneficial when the wind-chill temperature drops below 20°F (-6.6°C). For a horse in summer with a wet coat, wind-chill discomfort becomes a factor at temperatures below 60°F (15.5°C). Use common sense. If your horse has adapted to outside conditions, he probably does not need a blanket. However, for old horses, who are unable to regulate their body temperature well, or show horses without their natural haircoat, a blanket is a thing of comfort. Digestible energy is the principal dietary concern in cold weather. Protein, vitamin, and mineral needs increase slightly. In winter, it is important to feed a ration that helps the horse create internal heat. High-quality hay is best for this, and is a better choice than grain. This is because roughage is digested by bacterial fermentation in the cecum and colon, which produces a great deal of heat. If high-quality roughage is available and the horse has unlimited access to it, you will probably not need to feed extra concentrates. However, if high-quality roughage is not available or the horse loses body weight and condition, then feed some extra grain.

All grains are satisfactory, but corn has certain advantages. Corn generates twice as much energy as an equal volume of oats. Accordingly, you can feed less to produce the same amount of energy. This leaves more room in the digestive tract for hay. This is the main reason why corn is preferred by many horsemen as a winter feed. If the proportion of grain in the ration exceeds 40 percent, consider feeding a fat supplement (see *Fat and Oil Supplements*, page 417).

Water requirements for horses in cold weather are often overlooked. Water sources can freeze over. Occasionally, the water is too cold for the horse to drink, especially if he has bad teeth. A drop in water consumption results in a drop in food consumption and therefore in energy. It will then be difficult for the horse to keep up his weight and body temperature. Inadequate water consumption may cause the stool to become hard and difficult to pass. This is why constipation and large colon impactions are much more common in freezing weather.

Water heaters should be placed in outdoor tanks to keep the temperature in the trough above 45°F (7.2°C). Horses drink significantly more water in the winter if the water is warm. It is important to make sure the water heater is functioning properly by checking the trough daily. If the water heater shorts out, the shock may not be severe enough to injure the horse, but it will keep him from drinking. In extremely cold weather, remove ice several times a day.

Horses have been known to live on snow for limited periods. This is not ideal and should not be relied on to supply water needs.

Weight Gain and Loss

It can be difficult to determine if a horse is too fat or too thin. To detect weight changes before the horse develops a significant change in body condition, it is important to weigh the horse (or estimate the horse's weight, see the table on page 396) at least monthly and maintain a record.

Visual inspection is one way to estimate body condition. However, in the winter it can be quite difficult to tell if a horse is losing condition without feeling him. *The Body Condition Scoring System* on page 422, developed by Texas A&M University, gives you a consistent method with which to monitor body condition.

Obesity

Overfeeding is the most common cause of obesity. Horses will not adjust their appetites to balance energy expenditure. When given more calories than they need, they will readily consume them. Obese horses are less efficient individuals and have decreased exercise tolerance. They suffer from added stress to their joints, cardiovascular, respiratory, and reproductive systems. Equine metabolic syndrome is associated with obese, insulin-resistant horses (see *Equine Metabolic Syndrome*, page 228).

Keep in mind that the energy needs of idle horses are 50 percent less than those of hardworking horses. Be sure to adjust your horse's dietary energy in accordance with his level of activity.

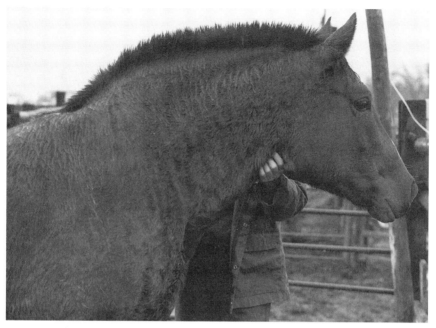

An extremely obese horse with a thick, heavy neck: score 8 to 9.

WEIGHT REDUCTION

Weight reduction is recommended for all horses with body condition scores above 5, with the exception of late-term pregnant and lactating mares, in whom a score of 6 is often desirable. Weight can be reduced by reducing calories and increasing exercise. When both are done together, the results are better because the body weight lost is mostly fat. The exercise helps retain muscle and lean body condition.

Obese horses are to some extent exercise-intolerant, so it is important to start an exercise program slowly and advance as the horse's condition improves. A one-hour trail ride at a walk and slow trot will burn only about 200 calories. Sweating does not indicate a large use of calories, but rather a lack of condition. At a slow trot with some cantering, the horse may burn up to 1,000 calories per hour. With intense work, a horse can expend several thousand calories an hour. (Compare this to the 16,000 calories required for daily maintenance.)

Step up the exercise gradually, building length of time and intensity as the horse's fitness level improves. Weight reduction should be slow as to not stress the horse or cause metabolic upsets. Start simple, walking and then trotting long enough for the horse to begin sweating, then walk to cool down. Daily exercise is preferred but is not always practical. However, the exercise must be consistent to be effective.

Dieting is accomplished not by changing the composition of the diet, as it is in people, but by reducing the quantity of feed. If you are feeding hay and

Body Condition Scoring System

Condition	Neck	Withers	Loin	Tailhead	Ribs	Shoulder
1, Poor	Bone structure easily noticeable, animal extremely emaciated, no fatty tissue can be felt	Bone structure easily noticeable	Spinous processes project prominently	Tailhead (pinbone) and hook bones project prominently	No fat cover over ribs	Bone structure easily noticeable
2, Very Thin	Faintly discernable, animal emaciated	Faintly discernable	Slight fat covering over base of spinous processes; Transverse processes of lumbar vertebrae feel rounded; Spinous processes are prominent	Tailhead prominent	Slight fat cover over ribs; Ribs easily discernable	Shoulder accentuated
3, Thin	Neck accentuated	Withers accentuated	Fat buildup halfway on spinous processes but easily discernable; Transverse processes cannot be felt	Tailhead prominent but individual vertebrae cannot be visually identified; Hook bones appear rounded but are still easily discernable; Pin bones not distinguishable	Slight fat cover over ribs; Ribs easily discernable	Shoulder accentuated

Condition	Neck	Withers	Loin	Tailhead	Ribs	Shoulder
4, Moderately Thin	Neck not obviously thin	Withers not obviously thin	Negative crease along back	Prominence depends on conformation; fat can be felt; Hook bones not discernable	Faint outline discernable	Shoulder not obviously thin
5, Moderate	Neck blends smoothly into body	Withers rounded over spinous processes	Back level	Fat around tailhead beginning to feel spongy	Ribs cannot be visually distinguished but can be easily felt	Shoulder blends smoothly into body
6, Moderately Fleshy	Fat beginning to be deposited	Fat beginning to be deposited	May have slight positive crease down back	Fat around tailhead feels soft	Fat over ribs feels spongy	Fat beginning to be deposited
7, Fleshy	Fat deposited along neck	Fat deposited along withers	May have positive crease down back	Fat around tailhead is soft	Individual ribs can be felt, but noticeable filling between ribs with fat	Fat deposited behind shoulder
8, Fat	Noticeable thickening of neck	Area along withers filled with fat	Positive crease down back	Tailhead fat very soft; Fat deposited along inner buttocks	Difficult to feel ribs	Area behind shoulder filled in flush with body
9, Extremely Fat	Bulging fat	Bulging fat	Obvious positive crease down back	Building fat around tailhead; Fat along inner buttocks may rub together; Flank filled in flush	Patchy fat appearing over ribs	Bulging fat

grain, start slowly by cutting back on the quantity of grain until the correct concentration of DE for the new level of activity is obtained. (For specific guidelines, see the online program for the Nutrient Requirements of Horses at www.nap.edu/catalog.) Since you want the horse to lose weight, slowly cut back another 10 to 15 percent while maintaining the same level of exercise. When feeding hay alone, follow the same formula. If you are feeding alfalfa hay, consider slowly switching to grass hay or a combination of both. If the horse is on pasture, reduce the amount of pasture time. Balance the diet based on the horse's age and activity level. Your horse's vitamin, mineral, and protein requirements must be met. It is simpler to control your horse's rations if he is fed separate from the herd.

In severe winter weather, weight loss should be postponed and enough DE supplied to maintain the horse's current weight.

A drastic reduction in feed intake should be avoided. In horses, even mild degrees of starvation increase the risk of high blood lipid levels with attendant neurological symptoms. Death can occur.

EMACIATION

Horses with low body condition scores (1 to 3) are severely undernourished. These horses are in negative energy balance, meaning they are not taking in enough energy to meet their daily requirements. Refueling must be done slowly. The gastrointestinal tract and metabolic condition of the horse will be unprepared for a large protein load, so feed is added slowly without a large amount of concentrate. Within two to three weeks, the malnourished horse

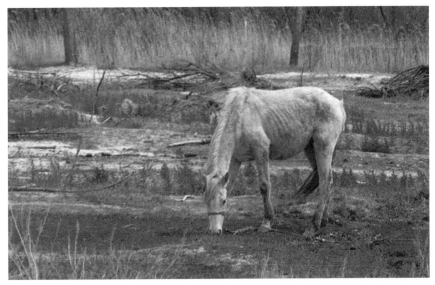

A thin, poorly nourished horse with no subcutaneous fat: score 1 to 2.

will begin to gain weight and add lean body mass, much like a growing horse.

Once the horse is gaining some weight, the feed ration can be increased to a more nutrient-dense diet. It would be wise to consult your veterinarian as you add concentrates to the horse's diet to avoid any of the complications that can occur, such as colic or laminitis.

THE HARDKEEPER

A horse who is perpetually thin or seems to require more food than others in a comparable situation is referred to as a hardkeeper. One or more of the following may be contributing factors.

- The quality or amount of ration fails to meet the horse's energy and/or nutrient requirements. Energy requirements increase as work increases. These requirements must be met by increasing the amount or energy density of the feed.

- The ration is complete but the horse is unable to extract all the dietary nutrients because of dental disease or a heavy burden of worms. Less commonly, the horse may have an intestinal disease or a deficiency of digestive enzymes, resulting in a malabsorption syndrome.

- The horse may not be taking in enough feed because a dominant individual is driving him away from the feeder. The horses should be fed from separate feeders spaced widely apart.

Occasionally there is no apparent cause. Some horses seem to be thin by nature. However, the horse who steadily loses weight and condition is a different matter. Something is wrong with the feed or the horse.

Treatment: Nutrient deficiencies should be corrected as described in this chapter. A good parasite control program will greatly assist in keeping the horse healthy (see *Controlling Internal Parasites*, page 63). All hardkeepers should be examined for abnormal tooth wear and other correctable causes of dental disease.

Finally, if the horse is moderately thin to thin, from no discernable illness or health problem (such as poor teeth or parasites) switch to a commercial horse feed or put the horse on pasture containing an abundance of high-quality forage. If pasture is unavailable and you are feeding hay, add cereal grain to the daily ration—half a pound (226 g) per 100 pounds (45 kg) of weight of the horse.

Wood Chewing and Cribbing

Wood chewing and cribbing are common vices that occur predominantly in stabled horses. Wood chewing usually does not cause digestive problems, because most of the wood is dropped and not swallowed. Occasionally splinters penetrate the soft tissues of the mouth and cause infections and abscesses.

Wood chewing, however, can be tremendously destructive to fences, stalls, and wooden siding.

Cribbing, while superficially resembling wood chewing, is a vice in which the horse sets his front teeth on a horizontal solid object such as the edge of a stall window, arches his neck, pulls back, and swallows large gulps of air.

The major problem with cribbing and wood chewing is wear of the incisor teeth, rarely to such an extent that the horse can no longer graze. In a few cases, the horse spends so much time chewing or cribbing that he fails to eat enough feed.

The causes of wood chewing and cribbing are not known. A hereditary predisposition for cribbing has been identified in some Thoroughbred families. Observation suggests that one or more of the following may be causative or contributing factors.

- Social isolation and lack of companionship
- Boredom
- Frustration
- Lack of opportunity to release tension and nervous energy
- Need for more fiber
- Imitative behavior
- Vestigial browsing behavior

Treatment: These habits are difficult to stop, but they can be minimized by turning the horse out to pasture, preferably with other horses. For stalled horses, you can try hanging a plastic jug from the ceiling to give the horse something to play with, or put up metal mirrors so the horse thinks he has a companion.

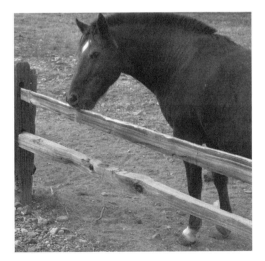

Wood chewing is a destructive vice that is readily copied by other horses.

If the horse is eating pelleted feed, switch to hay or continue the pelleted feed and add half a pound (226 g) of long-stemmed hay per 100 pounds (45 kg) weight of the horse. Make sure the diet contains all the necessary nutrients.

As a deterrent to wood chewing, string electric wires along the tops of fences. Wood can be painted with a nontoxic chemical substance to make it unpalatable. Avoid the use of creosote, one of the agents responsible for wood preservative poisoning (see page 439).

The usual method of preventing cribbing is to apply a 2- to 3-inch (51 to 76 mm) leather strap around the horse's throat at the narrowest part of the neck. Commercial cribbing collars are also available. When the horse tries to arch his neck to crib or swallow air, the strap becomes painful. Some straps have a metal piece at the gullet to increase the discomfort. The crib strap should be applied snugly, but not tight enough to interfere with breathing. Crib straps usually are effective, but some horses continue to crib in spite of the strap.

Another cribbing device that may be effective is a hollow bit in the form of a cylinder with perforated holes. The bit prevents the horse from creating an airtight seal with his lips.

Turning out often helps decrease the behavior, as long as the horse is only cribbing when confined. Be aware that horses pastured with a cribbing horse may imitate the habit and acquire the vice.

Forage Toxicities

Forage toxicities are the most common causes of poisoning in horses. Other causes of poisoning, and the treatment of acute poisoning, are discussed in *Poisoning* (see page 22).

FESCUE TOXICITY

Fescue poisoning is caused by an alkaloid-producing fungus that proliferates in fescue grass during the lush stages of growth. This tends to occur on fall pasture, particularly when autumn rains follow a dry summer. Fescue is less palatable than most other pasture grasses, and horses generally will not eat it if something else is available.

Toxicity produces reproductive problems among mares during the last three months of pregnancy. There is an increased frequency of prolonged pregnancy, retained placenta, *stillbirth*, and absent milk production (agalactia).

It is easier to prevent fescue toxicity than to treat it. Avoid feeding fescue hay to pregnant mares (or putting them on fescue pastures) during the last two to three months of gestation. If this is not feasible, supplement the fescue forage with alfalfa or legume hay.

SELENIUM TOXICITY

Selenium toxicity occurs in areas where selenium levels are high in the soil. These arid or semi-arid areas are marked by certain indicator plants that accumulate high levels of selenium. These "accumulator" plants are not palatable and are not eaten by horses except as a last resort. Other selenium "converter" plants (plants that convert an element such as selenium from a source from which it is usually unavailable to a soluble form that can be accessed), however, including grains and native grasses, absorb lower concentrations and are commonly grazed. Selenium is taken up by plants more readily in alkaline soils, found principally in the Great Plains and western Rocky Mountains. This is why the disease was known as "alkali disease" to early settlers, who incorrectly surmised that the high salt content in the soil and water were the cause of the symptoms.

Selenium toxicity falls into two categories: acute and chronic. The acute form is caused by the rapid ingestion of large amounts of selenium over a short period of time. This usually happens when too much selenium (in the form of selenium supplements) is added to the diet. Rarely, it is caused by the consumption of accumulator forages.

Horses with acute intoxication may die suddenly from cardiac and respiratory failure. A condition of aimless wandering and stumbling, called "blind staggers," is seen in cattle and sheep as a result of selenium toxicity and is thought to occur in horses as result of the consumption of locoweed plants containing high concentrations of selenium.

The chronic form of selenium poisoning, which is by far the most common manifestation of selenium intoxication in horses, occurs when a horse grazes forages containing converter plants for weeks or months. The horse becomes rundown and emaciated. Hair is lost, particularly over the mane and tail, giving this condition the name "bob-tail disease." Breaks and cracks develop in the hoof wall, resulting in foot tenderness and pronounced lameness. The hoof wall may partially or completely slough.

The daily selenium requirement for the horse is 1 mg per day. Amounts greater than 5 mg per kilogram are toxic. The diagnosis for selenium toxicity is commonly made by analyzing the horse's diet, which shows selenium concentrations in feed above these levels. Analysis of hoof and hair samples is also useful in confirming the diagnosis. Elevated serum selenium levels will be found in cases of both acute and chronic poisoning.

Treatment: Remove the horse from pasture. When the roughage or grain is high in selenium, switch to a feed lower in selenium. The new ration should contain 25 percent protein. Specifically, this is a high-protein ration. The horse also should be given 2 to 3 grams per day of the sulfur-containing amino acids DL-methionine and cysteine to bind the selenium.

To prevent selenium toxicity, limit the hours of grazing on problem pastures and use feedstuffs low in selenium. If in doubt, have the ration analyzed.

Several additives have been reported to be effective against high levels of selenium in the feed.

LOCOWEED POISONING

There are many toxic species of locoweed or milk vetch, all of which are members of the legume or pea family. They are distributed worldwide. Many horses develop an addiction to these plants and will seek them out even when better forage is available. A horse must consume large amounts of the plant (30 percent of body weight) over a period of several weeks or months to develop signs of poisoning.

The substances that cause locoweed poisoning include a neurotoxic indolizidine alkaloid called swainsonine, various nitroglycosides, and selenium. These substances cause different locoweed syndromes.

Locoism is seen most often on high desert ranges in the western United States during spring, when locoweed is most abundant. Affected horses become crazy (or "loco") and exhibit such signs as roaring, trembling, salivation, aimless wandering, staggering, respiratory difficulty, and paralysis. These are signs of brain involvement. Horses who recover from locoism may have permanent neurological deficits and are unsafe to ride.

Treatment: The only effective treatment is to remove the horse from pasture or prevent further consumption of rations containing poisonous plants. This must be done early in the course of the disease to be effective.

SORGHUM TOXICITY

Sorghum grasses, including milo, Sudan grass, and Johnson grass, are found in the Southwest and in much of the eastern United States, where they are sometimes used as forages. Not all varieties are poisonous. Johnson grass is the most toxic of the sorghums, while Sudan grass is the most frequent cause of poisoning.

Poisonous sorghums contain cyanogenic glycosides that are metabolized to cyanide. Levels of cyanide are highest in new-growth grasses. Since toxicity declines in the mature plant, pastures rather than hay are more likely to be associated with poisoning.

Acute cyanide poisoning (which is rare) is characterized by respiratory distress, flaring of the nostrils, staggering gait, involuntary urination and defecation, collapse, convulsions, respiratory arrest, blue mucous membranes, and sudden death. The most common condition associated with sorghum toxicity is equine sorghum cystitis ataxia, seen with the chronic consumption of low levels of cyanide. The signs are incoordination of the hind limbs, urinary incontinence, and paralysis of the bladder. Pregnant mares on sorghum pastures have been known to abort or give birth to deformed foals.

Treatment: Treatment of acute cyanide poisoning involves giving antidotes containing sodium nitrite and sodium thiosulfate. The management of sorghum cystitis is discussed in *Paralyzed Bladder* (see page 334).

Prevent exposure to toxicity by removing horses from sorghum pastures during periods of new growth. These tend to occur when a heavy rainfall follows a frost, after a warm spell, and when the grass has been heavily trampled.

Ryegrass and Dallis Grass Staggers

Ryegrass and dallis grass staggers are caused by *mycotoxins* produced by molds that invade these grasses. Dallis grass is a common pasture grass in the southern half of the United States. Ryegrass has a somewhat wider distribution. Ryegrass toxicity tends to occur in late summer or fall when pastures are short-grazed and the grass is dry and stubblelike.

Initially, a horse with grass staggers exhibits mild excitability and muscle tremors, which progress to dizziness, swaying, staggering, stumbling, and rigidity of limbs. These signs are attributable to neurotoxic biochemical effects that disappear when the horse is removed from the source of toxicity.

Treatment: Most horses recover on their own within a few weeks, but symptoms may persist for several months. Prevent exposure to toxicity by mycotoxins.

Ergot Poisoning

Ergot is a fungus that grows on grasses and cereal grains, especially rye. It appears as a black, banana-shaped mass about half an inch (13 mm) long replacing part of the grass or grain seed. Improperly stored grain can become contaminated with this fungus. Horses are less frequently and severely affected than other livestock.

Signs of acute ergot poisoning include muscle tremors, excitability, abnormal behavior, staggering, excessive salivation, diarrhea, and paralysis. Ingesting small amounts over a long time has been reported to cause sloughing of the ears, tail, and hooves. Long-term ingestion in pregnant mares can cause reproductive problems similar to those described for fescue toxicity (see page 427).

Treatment: There is no treatment for ergot poisoning. It can be avoided by keeping the seed heads mowed off in the late summer. Grain should be properly stored to prevent the growth of mold and fungus.

Moldy Corn Poisoning (Blind Staggers)

Epidemics of an encephalitis-like illness have occurred after horses eat moldy corn contaminated by a fungus that produces a nervous system mycotoxin called fumonisin. Moldy corn poisoning is one of the most common toxicities of horses. Outbreaks generally occur in the eastern and midwestern United States from late fall to early spring. Corn put into storage with greater than 13 percent moisture, and corn that is stored in damp areas, is most susceptible to mold. Infected kernels will appear pink to reddish-brown.

Symptoms appear after one week or more of continuous consumption of infected corn. Signs of brain involvement include profound *depression* and little response to stimuli, disorientation, circling, *head-pressing*, blindness, and occasionally, unprovoked frenzy. These signs appear suddenly and end in death, usually within one to four days. The diagnosis is made by identifying the mold or mycotoxin in the feed.

Another mold found in stored corn and other feeds produces a series of mycotoxins called aflatoxins. Horses are more resistant to these toxins than are other domestic animals. Accordingly, aflatoxin poisoning is rare in horses. Signs are like those of moldy corn poisoning. Liver damage is the major toxic effect.

Treatment: Discontinue feeding corn on suspicion of poisoning. Early cases are treated by eliminating the toxin in the gastrointestinal tract using activated charcoal and laxatives, as described in *Poisoning* (page 22).

BOTULISM

Horses are highly susceptible to botulism. Poisoning in foals is called shaker foal syndrome (see page 561). In adults, it is referred to as forage poisoning. Botulism is a paralytic disease that can be caused by seven potent neurotoxins (although types B, C, and D are responsible for nearly all cases of animal botulism), which are all produced by the bacteria *Clostridium botulinum*. Spores of this bacteria are found in soil and water contaminated by decaying plant and animal matter, and also in improperly processed hay and feeds containing animal matter or a high moisture content. Technology has enabled farmers to produce large hay bales—both round and square. By increasing the size of the bale, anaerobic conditions may be present that allow the botulism organism to grow. Paralysis develops after the horse ingests spores or the neurotoxin itself. *C. botulinum* also grows in infected wounds.

Weakness and paralysis appear several days after ingesting contaminated feed or water. Often, the first indication of paralysis is difficulty swallowing. Other signs include drooling, spilling feed and water from the corner of the mouth, and regurgitating food through the nose. Weakness and paralysis, which are progressive over several days, are apparent in a shuffling gait, a tendency to lie down often, and muscle tremors that occur with exercise. Collapse and *recumbency* are signs of advanced poisoning.

The outlook for recovery depends on the amount of toxin ingested. Some horses die from respiratory paralysis in one to two days. In others, the disease progresses slowly and treatment is possible. Suspect botulism when there is progressive paralysis that is not attributable to other causes. The diagnosis is confirmed by identifying spores in the feed, feces, or wound. Attempts to diagnose botulism are frequently unrewarding. However, a rapid (and, therefore, presumptive) diagnosis is the most important factor to the outcome.

Treatment: Confine the horse to restrict activity (which exacerbates the disease). Horses with tremors and muscular weakness should be sedated or tranquilized to conserve strength. Eliminate residual poison in the gastrointestinal tract as described in *Poisoning* (page 22).

Hyperimmune plasma is available to treat equine patients. The hyperimmune plasma greatly improves survival when given before the horse is in a state of obligate recumbency, meaning that he cannot get up. It does not reverse established paralysis. Thus, if the horse is recumbent and having difficulty breathing, the antitoxin has little effect.

Intravenous penicillin is beneficial in preventing secondary complications such as aspiration pneumonia. Aminoglycosides, tetracycline, and oral penicillin can exacerbate the release of endotoxins and should be avoided. The administration of metronidazole can predispose the horse to clostridial overgrowth in the intestines, and its use should be avoided.

The nursing care of the recumbent horse, which is of the utmost importance, is discussed in *Treating Brain Injuries* (see page 350). Horses who cannot swallow should receive prompt nutritional support via a stomach tube. Mineral oil should be given periodically to prevent fecal impaction. Wounds infected with *C. botulinum* should be treated aggressively with wound debridement and antibiotics, as described in *Wounds* (page 32).

There are many treatment options being explored to improve the outcome for the horse. As research progresses, more treatment options will become available. Ask your veterinarian.

Prevention: Horse feeds should be of the highest quality and free of excess moisture, insects, and dead animal parts. Hay should be baled at a moisture content below 15 percent to prevent decay and mold. These precautions will prevent the ingestion of spores in the hay. For vaccination, see *Shaker Foal Syndrome* (page 561). Vaccinating broodmares with inactivated toxin has proven effective in preventing shaker foal syndrome in areas with higher levels of botulism. Contact your veterinarian to see if this vaccine might be of use in your mare.

Yellow Star Thistle and Russian Knapweed (Chewing Disease)

Yellow star thistle and Russian knapweed are members of the sunflower family. Yellow star thistle is extensively established in northern California and along the Pacific Coast, and has now spread through the southern states to the Atlantic coast. Russian knapweed is a noxious weed in the Rocky Mountain states. Most poisonings occur late in summer or fall when pastures are dry and the plants may be the only available forage. In addition, because these plants are palatable, some horses may acquire a taste for them and seek them out. Large quantities of the green or dried plant must be consumed for several weeks before toxicity occurs.

Both plants produce a toxic chemical that permanently damages the part of the brain concerned with picking up and chewing feed. The resulting peculiar attempts at chewing account for the name "chewing disease," by which the problem is known among ranchers.

An affected horse generally holds his mouth open with his tongue hanging out and thus may appear to have a foreign body lodged in the throat. On closer inspection, you will see that the muscles of the lips and jaw are somewhat rigid, giving the horse a wooden look. He will have difficulty grasping feed with the lips, chewing it, and passing it to the back of the throat. Swallowing itself is not impaired.

Treatment: Brain damage is irreversible. The horse will die of dehydration or starvation if he is not euthanized to circumvent a painful death.

Prevent poisoning by eliminating pasture weeds with effective herbicides. These annuals should be killed or plowed under before they go to seed. Remove horses from pastures containing these weeds.

OTHER POISONOUS PLANTS

Pastures contain a variety of plants that are potentially toxic but often unrecognized. Even in well-cared-for pastures, plants can grow along fence lines and remain accessible to horses. Fortunately, horses do not normally graze on poisonous plants because they are not very palatable. But boredom may make noxious plants more palatable, and in the spring, horses are looking for anything green to nibble on. When there is scarce forage, overcrowding, or the introduction of a new horse into the herd, horses may also seek out and eat any green plant—including those that are poisonous.

Although numerous plants have been identified as being poisonous to horses, the commonly encountered ones, in addition to those described earlier in this chapter, fall into one of the following classes (the list is by no means complete).

- Those containing toxic alkaloids, glycosides, resins, and other substances that can produce sudden death—usually in a matter of minutes but occasionally in one to two days. They include larkspur, monkshood, chokecherry, sorghum grasses, foxglove, poison hemlock, water hemlock, milkweed, oleander, laurels, rhododendrons, death camas, yews, and black nightshade. Many of these plants are ornamentals and are unpalatable, and would not be consumed by horses except under unusual conditions.

- Those containing alkaloids and other substances toxic to the liver. Among these are the *Senecio*, one of the largest genera in the plant kingdom, containing the ragworts, stinking willie, rattlebox, and various groundsels. These plants are found over most of the United States. They grow in winter and early spring, and are therefore found in first-cutting hay. Cumulative ingestion over several weeks is necessary before the liver is affected badly enough to cause signs of liver failure. When this happens, however, the outlook is guarded.

- Those containing neurotoxins and other substances that affect the nervous system, producing salivation, head-bobbing, staggering, circling, weakness in the forelegs and/or hind legs, muscle tremors, reluctance to move, falling, and collapse. Some of these plants are sagebrushes of the western United States, milkvetches, horsetail, white snakeroot, bracken fern, and Johnson grass.

- The genus *Amsinckia intermedia*, which includes fiddleneck, fireweed, tarweed, buckthorn, and yellow bur weed, also produces liver failure. These are common weeds of wheat and other grain crops, found throughout the western United States. Trouble develops when contaminated grain is threshed and the screenings are fed to horses.

- A third genera that affects the liver, the *Crotalaria*, are commonly found in the southeastern United States. These plants, which belong to the pea family, include rattleweed and wild pea.

With a family horse, there is a tendency to feed yard waste to the horse who is hanging his head over the fence. See *Alternate Forages* (page 410) for information on feeding grass clippings. Horse owners need to be aware of the dangers of planting landscaping within reach of the horse. Not only could it have negative effects on the horse, but the equine pruning could damage the landscape. The table below lists just a few of the common poisonous trees, flowers, and shrubs.

Common Plants that Are Poisonous to Horses

Species Name	Common Name	Toxic Parts	Effects Reported
Acer rubrum	Red maple and its hybrids	Tree	Methemoglobinuria (blood components in the urine)
Aconitum spp.	Monkshood	Whole plant, alkaloids	Affects nervous system
Aesculus spp.	Horse chestnut, buckeye	Tree	GI, including diarrhea and colic
Aquilegia vulgaris	Columbine	Whole plant	Mild cyanide poisoning
Brugmansia spp.	Angels trumpet	Shrub	Nervous system
Buxus sempervirens	Boxwood	Shrub	Alkaloid poisoning, severe diarrhea

Species Name	Common Name	Toxic Parts	Effects Reported
Cestrum diurnum, *C. nocturnum*	Day- or night-blooming jasmine	Shrub	Hepatotoxin
Coronilla spp.	Crown vetch	Whole plant	Paralysis
Delphinium spp.	Larkspur	Whole plant	Potent, cardiac impairment
Digitalis purpurea	Foxglove	Whole plant	Cardiac impairment
Euonymus atropurpurens	Burning Bush	Shrub	Abdominal pain, constipation
Euonymus europaeus	Common spindletree	Whole plant	Abdominal pain
Frangula alnus	Alder buckthorn	Leaves, bark, fruit	Diarrhea
Gelsemium sempervirens	Carolina jessamine	Vine	Nervous system
Gymnocladus dioica	Kentucky coffee tree	Tree	Colic, narcotic
Hydrangea spp.	Hydrangea	Flower	Colic
Hypericum spp. liver disease	St. John's wort	Whole plant	Photosensitivity,
Iridaceae	Iris, narcissus, daffodil	Bulb	Diarrhea
Juglans nigra	Black walnut	Bedding from shavings	Laminitis
Kalmia spp.	Laurel	Shrub	Cardiac impairment
Laburnum anagyroides	Laburnum	Pods, seeds	Curarelike effect (muscle paralysis)
Lantana camara	Lantana	Leaves, fruits	Liver failure
Lathyrus	Sweet pea	Seeds, vines	Neuromuscular degeneration
Leucothoe davisiae	Black laurel	Flowers, nectar	Colic, cardiac impairment
Ligustrum spp.	Privet	Shrub	Colic
Liliaceae	Field garlic, bluebell, fritillary, lily of the valley, meadow saffron	Bulb	Oxidizes hemoglobin
Linum spp.	Purging (fairy) flax, common flax	Seed	Cyanogenetic

continued

Common Plants that Are Poisonous to Horses (*continued*)

Species Name	Common Name	Toxic Parts	Effects Reported
Lonicera xylosteum	Honeysuckle	Berries and leaves	Gastrointestinal irritant
Lupinus spp.	Lupines	Whole plant	*Teratogenic* (harms the embryo or fetus)
Nerium oleander	Oleander, rose laurel	Leaves, flowers, seeds	Cardiotoxic
Nicotiana	Tobacco	Stocks, leaves	Teratogenic, stimulant
Papaver spp.	Poppy	Wilted plant	Opiate
Parthenocissus quinquefolia	Virginia creeper	Leaves, berries	Colic
Prunus spp.	Chokecherry	Fruit	Cyanide poisoning
Quercus spp.	Oak	Leaves, acorns	Tannic acid poisoning
Ranunculus spp.	Buttercup	Whole plant	Irritant, colic, inflammation
Rhododendron spp., Azalea, Kalmia	Rhododendron, azalea, kalmia	Leaves, flowers	Colic, respiratory depression
Ricinus communis	Castor bean	Seeds, flowers	Hemorrhagic diarrhea
Robinia pseudoacacia	Black locust	Bark, seeds	Gastrointestinal irritation, cardiovascular irregularity
Taxus baccata	Yew	Whole shrub	Cardiac failure

Treatment: Suspect plant poisoning with any unexplained illness of abrupt onset, especially when accompanied by nervous system signs, colic, diarrhea, sudden collapse, or death. Immediately prevent further access to contaminated feed or pasture. With acute poisoning, begin treatment by eliminating plant toxins from the gastrointestinal tract, as described in *Poisoning* (see page 22).

Prevention: Eliminate potentially dangerous pasture plants by digging them out or applying weed killer. Check along fence rows, ditches, and around watering spots, where poisonous plants are most often found. Mow annual weeds before they go to seed. Carefully inspect the hay you feed, and don't feed hay baled with weeds.

Avoid turning hungry horses into unfamiliar pastures, as they are likely to eat the first plants they see. Young horses, in particular, are quite inquisitive and are likely to ingest dangerous plants.

Be familiar with which plants are toxic, and if they are present on your property do not allow your horses anywhere within lips' reach. Do not feed plant clippings. Garden clippings containing plant cuttings should not be thrown into areas where horses are accustomed to eating hay.

BLISTER BEETLE POISONING

There are more than 200 species of blister beetles. Most of them are found in the southern and southwestern United States, from Florida through Texas to Arizona, and as far north as Illinois. All contain a poisonous substance called cantharidin, which is toxic to the kidneys and the digestive tract. Cantharidin on the skin and mucous membranes produces a severe burning sensation followed by redness and blistering. Rubbing the eyes after handling the beetles can cause blindness. A burning sensation on urination occurs after ingesting ground beetle extract. This is the basis (unfounded) for its use as an aphrodisiac called Spanish fly.

Blister beetles vary in size from .25 to 1 inch (6 to 25 mm) in length. They are either black, black with orange stripes on the wings, gray, or yellow-tan with black spots. A characteristic feature is that the head and neck make up about one-quarter of the length of the insect and about half the width of the body.

Blister beetles live in flowering grasses such as alfalfa and clover. When alfalfa is cut and baled in two stages, the beetles escape from the winnows and are not incorporated in the hay bale. But when alfalfa is cut and baled in one operation, the beetles are crushed and their dead bodies are baled with the hay. Because they tend to congregate in large groups, hundreds of beetles may be trapped in a single flake.

The severity of the toxic reaction depends on the number of beetles eaten by the horse. When the horse eats more than a few beetles, the signs are those of acute shock, followed in a matter of hours by death. When small numbers are consumed, the horse may exhibit abdominal pain and colic accompanied by fever, profuse sweating, listlessness, rapid heartbeat, and watery or bloody stool. Bloody urine may be passed in the later stages. Often the horse dips his muzzle in and out of the watering trough to wash the burning from his mouth.

Treatment: Discontinue feeding contaminated alfalfa. Eliminate the toxin in the gastrointestinal tract using activated charcoal and laxatives, as described in *Poisoning* (page 22). Mineral oil (4 quarts, 3.8 l) should be given repeatedly by stomach tube. Give large volumes of IV fluid to combat dehydration and to protect the kidneys. If the horse survives the first few days, complete recovery is likely, but renal failure may be chronic. Treat all potentially exposed horses, whether symptomatic or not, with mineral oil.

Prevention: Inspect alfalfa hay for the presence of blister beetles. However, due to the erratic distribution of beetles within baled hay, beetles can be easily missed in a random inspection. Since it is generally not possible to examine all hay, it is important to harvest hay in such a manner that blister beetles will not be crushed and incorporated in the harvest. Blister beetles usually are not present in alfalfa cut before the last part of July. Cutting the hay before it flowers lessens the chance of beetles and also increases the nutritional value of the alfalfa.

Eliminate insects by spraying alfalfa with an insecticide such as carbaryl (Sevin). Sevin also kills grasshoppers and other insects. This provides an additional benefit, since the larvae of blister beetles feed extensively on grasshopper eggs. Pastures containing beetles may be safely grazed, because the live beetles escape and are not consumed by the horse.

CATTLE FEED POISONING

Commercial feeds manufactured specifically for cattle may contain substances that are harmful to horses. Monensin sodium (Rumensin) is a liposaccharide antibiotic widely used to increase the efficiency with which the animal converts feed into meat or milk, and to control coccidiosis in cattle. It is often added to grain mixes intended for poultry and cattle, and it may be incorporated into pasture feed blocks intended for cattle only.

Rumensin is highly toxic to horses and will cause acute heart failure and death. The signs of acute poisoning are like those of acute selenium intoxication (see page 428). Death can occur in 12 hours.

Some cattle feeds contain high levels of urea. Urea is an inexpensive source of nitrogen. Although it can be toxic to horses when fed at high levels, the amount in cattle feed generally is not dangerous for horses. However, urea provides no benefit over other sources of nitrogen.

Treatment: There is no treatment for monensin poisoning; horses must be euthanized. As a precaution, do not allow your horse access to commercial cattle feeds.

LEAD POISONING

Lead poisoning is uncommon but can occur with prolonged low-level ingestion. Horses can get access to lead-based paints by chewing on old painted surfaces or if paint chips fall into their food or stalls. Pastures close to ore-producing or industrial smelting operations may become contaminated with pollutants such as lead. Old car batteries can be a source of lead poisoning, so keep old cars out of the pasture.

An early sign of lead poisoning is an abnormal inspiratory sound heard during exercise. It is due to paralysis of recurrent laryngeal nerves. Difficulty in swallowing and regurgitation of food through the nose indicates further cranial nerve involvement. Lameness, weakness, and knuckling at the fetlock are signs of peripheral nerve involvement.

A horse with chronic lead poisoning exhibits emaciation, colic, and anemia. There may be a blue "lead line" along the gums at the base of the teeth. The diagnosis is confirmed by a whole blood lead concentration showing a level of 0.30 parts per million (ppm) or greater. Levels over 1.0 ppm indicate a poor prognosis.

Treatment: In mild cases, removing the horse from the pasture or source of contamination may allow for recovery. In more severely affected horses, a lead-binding chelating agent can be used to quickly wash out excess lead from the body. The chelating agent is given intravenously daily in divided doses for several days.

FLUORIDE TOXICITY (FLUOROSIS)

Exposure to inorganic and organic fluoride occurs through contamination of forage, soil, and water. Common toxic sources of fluoride include rock phosphates, phosphatic limestone, or fertilizer-grade phosphates that have not been defluoridated. Wells located near phosphatic rock may contain toxic fluoride concentrations.

A total daily dietary concentration (dry basis) of greater than 40 ppm is considered potentially toxic when consumed by horses for long periods. Water containing more than 4 ppm is marginally safe, and water containing greater than 8 ppm should be avoided.

Signs of fluorosis are primarily related to the musculoskeletal system. There is increased bone thickness, first noted as bumps on the inside of the legs below the knees, then found on the jaw and elsewhere. Intermittent lameness and stiffness appear as the disease progresses. There is a generalized debilitation and unthrifty appearance, with the horse losing weight despite adequate amounts of good-quality feed.

In young horses, fluorosis affects tooth enamel and dentine, and the teeth develop a characteristic mottled or stained appearance. Dental deterioration and abscesses occur as the disease worsens.

Treatment: There is no specific treatment for fluorosis. The disease will not progress once the horse is removed from the source of contamination. However, lameness, tooth damage, and bone changes are permanent.

WOOD PRESERVATIVE POISONING

Lumber treated with a phenolic preservative to prevent soil fungus and insect degradation is often used in the construction of farm and stable facilities. The usual chemicals involved are pentachlorophenol (PCP) and creosote.

Exposure to phenolic chemicals occurs by skin contact with treated lumber, and more commonly by direct consumption of the chemical through licking or chewing on treated wood.

PCP speeds up metabolism and produces a high body temperature. Signs of acute poisoning include rapid gasping, intense sweating, rapid heart rate, weakness, and coma. Chronic low-level consumption produces anemia and weight loss. The diagnosis can be suspected by the history of licking or chewing at treated wood. It can be confirmed by a PCP blood level.

Treatment: Remove the horse from the source of contamination. There is no specific antidote. A horse with acute intoxication should be treated for overheating as described in *Heat Stroke* (see page 19). Poisoning can be prevented by not using oily, freshly treated wood in areas used by horses.

16

Sex and Reproduction

The Mare

The *mare*'s reproductive system is composed of the two ovaries, fallopian tubes (the uterine horns, also called oviducts), uterus, vagina, and vulva. The ovaries are bean-shaped and vary in size from 1.5 inches (38 mm) across during the nonbreeding season to 3 inches (76 mm) during *heat*. In addition to producing the eggs (ova), the ovaries produce the sex hormones, which prepare the reproductive tract for mating, fertilization, and pregnancy.

The surface of each ovary is made of a capsule of fibrous connective tissue, which prevents egg follicles from developing on its surface. As a follicle inside the ovary enlarges and prepares to ovulate, the follicle migrates toward a chutelike recess in the ovary called the *ovulation* fossa.

The uterus is composed of a cervix, body, and two horns. The cavity of the uterus is lined by a layer of tissue called the *endometrium*. The body of the uterus is about 10 inches (25 cm) long. Each horn is an additional 8 inches (20 cm).

The fallopian tubes carry the eggs from the ovulation fossa down into the horns of the uterus. This process takes five to six days. However, an unfertilized egg can live for only 12 hours. Accordingly, the egg must encounter a viable sperm in the fallopian tubes within 12 hours of ovulation for fertilization to take place. When it does, the fertilized egg is called an *embryo*.

The newly fertilized embryo arrives in the uterus at about six days postovulation. It now begins wandering about in the uterus, passing from one horn to the other, and then back into the uterus, finally implanting in the body of the uterus at the base of one of the horns at 16 days of gestation. This wandering back and forth stimulates the endometrium to stop producing a hormone called PGF2α. This hormone, a prostaglandin, acts on the ovaries to cause the *corpus luteum* to regress (return to its previous state). If the corpus luteum does regress, *progesterone* levels would fall dramatically and the endometrium would shed, causing the embryo to die. Thus, by wandering about in the uterus for 16 days, the embryo suppresses the production of prostaglandin and ensures its own survival. This process is called maternal recognition of pregnancy.

There are three physical barriers that guard the uterus from bacterial infection. The first is the cervix, projecting into the back of the vagina, which, in the sexually quiescent mare, is about the same length and diameter as an index finger. The cervix shortens and widens during the receptive phase of heat, allowing sperm to enter the uterus after breeding. The second barrier is the vulvovaginal sphincter. This is a muscular ring located inside the vaginal opening where the hymen is located in a maiden mare. The third barrier is the arrangement of the vulva, or lips of the vagina, which close the entrance to the vagina. The vagina in an adult mare is about 18 inches (46 cm) long.

NATURAL BREEDING SEASON

Mares are seasonal breeders. The natural breeding season is the time of the year when a mare comes into heat naturally. The operational breeding season is a heat season caused by human intervention in and manipulation of the mare's environment.

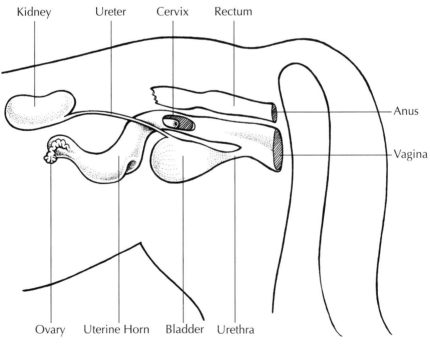

The mare's reproductive system.

The natural breeding season is determined by several factors, including hours of daylight, temperature, nutrition, rainfall, climate, and latitude. After a period of ovarian inactivity (called *anestrus*) that lasts through the winter months, the natural breeding season in the Northern Hemisphere begins in April and continues through September. In high northern latitudes the breeding season is shorter, while in deep southern latitudes mares may cycle all year long. It has been shown that the number of daylight hours has a direct effect on ovarian activity. This effect is mediated through the optic nerves and the pineal gland. As day lengthens, melatonin secretions from the pineal gland begin to decline. Falling levels of melatonin signal the hypothalamus to release *gonadotropin*-releasing hormone (*GnRH*). GnRH is barely detectable during deep winter anestrus, but within two to three weeks of exposure to increasing day length, levels begin to rise. GnRH triggers the pituitary gland to release first follicle-stimulating hormone (FSH), which wakes up the ovaries, and then luteinizing hormone (*LH*), which triggers ovulation.

Levels of both FSH and LH follow a distinct seasonal profile, with LH rising more slowly than FSH in the spring and dropping more quickly than FSH in the fall. The discrepancy between the timing and presence of these two hormones is the reason why anovulatory heat cycles (heat cycles without ovulation) are seen in early spring and late autumn.

December 22, the winter solstice, is the day with the shortest period of daylight. Seventy percent of mares are in deep anestrus at this time; about 85 percent are by mid-January. In March, some of these mares begin to develop cyclic ovarian activity. The first cycles may not be accompanied by ovulation; but by the middle of April to the first of May, with the increased number of daylight hours, more sun, warmer temperatures, and green grass, nearly all mares are cycling consistently. Conception rates peak in June.

The advantage of the natural breeding season is that when a mare is bred in summer, she foals in the spring, when conditions are most hospitable for raising a *foal*.

OPERATIONAL BREEDING SEASON

Thoroughbred racing associations and breed registries have designated January 1 as the universal birth date for horses born in the northern hemisphere; all foals born at any time during the year automatically become yearlings on January 1 of the following year. In the southern hemisphere, the universal birth date is August 1. The effect of this universal birth date is to emphasize early births for larger, stronger yearlings. A colt born in January, for example, has an athletic advantage over one born in June. But to produce foals early in the year, breeding must begin in the winter months. This is why the operational breeding season was developed.

The operational breeding season begins February 15 and ends July 15. What makes it possible is an artificial light program. By exposing the mare to increasing photoperiods of natural plus artificial light, winter anestrus can be shortened and the mating season started earlier than would be the case naturally.

Since it takes at least 60 days to induce early ovulation with artificial light, if the breeding season is to start on February 15, a lighting program should be initiated between November 15 and December 15. The best results are obtained when the mare is exposed to 15 hours of continuous light a day, adding artificial light to the end of the natural day. The full 15 hours can be provided from the first day of the program, or artificial light can be added at the rate of 30 minutes a week until 15 hours of continuous light are achieved.

Artificial light schedules must be consistent. Irregular schedules will not induce heat and may even throw the mare back into anestrus. A 200-watt incandescent bulb or a 400-watt fluorescent lightbulb is an effective light for a stall. For pens and paddocks, incandescent, mercury vapor, sodium, or quartz lights are suitable if the intensity of light is such that a newspaper can be read at any spot within the enclosure. The lighting system can be equipped with an automatic timer. It is important to note that show mares kept in a barn year round may be difficult to cycle.

The Estrous (Heat) Cycle

The estrous or heat cycle is the period from one ovulation to the next. The length of the cycle is 21 to 23 days. This may vary by a few days, especially at the beginning and the end of the breeding season.

When a *filly* reaches puberty, she becomes sexually mature and begins to produce eggs. This usually happens between 10 and 24 months of age, with 18 months being the average. At this time she can become pregnant. However, most horse breeders believe that a 2-year-old mare is too immature to be bred. After she is 1 year old, separate fillies from *stallions* to prevent accidental pregnancy.

The reproductive cycle of the mare is divided into two phases: *estrus* and diestrus. Estrus is the phase in which the mare is actively interested in and receptive to the stallion. This is also when she ovulates. Diestrus is the period of sexual disinterest, which begins 24 to 48 hours after ovulation and lasts 14 to 16 days. It is followed by a return to estrus.

ESTRUS

The duration of estrus varies. Early in the year it lasts six to eight days, but by midsummer it decreases to about four days. The hormonal effects that govern estrus and ovulation are complex. In brief, the pituitary gland releases FSH, which causes egg follicles within the ovary to grow and produce increasing amounts of estrogen. Estrogen prepares the reproductive tract for mating and fertilization, and is also responsible for the behavioral changes of the estrus mare.

When the egg follicle approaches maturity, the pituitary releases LH, which causes the follicle to ovulate. Ovulation usually occurs about 24 hours before the end of heat.

A mare in standing heat who is receptive to breeding displays typical estrus behavior in the presence of a stallion. She presents her hindquarters to the stallion and, if separated by a partition, leans back against it. The receptive attitude includes a squatting posture, raised tail, flexed pelvis, urination, and spasmodic "winking" of the labia with presentation of the clitoris.

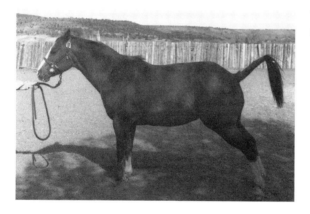

The typical stance of a mare in standing heat.

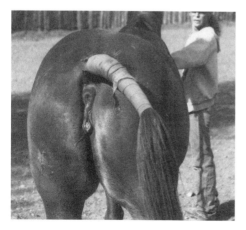

Winking of the labia with presentation of the clitoris.

Diestrus

Diestrus begins with an abrupt change in behavior in which the mare refuses the stallion and exhibits her rejection by laying back her ears, wheeling, squealing, kicking, and occasionally biting and pawing.

Twenty-four hours after ovulation, the follicular space in the ovary fills with blood. The blood undergoes a process called lutenization over the next five days, and becomes the mature corpus luteum. The corpus luteum is a yellow mass within the ovary that produces the hormone progesterone. A critical function of progesterone is to prepare the lining of the uterus to receive, support, and maintain the embryo. If the corpus luteum fails to develop, the embryo will be lost.

What happens to the corpus luteum depends on whether the mare becomes pregnant. If she does not, the corpus luteum remains active for only 12 to 14 days. It then undergoes rapid regression (return to an inactive state). This is followed in three days by a new estrous cycle.

If the mare does become pregnant, the uterus sends a message to the corpus luteum to continue progesterone production until the placenta takes over this task. This transition occurs between days 70 and 90 of gestation.

Determining Estrus

The accuracy of predicting ovulation is improved with *ultrasonography*, rectal palpation of the reproductive tract, and assessing the behavior of the mare. The estimate must be within 24 hours of ovulation. This time frame is especially important if you are using cooled or frozen *semen*. There should be less than 12 hours between exams to determine ovulation.

Teasing

The teasing behavior of the stallion and the mare indicate to the experienced stallion manager when the mare is receptive and about to ovulate. The most

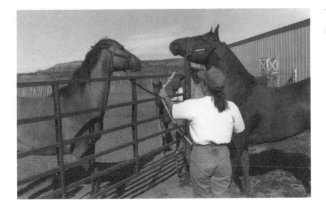

The laid-back ears of a mare in diestrus.

decisive indicator of receptivity is when the mare presents her hindquarters to the stallion, stands in the braced position, and swishes her tail to the side. This positive teasing response normally indicates the mare is cycling. For more information on teasing procedures, see *When to Breed* (page 469).

Rectal Palpation

The estrous cycle produces changes in the mare's reproductive tract that indicate whether she is experiencing the hormonal effects associated with estrus. These changes can be identified by rectal palpation. Experience is required to interpret the findings. The organs affected by the sex hormones are the uterus, ovaries, vagina, and cervix.

The horns of the uterus exhibit a degree of firmness (tone) that changes with the heat cycle. During diestrus, the uterus feels quite firm and does not indent on pressure. As estrus and ovulation approach, the wall of the uterus becomes less firm to finger pressure and does not spring back after indentation.

The ovaries are about twice as large during estrus as they are during anestrus. As ovulation approaches, one follicle becomes larger and begins to soften. Ovulation can be expected when this dominant follicle is about 1.5 inches (4 cm) across. After ovulation, an ovulatory depression can be felt at the site of the follicle (the corpus hemorrhagica), which is followed in five days by the development of the corpus luteum. The corpus luteum lies within the ovary and so cannot be palpated.

During anestrus and diestrus, the cervix is a long, firm, muscular tube about the size of an index finger and the canal is tightly closed. Under the influence of estrus, the cervix softens. It becomes shorter by about half as the width doubles. The cervix opens to allow sperm to enter.

Determining the moment of ovulation is one of the most important indications for rectal palpation. The egg is viable for only a few hours after ovulation, so the best time to breed is just before ovulation. Accordingly, many

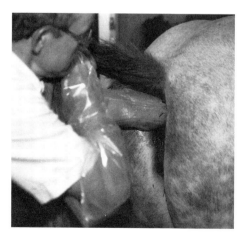

Rectal palpation helps determine if the mare is cycling.

unnecessary breedings can be avoided by knowing that the mare has already ovulated. Collapse of the follicle, indicative of postovulation, can be felt as a crater or pit in the ovary.

Ultrasonography

Ultrasonography uses visual imaging and is a much more sensitive tool than rectal palpation. It is commonly used in artificial insemination programs to measure the size of follicles. Pathologies of the uterus that can't be identified by palpation, such as endometrial cysts and abnormal uterine fluid, can be visualized using ultrasound. Ovaries that can't be palpated can also be identified.

Transrectal ultrasound examination helps confirm the findings of rectal palpation. The uterus during estrus shows characteristic folds caused by estrogen-induced swelling of the endometrium. These folds disappear just before ovulation. A follicle about to ovulate changes shape from spherical to teardrop and leaks fluid toward the ovulation fossa.

Follicles that do not ovulate, a persistent corpus luteum, twin pregnancies, tumors, and other abnormalities also can be seen on ultrasonography.

Abnormal Heat Cycles

Mares are notorious for a profound and frustrating inconsistency in their heat cycles. The average interval is 21 to 22 days, but some mares cycle at shorter, longer, or less regular intervals. Maiden mares, and mares over 15 years of age, are most likely to have irregular heat cycles, especially at the beginning and end of the breeding season.

When a mare fails to breed or fails to conceive after breeding, the cause should be investigated. The first step is to determine if the mare is cycling (having estrous periods). If it is determined by teasing, rectal palpation, or ultrasonography that the mare is not cycling normally, or is cycling but is not reacting normally to the hormonal influences of estrus, the problem may be anestrus, transitional heat period, persistent corpus luteum, silent heat, or (rarely) nymphomania.

ANESTRUS

Anestrus is lack of estrus, or failure to cycle. Seasonal anestrus is a physiologically normal state of ovarian inactivity that occurs in the winter months. Pregnancy is the most common cause of anestrus during the breeding season. A mare who has had an ovariectomy (a fact that may not be known to a new owner) does not have ovaries and will not cycle. Mares may also have a lactational anestrus while they are nursing.

Absence of cyclical activity and failure to ovulate are closely associated with diseases that affect the uterus. A mare with pyometra or *endometritis* often will not cycle because the damaged endometrium does not produce prostaglandin. Lacking prostaglandin, the corpus luteum persists for long periods during which the mare does not ovulate (see *Persistent Corpus Luteum*, page 451).

Gonadal dysgenesis, ovarian hypoplasia, and testicular feminization are rare diseases related to chromosomal abnormalities. Mares with gonadal dysgenesis and testicular feminization do not have functional ovaries. Mares with ovarian hypoplasia may exhibit occasional or very irregular cycles. These abnormalities can be diagnosed by rectal palpation and ultrasonography. Occasionally, *chromosome* analysis is required. Fertility is not possible in mares with any of these disorders.

The most common tumor of the ovary is a benign granulosa-theca cell tumor. This tumor, which is found most often in mares 5 to 7 years of age, produces large amounts of the hormones estrogen, inhibin, and *testosterone*. Estrogen exerts negative feedback on the pituitary gland, which ceases to produce FSH and LH and thus shuts down the ovaries. On rectal palpation and ultrasonography, the ovary with the tumor is large and the other ovary is small, firm, and inactive. Despite the fact that these mares do not cycle, they may exhibit strong estrus behavior due to high levels of circulating estrogen. Treatment involves removing the diseased ovary.

Tumors of the hypothalamus or anterior pituitary gland can cause cyclic failure by interfering with the production of the sex hormones. These tumors are rare.

Anabolic steroids and testosterone adversely affect the ovaries. Mares receiving these drugs (usually to enhance racing performance) have smaller ovaries and generally do not ovulate. Negative effects can persist for up to 6 months after the steroids are stopped. These mares are often aggressive and difficult to cover. Accordingly, performance-enhancing drugs should be avoided when breeding is anticipated.

Debilitation anestrus occurs among run-down, underfed, emaciated mares who are habitually overworked. Chronic diseases, especially a heavy burden of parasites, contribute to a run-down state. Old mares with teeth that are not taken care of are subject to nutritional deficiencies and weight loss. Rectal palpation reveals small, firm, inactive ovaries. The uterus is flaccid. The mare shows no signs of estrus when teased. The estrous cycle can often be restored by correcting the cause of debilitation.

Early in the breeding season, some maiden and barren mares exhibit an abnormally long winter coat (hirsutism). This winter coat must be lost before the mare begins to cycle. Thus, a hirsute coat indicates that estrus will be delayed.

TRANSITIONAL HEAT PERIOD

At the beginning (and end) of seasonal estrous, many mares are inconsistent in their heat cycles, exhibiting signs of heat without ovulating. Although actually not an abnormal heat cycle, this transitional heat period becomes a problem for farm managers who would like to have their mares bred early in the spring so they can foal as close to the universal birth date (January 1) as possible.

Ultrasound findings in a mare in transitional estrus include multiple follicles 2 to 3 cm (.78 to 1.2 inches) across that do not produce eggs. These follicles produce the estrogen that causes the observed signs of heat. The reason these mares do not ovulate is the lag in production of LH (discussed in *Natural Breeding Season*, page 442). Pituitary and plasma levels of LH are not yet high enough during transition to trigger ovulation. Instead of an orderly progression to a dominant follicle that matures and ovulates, the follicles all collapse together, after which a new cycle begins. Ultimately, a dominant follicle (35 mm or larger) develops at a time when LH stores are adequate. This results in ovulation, which ends the transitional period.

Treatment: Follicles that do not ovulate do not require treatment unless you are breeding for the universal birth date. The increase in the spring photoperiod will start the breeding season spontaneously in May or June.

The most effective method of hastening the breeding season is to institute an artificial light program (see page 443). Keep the mare in good condition and feed her just enough additional energy so that she gradually gains weight. Regular teasing with a stallion is helpful in bringing on early estrus.

A daily progesterone injection or oral altrenogest may be also used to shorten the transition period and advance the first ovulation. Results are inconsistent, but if successful, a normal estrus occurs three to five days after the injections are stopped. Normal cycles follow, with a 50 percent conception rate on the first service.

PROLONGED ESTRUS

This is a variation of transitional estrus in which the mare shows sustained receptivity to the stallion. A large percentage of mares, especially maiden and barren mares, exhibit this behavior. The cause is failure of the anovulatory follicles to collapse, resulting in a persistently high output of estrogen.

Due to the high estrogen influence, the mare may allow the stallion to mount and breed for 30 days, or even continue to do so for up to two to three months. This presents problems. If you are not familiar with the condition, you may conclude that since the mare continues to breed without becoming pregnant, she must be infertile. Another problem is that multiple acts of coitus increase the likelihood of developing a bacterial infection of the mare's reproductive tract.

Treatment: Wait one month before breeding. During this time, most mares will begin to ovulate and can be successfully bred. If immediate breeding is desired and the mare has a mature follicle more than 1.4 inches (35 mm) across, ovulation can often be induced by an injection of deslorelin or recombinant equine luteinizing hormone (rELH). Ovulation should occur within 48 hours. Breed the mare immediately after the injection, in anticipation of ovulation.

In the absence of a preovulatory follicle, a course of progesterone, as described for *Transitional Heat Period* (page 449), may induce estrus and advance the date of ovulation.

SPLIT ESTRUS

This uncommon condition is more frequent during the transition period. The hormonal basis is not known. The mare presents to the stallion for a few days, goes out of heat for several days, and then returns to estrus and ovulates.

Treatment: Split estrus appears to be influenced by stress, transportation to the *stud*, and improper teasing methods. The advent of the natural breeding season should resolve the problem.

PERSISTENT CORPUS LUTEUM (PROLONGED DIESTRUS)

Persistent corpus luteum is a state in which the corpus luteum continues to produce progesterone and doesn't regress. It is a common cause of lack of estrus behavior during the breeding season. It can last one to three months, with an average of 60 days.

A persistent corpus luteum results in prolongation of the diestrus stage of the heat cycle. Some mares with a persistent corpus luteum will ovulate during diestrus. However, they will not show estrus behavior or stand for the stud. The reason for this is that high levels of progesterone produced by the corpus luteum block the behavioral effects of estrus.

The cause of persistent corpus luteum is insufficient prostaglandin (PGF2α) from the *endometrium* of the uterus. What causes this to happen in each specific case is generally not known. In a mare who is not pregnant, the endometrium synthesizes and releases PGF2α, which travels to the ovary and there causes regression and disappearance of the corpus luteum. It follows that conditions that interfere with endometrial PGF2α production or release will be associated with a persistent corpus luteum and high levels of progesterone. An endometrium that has been partially destroyed by pyometra or endometritis is an example.

The embryo forces the uterus to recognize pregnancy and inhibit PGF2α release by contacting the entire surface of the endometrium during the initial mobility phase (described on page 441). Loss of the embryo after this uterine recognition process may prolong diestrus for several days, assuming that remnants of the embryo remain in contact with the endometrium. Thus, a prolonged diestrus without other signs may be the only indication of a missed pregnancy.

Another cause of persistent corpus luteum is established pregnancy complicated by early embryonic death, *abortion*, or fetal reabsorption after day 36 of pregnancy. By day 37, specialized fetal cells called *endometrial cups* interlock with the endometrium, forming the earliest attachment of the developing *fetus* to her mother. The endometrial cups produce measurable amounts of equine chorionic gonadotropin (eCG; formally known as pregnant mare serum gonadotropin, or PMSG). This eCG has the effect of stimulating and prolonging the corpus luteum, making it seem as if the mare is still pregnant. The mare will not return to estrus until the endometrial cups cease to function, which does not occur for several months.

When the embryo is lost before day 36, the corpus luteum regresses within several days, and the mare returns to estrus.

The diagnosis of persistent corpus luteum is made by rectal palpation that reveals a nonpregnant uterus with a long, closed cervix and increased uterine tone. The corpus luteum is not palpable because it is buried in the ovary. However, it can usually be seen by ultrasound. A high serum progesterone in the pregnancy range confirms the diagnosis.

Treatment: An injection of PGF2α causes the corpus luteum to regress, provided that the corpus luteum has been present for at least 4 to 5 days. The mare will return to estrus in 3 to 5 days. A corpus luteum less than 4 to 5 days old will not respond to PGF2α. Administer a second dose 7 to 10 days later.

Vaginal douching with sterile saline and antibiotics to stimulate release of PGF2α from the uterus is not as effective as giving PGF2α by injection. Curettage of the uterus is of questionable value.

Administering estrogen is not effective and will actually prolong the corpus luteum.

SILENT HEAT

Silent heat, also called behavioral or psychological anestrus, is a behavioral disorder in mares characterized by normal estrous cycles but lack of receptivity to the stallion. Veterinary examination discloses the presence of heat and ovulation, but the mare fails to show the normal behavior signs of estrus.

Silent heat is common in nervous mares, shy mares, maiden mares, and mares with foals. Occasionally, what appears to be lack of heat is actually the handler's lack of familiarity with the subtler signs of estrus. Some estrous mares exhibit diminished estrous behavior and require prolonged and intense teasing to demonstrate receptivity to the stallion.

Lactation anestrus occurs in mares who are extremely possessive of their suckling foals and may not breed when the foal is by their side. Attempt a teasing program to identify silent heat or breed the mare every other year. A common cause of silent heat is ineffectual teasing practices. Mares should be teased frequently (once a day or every other day) on a regular schedule. Regular teasing helps bring the mare into heat. Irregular teasing may delay the development of heat behavior and can lead to missing the moment of receptivity to the stallion.

Treatment: Intense stimulation and much patience are required when teasing mares with diminished estrus behavior. Techniques such as changing stallions, changing location, and flank and vulvar presentation may be required before mares with prolonged reaction time will exhibit estrus behavior. Most mares, however, when intensively teased at full heat, will show some signs of estrus to the experienced handler and can be successfully bred.

Repeated rectal palpation with or without ultrasounds can be used to time ovulation. An ovulating mare who continues to refuse the stallion can be twitched and hobbled, permitting the stallion to mount and breed at the correct moment. Artificial insemination is another alternative. Reluctant maiden mares often improve after their first successful breeding.

NYMPHOMANIA

Nymphomania is a rare condition characterized by an exaggerated and wanton display of estrus. The cause is unknown. Nymphomaniac mares do not have any genital tract abnormalities and cycle normally. There is a strong association with neurotic behavior, apparently influenced by rising and falling levels of estrogen.

In the mild form of nymphomania, the mare's behavior is limited to estrus and abates during diestrus. In the severe form, the mare exhibits strong estrus responses (squirts urine, swishes her tail, squeals when touched about the hindquarters), often throughout the estrous cycle, and is extremely aggressive toward horses and people. It is dangerous to perform rectal examinations on nymphomaniac mares, whether mild or severe.

Breeding is difficult or impossible because of the mare's violent aggression when presented to the stallion or when handled about the hindquarters.

Treatment: Mares with mild nymphomania often respond to removal of the ovaries. Mares with severe nymphomania do not respond to any form of treatment. Euthanasia is recommended in severe cases.

Preparing the Mare for Breeding

Only 60 percent of mares bred annually in the United States produce live foals. The main reasons for this low reproductive efficiency are poor preparation for breeding, uterine infections, and abnormal estrous cycles.

Good preparation begins with selecting a suitable stallion, completing all arrangements for transporting the mare to the breeding farm, and having a prebreeding physical examination, during which problems that may prevent breeding or interfere with fertility can be identified and treated. All of this should be done well before the breeding season begins.

The general health and age of the mare are important considerations. Mares over 15 years of age are more likely to have infertility problems. Bad teeth, nutritional deficiencies, and chronic laminitis (often seen in older mares) are physical handicaps that can interfere with the ability to carry a foal.

Most stallion owners require a health certificate or a statement of gynecological health status called the breeding soundness examination (BSE), with a negative uterine culture and an up-to-date vaccination certificate. Proof of serological negativity will be required for equine infectious anemia—either a Coggins test (AGID) or C-ELISA. If you plan to cross state lines, an interstate health certificate is mandatory. Your veterinarian can provide you with the necessary documents after the mare's breeding soundness examination.

To ensure that all vaccinations are current, consult the immunization schedule on page 100. Additional vaccinations may be needed if the mare will be exposed to endemic diseases for which she has not been vaccinated. Discuss this with your veterinarian.

The effect of nutrition on fertility is very pronounced in mares. Both overly fat and excessively thin mares have a difficult time conceiving. The ideal mare should be in good condition or slightly lean coming out of winter anestrus. Her diet should contain all the necessary nutrients and minerals for the adult horse, as described in chapter 15, "Nutrition and Feeding."

Four to six weeks before the breeding season, increase the mare's maintenance ration so she gradually gains weight. This can be accomplished by reducing roughage slightly and adding 2 to 3 pounds (.9 to 1.3 kg) of grain to the daily ration. The process is called flushing and is thought to improve the mare's chances of conceiving. However, do not add grain to the ration if the mare is already overweight.

Mares taken straight from the racetrack or show circuit just before breeding have a difficult time conceiving. A letdown period of at least 60 days should be allowed for the mare's reproductive system to establish regularity. Mares on testosterone or anabolic steroids do not display estrus. Anabolic steroids should be withdrawn at least six months before the breeding season.

All mares should be on a good parasite control program, as described in chapter 2, "Parasites." No additional deworming is required in preparation for breeding. Correct any dental problems. Remove the mare's shoes and trim her hooves before she is presented to the stallion.

THE BREEDING SOUNDNESS EXAMINATION

This is an overall physical examination with special emphasis on the reproductive organs. The soundness exam is routinely performed before each breeding season, at the end of the breeding season in the case of a barren mare, before buying a *broodmare* or a maiden mare, and whenever a problem is suspected.

If the mare has produced foals, the exam should include a good breeding history. This includes notes on the health of each foal, prior *foaling* or breeding difficulties, and any prior injuries or infections, as well as a record of the mare's estrous behavior, teasing behavior, and past heat patterns.

The exam will include a standard rectal palpation exam. Other procedures that may be performed include an endometrial culture and cytology exam, endometrial biopsy, transrectal ultrasound, and endocrine assays. Chromosome analysis or cytogenic studies might be indicated for infertile maiden mares. Fiber-optic examination of the uterus is available in some referral centers. Not all of these procedures are needed for every mare; their use depends on the reasons for the examination.

The reproductive examination begins by inspecting the perineum for the defect known as windsucking or pneumovagina. The windsucking perineal conformation allows air and fecal material to enter and pool in the vagina, resulting in a persistent source of bacterial infection. The top of the vulval opening should be no higher than 1.5 inches (4 cm) above the vaginal floor. A long vulva that extends well above the pelvic brim, associated with a sunken anus, creates a sloping perineum that predisposes the mare to pneumovagina. Mares with pneumovagina frequently lose the protective value of the vulvovaginal sphincter. This entire process can occur simply with aging, abetted by weight loss, loss of vaginal fat, and the presence of vaginal tears associated with prior deliveries. Thus, pneumovagina is most frequently seen in elderly, thin, broodmares who have foaled before.

The windsucking test involves spreading the lips of the vulva and listening for the characteristic noise of air rushing into the vagina. The test is also performed by applying uniform pressure with the hands on each side of the labia.

The windsucking perineum is the most common cause of genital tract infection, and the primary cause of infertility in mares. When present, it should be corrected surgically. The procedure, called a Caslick's operation, consists of removing the mucous membrane from the lips of the vulva and then stitching the lips together, allowing sufficient room for the mare to pass urine. The closure must be opened for each foaling and then resutured.

The next step in the breeding soundness exam is to perform rectal palpation. This is accomplished by inserting a well-lubricated, shoulder-length glove into the rectum. Both ovaries, the entire uterus, and the cervix are palpated. Because the rectum is easily ruptured, rectal palpation should be done only by experienced personnel.

The uterine culture examination is an important part of the prebreeding exam and should always be performed as a sterile procedure. The mare's tail is wrapped and the vulva and perineum cleansed with surgical soap. Cultures are taken using a swab inserted through the vagina and cervix.

In the maiden mare, a persistent hymen may be found at the vestibulovaginal junction. When the hymen is completely intact, it is said to be imperforate. More often, there are transverse bands across the vaginal canal, indicative of a partially intact hymen. When an intact hymen is not opened

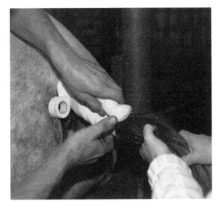

The vaginal speculum examination is a sterile procedure. Wrap the tail to prevent hair from contaminating the field.

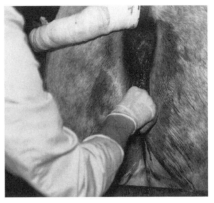

Wash the vulva and perineum with a soap solution and rinse thoroughly.

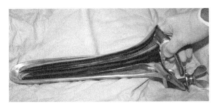

The vaginal speculum.

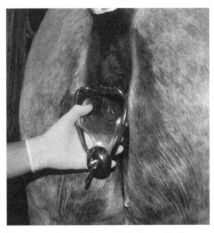

The speculum is inserted. Any discharge indicates infection.

before breeding, slight bleeding will occur with the first mating. A thin or partially intact hymen can be broken by gentle finger pressure. A thick hymen will need to be cut. The mare can be bred two to three weeks after opening an imperforate hymen.

The color of the vaginal mucosa indicates the presence or absence of estrus. A glistening pink to red mucosa indicates true estrus. Anestrus is reflected by a pale, dry mucosa. Vaginal cultures are routinely taken from the clitoral sinuses.

The routine examination concludes with manual palpation of the vagina. The speculum is removed. After sterile preparation of the vaginal opening and vault, a gloved hand is inserted into the vagina. The cervix is carefully palpated. In mares who have given birth before, the cervix is occasionally explored with a finger to palpate and measure the length of the cervical canal and perhaps to evaluate for any damage.

The Extended Examination

Endometrial culture and cytology, endometrial biopsy, and manual or endo-scopic examination of the uterine cavity are indicated when there is a history of infertility or a finding that requires a further medical work-up. All of these procedures are performed using sterile techniques. Manual palpation of the uterus is performed by dilating the cervical canal and introducing a gloved hand into the uterine cavity. Hysteroscopy is a procedure in which a fiber-optic endoscope is inserted into the uterine cavity to visualize the endometrium, take tissue samples, and perform simple surgery.

Any sort of vaginal discharge or yellow fluid on the vaginal floor suggests endometrial infection and the need to assess the uterine cavity by either cul-ture and cytology or endometrial biopsy. A culture from the uterine cavity is a better indicator of endometritis than is a culture from the cervix, since the lat-ter is more likely to be caused by a vaginal infection than a uterine infection.

When foreign bodies such as instruments and gloved hands are inserted into the cavity of the uterus, there is a risk of introducing infection. Accordingly, such invasive procedures are usually reserved for mares in whom the likelihood of finding and treating a problem outweighs the risks of creat-ing one. On some stud farms, uterine cultures are taken routinely on all maiden mares before breeding.

A typical candidate for an intrauterine sampling procedure is an infertile mare, a mare with a history of repeated abortions or early embryonic deaths, or a mare with a history of abnormal heat cycles. Other candidates for endometrial culture or biopsy include mares presenting for a fertility evalua-tion as part of a pre-purchase agreement, and mares scheduled for a Caslick's operation (or some other genital procedure), to be sure the rest of the repro-ductive tract is free of disease.

Endometrial cultures and cytology samples are taken together. A sterile swab inside a plastic case is inserted through the cervix into the uterine cavity. The swab is extended, samples are taken, and the swab is retracted into the case before being removed from the uterus. The extracted swab is then re-extended and part of the sample is sent for culture while the remainder is looked at under the microscope for cells and bacteria—which, if present, indicate endometrial inflammation (see *Endometritis*, page 489). If the culture grows bacteria or yeast, cytology is still needed to show that the organism present was actually causing the inflammation and was not just a contaminant.

In the healthy endometrium, microscopic examination shows a field of uterine cells mixed with less than 1 percent white cells, or polymorphonu-clear leukocytes (*PMNs*). The finding of numerous PMNs (more than 1 per-cent) indicates inflammation. When inflammation is extensive, the gross appearance is like that of pus.

As an alternative to the swab technique, the uterus can be flushed with sterile saline, and the washings cultured and examined microscopically.

Endometrial biopsy provides additional information. It is more precise than culture and cytology and helps establish the diagnosis of uterine infection when these two studies are equivocal. Most important, it quantifies the degree of scarring or *fibrosis* in the wall of the uterus, which correlates with infertility. The biopsy is obtained as described for taking a uterine culture, except the instrument takes a bite of tissue from the wall of the uterus.

Inflammation is determined by counting the number of inflammatory cells. Fibrosis is graded according to the amount of scar tissue surrounding the endometrial glands. Extensive scarring correlates closely with early embryonic death; therefore, a mare with extensive scarring is not a good choice for breeding.

The Stallion

The age at which a stallion reaches sexual maturity and begins to produce sperm varies from 1 to 2 years, with an average of 16 months. However, few stallions are used at stud at or before 2 years of age. Even then, the number of services is usually restricted to two per week. At 36 months of age, the stallion reaches his full reproductive capacity. A fertile stallion at 4 years of age can be used two or three times a day if he is given occasional periods of sexual rest.

MALE ANATOMY

The stallion has two testicles enclosed by the scrotum and located in the prepubic region. The testicles produce sperm and also the male hormone testosterone, which is responsible for the secondary sex characteristics of the stallion. The temperature within the scrotum is two to three degrees below body temperature. This lower temperature is necessary for sperm production.

The *epididymis* is a coiled tube resting on top of the testicle. It connects the testicle with the spermatic cord. In addition to its transport function, the epididymis serves as a reservoir for sperm during the last five to ten days of their maturation. (Sperm maturation takes 21 days.) If mature sperm are not ejaculated within a few days of maturation, they die and are reabsorbed.

Sperm are transported up the spermatic cord into the ampulla, and then to the urethra. Also entering the urethra and mixing with the sperm are the secretions of the three accessory sex glands: the seminal vesicles, the prostate, and the bulbourethral glands. These glands produce seminal fluid, which provides energy and protective buffers for the sperm. The combination of sperm and seminal fluid is called semen.

The sheath surrounding the penis is the *prepuce*. The prepuce is actually a double layer of sliding skin. The internal layer contains sebaceous glands whose secretions, together with flaking epithelial cells, form a thick, waxy material called smegma. Smegma tends to collect in the folds of the prepuce and, if not periodically removed, may become a source of infection.

The penis is a cylindrical structure about 20 inches (51 cm) long when relaxed. During erection, cavernous erectile tissue within the penile shaft engorges with blood and the penis becomes twice as long and enlarges in diameter. At the end of the penis is the bell-shaped glans. In the horse, the urethra projects slightly beyond the tip of the glans. This extension is the urethral process.

There is a pocket within the glans above the urethra called the urethral diverticulum. A build-up of puttylike smegma in this pocket, called a bean, compresses the urethra, causing spraying and frequent urination. The condition is treated by manually everting the urethral diverticulum and removing the accumulated smegma. The entire sheath and glans should be cleaned as described in *Cleaning the Sheath* (see page 112).

The glans of the penis contains additional erectile tissue that engorges after the penis enters the vagina. This marked enlargement of the glans is called "belling" or "flowering." When belled, the penis is seated against the cervix in such a way that the urethral process is coupled with the opening of the cervical canal (called the cervical os). Thus the semen is ejaculated directly into the uterus. If belling does not take place, ejaculation cannot occur. See page 331 for an illustration of the urogenital system of the stallion.

A stallion with an exceptionally short penis may be unable to successfully seat the glans during belling. At the opposite extreme, a stallion with an exceptionally long penis may bruise or tear the mare's cervix. This can be prevented by using a breeding roll, as described in *Covering the Mare* (see page 471).

Ejaculation is controlled by nerves within the base of the penis that ultimately connect with the sex center in the brain. During coitus, muscles within the penis and the urethra contract to expel the semen. An ejaculation consists of about six to eight pulsations. Most of the sperm are present in the first four pulsations.

PREPARING THE STALLION FOR BREEDING

Nutritional requirements vary according to the size, condition, activity, and temperament of the stallion. Contrary to popular belief, a stallion's protein requirements do not increase during the breeding season. Furthermore, there are no dietary supplements known to improve sperm concentration or sex drive. Nevertheless, stallions are often overfed and oversupplemented, despite the fact that excess dietary energy is associated with obesity, laminitis, and lack of libido.

The stallion should be fed the maintenance ration for the adult horse, as described in chapter 15, "Nutrition and Feeding," with adjustments for activity and recent weight gain or loss. To ensure that dietary protein and other nutrients are of the highest quality, choose only the best feeds. The diet should provide adequate amounts of vitamin A for healthy sperm production. Water and trace-mineralized salt should be offered free-choice.

A program of good oral hygiene will prevent dental disease and maximize the benefits of the feeding program.

It is not necessary for a breeding stallion to be in top athletic condition. In fact, if the stallion is being intensively trained or in competition, a period of physical letdown is advisable before using the horse at stud. Extensive physical work may depress the libido and sperm production.

A stallion should be given daily exercise to maintain his cardiovascular fitness and stamina for breeding. Regular exercise enhances fertility by developing muscle tone, improving sex drive, and preventing obesity. Well-exercised stallions are generally less nervous, have fewer stallion vices, and are more confident around mares, and are therefore more consistent in breeding.

Since the stallion will likely be exposed to many outside mares each breeding season, it is essential that all vaccinations are up to date *before* the season begins (see *Immunization Schedules*, page 100). Vaccinations for influenza type A1 and A2 should be given twice a year or every two to three months, depending on the prevalence of the influenza in your areas. Annual or semiannual boosters offer adequate protection against rhinopneumonitis. Maintain protection against eastern, western, and Venezuelan encephalomyelitis, and West Nile virus. Annual boosters are required, ideally given one month before the height of the mosquito season. An annual rabies vaccine is desirable in rabies-endemic areas.

Chronic parasite infections cause weight loss, anemia, diarrhea, and reduced fertility. The stallion should be on a routine deworming program, as described in chapter 2, "Parasites." Anthelmintic drugs have no deleterious effects on sperm production or reproductive performance.

Hoof and foot care are important. Pain and lameness in the back feet can make it difficult for the stallion to mount. The hooves should be trimmed every four to six weeks. Remove the front shoes to prevent injury to the mare.

Sperm production and libido are depressed during the winter season. An artificial light program, as described for mares (see *Operational Breeding Season*, page 443), has been shown to somewhat improve both, but the effect is short-lived and may be associated with a rebound *depression* when high fertility is desired. Accordingly, an artificial light program is not suggested for stallions. One option to breed mares in the winter season is to use fresh cooled or frozen semen.

The Breeding Soundness Examination

A breeding soundness examination is a general physical exam undertaken before the breeding season, with special emphasis on the reproductive tract. The medical history includes notes on past breeding performance and any recent illnesses. A history of any injury to the testicles or penis is important, because such an injury could interfere with fertility or reproductive performance. A musculoskeletal injury can prevent the stallion from mounting the mare. A history of being given performance-enhancing drugs is significant, as well, because anabolic steroids and testosterone are known to cause testicular degeneration.

Veterinary examination of the stallion's reproductive tract is the main focus of the examination. Ultrasound, urethral endoscopy, and videoendoscopy may be used to predict the quality of the stallion's fertility.

Both testicles should be present in the scrotum and should be of normal size, texture, and consistency. When only one testicle is present, the stallion may still be fertile but should be considered unsuitable for stud because this condition is thought to be inheritable. Testicular size is closely related to sperm production and fertility. A stallion with very small testicles is less likely to be potent. (Note that the testicles do not begin to develop before 15 months of age and will continue to increase in size until the horse is 4 to 5 years old.) Excessive fat in the scrotum is a sign of poor condition.

The penis and prepuce should be examined for scars, pustules, and growths. Cultures are taken from the urethra, urethral diverticulum, and the shaft of the penis. After ejaculation, the urethra is again cultured, as is the semen, because even stallions with a complete BSE can spread disease.

The condition of the prostate, seminal vesicles, and secondary sex glands are determined by rectal palpation or endoscopy. Finally, the inguinal canals are examined for hernias.

Collecting and analyzing semen is a most important part of the breeding soundness examination. This highly technical aspect of stallion management should be done by an equine veterinarian. The number of sperm per milliliter and the quality of the semen sample help the veterinarian predict the number of mares a stallion can cover efficiently. When the semen contains less than 60 percent live sperm cells, there could be a problem with the epididymis or the testicles. Blood in the sample may be associated with infection and infertility. A pH above normal (alkaline) may be caused by an infection within the urethra or the secondary sex glands. The same is true for an increase in the number of white blood cells.

HANDLING THE STALLION

Handling a stallion requires special skills that include self-confidence, an understanding of stallion psychology, and the ability to anticipate a stallion's behavior and make quick decisions. An inexperienced horseman should not handle stallions; the handler and horses may be injuried.

Owning and breeding a stallion requires commitment, time, and discipline. Stallions, for the most part, are kept isolated from the general herd and may develop vices as a result. This is a serious business requiring a great deal of thought and preparation. This is one area in which the horse owner would benefit from some formal education. Many universities with an equine science program offer stallion handling classes. This prepares the horseman for the special skills and facilities that are necessary to maintain a stallion on the premises.

Genetic Testing

Due to rapid advances in biomedical research, along with an equine industry push to support research for certain breed-related genetic birth defects, there has been an explosion in the availability of DNA testing. These tests help breeders avoid genetic diseases, breed healthier horses, and prevent carrier genes from being passed on to successive generations. The popularity of certain color breeds has also spurred the development of tests for color gene—although testing for the overo lethal white syndrome gene is serious, since it is a birth defect. Testing for most color genes determines the probability of getting a certain color foal.

It's also important to test the blood type of mare and stallion, to avoid neonatal isoerythrolysis (see page 562). Blood tests will require a veterinarian. The DNA tests require just hair with the follicle attached; your veterinarian can recommend a testing facility.

Both the stallion and the mare should be tested for genetic birth defects to determine carrier status. Your veterinarian can assist you with finding laboratories that conduct the tests that need to be done before breeding. The table on page 463 lists several hereditary birth defects that can be prevented by testing potential mates. These tests are all offered by commercial laboratories, and new tests are being developed rapidly as research advances.

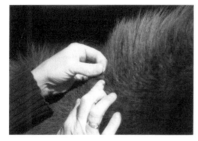

When pulling hair for DNA testing, it is important to pull out the whole hair follicle and not simply break the hair off.

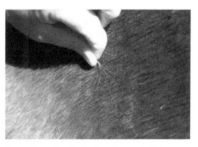

Examine the hair that's pulled to make sure the follicle is present. It will appear as a white end on the hair shaft.

	Genetic Tests for Horses		
Test	**Sample**	**Purpose**	**Breed(s) seen most often**
Blood typing	Blood	Rule out blood group incompatibilities and prevent neonatal isoerythrolysis	Thoroughbred
DNA	Hair follicle*	Determine parentage (some breed registries require DNA testing)	
Diseases			
Glycogen branching enzyme deficiency	Hair follicle* on mare/ stallion and muscle or liver biopsy on foal or PCR test	Detect carriers of this fatal enzyme deficiency	American Quarter Horse and related breeds
Hereditary equine regional dermal asthenia	Hair follicle*	Detect carriers of this genetic skin disease	American Quarter Horse (prevalent in cutting horse lines), American Paint Horse, Appaloosa
Hyperkalemic periodic paralysis disease	Hair follicle*	Detect carriers of this paralyzing birth defect	American Quarter Horse (linked to the *Impressive* line), American Paint Horse, Appaloosa
Junctional epidermolysis bullosa	Hair follicle*	Detect carriers of this fatal skin disease	Belgian Draft Horse and derivative breeds
Overo lethal white syndrome	Hair follicle* on foal, dam, sire	Detect carriers of this fatal bowel disease, which is linked to the overo pattern	American Paint Horse, Thoroughbred, Quarter Horse, Miniature Horse
Severe combined immunodeficiency disease	Mucosal swab or blood	Detect affected horses, carriers, and those clear of the gene	Arabians and Arabian-related horses

continued

Genetic Tests for Horses (*continued*)			
Test	Sample	Purpose	Breed(s) seen most often
Colors and patterns			
Agouti (bay/black)	Hair follicle*	Color	
Cream dilution	Hair follicle*	Color	
Red factor/ black factor	Hair follicle*	Color	
Sabino1	Hair follicle*	Pattern	Tennessee Walking Horse, American Miniature Horse, American Paint Horse, Azteca Missouri Foxtrotter, Shetland Pony, Spanish Mustang, Pony of the Americas
Silver factor	Hair follicle*	Color	
Tobiano	Hair follicle*	Pattern	American Paint Horse

*Sample is collected by pulling (not cutting) 20 to 30 mane or tail hairs.

COLOR GENETICS

Although genetic tests for hereditary defects are very reliable, tests for the genes that govern color and pattern are helpful only in making better predictions. This is because the interplay of color genes is very complex, and because there are factors other than genetics that influence coat color and pattern.

The coat color of all horses is determined by two possible base pigments: red or black. Breeders of black horses often want to test for the red factor gene to determine if a horse is *homozygous* (possessing two identical forms of a particular gene, one inherited from each parent) for black. Homozygous black horses always produce offspring with black as a base color; they never produce red offspring. Cremellos, palominos, and red duns are red-based horses and will test homozygous for the red factor gene.

The cream dilution gene controls the amount of base color dilution in a horse's coat. *Heterozygous* (possessing two different forms of a particular gene, one inherited from each parent) cream dilution produces buckskins, smoky blacks, and palominos, while homozygous cream dilution produces cremellos perlinos and smoky creams.

Currently, the test for the tobiano coat pattern looks for a gene that is strongly linked to the tobiano pattern but is not the actual gene. Therefore, the pattern of the foal may still be a complete surprise.

The agouti (bay/black) gene controls the distribution of black pigment. This can be translated into black points (ear rims, legs, mane, tail), or uniformly distributed color, such as black horses, grullos, or roans.

Sabino is a group of white spotting patterns, usually legs, belly, and face, with extensive roaning. Other breeds in addition to those listed on the table on page 464 (including Clydesdales and Arabians) may have sabino patterns but test negative for the sabino 1 gene.

Silver dilution is a *dominant* trait, meaning only one parent is needed to pass on the gene. Similar to the agouti gene, it will affect only black pigmented horses, not red.

In a horse with the overo coat pattern, the white does not usually cross the back between the withers and the tail. One or often all four legs are dark, the white is irregular, head markings are distinctive, the horse is often bald-faced, and the tail will be a solid color.

Breeding

The three basic methods for breeding horses are pasture breeding, hand breeding, and artificial insemination.

PASTURE BREEDING

This involves putting a stallion out with a herd of mares in a large area and letting nature take its course. It is most important that all horses be in good health and free of sexually transmitted diseases. Management is limited to preparing the stallion and the mares for the breeding season, introducing new members to the herd, and watching for problems.

Pasture breeding for one mare and one stallion requires no more space than a large paddock. For a herd of 15 to 20 mares, 40 fenced acres (16 hectares) is a reasonable area.

Pasture breeding is excellent training for young stallions, who learn the code of mating through contact with experienced mares. It may possibly improve conception rates for the marginally fertile stallion. Mares free of reproductive tract disease but with a history of *infertility* of undetermined cause will occasionally become pregnant when turned out into a natural setting with a seasoned pasture-breeding stallion.

However, it does have some disadvantages. The stallion's natural proclivity to guard his herd and protect his mares makes it difficult to routinely handle individual horses. In addition, introducing new mares into the herd can create jealously among the resident mares. In some cases, it is actually the

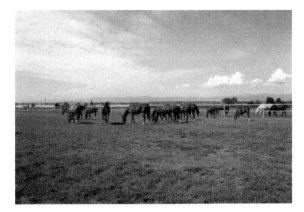

Pasture breeding is cost-effective and produces relatively high rates of conception.

stallion who rejects the new arrival. The new mare must quickly be removed from the pasture to prevent injury. The majority of such problems can be avoided by using proper introduction techniques.

The main disadvantage of pasture breeding is the increased likelihood that a valuable stallion will be injured by a mare's kick. Although the chances of this are small, such an injury could render the stallion unserviceable. Another disadvantage is that unless activity is closely monitored, you will not know the exact breeding date.

Another potential disadvantage of pasture breeding is the limit imposed on the number of mares a stallion can cover during the breeding season. By skillfully manipulating the size of the herd, removing pregnant mares and replacing them with mares who are not pregnant, it is possible to breed 30 to 40 mares in a season. In a hand-breeding operation, it is possible to breed at least twice that number. With artificial insemination, up to 200 mares can be covered in a season. However, when time and expertise are limited and there is ample space, nutritious forage, and a small number of healthy resident mares served by a fertile and sexually confident stallion, pasture breeding is cost-effective and convenient, and produces relatively high rates of conception.

Hand Breeding

Hand breeding involves bringing the mare to the stallion and restraining her by various methods while the stallion breeds her. Usually the mare is placed in breeding stocks while the stallion is led to her, allowed to tease (encouraging her receptiveness), and then allowed to breed. It has the advantage of enabling the horse's owner to directly manage the breeding process. It also provides the opportunity to select breeding individuals for various complementary characteristics. It is safer from the point of view of sexually transmitted diseases. Injuries to the mare or stallion are less likely. Fertility problems can be identified early in the season when there is still time to achieve pregnancy.

Along with artificial insemination, hand breeding is the only practical method of servicing outside mares visiting on the farm for only one or two estrous cycles.

ARTIFICIAL INSEMINATION

Artificial insemination (AI) is the procedure by which semen is collected from the stallion and introduced into the reproductive tract of the mare. When properly performed, AI increases the number of mares who become pregnant on the first cycle. Other advantages of AI are a low risk of spreading reproductive infections and the elimination of breeding injuries.

The chief disadvantage of AI is that it requires special facilities and equipment as well as personnel experienced in collecting, handling, and storing semen.

Fresh semen is divided into aliquots containing about 500 million progressively motile sperm in each aliquot. It is inseminated into one or more mares shortly after collection.

Cooled semen from some fertile stallions will remain viable for three to four days, and can be shipped and used to inseminate mares who would otherwise be unable to breed to that stallion. The mare to be bred must be palpated or scanned with ultrasound after she comes in heat to determine if she has a follicle large enough to be forced to ovulate (see *Forced Ovulation*, page 478).

Frozen semen can be stored for weeks, months, or even years, and then thawed and inseminated into one or more mares.

In the hands of skilled personnel, conception rates using fresh semen or cooled transported semen approach per-cycle pregnancy rates similar to those of live cover. Under ideal conditions, pregnancy rates from frozen-thawed semen range from 30 to 40 percent.

AI using freshly collected semen is allowed by almost all breed registries in the United States. Many registries permit the use of cooled transported semen; however, only a few allow frozen-thawed semen. It is important to check the rules of the breeding association before going to the expense of collecting semen.

Collecting the Semen

Most stallions can be easily trained to use an artificial vagina. Several models are available. All consist of a hollow inflatable rubber bladder surrounded by a cylinder. At the end of the bladder is a funnel that empties into a container for collecting the semen. The bladder is inflated with warm water at a temperature between 110 and 115°F (43 and 46°C). Sterile disposable liners are available that protect against chemical and detergent contamination of the semen. An optional filter retains the gel fraction of the semen and allows the sperm-rich portion to pass into the sperm receptacle. A sterile nonspermicidal lubricant, such as K-Y Jelly, is used to lubricate the interior of the bladder.

The artificial vagina is used in conjunction with a phantom mare or a live "jump" mare. A phantom mare can be made by welding two oil drums together and mounting them on a steel pipe, or one can be purchased. The phantom is padded with several layers of foam and covered with canvas or leather.

A jump mare is a mare in estrus, or more commonly, a mare whose ovaries have been surgically removed and who is then given estrogen to create artificial heat.

The stallion is brought into the breeding area and shown the phantom or jump mare until he has an erection. The erect penis is washed, as described on page 112. The stallion is then allowed to mount the phantom or jump mare. The stallion handler now directs the erect penis to the side and into the artificial vagina. Ejaculation occurs in the usual manner.

After dismounting, the penis is washed again with warm water to remove the lubricant. The filter containing the gel is removed (or the gel fraction is aspirated), leaving the sperm fraction in the receptacle. The resulting semen is mixed with an appropriate semen extender that contains an antibiotic. Subsequent handling depends on whether the semen will be used fresh, cooled and transported, or frozen.

Inseminating the Mare

The insemination procedure is performed under antiseptic conditions. The mare's tail is wrapped and the perineum thoroughly washed and dried. An 18- to 20-inch (45 to 50 cm) sterile plastic disposable insemination pipette is inserted through the cervical canal and into the body of the uterus. The volume needed to deliver the required number of sperm typically ranges from 5 to 20 ml. Most breeders inseminate at day two or three of estrus, based on palpation and teasing results and continue every other day until ovulation occurs, as determined by rectal palpation or ultrasound exam (see *Determining Estrus*, page 446). However, in the case of shipped cooled semen, the window for insemination is greatly narrowed due to the effort and expense of shipping the semen.

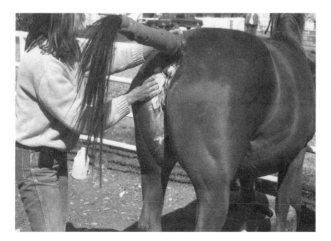

Before inseminating the mare, the tail is wrapped, and the perineum washed and dried.

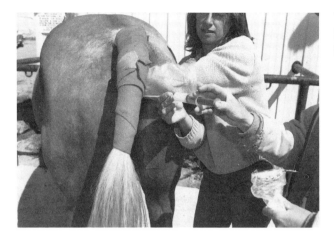

The semen is injected directly into the uterus.

WHEN TO BREED

A mare reaches puberty at about 18 months but does not achieve physical maturity until 3 years of age. Since it is desirable for her to be physically mature when she carries her foal to term, most people do not breed a mare until she is at least 3 years old.

When a mare in heat is receptive to the stallion, she exhibits certain characteristic signs. They include frequent urination, a raised tail, and a winking of the vulva as the lips of the vagina contract and relax. Rectal palpation reveals a mature follicle greater than 35 mm in size. As the mare ovulates, the follicle ruptures, releasing an egg into the oviduct.

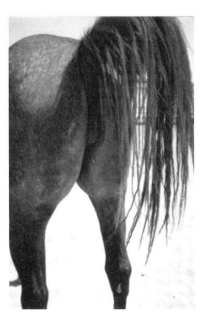

The typical stance of a mare in heat, spreading her hind legs, lifting her tail, and winking.

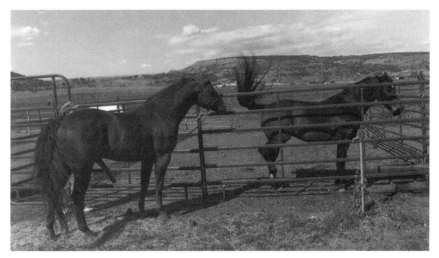

An unreceptive mare swishing her tail and kicking at the fence.

The best time to breed a mare is just before ovulation (see *Determining Estrus*, page 446). Ovulation usually occurs 24 hours before the end of estrus, but this varies. To maximize the chances for conception, most breeders recommend covering the mare on the third day of estrus and then every other day thereafter for as long as she remains receptive. On this schedule, motile sperm are present in the mare's reproductive tract at all times when ovulation is likely to occur.

Ovulation can be timed precisely using daily rectal palpation and ultrasound exams. The advantage here is that only one cover will be necessary—timed just before or within 12 hours after ovulation. When covering occurs 24 hours or more after ovulation, the mare will not conceive.

Teasing

The best way to determine when the mare is in heat is to bring her together with the stallion, or a teaser stallion who assumes that role. The mare's response at the sight and sound of the teaser will determine her level of receptivity. In some breeding programs mares are teased daily, while in others they are teased every other day.

When the breeding farm is large or the stallion is very valuable, it is customary to use another male to do the teasing. The temperament of the stallion teaser is an important consideration. He should be easy to handle but aggressive enough to elicit the signs of heat. The ideal teaser courts his mares consistently and does not lose interest halfway through the procedure. The teaser is allowed to cover one or two mares a season to maintain his sexual interest.

A common method of teasing involves trying a mare with a stallion across a teasing barrier. This can be a heavy stall door or a tubular steel gate. The barrier should be short enough to allow the stallion to get his head and neck

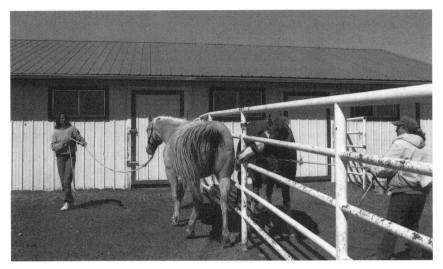

Trying a mare with a stallion across a teasing barrier.

over, and well padded to protect the horses if they kick or strike. The safest teasing wall is one equipped with extensions to protect the handlers.

The stallion is led up to the mare who stands, for example, behind a stall window. The horses are introduced nose-to-nose. If the mare is not receptive, she will lay back her ears and swish her tail violently from side to side. It is most important to maintain control of the mare and anticipate the possibility that she may strike out or swing around and kick at the barrier.

If the mare is receptive, she will lean toward the stallion, spread her back legs, urinate, and show winking of the vulva.

Another method of teasing involves leading the stallion past a series of paddocks containing estrous mares. The stallion investigates each one in succession, and the manager makes notes on the readiness of each individual mare.

COVERING THE MARE
Getting Ready

Before the mare is brought to the stallion, she should be encouraged to empty her bladder. Her tail is then wrapped with a disposable sleeve or bandage. It is important to include all the hair at the base of the tail in the wrap. Loose hair can get caught between the vagina and the penis and lacerate the penis.

The mare's vulva and perineum are then surgically prepped with a mild soap or dilute surgical scrub, using sterile disposable gloves. Rinse thoroughly with lukewarm water to remove residual soap. Dry the hindquarters with clean paper towels. The mare is now ready to be taken to the breeding area.

The stallion is brought into the breeding area and allowed to see the mare, if necessary, to encourage erection. The extended penis is gently lathered with water or a mild soap solution. Do not use antiseptic solutions such as Betadine or chlorhexidine, which can inflame the skin. Remove smegma from the urethral opening and folds of the prepuce. Rinse the penis with lukewarm water.

The Cover

Mating should take place in an area free of distractions. If the mare has a foal at her side, the foal should be kept in a holding pen where she can be seen by her mother. The procedure for hand breeding requires two or three people. Each person has assigned responsibilities and must know exactly what to expect.

For the safety of the stallion and handlers, the mare should be restrained during the cover. It is impossible to be 100 percent certain that a mare will stand submissively. There is always a distinct possibility that she will panic and kick out at the stallion.

A holding or palpation chute is an effective restraint, but since the stallion cannot mount or dismount at an angle, there is a danger that he will become trapped and injured if he falls off during the mating.

Most breeders prefer to restrain a mare with breeding hobbles. A lip twitch may also be used (see *Handling and Restraint*, page 6). Breeding hobbles consist of a leather strap that buckles around the mare's neck just in front of her shoulders. A rope extends from the lower part of this neck strap down

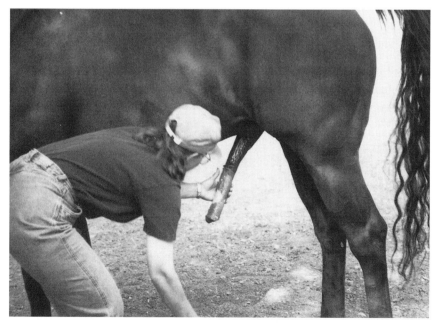

It is most important to wash the stallion's penis before and after the cover, to prevent sexually transmitted diseases.

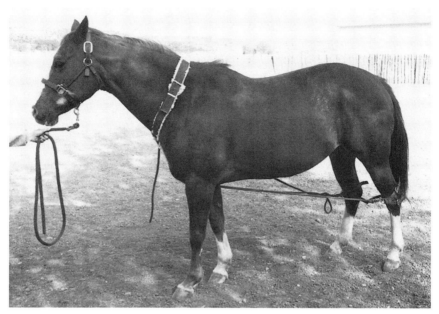

Breeding hobbles prevent the mare from kicking the stallion during the dismount.

between her front legs and attaches beneath her abdomen to another set of straps that buckle around the hocks. The connection between the front and rear restraints is secured with a quick-release knot. While in hobbles, a mare can walk forward but cannot kick.

An especially difficult mare can be fitted with a leather strap that holds up one front leg. The mare will be unable to kick when standing on three legs, but she will lose her balance and fall as the stallion mounts unless the strap is quickly released. This restraint will not prevent the mare from kicking on the dismount, when kicking is most likely.

When the mare is a known kicker, she should be fitted with kicking boots. These boots are made of heavy felt designed to soften the impact. Even when using a kicking boot, the shoes should always be removed.

If a small or maiden mare is going to be bred to a stallion with a large penis, he could tear the vagina or cervix. To prevent this injury, a breeding roll can be used. A breeding roll is a padded cylinder about 5 inches (13 cm) in diameter and 18 inches (46 cm) long. It is covered by a sterile sleeve and placed between the mare and stallion just above the stallion's penis as he mounts. The roll prevents the stallion from penetrating too deeply.

Some stallions have a habit of savagely biting the necks of their mares during mounting and coitus. Painful bites can be prevented by putting a leather neck shield on the mare or by fitting a cage muzzle over the stallion's mouth and nose.

The stallion and mare are restrained with a lead shank, chain, and halter. The shanks should be long enough so that the handlers can step back quickly.

The exact positions of the mare and her handler and the stallion and his handler are of critical importance for safety and control. *At no time should any handler stand between the two horses or directly in front of or directly behind either horse.* The mare handler should stand at the mare's shoulder on the same side as the stallion (usually the mare's left side). The duties of the mare handler are to steady the mare, allow her to see the stallion, and prevent her from moving out from under the stallion as he mounts.

The stallion handler stands at the left of the stud's shoulder and leads him calmly and directly to the mare's left shoulder. A 45-degree-angle approach allows the mare to see and prepare for the stallion and is recommended for safety.

As the two horses make contact, either may attempt to bite or strike. Mares can strike with blinding speed. Both handlers must be positioned out of the strike zone and be prepared to move back quickly. Control is obtained by yanking down hard on the lead shank and backing the horses away. When a mare strikes out or kicks at a stud, she is either not in standing heat or is going to be very difficult to cover.

A vigorous stallion, when presented to a quiet mare in standing heat, should greet her vocally, sniff and nuzzle her, display the flehmen response by curling his upper lip, then drop his penis and obtain an erection—all within three minutes. After the initial friendly greeting, in which the stallion is allowed to sniff and nuzzle the mare, he is backed away. This greeting and identification procedure is repeated two or three times as the stallion works down the mare from shoulder to flank. The receptive mare, now suitably coaxed, spreads her legs, flexes her pelvis, and takes a breeding stance.

The stallion should remain at the left side of the mare until he is fully erect and ready to cover. This takes about 15 seconds for the experienced stud. After receiving a cue to mount, the stallion rises up slightly to the side of the mare and quickly positions himself behind her buttocks for intromission and ejaculation. A third handler (optional), standing beside the mare's left hip, can hold the mare's tail to one side and guide the stallion's penis into the vagina. Guidance is particularly helpful when the mare is tall. This handler should immediately step back after intromission is accomplished.

Breeding averages 20 seconds. The normal ejaculatory pattern consists of five to six intravaginal thrusts, followed by three to five short thrusts synchronous with ejaculation. As the stallion ejaculates, his tail moves up and down. This is called flagging. It may not be seen in a horse with a high tail carriage, but the pulsations can be felt by placing a hand under the stallion's penis.

The stallion is allowed to dismount at his leisure. As the stallion begins to dismount, the mare handler should turn the mare's head quickly to the left. This causes her hindquarters to move to the right and away from the stallion,

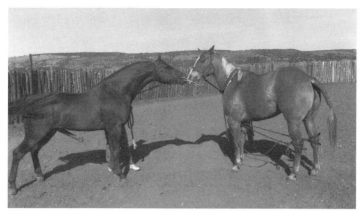

The horses make contact. The mare is receptive.

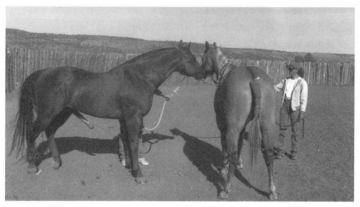

The stallion works down from shoulder to flank.

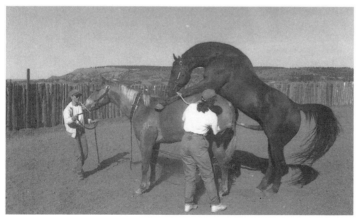

The stallion must be absolutely ready and fully erect before being given the signal to mount.

which places the stallion out of line if she kicks. At the same time, the stallion is backed from the mare.

The stallion is now returned to the wash area to have his penis and sheath cleaned and rinsed again. Washing immediately after each service is a most important step in preventing the transmission of sexual diseases.

BREEDING ON THE FOAL HEAT

The first postpartum heat occurs from day 7 to day 12 after foaling. In some cases, this interval is too short for the uterus to involute (return to breeding status) and the reproductive tract to return to a normal state of readiness for the next pregnancy. Most breeders simply wait until the second heat cycle at 30 days postpartum, at which time the chances for successful pregnancy are greater.

Breeding on the foal heat, however, becomes an important issue when the goal is to maintain a 12-month interval between foals to continue to produce foals close to the universal birth date (see *Operational Breeding Season*, page 443).

The mare has a relatively long gestation period, averaging 340 days. This leaves only about 25 days between the birth of one foal and the conception of the next, if the mare is to produce foals annually. Since the second heat occurs 30 days postpartum, it falls outside this window of opportunity.

Recent ultrasound studies of the uterus reveal that although *involution* of the uterus is not complete until day 21 postpartum, fertility can actually be achieved earlier. It is the presence or absence of uterine fluid that determines reproductive readiness. Persistent fluid makes it difficult for the embryo to implant in the uterus and decreases the chances of pregnancy. Ultrasound monitoring of postpartum uterine fluid reveals that after 15 days, there is little or no fluid detectable in the uterus in the majority of mares. Thus, if the embryo enters the uterus on day 15 or later, the embryo should survive.

After conception occurs, there is a five-day interval before the embryo enters the uterus. Thus, if ovulation and conception can be postponed until day 10 or later, there is a good chance the uterus will be receptive to maintaining the pregnancy. In point of fact, ovulation can be delayed until day 10 or later using a combination of progesterone, estrogen, and prostaglandin. Alternately, the interval between the foal heat and the second postpartum heat can be shortened to less than 30 days by administering prostaglandin alone.

A workable approach that meets all objectives is to monitor the mare by rectal palpation and ultrasound for ovulation and uterine fluid. If it is apparent that the mare will not ovulate until day 10 or later and there is little or no fluid in the uterus, she can be bred on the foal heat with the expectation of achieving a normal per-cycle pregnancy rate. When ovulation is expected to occur before day 10, or if there is significant fluid accumulation in the uterus, breeding is postponed. Seven days after ovulation, the mare is injected with prostaglandin PGF2α, which shortens diestrus and brings her back into heat ahead of schedule and in time to meet the universal birth date.

Twins

Although double ovulation occurs commonly, only about 1 percent of conceptions result in twin pregnancies. Twin pregnancies are considered a disaster in horses. The mare's endometrium does not have the surface capacity to support two pregnancies, and one or both fetuses suffer the effects of placental insufficiency.

The majority of twin conceptions result in early embryonic death with loss of both embryos—an event that may be seen only as a prolongation of diestrus. Among fetuses that survive beyond 150 days, 90 percent end in abortions or stillbirths.

Treatment: To preserve treatment options, it is necessary to diagnose twin pregnancy before 30 days of gestation. Rectal palpation and transrectal ultrasound, starting at three weeks post-conception, will identify many (but not all) twin pregnancies.

When twin pregnancies are diagnosed, the decision must be made whether to continue the pregnancy, terminate the pregnancy and re-breed the mare on the next estrus, or selectively terminate one embryo. Re-breeding on the next estrus is possible only when the pregnancy is terminated before 37 days of gestation. If it is terminated after 37 days, the endometrial cups (discussed in *Persistent Corpus Luteum*, page 451) will prevent the mare from returning to estrus for several months. This nearly always means the mare can't be re-bred until the next season.

Terminating the pregnancy is discussed in "Terminating a Pregnancy" (see page 500). Converting the pregnancy to a singleton by selective termination of one embryo is another alternative. This is commonly done by rectal palpation, then manually grasping one of the embryonic vesicles through the wall of the rectum and crushing it. Selective termination does traumatize the uterus and may result in the loss of both pregnancies. Medications can be given to minimize the effects of the trauma and maximize the mare's chances of maintaining the remaining embryo.

The last alternative is to allow the pregnancy to proceed to term, while supporting the mare with progesterone during the second half of gestation. However, very few twin pregnancies produce live foals.

Prevention: Monitoring mares with frequent rectal exams during the pre-ovulatory stage of estrus will identify most double follicles. Monitoring is particularly important for mares with a history of double ovulation. If ultrasound shows two follicles maturing at the same time, an alternative is to postpone breeding until the next estrus. When two follicles mature and ovulate at *different* times, a double pregnancy can be avoided by not breeding until 12 to 18 hours after rupture of the first follicle. Alternatively, the mare can be bred without consideration of the number of follicles, and if a twin pregnancy occurs, one embryo can be selectively terminated.

Infertility in the Mare

Mares who do not conceive after one or two cycles are called repeat breeders. Repeat breeders usually cannot conceive because of a genital tract infection.

The main cause of mare infertility and fetal loss during pregnancy is infection in the uterus. The wind-sucking perineal conformation, described in *Breeding Soundness Examination of the Mare* (page 454) and the sexually transmitted diseases discussed in this chapter, are responsible for the majority of uterine infections.

The second leading cause of mare infertility is abnormal heat cycles (see page 448).

REFUSAL TO MATE

Behavioral mating problems are less common in mares than they are in stallions. The role of the mare in coitus is passive. The main reason the mare refuses the stallion is simply because she is not in standing heat.

Maiden mares, nervous mares, and mares with a foal at their side can be more difficult to breed. Nursing mares can be reassured by placing the foal where the mare can see her baby during the breeding process.

A fastidious mare who refuses to respond to a particular stallion may respond when placed with another stallion she knows and likes. A maiden mare who fears stallions in general should be bred to a gentle, experienced, self-confident stud who is not easily put off. She will usually accept this stallion and present no further difficulties.

If the mare continues to be recalcitrant, she can be hobbled or restrained by tying up a front leg. Tranquilization can be considered. If these measures fail, artificial insemination remains an option.

Assisted Reproduction Techniques

Horses are not bred for their reproductive efficiency. Consequently, only about half of all mating cycles result in live foals. There are a number of newer techniques available to increase these odds. Most are complex, require highly specialized training, and are expensive.

FORCED OVULATION

A mare's follicle must rupture and release its egg within 48 hours after breeding. This ovulation is difficult to predict. Artificially forcing the ovulation makes it entirely predictable. There are three products commonly used for forced ovulation. All are available only by prescription from a veterinarian.

Human chorionic gonadotropin (HCG), given by injection, causes ovulation in 48 hours or less if the ovary contains a follicle 35 mm or greater in diameter. Ultrasound is an important tool for determining follicle size.

Deslorelin (Ovuplant) is a synthetic HCG that is used for forced ovulation. Placed under the mare's skin after the follicle reaches 30 mm in diameter, ovulation occurs in less than 48 hours. This product is not available in the United States as an implant; it comes only in injectable form.

Recombinant equine luteinizing hormone is an artificially engineered form of the luteinizing hormone, and in most cases causes ovulation takes place within 48 hours.

ESTRUS (HEAT) CONTROL

There are several ways to schedule a mare into heat. Regu-Mate (altrenogest), a synthetic hormone, is available by prescription. When fed for 15 days, the mare will not come into heat. Most mares will then cycle four to five days after the Regu-Mate is discontinued. It can also by given for ten days with a prostaglandin injection on the last day. Heat should occur in four to five days.

A new method of estrus suppression involves placing a uterine glass ball in a mare's uterus at the end of her heat cycle. It is not yet known why this works to suppress estrus, and it is only effective about 50 percent of the time. It must be placed in the uterus by your veterinarian and removed toward fall, when the mare would naturally stop cycling.

Various prostaglandins are available from your veterinarian. Two injections 14 days apart will result in a heat cycle within six days.

EMBRYO TRANSFER

Equine embryo transfer is becoming increasingly commonplace in the equine industry, even though it is expensive. Embryos are recovered from bred donor mares and placed in a recipient mare, who carries the foal. This is not an acceptable method of breeding for all breeds of horses. Be sure to check with the specific breed registry.

There are several reasons to use this method: a performance mare can't necessarily take time off; a mare may be unable to carry a foal to term; and young fillies and old mares may still be good donors. This technique can be used to optimize the number of foals from a genetically superior mating. Both mares must be healthy, reproductively sound, and cycling regularly. The donor and recipient mare must be synchronized in their estrous cycles. The recipient mare must have ovulated no more than one day before and three to five days after the donor mare. The donor mare's uterus will be flushed with a phosphate-buffered saline solution seven days after breeding.

The collected embryo is evaluated for size, grade, morphology, and developmental state. The embryo, in a straw attached to an insemination gun, is placed into one uterine horn, aided by rectal palpation. At day 12 (5 days after transfer) the recipient mare is examined by ultrasound for pregnancy, and again at days 14 and 30.

Infertility in the Stallion

Low fertility rates are a common problem in horses. The stallion, the mare, or both may be implicated. Stallion infertility is the inability to fertilize an ovum. The reasons include impotence (low libido), physical ailments that prevent coitus, and diseases of the male system that adversely affect semen quality.

LOW LIBIDO

Lack of sexual interest and arousal is the most common behavior problem in stallions. A young stallion who services just a few mares each season often exhibits slow breeding characteristics with long delays in arousal, mounting, and ejaculation. This is considered normal. It improves with use and experience.

A common behavioral cause of the loss of libido is a painful or traumatic breeding experience. Rough handling, excessive punishment, or severe discipline can discourage a stallion from expressing normal sexual urges.

Breeding fatigue is another common cause of loss of sexual interest and arousal. Although some stallions are able to service two or three mares a day for prolonged periods without becoming sexually fatigued, for many others this schedule is too strenuous. In fact, nearly all stallions show a gradual decline in sexual interest toward the end of the breeding season. On occasion, a vigorous stallion will suddenly stop breeding, exhibiting what is called a stale or sour attitude.

Rarely, lack of libido is caused by a testosterone deficiency. A stallion recovering from a protracted illness may need several months to regain his normal hormone balance and sex drive. A medically induced cause of testosterone deficiency is the administration of male hormones to enhance racing performance. The administered testosterone suppresses the pituitary gland, which stops producing gonadotropin. In the absence of gonadotropin, the testosterone level remains low until the pituitary recovers. This can take months.

Treatment: Young stallions typically show remarkable improvement after breeding their first mares. The best way to expedite a successful mating is to try the stallion repeatedly using minimal restraint and lots of patient encouragement. Select an experienced mare who shows strong signs of estrus, who is well-liked by the stallion, and who stands quietly when mounted. A similar approach applies to the experienced stallion who may have been traumatized.

A time-honored method of developing stallion libido is to turn the stud out to pasture with one or more broodmares, as described in *Pasture Breeding* (page 465). In the sexually fatigued stallion, a vacation from breeding usually restores low libido. A prolonged period of rest is usually required.

Impotence caused by hormonal rather than behavioral factors is difficult to treat with hormone replacements. Unfortunately, the dose of testosterone that stimulates the male libido also depresses sperm formation. One alternative is a subcutaneous injection of gonadotropin-releasing hormone (GnRH) just before breeding. GnRH releases stored testosterone. This may temporarily increase sexual arousal without the undesirable side effects associated with injected testosterone.

MALE FUNCTIONAL PROBLEMS

The stallion may begin courtship with a good libido, become aroused in the presence of an estrous mare, and yet not be able to perform the act of coitus for various functional reasons. Some of these problems have a medical basis, others a medical and behavioral basis, and some are behavior and management problems.

Penile trauma can cause temporary or permanent loss of the ability to erect the penis. The injury may be a severe laceration, penile rupture, or paraphimosis (the foreskin becomes trapped behind the glans penis). The usual cause is a kick to the erect penis from the mare during a cover. The use of stallion rings can result in penile trauma. A poorly constructed phantom mare and misuse of the artificial vagina are other causes of penile lacerations and abrasions.

Premature erection is a condition in which belling of the head of the penis occurs before intromission, making the penis too large to enter the mare. The situation can be accommodated by lubricating the vagina well and manually directing the penis through the vulva.

Mounting problems are characterized by repeated attempts to mount, mounting and dismounting, and dismounting before ejaculation. The usual causes are joint and back pain. Osteochondritis of the hocks, spine, or pelvis is frequently the problem. Stallions suffering from chronic laminitis or hoof disease experience pain when standing up on their back legs. A common cause of painful mounting is abrasion on the inside of the knees acquired from frequent mounting, particularly of a phantom mare. Nonpainful causes of failure to mount include muscle disease and nerve and spinal cord injuries.

A horse with a painful mounting problem often improves when placed on a course of phenylbutazone (Butazolidin) for 7 to 10 days.

Ejaculatory failure is intromission without ejaculation. The signs of ejaculation (flagging, urethral pulsations, and belling of the glans penis) do not occur. The stallion exhibits poor or irregular thrusts, dismounts as ejaculation appears imminent, or thrusts repeatedly to the point of exhaustion.

Ejaculatory failure has been treated successfully by administering drugs that contract the smooth muscles in the genital tract. However, ejaculatory failure is often the final, frustrating expression of other factors, including low libido, penile pain, and difficulty mounting.

Treatment: Treatment of the physical problem may not be sufficient to enable the stallion to regain all of his potency. If the horse has learned to associate the act of sexual intercourse with pain, frustration, danger, or punishment, the therapy must also teach the horse that sex is painless, safe, pleasurable, and rewarding. This involves a sex therapy rehabilitation program. Some techniques that have proven effective include training the stallion to use an artificial vagina, which can be made more or less stimulatory by adjusting the temperature and pressure; allowing the stallion to socialize with mares more freely; changing broodmares and breeding locations; engaging in longer periods of teasing; waiting patiently for time to heal all wounds; and converting to pasture breeding.

Finally, conception can proceed through artificial insemination even if the horse remains functionally impaired. Semen can be collected while the stallion is standing, using an artificial vagina. Neither mounting nor full erection is necessary for ejaculation. Accordingly, if a valuable stallion is unable to provide live cover for any number of reasons, artificial insemination remains a good alternative.

SEMEN QUALITY PROBLEMS

Absence of sperm is seen in horses with several conditions that are not difficult to diagnose. They include undescended testicles, testicular hypoplasia, testicular degeneration, acute orchitis, testicular growths, and injuries resulting in testicular atrophy or loss. All are discussed in *Diseases of the Male Reproductive System* (see page 492).

A frequent cause of reduced sperm numbers (and quality) is overuse. Stallions vary widely in their ability to produce sperm in response to breeding demands. Mature breeding stallions can be used more frequently than young stallions. However, excessive use can reduce semen quality in even the most fertile stallion. A good policy is to give all stallions a period of sexual rest during the season.

Semen contaminated by blood (hemospermia) or urine (urospermia) is abnormal. Blood in semen is frequently associated with *Pseudomonas aeruginosa*, a bacteria known to cause infection in the male genital tract. Red blood cells are recognized by the pink to red color of the ejaculate. Blood in the semen is believed to interfere with fertility, although this is not proven. Urine in the semen is recognizable by the yellow color and large volume of the sample. The effect of urine is to greatly reduce sperm motility.

A large number of bacteria of one species (especially a *pathogenic* species) is highly suggestive of urethritis or an accessory sex gland infection. The presence of numerous white blood cells in the semen confirms this diagnosis.

Horses with any of these semen quality problems should undergo diagnostic studies, beginning with bacterial culture of the sheath, the urethra (both before and after ejaculation), and seminal fluid. If further information is needed, other studies, such as a diagnostic ultrasound of the accessory sex glands and a transurethral fiber-optic exam of the male genital tract, can be performed. The horse should be placed at sexual rest pending diagnosis and treatment.

Nutritional deficiencies can be a cause of semen quality problems. A male who is grossly undernourished and on a very low plane of nutrition will frequently experience loss of libido and his testicles may atrophy. Any chronic disease associated with weight loss and debilitation reduces sperm production and adversely affects libido. Overweight studs are sluggish and lazy, but this does not affect *spermatogenesis* and has not been proven to reduce libido.

Anabolic steroids and testosterone can cause testicular degeneration. This effect may be temporary or permanent. Most adult stallions need several months to recover sperm production after the steroids are stopped. A few remain permanently sterile.

Thyroid deficiency is not a cause of reduced sperm production. In fact, adult hypothyroidism is a rare condition in horses, although a few cases have been described in Standardbreds and Thoroughbreds. Pituitary and other hormonal causes of reduced spermatogenesis are difficult to identify and treat. In general, hormonal therapies have been disappointing and appear to be of questionable value.

Genetic and chromosomal abnormalities are rare causes of infertility. Due to the complexity of the controlling genes, they are difficult to diagnose. Genetic work-ups must be done at schools of veterinary medicine.

Vitamin supplements have no beneficial effect on spermatogenesis or libido. Vitamin A is necessary for sperm formation, but unless a vitamin A deficiency exists (rare if the horse is receiving standard feeds), supplementing with vitamin A has no proven value.

Sexually Transmitted Diseases

Sexually transmitted diseases are a significant cause of sterility and abortion. There is a normal flora of bacteria on the penis and prepuce of the stallion and in the vulva and vestibule of the mare that inhibit the growth of virulent bacteria. When local conditions are disturbed, pathogenic bacteria become established and cause infection. Once a bacterial infection becomes established, it can be passed back and forth during coitus.

Disturbances in the normal flora of the skin of the penis can be caused by the presence of smegma that accumulates beneath the sheath and in the urethral diverticulum. Although it is important to keep the penis clean, excessive washing, or the use of detergents and antiseptic solutions such as Betadine or chlorhexidine, removes friendly bacteria and inflames the skin.

Seventy-five percent of uterine infections and a majority of septic abortions in mares are caused by *Streptococcus equi ssp. zooepidemicus*. Other bacteria commonly found around stables and paddocks, and capable of causing infection when sexually transmitted, are species of *Staphylococci, Pseudomonas aeruginosa, Klebsiella pneumoniae, Actinobacter,* and *E. coli.*

When present, the windsucking vagina and the urovagina make it virtually impossible to maintain a normal bacterial flora in the vagina.

Sexually transmitted infections cause vaginitis, endometritis, and pyometra in mares. In stallions, they cause urethritis, orchitis, epididymitis, and infections of the accessory sex glands. A stallion can harbor pathogenic bacteria and transmit the disease without having a symptomatic infection.

Treatment: Early diagnosis of bacterial infection may prevent chronic disease and sterility. Treatment is discussed in *Diseases of the Male Reproductive System* (see page 492) and *Diseases of the Female Reproductive System* (see page 487). A period of sexual rest for at least two months is important to prevent relapse. It is essential to reinvestigate the mare or stallion with appropriate diagnostic tests to be sure the infection has been eliminated before returning the horse to breeding.

Prevention: Lax breeding practices contribute to the transmission of sexual diseases. Although it is common practice to wash the mare's vulva and buttocks before breeding, failure to wash the stallion's penis and sheath before and after mating is a critical omission and can lead to a sexually transmitted infection in all the mares he services.

Good hygienic technique involves wearing sterile disposable gloves when washing the genitalia. Change gloves between horses. Each horse should have a separate wash bucket with a clean plastic liner filled with warm soapy water. Use only clean linen or paper towels, and discard after use.

A breeding soundness examination (discussed on page 454) should be done on all horses before the breeding season. This exam includes endometrial, urethral, and semen cultures. These cultures should identify infected horses.

CONTAGIOUS EQUINE METRITIS

Contagious equine metritis (CEM) is a highly contagious venereal disease caused by the bacteria *Taylorella equigenitalis*. No cases have been reported in the United States or Canada since 1983, but the disease is of concern to breeders who import horses from Europe and Japan. Federal regulations impose restrictions on the importation of horses from these areas.

CEM is a significant cause of infertility in mares. Early abortions do occur, but this does not happen often because most CEM-positive mares usually are unable to conceive. In the mare, signs of CEM occur two to six days after breeding. They include a copious gray to creamy discharge that mats the tail and hindquarters. However, many mares do not show signs of infection. These mares are asymptomatic carriers.

A stallion who harbors *T. equigenitalis* usually does not show signs of infection. The first indication of disease is a high incidence of reproductive failure in the mares he services.

In mares, the diagnosis of CEM is made by taking cultures from the clitoral fossa at any stage of the estrous cycle. CEM survives for long periods in this location. A blood test for CEM is reliable in mares three to six weeks after exposure, but serological *titers* decline quickly and there is no blood test that will detect the carrier state. In stallions, the bacteria survive in the smegma of the prepuce, the urethral fossa, and the surface of the penis. Stallions are checked by taking cultures from these areas. There is no blood test available for diagnosing CEM in stallions.

Treatment: Due to the probability of the horse developing the carrier state, antibiotics are not usually used to treat this infection. However, your veterinarian may wish to treat it in certain circumstances. Treatment in mares with acute infection involves the use of antibiotics orally or by intrauterine infusion. The carrier state in females, however, is difficult to eliminate. Recommendations include washing the genitalia daily with 2 percent chlorhexidine solution and applying 0.2 percent nitrofurazone cream to the clitoral fossa. Surgery to remove the clitoris may be advised to eliminate a continued focus of infection.

It is relatively easy to eliminate the carrier state in males. The penis should be cleaned daily with 2 percent chlorhexidine. After drying, nitrofurazone cream is applied to the penis.

Prevention: Prevention involves the use of strict hygiene before and after breeding. Because outbreaks of *T. equigenitalis* are of great concern to the horse industry and animal health regulators, this disease must be reported in the Northern Hemisphere and is a notifiable disease in the United Kingdom and other countries.

EQUINE VIRAL ARTERITIS

This RNA virus primarily targets the endothelium (a layer of flat cells) of the small blood vessels and macrophages (a type of white blood cells), but can replicate in different types, as well. It infects horses, donkeys, and mules. Equine viral arteritis (EVA) is transmitted by venereal and respiratory routes.

Clinical symptoms vary in severity, depending on the age, breed, and immune status of the infected animal. Incubation is 3 to 14 days and infected horses may or may not present symptoms. The most common signs include fever, depression, *anorexia*, rhinitis with serous nasal discharge, edema, and hives.

Infection is persistent in stallions and can cause abortion in pregnant mares. Abortion occurs 10 to 33 days after infection, sometimes with no preceding signs. There is no residual infertility in the mare. Except for the acute phase in the stallion, he also has no infertility problems.

Stallions in the chronic phase of the disease will excrete the virus months and years after infection. EVA infects the entire male urogenital tract. It can be well preserved in frozen and cooled semen, so transmission can occur during artificial insemination as well as a natural cover.

If EVA is suspected, several blood tests are available for diagnosis. The viral neutralization test will sometimes give a false positive due to a cross-reaction from a previous vaccination. Polymerase chain reaction (PCR) is more specific and has fewer false positives. Mare owners need to know what their options are if the stallion that they want to breed their mare to has a positive titer to EVA. They may choose to vaccine their mare, go ahead and breed and then monitor for signs of disease, or not breed to this stallion.

Treatment: Supportive care must be provided to the horse during the acute phase of the illness.

Prevention: This disease can be prevented with serologic surveillance, aggressive vaccination, and sound management practices. Artificial insemination is the best way of protecting stallions from visiting mares, but it will not protect mares from infected stallions. These vaccines are under tight control and their use may prevent international transportation of the horse.

COITAL EXANTHEMA

This is a highly contagious viral disease caused by equine herpesvirus type 3. It is spread from mare to stallion by genital contact. It is rare in the United States, and is not a cause of infertility or abortion. However, it can lead to infertility by causing a bacterial infection or behavioral issue due to painful intercourse.

During the acute stage in mares, painful blisters appear quite suddenly on the surface of the vulva and perineum. There is a whitish discharge on the buttocks and tail. The blisters become ulcerated and later scab over.

In the stallion, blisters 1 to 1.5 cm (.4 to .6 inches) in size form on the glans and body of the penis. These vesicles also develop into pustules and ulcers, leaving depigmented spots after healing. In a horse with a severe infection, the penis becomes inflamed and swollen.

Treatment: The disease runs its course in about two to three weeks. Recovery from infection does not confer immunity; future relapses can occur during serious illnesses and times of stress.

It is important to avoid secondary bacterial infection of the penis. Wash the penis with a mild soap (such as Ivory) and rinse thoroughly. An antibiotic ointment may be useful in preventing infection and helps to soften scabs. Insect control is a major factor, because flies can seriously aggravate open sores on the penis. Inflammation of the vulva is treated in a like manner.

The stallion should be rested until the skin of the penis is completely healed (three to four weeks). The mare can usually be bred on the next heat cycle.

DOURINE

This disease is caused by a trypanosome (a type of protozoan) transmitted during sexual intercourse. Dourine has been eradicated in many countries, including the United States, but still occurs in South Africa, Asia, Brazil, the former Soviet Union, and, rarely, in Germany. This trypanosome is unusual in that it is a tissue parasite rather than a blood parasite.

In the mare, the initial signs are swelling of the vulva and a vaginal discharge; in the stallion, a urethral discharge accompanied by swelling of the penis, prepuce, and scrotum. As the disease progresses, large round patches of raised skin appear in plaques all over the body. Dourine is often fatal.

The infection is confirmed by the use of blood tests. The most widely used and most reliable test is the complement fixation test (CF). Animals being imported from an endemic area must test CF negative. This is a reportable disease.

Treatment: Treatment is impractical because results are poor. Euthanasia is mandatory to prevent epidemic spread.

Diseases of the Female Reproductive System

Infections in the female reproductive system adversely affect fertility and the ability to carry a foal to term.

VAGINITIS AND VULVITIS

Infections of the vulva and vagina are common and occur after coitus, foaling, vaginal examination, and birthing injuries. The acquired perineal conformation described as windsucker or pneumovagina (see page 455) is the major cause of vaginitis and all other genital tract infections in the mare. In horses with this condition, the perineum is sloping, the anus is sunken, and the lips of the vulva and vulvovaginal sphincter do not form a protective seal against fecal contamination of the vagina.

The urovagina is an acquired perineal conformation defect similar to pneumovagina. Urine refluxes from the urethra and pools in the dependent portion of the vagina near the cervix. This invariably results in vaginal and cervical infections. Urine scalds may be visible around the buttocks and the perineum.

Vaginitis and vulvitis are mild infections which by themselves do not cause infertility. The importance of vaginitis is that it can progress to endometritis, particularly when there is a continuing source of contamination.

Treatment: Uncomplicated vaginitis usually clears spontaneously. Vaginal washes with an antiseptic such as 2 percent chlorhexidine hasten this process.

Treating urine scalds involves periodically applying zinc oxide ointment. All predisposing perineal deformities should be surgically corrected.

Vaginal Bleeding

A maiden mare with an intact hymen will experience vaginal bleeding after coitus. Ordinarily, the bleeding is not severe. An intact hymen should be opened before the breeding season.

A mare who bleeds profusely after a covering may have sustained a tear in the vagina or a laceration of the cervix. A cervical tear is most likely to occur when the mare is bred to a stallion with a large penis. Coital injuries can be minimized by knowledgeable stallion handling and the use of a breeding roll, as described in *Covering the Mare* (see page 471).

Postpartum vaginal bleeding is discussed in *Perineal and Vulvar Lacerations* (see page 534).

Treatment: Veterinary repair is indicated for a cervical tear.

Diseases of the Cervix

Infection of the cervix (cervicitis) follows infection of the vagina. Occasionally, an infected cervical canal becomes scarred and constricted, interfering with uterine drainage and predisposing the mare to pyometra.

Lacerations of the cervix occur during foaling and, less commonly, during coitus. A lacerated cervix results in cervical incompetence. An incompetent cervix remains partially open. This nearly always leads to infection of the uterus. If the mare is able to become pregnant, the incompetent cervix results in abortion.

Treatment: Lacerations of the cervix should be repaired. Standing sedation will be required for the surgery. The repair is best done about one month after foaling. When a broodmare presents with an incompetent cervix, a purse string suture can be taken around the cervix a few days after service. This may prevent the cervix from opening up prematurely. If the pregnancy goes to term, the suture must be removed before foaling.

Uterine Infections

Uterine infection is the most common cause of infertility. The two major predisposing causes of uterine infection are poor vulvar conformation and sexually transmitted diseases. In addition, contamination of the uterus occurs whenever the cervical barrier is breached by foaling, vaginal palpation, and all procedures in which instruments are introduced into the uterine cavity.

All mares experience some degree of bacterial contamination after service and foaling. A mare with an intact defense system clears the contamination within a few days. These defenses include all the physical barriers to uterine contamination (a closed vulva, an intact vulvovaginal sphincter, and a tight cervix); hormonal and immune mechanisms that establish a resistant endometrium; and, most important, the uterine tone and muscular contractility that cause infected secretions to be expelled rapidly from the uterine cavity.

An older, barren mare who has given birth many times previously (and who may also have acquired a pneumovagina) is an example of the individual who, because of repeated assaults on her defense mechanisms over the years, is no longer capable of clearing her uterus spontaneously and thus is more likely to harbor infection.

Treatment: Treatment for recurrent uterine infections is not usually successful. Therefore, the recommendation is to retire the mare from breeding.

ENDOMETRITIS

Endometritis is an infection of the cavity of the uterus. It is classified as acute or chronic, depending on the severity and duration of the infection. A mare with endometritis usually appears to be in good health, yet fails to conceive after several matings. Occasionally, she exhibits a pattern of unexplained fetal loss during pregnancy. A vaginal discharge is sometimes present or can be detected on vaginal exam. A rectal exam is often normal, but may show an enlarged uterus containing fluid. This can be confirmed by ultrasound.

Bacterial Endometritis

There are no bacteria present normally in the uterus of a cycling mare. The findings of a pathogenic strain (*Streptococcus equi ssp. zooepidemicus*, *E. coli*, *Klebsiella pneumoniae*, *Pseudomonas aeruginosa*, *Staphylococcus species*, and rarely, *Tayorella equigenitalia*) on one or more cultures is significant. Anaerobic bacteria such as *Bacteroides fragilis* appear to be significant causes of endometritis, especially in postpartum and foal heat mares. Cytology and endometrial biopsy will confirm the diagnosis. For more information on these procedures, see *Breeding Soundness Examination of the Mare* (page 454).

After a long-standing endometrial infection, the uterus becomes fibrotic (scarred). Fibrosis interferes with placental attachment. An endometrial biopsy will show the extent of fibrosis, which can then be graded. Mares in category 1 have normal findings (or slight changes), with a 70 percent chance of producing a live foal. Mares in category 2 have reversible or moderately severe changes, with a 30 to 70 percent chance of producing a live foal. Mares in category 3 have widespread fibrosis and less than a 10 percent chance of producing a live foal.

Treatment: The objective of treatment is to eliminate infection and produce a live foal. The treatment of mares with chronic low-grade inflammation and no symptoms of active infection can be deferred until the time of breeding. Mares with severe acute endometritis characterized by purulent vaginal discharge should be treated intensely before they are bred.

Antibiotics, selected based on sensitivity tests, have been the mainstay of treatment in the past. Antibiotics can be given either systemically or by local infusion into the uterus. The advantage of local infusion is that it puts the antibiotic in the spot where it can do the most good. The disadvantage is that infusion runs the risk of introducing new strains of bacteria, which are likely to be resistant to the antibiotic initially selected. Unfortunately, the development of antibiotic-resistant strains of bacteria is a common problem. Even antibiotics are given systemically, *superinfection* with resistant bacteria, as well as yeast and fungi, remains a possibility. For these reasons, antibiotics are being used less frequently and selected based on the culture and sensitivity result performed by the veterinarian. Based on the observation that natural defenses and the ability to clear the uterus of contamination correlate with successful pregnancy, irrigation of the uterus with saline and oxytocin (and no antibiotics) has become the standard treatment of many veterinarians. Mechanically flushing the uterus appears to successfully eliminate infected fluid, debris, and toxic products.

A balloon catheter is placed through the cervix into the uterine cavity with a 100 ml inflatable cuff to seal the cervix. A liter (34 ounces) of saline is introduced, agitated, and siphoned off. The initial flush may be submitted for cytology and culture. The mare is given 10 IU of oxytocin after the final flush to aid in removing any remaining fluid. Exercise will aid in uterine drainage after *lavage*; therefore, the mare should be turned out and not left standing in a stall.

Because uterine lavage is labor intensive, ultrasonography should be used to monitor its effectiveness and the need for continued therapy. The appearance of the recovered fluid (going from cloudy to clear) indicates the degree of progress and the need for further irrigation. On average, the lavage is repeated for three to five days, or as prescribed by the veterinarian.

In mares with a low-grade infection, flushing is initiated just before breeding and then again six hours after breeding. The sperm are well up into the oviducts within two hours, so there is little likelihood of interfering with conception.

Since natural defenses are most efficient during estrus, when the output of estrogen is greatest, shortening the second half of the estrous cycle to increase the frequency of estrus is an adjunctive step that has proven to be advantageous. This is accomplished by giving prostaglandin five to six days after ovulation to regress the corpus luteum and shorten the length of diestrus.

To prevent reinfection after treatment, it is important to correct any anatomical problems such as poor vulval conformation, pneumovagina, or incompetent cervix.

Fungal Endometritis

Treating equine fungal endometritis is difficult. Mares affected are usually 10 years old or more with a history of infertility, and tend to become reinfected.

A number of fungi have been isolated from the mare's reproductive tract; *Candida spp.* and *Aspergillus spp.* are the most common. Predisposing factors include immunosuppression, malnutrition, tissue trauma, endocrine *dysfunction*, poor vulvar conformation, and changes caused by antibiotics.

To diagnose this condition, a veterinarian will rely on *cytology*, endometrium or uterine culture, and tissue biopsy.

The danger in treating fungal infections is that bacteria will then have decreased competition. Pathogenic bacteria will overgrow and cause a bacterial infection. The mare's anatomy should be considered, to prevent fecal contamination (See *Breeding Soundness Examination of the Mare*, page 454).

Treatment: This involves large volume uterine lavage to decrease uterine fluid, decrease fungal and bacterial numbers, and expose organisms to antifungal solutions such as 2 percent acetic acid (white vinegar), 0.1 percent povidone-iodine solution, or 20 percent DMSO. Acidic or alkaline environments are not conducive to fungal growth. Follow up with oxytocin to increase uterine contractions. Infuse specific antifungal agents determined by the culture results. Concurrent antimicrobials should be used as well to prevent the overgrowth of bacteria.

The prognosis for a mare with fungal endometritis is guarded to poor for future fertility.

Prevention: Before coitus, the mare and the stallion should be washed as described in *Breeding* (see page 465). This reduces the frequency of contamination and the transmission of sexual infections. Invasive diagnostic procedures that breach the cervix should be restricted to medical necessity and should be performed with antiseptic techniques. Strict hygiene during foaling also is of utmost importance.

PYOMETRA

Pyometra is the accumulation of pus in the uterus. Some cases are related to cervical incompetence, which predisposes the mare to ascending infection; others to cervical scarring that blocks the cervical canal and thus interferes with the protective flushing mechanism by which the uterus rids itself of infection. Other predisposing factors include *Pseudomonas aeruginosa*, or fungi. In many cases, however, there is no explanation for the pyometra.

When scars or adhesions plug the cervix, several quarts of fluid (up to 60 quarts, 57 l) can accumulate in the distended uterus. Rectal palpation and transrectal ultrasound and analysis of the uterine fluid will easily diagnose this problem. When the cervix is not obstructed, a vaginal speculum exam may reveal pus in the vagina.

Mares with pyometra generally do not appear ill and rarely exhibit signs of toxicity. However, they usually don't come into heat at regular intervals because of a persistent corpus luteum (see *Abnormal Heat Cycles*, page 448), and this is why a medical opinion is usually sought. A persistent corpus luteum can be diagnosed by obtaining a serum progesterone level, which is positive when elevated.

Acute metritis is a severe and often fatal disease of the entire uterus caused by a postpartum infection of the mare's reproductive tract during or shortly after foaling. It is discussed on page 536.

Treatment: This involves draining and flushing the uterus with large volume warm saline lavages with oxytocin. Broad-spectrum antibiotics are added to treat the accompanying endometritis. Despite aggressive treatment, relapse is common. Endometrial biopsy is performed in all cases to determine the amount of salvageable endometrium. In the majority of mares, the extent of endometrial scarring and atrophy make successful breeding unlikely.

Diseases of the Male Reproductive System
The Penis
Skin Disorders

A buildup of smegma and bacteria within the prepuce and urethral diverticulum can lead to inflammation of the surrounding skin. This happens in both stallions and geldings. In addition, bacterial infection can occur when the resident flora of the penile skin is destroyed by excessive washing, particularly with antiseptics such as Betadine or chlorhexidine.

Regardless of the cause, the skin of an inflamed penis and prepuce appears fluid-filled and swollen. The penis may be extended.

The larva of the Habronema stomach worm may be deposited on the sheath or skin of the penis by stable flies and horseflies. These summer sores (Habronema granulomas) often cause intense itching and may interfere with urination and ejaculation. Treatment is discussed in *Insect Bite Allergies* (see page 122).

Squamous cell carcinoma is the most common growth affecting the penis. Smegma accumulation is a predisposing cause. The tumor begins as a rough, thickened patch of skin that becomes ulcerated and infected. Malignant squamous cell carcinomas can metastasize. Sarcoids, papillomas, melanomas, and lipomas are other tumors of the penis. Biopsy is the only way to make an exact diagnosis.

Treatment: Clean the penis and sheath with warm soapy water to remove smegma. Use a mild soap such as Ivory. If the penis is infected (red, swollen, or tender to the touch), apply a topical antibiotic ointment. Insect control is important, because flies can seriously aggravate an inflamed penis (see *Controlling External Parasites*, page 63). Bacterial infection can be prevented by periodically cleaning the sheath, as described on page 112.

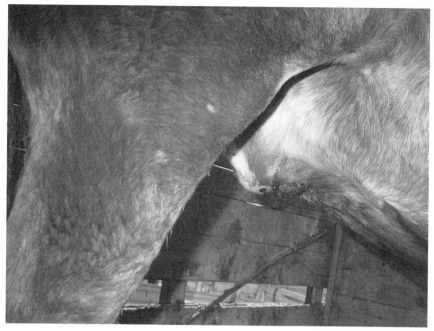

Squamous cell carcinoma, seen here as a white patch, is the most common tumor of the penis and sheath.

Penile tumors can be treated by cryotherapy (freezing), by a circumcision-like removal of skin, or by removing the entire penis. The decision depends on the size, location, and degree of malignancy of the tumor.

Phimosis

Phimosis is the inability to protrude the penis through a constricted prepuce. Constrictions almost always follow sheath infections, which invariably heal with scarring. Rarely, the constriction is congenital or is caused by a growth.

Treatment: Treatment involves cleaning the sheath cavity with 3 percent hydrogen peroxide solution (dilute 1:10) and then instilling a topical antibiotic such as triple antibiotic ointment. Antiseptics such as Betadine and chlorhexidine make the problem worse and should not be used. Surgical opening of the constricted prepuce may be required.

Paraphimosis

In horses with this condition, the extended penis is unable to return to its former position inside the sheath. There are three types of paraphimosis. In the first, the retractor muscles are paralyzed. This usually follows the administration of a phenothiazine tranquilizer. In the second, the penis remains engorged because the erectile tissue clots. This follows kicks to the penis during breeding. The third type of paraphimosis is actually phimosis, in which the penis manages to extend through a tight prepuce that then forms a constricting band around the shaft of the penis, causing sustained engorgement.

Treatment: Paraphimosis is an emergency. The penis must be returned to its sheath as quickly as possible to prevent further swelling and inflammation that makes reduction increasingly difficult. Ice packs and pressure are used to slowly reduce swelling as the penis is worked back up into the sheath. A purse-string suture through the prepuce prevents the penis from re-extending. The penis is supported with a gauze sling tied around the horse's body. Infection is treated with antibiotics. Sexual rest is essential. An antidote to phenothiazine-induced paralysis is available.

If the penis cannot be manually reduced, two surgical options remain. One is a penis suspension in which a bandage or sling is wrapped around the horse's body to include the penis, which is thus suspended in a horizontal position. This helps prevent further damage to the retractor penis muscle so that it will be able to function if reduction efforts are successful in reducing the swelling and inflammation that resulted in or from the original problem. Some horses will not tolerate a sling, others will. It is certainly worth a try, because the option is penectomy—surgical removal of the penis.

THE URETHRA
Urethritis

Sexually transmitted diseases are the most common cause of infection of the urethra. Sheath infections, Habronema granulomas, and growths of the penis are other causes. A stallion with urethritis often passes blood in his ejaculate. Blood in the semen is believed to interfere with fertility, although this has not been proven. The signs of urethritis include a urethral discharge and frequent painful urination. These signs may be absent.

Treatment: The primary cause of the urethritis must be determined. The presence of infection can be confirmed by culturing urethral swabs. Response is good with systemic antibiotic therapy and urethral lavage with a nonirritating antimicrobial agent, accompanied by sexual rest.

The accessory sex glands may be involved. This is determined by collecting and examining separate phases of the ejaculate. Fiber-optic endoscopy can be used to directly visualize the urethra and the openings of the accessory sex glands, as well as the neck of the bladder. This helps to determine the cause of blood in the ejaculate and to rule out stones and tumors. See *Uroliths* (page 335) for treatment of stones.

If the cause is Habronema granuloma, the hypersensitivity can be treated with a topical or systemic corticosteroid and the larvae can be destroyed with an organophosphate or ivermectin. If the treatment therapies are unsuccessful, surgical amputation of the urethral process may be indicated.

Urethral Obstruction

Strictures and stones are the most common causes of urethral obstruction. Stones in the urinary tract are discussed in *Uroliths* (see page 335). Strictures of the urethra occur from stallion rings, Habronema sores, and sexually transmitted bacterial infections. The tip of the urethra protrudes during erection and can be lacerated by the tail hairs of the mare. A laceration of the urethra frequently goes on to form a stricture. Kicks to the penis can result in posttraumatic urethral scarring.

Smegma may accumulate in the urethral fossa in sufficient amounts to press on the end of the urethra and cause obstruction. This is called a bean. It is more common in older horses. The chief sign is spraying. Rarely, a tumor of the penis obstructs the urethra.

The signs of urethral obstruction include *colic*, urine spraying, dribbling, extension of the penis, and frequent difficult urination.

Treatment: A catheter is placed to relieve a blockage. Further treatment is directed at the initiating cause. Clean lacerations of the urethra are repaired at the time of injury. Badly traumatized wounds are left not sutured and allowed to heal around an indwelling catheter.

THE TESTICLES
Orchitis

Inflammation of a testicle is called orchitis. It is sometimes accompanied by epididymitis, which is inflammation of the coiled tubules on top of the testicle. Sexually transmitted bacterial infections are the most common cause of both conditions, especially those produced by *Streptococcus equi ssp. zooepidemicus*. The infection starts in the urethra and works its way up to the testicle. Viruses and parasites are rare causes of orchitis.

Signs of orchitis (and associated epididymitis) include a hard, swollen, painful mass in the scrotum. There is a characteristic hopping gait. The semen contains bacteria, pus, and abnormal sperm. Ultrasound of the testicle is helpful in distinguishing between infection, trauma, and tumor, and to determine if the epididymis is involved.

Treatment: Ice packs are applied to the scrotum to reduce pain and swelling. The testicles are elevated using an external support. Antibiotics are selected based on semen culture and sensitivity tests. They are given intravenously and continued for one to two weeks after the swelling and pain subside. Anti-inflammatory drugs and corticosteroids can help to reduce pain and swelling.

Testicular degeneration often follows acute orchitis. Fertility thus depends on the health of the remaining testicle. A testicular abscess or chronic infection may necessitate unilateral castration to clear the reproductive tract of infection and to preserve fertility.

Acute epididymitis results in scarring of the tubules. This blocks the passage of sperm. The only effective treatment is to remove the epididymis and testicle.

Testicular Injury

The usual cause of a testicular injury is a kick during mating. A severe blow results in hemorrhage and marked swelling of the testicle. Later, the testicle atrophies and becomes small and hard.

Treatment: Treatment and prognosis are like that for *Orchitis* (see page 495).

Undescended Testicle

A horse with one or both testicles missing from the scrotum is said to be *cryptorchid*. Testicular descent from the abdomen to the scrotum occurs in utero at about 300 days of gestation. An interruption in the normal sequence of events can leave a testicle in the abdomen (10 percent of cases) or in the inguinal canal (90 percent). Retained testicles are associated with an increased incidence of tumors.

Two to three days after birth, the rings in the abdominal wall close tightly. A testicle that has not passed through the inguinal ring at this time remains in the abdomen. One that makes it through the ring and remains in the inguinal canal may yet descend. It is reported that descent can occur as late as up to 4 years of age.

Undescended testicles continue to produce testosterone but don't produce sperm. Thus, a horse with two cryptorchid testes has all the behavioral characteristics of the stallion but is not fertile. A horse with one normal testicle is fertile but usually is not bred because the condition is considered to be hereditary.

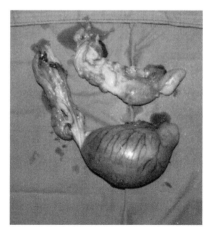

These are two equine testicles. The larger one is normal. The smaller one was an undescended testicle found in the inguinal canal.

An undescended testicle can often be felt in the inguinal canal or can be located by rectal palpation. Ultrasonography is useful in horses with one descended testicle because hormone tests cannot differentiate between animals with two testicles, one descended and one cryptorchid, and an animal with only one testicle. Ultrasound can also help locate a testicle that can't be palpated.

Treatment: Castration is indicated for all cryptorchid horses. It is important to find and remove the cryptorchid testicle. This can be technically difficult if the testicle is in the abdomen or is located out of the usual path of descent (ectopic). Removal of the cryptorchid testicle involves surgery with general anesthesia. *Laparoscopy* is a procedure that may be available that will minimize cost and complications. The descended testicle should not be removed until the owner and the veterinary surgeon are prepared to find the retained testicle.

There is a specific syndrome in which the horse is said to have been gelded but continues to act like a stallion. The cause is a retained testicle missed at castration. A serum testosterone level before and after administering HCG, or a single estrone sulfate measurement, will determine whether functioning testicular tissue is present. If the test is positive, one testicle was not removed and the horse should undergo an exploratory operation.

Testicular Hypoplasia

This is a developmental disorder in which one or both testicles are small and flabby, failing to reach normal size by maturity. Small testicles are the norm in colts and young stallions. The testicles do not achieve adult size until about age 4. In a normal 3-year-old, the scrotal width should be greater than 3 inches (76 mm). If it is less than 3 inches, hypoplasia is likely.

Hypoplastic testicles are associated with impaired sperm production. An ejaculate will show either no sperm or a low concentration of sperm with numerous abnormal spermatocytes. The diagnosis can be confirmed by testicular biopsy.

Testicular hypoplasia should be distinguished from testicular degeneration (described on page 498) because the outlook for future fertility is better with testicular degeneration. In cases of testicular degeneration, the testicles were normal before they became small.

Treatment: There is no treatment for this condition.

Testicular Neoplasms

Benign and malignant testicular tumors are uncommon in horses. These tumors rarely cause an enlargement of one testicle and therefore may go unnoticed for some time. Bilateral tumors are rare. The diagnosis is suspected on examination of the testicles. Ultrasound may provide additional information. Fine needle aspiration is the easiest way to obtain tissue for a diagnosis.

Treatment: Malignant tumors tend to grow slowly and can often be cured by orchiectomy (removal of the testicle). Benign tumors are almost invariably cured by orchiectomy. The effect of the tumor on sperm production varies, and this frequently influences the timing of surgery. If the semen quality is good and the stallion is booked, surgery is often deferred until the end of the breeding season.

There is a higher incidence of tumors in undescended testicles. Early removal of these testicles is the best method of prevention.

Torsion of the Spermatic Cord

A 360-degree twist of the testicle within the scrotum shuts off the blood supply to the testicle. Because this torsion is acutely painful, most stallions present with signs of colic. Young stallions are most commonly affected, often during or immediately after strenuous exercise. The testicle will die unless the problem is corrected within a few hours. Signs of torsion are indistinguishable from those of acute orchitis.

Treatment: The veterinarian should be called at once when you see or suspect a swollen, painful testicle. Emergency surgery is indicated when there is a possibility of salvaging the testicle. Unfortunately, in most cases, too much time has elapsed and irreversible damage has occurred. Atrophy of the testicle is the usual outcome.

Testicular Degeneration

Testicular degeneration is an acquired condition in which the sperm-producing tissue of the testicles is damaged, resulting in reversible or permanent sterility. A common cause of reversible testicular degeneration is high fever. For testicles to produce sperm, the temperature in the scrotum must be at least 2 to 3 degrees below body temperature. Fever raises scrotal temperature. The problem will be further compounded if the horse lies down, bringing the testicles up close to the body. Diseases commonly associated with fever and temporary sterility include equine infectious anemia, pneumonia, laminitis, equine viral arteritis, equine influenza, strangles, and ehrlichiosis.

Prolonged high environmental temperatures with high humidity have been implicated in causing testicular degeneration, as have scrotal hernias in which the heat of the intestines raises the scrotal temperature. In all these conditions, the testicles become small and flabby, like those of a horse with testicular hypoplasia.

A type of testicular degeneration that can be either reversible or permanent is caused by the injection of anabolic steroids and testosterone given to enhance racing performance. Early administration (during the first year of life), and continuous administration over the stallion's racing career, appear to increase the likelihood of permanent damage.

Irreversible sterility follows diseases that destroy the testicles, including testicular trauma and acute bilateral orchitis. These testicles become small as glandular tissue is replaced by fibrous connective tissue.

Treatment: Temporary sterility often improves once the cause is removed. It takes 50 to 60 days for regenerating sperm to reach the ejaculate, so any improvement in sperm quality will not be seen for at least two months. Frequent semen examinations are required to monitor progress. Sexual rest is necessary. Feed a balanced ration that is high in protein and vitamin A.

Preventing Heat

Estrus synchrony for breeding management, pain or colic during estrus, and cycle-related behavior or performance problems are the most common reasons to suppress the *estrus cycle* of a mare. Altrenogest (Regumate), a synthetic progestin, is highly effective for suppressing estrus when administered daily. Estrous behavior disappears two to three days after the start of treatment and does not return until treatment is stopped. However, there are some disadvantages: the oil solution is messy to handle, it's expensive, daily dosing is inconvenient, and human safety (especially for women who have had breast cancer) must be considered when handling the product. Progesterone weakens the cellular defense mechanisms of the uterus against infection. Veterinary consultation is advisable before starting a mare on progesterone, particularly because timing is very important for the success of the treatment. Use in a mare with uterine inflammation is contraindicated.

There is a variety of other drugs and implants, but none are labeled for use in horses. There is about a 50 percent success rate with the use of the uterine glass ball (see page 478 for more information).

Preventing Pregnancy

When stallions and cycling mares are kept on the same premises, accidental pregnancies can occur. Stallions are remarkably adept at getting to mares in heat. Confining stallions to box stalls except when under direct supervision is probably the most practical way to prevent accidental matings.

An *intact* male who will not be used at stud is usually gelded. This controls stallion behavior and makes the horse easier to handle. However, some horsemen prefer to own and ride a stallion.

Due to the seriousness of the surgery, removal of the ovaries is seldom done to sterilize a mare.

When accidental or unwanted pregnancy does occur, the two available options are to terminate the pregnancy or allow the mare to carry the foal to term.

TERMINATING A PREGNANCY

Indications for elective abortion include mismating, accidental or unwanted pregnancy, hydrops amnion (when the uterus fills with an abnormal amount of fluid), and twins. The rationale for avoiding twin pregnancies, as well as the methodology for converting a double pregnancy to a singleton, is discussed in *Twins* (see page 477).

Elective abortion should be done during the first four months of pregnancy. After four months, it is safer and better to allow the mare to carry her foal to term.

The two techniques for elective abortion are prostaglandin injection and intrauterine infusion. The choice of method will depend on the stage of pregnancy.

Prostaglandin (PGF2α) Injection

High levels of progesterone are needed to maintain a pregnancy. Progesterone is manufactured by the corpus luteum in the ovary. A single injection of PGF2α given after the formation of a mature corpus luteum (five days after ovulation) and before the formation of endometrial cups (37 days), will cause rapid regression of the corpus luteum, loss of pregnancy, and return of the mare to heat. Before five days postovulation, PGF2α will not cause abortion because the corpus luteum has not matured.

After 37 days, PGF2α must be administered daily for four days. Even though the mare will abort, she will not return to estrus until the endometrial cups cease to function, which takes 120 to 150 days. These mares usually cannot be rebred until the next season.

Intrauterine Infusion

Dilatation of the cervix followed by infusion of a saline-antibiotic solution into the pregnant mare's uterus will cause abortion within 48 hours. The infusion irritates the uterus and causes contractions. In addition, the irritation releases PGF2α. Both mechanisms appear to be involved in causing the abortion.

Just as with PGF2α, intrauterine infusion must be done within 37 days of gestation; otherwise, the mare will not cycle for four to five months.

OVARIECTOMY

Removal of both ovaries (ovariectomy) is a major operation and therefore is not often done for sterilization. A complete hysterectomy (removal of the uterus as well as the ovaries) is not done to sterilize mares. The usual reasons for ovariectomy are to remove an ovarian neoplasm, to eliminate estrous behavior in a mare who is not going to be bred, or to modify aggressive or nymphomaniac behavior.

Ovariectomy can be done by the vaginal, flank, or midline abdominal approach, depending on the size of the ovaries, the temperament of the mare, and the preferred technique of the veterinary surgeon. The vaginal approach is the most common because it can be done under local anesthesia with the mare standing, is less expensive, and perhaps has fewer complications. Laparoscopic procedures have significantly reduced the risks associated with this surgical procedure.

Two days before surgery, the mare should be given mineral oil by gastric tube to remove fecal balls in the colon that might feel like ovaries to the veterinary surgeon. Withhold feed for 24 to 48 hours but allow unlimited access to fresh water.

After the operation, your veterinarian may suggest cross-tying the mare for one week to prevent stress in the incision area caused by getting up and down. The mare can return to full activity in two weeks. Postoperatively, antibiotics and anti-inflammatory drugs are often prescribed. Postoperative complications, although uncommon, include intra-abdominal bleeding and shock (during the first 24 hours), wound infection, rupture of abdominal contents through the vaginal or abdominal incision, and peritonitis.

GELDING (CASTRATION)

The primary indication for gelding is to prevent aggressive or stallion behavior in a horse who is not going to be bred. A gelding is always more tractable than a stallion and tends to perform better for pleasure and show riding. A gelding is easier to keep with other horses and shows little or no interest in estrous mares.

Castration may be indicated for medical reasons, including testicular disease, undescended testicles, and inguinal hernia.

Castration can be performed at any age, including the first few weeks of life, without complications. Although male colts can be neutered at 3 to 4 weeks of age without harm, most horses are not *castrated* before 12 to 18 months of age to allow for physical development. When the stallion is castrated after sexual maturity, his libido and sex drive usually persist for four to six months, but can remain for up to a year.

A complete physical examination should precede the surgery. Infectious diseases, anemia, and unthriftiness caused by parasites or malnutrition should be corrected before surgery is done. A tetanus toxoid booster is given to all immunized horses, and tetanus antitoxin is also given if the horse was not previously immunized.

The operation can be performed under local anesthesia and intravenous sedation with the horse standing or lying on his side or back. Postoperative complications are uncommon. They include bleeding, peritonitis, prolapse of abdominal contents through the inguinal ring, spermatic cord infection, and abscess of the scrotum.

After surgery, your veterinarian may ask you to confine the horse in a clean stall or paddock (away from flies, if possible) for 24 hours. The horse then may return to light work for several weeks, as determined by your veterinarian's recommendation. Exercise the horse for 15 to 30 minutes twice a day to prevent scrotal swelling.

Consult your veterinarian if the horse exhibits colic, fever, unusual swelling at the site of the operation, or drainage of purulent material.

PREGNANCY AND FOALING

17

Gestation is the period from conception to birth. As reckoned from the first day of successful mating, it averages 340 days with a range of 320 to 370 days. A gestation period of 370 days is considered long, but *mares* have been known to deliver healthy *foals* after 399 days. Foals born before 320 days are considered *premature foals*. If the foal is born before 300 days, he will usually be too young to survive.

Failure to show heat 18 to 22 days after mating is suggestive but not conclusive of pregnancy. Regular stallion teasing every 1 to 2 days for up to 40 days is required to establish failure to show heat.

Rectal palpation as early as 20 to 30 days is an early reliable indicator of pregnancy, as long as the examiner is highly skilled at pregnancy palpation. Transrectal palpation performed between days 40 and 50 is 95 percent accurate. Findings that confirm pregnancy are a uterine horn that is firm and tubular and a cervix that is firm and contracted. The ovaries should contain follicles no larger than 1 inch (2.5 cm) across. The uterine wall is thinner at the site of the implanted embryo.

Transrectal ultrasound has improved the determination and prognosis of a successful pregnancy. Between days 14 and 50, ultrasound is 95 percent accurate in diagnosing pregnancy. It is important in the diagnosis of twins. Mares with a history of twins or double ovulation should be scanned between days 12 and 15 to effectively manage the pregnancy reduction to a singleton.

All embryos should be detectable by day 24. Failure to detect an embryo by that time is an indication that the pregnancy will fail. The fetal heartbeat is visible on ultrasound by day 26. Ultrasound is a useful tool in determining fetal age, some gender determination can be done at the right gestational age, and even the cervix can be examined for proper closure.

The mare immunological pregnancy (MIP) test is the most frequently used serum pregnancy test. It is accurate and inexpensive, but the information is not available as soon as it would be with a transrectal ultrasound. The MIP test detects elevated levels of the hormone equine chorionic *gonadotropin* (eCG) in the mare's serum between days 40 and 120 of gestation. This test is 95 percent accurate. It will not detect pregnancies at less than 40 days of gestation. In addition, if the pregnancy is lost after day 37, the test will remain falsely positive due to the activity of the endometrial cups, as discussed in *Persistent Corpus Luteum* (see page 451).

Plasma progesterone levels and milk progesterone levels in lactating mares are elevated as early as the sixteenth day of gestation. Tests for these are 90 percent accurate.

Care and Feeding During Pregnancy

During the first eight months of pregnancy, feed the mare her usual ration of high-quality feed. Trace-mineralized salt, which, in selenium-deficient areas should contain selenium, should be fed free choice as the only salt available.

During the last three months of pregnancy, there is a significant increase in the size of the foal. The mare can be expected to gain about half a pound (227 g) per day. This weight represents growth of the foal. Since the mare's weight increases by about 15 percent during the last three months, increase the amount of feed accordingly to maintain body *condition*.

The nutrient requirements for a 1,100 pound (500 kg) mare during the last three months of pregnancy are given in the table on page 395. In essence, the mare's daily ration will require a total of 16 percent protein and digestable energy (DE), as well as twice as much calcium, phosphorus, and vitamin A.

If you are feeding high-quality alfalfa or legumes, either as hay or pasture *forage*, most of these additional requirements can be met by the mare's natural tendency to eat more feed. A grain or protein supplement is not required when you are feeding top-quality hay. However, additional calcium and especially phosphorus are needed and should be provided by mineral supplements, because grass and legume hays generally do not contain sufficient amounts of either. To the trace-mineralized salt, add a calcium-phosphorus mixture such as dicalcium phosphate or another calcium-phosphorus mineral supplement, as shown in the table on page 404. Alternately, instead of feeding alfalfa, you can use a ration determined by using the online program Nutritional Requirements of Horses, www.nap.edu/catalog.

It is particularly important for the mare to be well nourished at the end of pregnancy in order to maintain milk production and prevent weight loss during lactation. She should be moderately fleshy to heavy with a body condition score of at least 6 (see *Body Condition Scoring System*, page 422).

Note that mature grass pastures and hays do not contain enough protein or dietary energy for significant weight gain during pregnancy and lactation. Mares on such pastures should be given a supplemental grain mix that contains at least 16 percent crude protein; they'll need .5 to 1 pound (226 to 453 g) per 100 pounds (45 kg) of body weight of this supplemental fed each day to effect weight gain and a body score of 6 to 7. In addition, larger quantities of calcium will be needed than when feeding legume hays.

Water requirements increase greatly during pregnancy. The mare should have free access to clean, fresh water at all times.

Exercise

A moderate exercise program maintains muscle tone and condition. A physically fit mare is more apt to deliver a healthy foal and to have fewer *postpartum* complications. Mares on pasture get adequate exercise. Those confined to a stall or paddock should be taken out and exercised twice a day.

A mare can be ridden up to the last month of pregnancy. However, intense physical exercise should be avoided. Overexertion and stress have been linked to fetal loss. Transporting a mare over a long distance causes emotional and physical stress, and should be avoided if at all possible, especially during the last two months of pregnancy.

Vaccinations

Certain vaccinations are suggested during pregnancy (see the table on page 100). Vaccinations boost the immunity of the *broodmare* and ensure that high levels of antibodies will be present in her *colostrum*.

The risk of fetal loss following exposure to the rhinopneumonitis virus is significant. Vaccinations provide immunity for only two months. It is recommended that vaccinations for rhinopneumonitis be given during the fifth, seventh, and ninth months of gestation. Some practitioners recommend vaccinating mares in the third month as well. A modified live virus vaccine and a killed (inactivated) vaccine have been approved for pregnant mares. Only the killed vaccine is labeled for use in preventing fetal loss.

Tetanus, equine encephalitis, equine influenza, and West Nile virus boosters should be given three to six weeks before the foal is due. Potomac horse fever and rabies vaccinations should be given in certain geographic areas. Ask your veterinarian what is best for your mare.

If a pregnant mare develops equine viral arteritis, there is a 50 percent chance she will lose the fetus. Preventive vaccination before pregnancy may be indicated in certain high-risk areas, and especially when breeding to carrier stallions.

Deworming

All horses should be on a regular deworming program, as described in chapter 2, "Parasites." Internal parasites drain the mare of nutrients, damage tissue, decrease her resistance to infection, and have a harmful effect on the fetus. Accordingly, the mare should be on the same deworming schedule as other horses on the premises. Because of the risk of abortion, benzimidazole dewormers are not recommended during the first trimester, and organophosphate dewormers are not recommended past the middle trimester. It is routine practice not to administer dewormers during the last six weeks of gestation.

On the day of *foaling*, ivermectin should be given to prevent the passage of threadworms to the foal in the mare's milk. Threadworms cause respiratory and intestinal damage in foals. A foal at risk for threadworms should be dewormed at 3 weeks of age.

Fetal Loss

The risk of fetal loss may be as high as 30 percent. Loss of pregnancy is highest during the period when the fetus is an embryo. It is more common in mares over 18 years of age and in mares with a history of infertility or prior abortion.

Early Embryonic Death

Early embryonic death is defined as the loss of the embryo before day 40 of gestation. Fetal loss can actually occur even before the embryo implants in the wall of the uterus, because of unfavorable environmental conditions or a genetic defect in the fertilized egg. Ultrasound scanning in early pregnancy reveals that this is common. These early embryos are small and are reabsorbed.

Ultrasound scanning of the cervix after implantation reveals that the cervix is open at the time of early embryonic loss. This suggests that many of these embryos are lost through the cervix rather than by true reabsorption.

When pregnancy loss occurs after 37 days, the endometrial cups (discussed in *Persistent Corpus Luteum*, page 451) continue to produce equine chorionic gonadotropin (eCG), which prevents the mare from coming back into heat for 120 to 150 days. This condition has been referred to as false pregnancy.

Abortion

Abortion is the death of a fetus after organ development (45 to 55 days), but before 300 days when the fetus is capable of independent existence outside the womb. A dead foal delivered after 300 days is a *stillbirth*.

Suspect chronic *endometritis* or a progesterone deficiency in mares who abort on successive pregnancies. A mare who aborts (or has a history of early embryonic death) should have an infertility examination to determine the cause of the problem. The fetus should be submitted for necropsy, if possible, along with the placenta, to determine the cause of the abortion. Chromosomal abnormalities and genetic defects incompatible with life usually cause abortion before 90 days of gestation. It is estimated that 1 percent of foals are born with minor abnormalities.

When abortion occurs after the second month of pregnancy, laboratory examination of the fetus and placenta will reveal the cause in about 50 to 60 percent of cases. When postmortem tissue examination is not done, the cause will be known in less than 10 percent of cases. Most diagnostic laboratories prefer to have the complete fetus and placenta submitted chilled (not frozen) as soon as possible after the abortion. It is particularly important to include the placenta, since abnormalities of the placenta are common causes of sporadic abortion. Until a cause is established, assume that all abortions are infectious and handle the tissues with sterile precautions.

Viral Causes of Abortion

The rhinopneumonitis virus (the EHV-1 form) is the number one cause of abortion in late pregnancy. It is highly contagious and natural or acquired immunity is not well-maintained. Repeated infections keep the virus active in the horse population. Abortion storms, involving nearly all pregnant mares on a single farm, have been reported.

Pregnant mares are likely to be exposed in the fall, in the first half of pregnancy, during the respiratory virus season. The typical signs include a runny nose, conjunctivitis, and a dry cough. The virus enters the bloodstream, crosses the placental barrier, and invades the fetus. Death and abortion, however, do not occur until one to three months after exposure. Therefore, the majority of mares tend to abort in late pregnancy. EHV-1 infection does not impair future fertility. Vaccination will prevent many (but not all) EHV-1 abortions. All horses on the farm, not just the mares, should be vaccinated to reduce the risk to pregnant mares. If your horse is kept at a boarding facility, this may be difficult.

Equine viral arteritis (EVA) is another respiratory virus that causes abortion. It is shed primarily through respiratory secretions, but can be transmitted to a broodmare in the semen of an infected stallion. During the acute respiratory illness, the virus crosses the placenta and infects the fetus, resulting in death and abortion shortly thereafter. About half of infected mares will abort.

Stallions, but not mares, can develop a carrier state. Thirty to 50 percent of stallions become carriers. A carrier stallion sheds virus in his semen, either temporarily or permanently. If a mare is venereally infected, she can develop a respiratory infection and pass it on to other horses with whom she comes in contact. A serological blood test is available that becomes positive two weeks after infection.

Abortions can be controlled to some extent by screening all *seropositive* stallions to look for the carrier state. This is done by culturing the virus. A *seronegative* mare (susceptible to EVA) should not be bred to a seropositive stallion unless it has been conclusively established that the stallion is not a carrier, or unless the mare has been given a series of EVA vaccinations. Virus isolation tests on semen are the only ways to determine if a seropositive stallion is infectious. For more information, see *Equine Viral Arteritis* (page 87).

Equine infectious anemia (EIA) is a rare cause of abortion because the disease is so well contained through testing and isolating infected horses. A negative Coggins test is a prerequisite for breeding. EIA is transmitted through the bites of bloodsucking flies. Infection can occur during pregnancy. Infected mares do not always abort unless they are very ill, and may actually give birth to normal, healthy foals.

EIA is a lifetime infection. There is no vaccination or treatment to prevent or cure the disease. Seropositive horses must be isolated indefinitely, because they remain a reservoir for the virus.

Bacterial Causes of Abortion

The bacterial causes of abortion in the mare are a result of bacterial inflammation of the placenta (*placentitis*). About 25 percent of abortions are caused by bacteria. The most frequent cause of placentitis is *Streptococcus equi* subspecies *zooepidemicus*. Most of these abortions occur before the eighth month of gestation. A few mares may carry the foal to full term, but these foals are born premature and weak. The prognosis is very grim for a live foal born with a preexisting *Streptococcus equi* subspecies *zooepidemicus* infection.

E. coli is also a frequent cause of placentitis and abortion. This occurs prior to seven months of gestation. Other bacteria frequently found to be a cause of abortion include *Pseudomonas aeruginosa*, *Enterobacter species*, and *Klebsiella pneumoniae*. These infections are often the result of poor vulvar conformation. The early signs of infection or placentitis may be detected by rectal palpation and treated to prevent abortion. Vulvar discharge is really the only visible sign, unless the mare is palpated. In all cases of abortion, only laboratory examination of tissue samples submitted by your veterinarian can tell you the cause. However, only 65 percent of the causative organisms will be specifically identified. Discussion between you and your veterinarian should include any additional steps to protect your mare from reoccurrence. Leptospirosis is a disease caused by a spiral-shaped bacterium that attacks both humans and animals. It is an uncommon cause of abortion during late gestation. The aborted fetus often appears jaundiced, suggesting the diagnosis.

Leptospirosis is transmitted by contact with the infected urine of rodents, wild animals, sheep, and cattle. Infection in the mare, often mild and inapparent, precedes abortion by about two weeks. After recovery from illness, bacteria can be shed in the urine for two to three months. During this time, the mare should be isolated. Antibiotics are not effective in eliminating the carrier state.

Fungal Causes of Abortion

Aspergillus fumigatus and other fungi account for a small number of cases of placental infection (15 percent). The mechanism of transmission is like that described for bacterial placentitis. Fungal placentitis tends to produce less initial inflammatory reaction than bacterial placentitis. As a result, abortion (or stillbirth) occurs quite late in gestation (within one month of term).

Uterine Causes of Abortion

Placental insufficiency results in a malnourished fetus that is either aborted or born weak. A poorly developed placenta is the result of preexisting conditions within the uterus (such as chronic endometritis) that interfere with placental attachment and reduce the surface area for the placenta to attach to the uterus.

Twin pregnancies account for 20 to 30 percent of all observed abortions. The mare's uterus simply does not have the surface area to allow two placentas to attach and grow normally. One twin generally develops more rapidly and acquires most of the space. The other twin dies and brings on the abortion of both. Ninety percent of mares who do not abort early in pregnancy do so after 150 days. It is therefore unusual for a mare to go to term with twin pregnancies. When this does happen, usually one twin is born mummified and the other is small and weak. Twin pregnancy is best prevented and treated as described in *Twins* (see page 477).

Twisting of the umbilical cord can cause sudden death if the umbilical cord shuts off the blood supply to the fetus. An abnormally long umbilical cord lends itself to this. The incidence is reported to be about 1 percent, but the actual incidence may be somewhat lower because torsion of the cord is often blamed for abortion when there is no other explanation.

Incompetent cervix means the cervix, having been weakened by a laceration during a previous foaling, does not seal the uterus. Infection or air can then gain access to the uterine cavity.

If the incompetence is detected before infection develops within the uterus, the cervix can be repaired surgically. The cervix is more likely to tear again during foaling, and these mares should be examined closely. The suture must be removed before foaling.

Injuries, such as kicks, seldom cause abortion. The foal is well protected by a shock-absorbing cushion of fluid.

Hormonal Causes of Abortion

Progesterone deficiency caused by inadequate production from the corpus luteum has long been considered a cause of unexplained early pregnancy loss, although the condition has not been well documented in horses. However, some mares with a history of habitual abortion will deliver a live foal when supplemented with progesterone. To be effective, progesterone should be administered throughout the first four months of gestation. After four months, the placenta takes over the function of manufacturing this hormone, and extra progesterone is no longer required. There are no known adverse effects of giving progesterone. Your veterinarian will select a progesterone supplement that is effective for your mare.

Estrogen deficiency is not a cause of abortion.

Physical and emotional stress lowers plasma progesterone levels and releases steroids, which may be the reason why a higher rate of abortion has been noted in mares subjected to stressful events, such as prolonged and difficult transportation, intense physical work, episodes of colic, surgery, and a change from a wet and cool environment to a hot and humid one.

Toxic Causes of Abortion

Forage toxicity—the consumption of certain pasture grasses and poisonous plants—has been linked to abortion, difficulty foaling, and the birth of deformed foals. Among these forages are fescue toxicity, ryegrass poisoning, sorghum toxicity, and locoism. The toxic effects of these plants and grasses are not limited to abortion. For more information, see *Forage Toxicities* (page 427).

Mare reproductive loss syndrome results in the death of the embryo between 6 and 12 weeks, although a few mares may experience later term loss of the fetus. The cause of the early death is pasturing mares during a cyclical upswing of the eastern tent caterpillar. Every 10 to 20 years, the eastern tent caterpillar naturally has a sudden population explosion. This caterpillar feeds on cherry trees, but ends up being ingested with forage when it falls to the ground.

Removing mares from pastures with cherry trees in the two or three years prior to peak eastern tent caterpillar populations decreases exposure and therefore decreases risk. Removing all cherry trees from the horse farm will result in a similar decline. Spraying to eliminate the caterpillar has variable effectiveness in preventing embryo losses.

Chemicals and drugs implicated in causing abortion include phenothiazines, lead, some dewormers (benzimidazoles in the first trimester; organophosphates in the second and third trimesters), and organophosphate insecticides.

Life-Threatening Complications of Pregnancy

Catastrophic events during pregnancy are not common, but when they occur, it is crucial to recognize them immediately.

RUPTURED PREPUBIC TENDON

The prepubic tendon is attached to the pubic bone and serves as a common tendon for the abdominal muscles. In susceptible mares, the tendon slowly gives way from the weight of the pregnant uterus. Draft mares and fat, idle mares are most often affected. The signs of impending rupture are an excessive accumulation of fluid in the underside of the belly (ventral edema) with a sagging, pendulous abdomen. Sudden, complete rupture is accompanied by shock, collapse, and death.

Treatment: When the tendon gives way gradually, confine the mare, limit exercise, and support the abdomen with a sling until the foal is mature enough to be delivered vaginally or by cesarean section. The damaged tendon cannot be repaired. If the mare survives, she can no longer be bred.

Ruptured Uterus

The uterus generally ruptures if active labor is arrested by a large foal, twin foals, an abnormal presentation, or some problem that causes difficult and prolonged labor. Rupture can also occur as a sequel to torsion of the uterus (see page 512).

When the uterus ruptures completely, the foal, along with the placenta, may be extruded into the abdomen. Sudden vaginal or abdominal bleeding with shock during foaling are signs of rupture of the uterus and indicate the need for rapid delivery or emergency cesarean section. A partial tear of the uterus may go unnoticed during foaling and then cause postpartum peritonitis several hours later.

Treatment: Some partial tears can be sutured through the birth canal after delivery. If this is not possible, the repair is usually done through a midline incision under general anesthesia.

Rupture of the Uterine Artery

The middle uterine or utero-ovarian arteries, one on each side of the uterus, are the major blood vessels that supply the uterus. One of these major vessels, usually on the right side, may rupture during the birthing process. This may also occur if the mare's uterus *prolapses* or everts outside through the vaginal canal. Another cause of rupture can be uterine torsion, which is a twist or turn of the uterus.

There are two different sets of symptoms. In the most severe cases, the mare shows sudden, severe *colic* signs with increased pulse and respiratory rates, weakness, and pale mucous membranes. This is caused by the pulsing artery suddenly hemorrhaging a large quantity of blood into the abdominal cavity.

The other type of rupture contains the hemorrhage within the broad ligament associated with that particular uterine artery. This is usually diagnosed during a postpartum breeding examination. The mare shows little or no pain and this type of contained rupture is often unnoticed.

Treatment: In mares with a sudden onset of pain, treatment often cannot begin quickly enough to prevent death from such massive blood loss. Pain management is started immediately with sedation. The mare must be kept in a quiet stall and given massive volumes of fluids, including blood. The outlook is usually poor.

In mares with blood contained within the broad ligament, the blood clot can be 8 to 12 inches (20 to 30 cm) in diameter. These mares usually live and recover, even becoming pregnant again. However, they are prone to rupture of the artery again during the subsequent foaling, with fatal consequences from the hemorrhage. A valuable mare with this condition may be a candidate to be an embryo transplant donor (see *Embryo Transfer*, page 479), as she would not have to bear the stress of pregnancy with the threat of death.

TORSION OF THE UTERUS

Torsion is a rotation of the uterus about its long axis. This is rare. A hard fall, an episode of violent rolling, or an excessively active fetus have been implicated as possible causes. When the uterus rotates 180 degrees, the broad ligaments become stretched. This interferes with the blood supply to the uterus and the fetus. A 360-degree rotation, which is even more rare, cuts off the blood supply and results in the death of the fetus within hours. The mare goes into shock and collapses.

Torsion nearly always occurs in the last trimester, when the uterus increases rapidly in size. An incomplete rotation produces colic, frequent urination, listlessness, and loss of appetite—signs often mistaken for early labor. Accordingly, any mare who exhibits colic in late pregnancy should have an immediate veterinary consultation. Rectal palpation will confirm the diagnosis or torsion of the uterus and also indicate the direction of the twist.

Treatment: Rolling the anesthetized mare in the direction of the torsion may correct the rotation. However, in most cases, it is necessary to make a flank incision and twist the uterus back into its normal position. If the mare is close to term, the next step is to induce labor. Death of the uterus and the fetus requires emergency cesarean section to save the life of the mare.

Preparing for Foaling

When foaling takes place in a pasture, the acreage should be large enough to allow the mare to withdraw from the herd, which she will do instinctively at foaling time. This is especially important because other horses in the herd may harass or even attack a newborn foal at a time when the mother is unable to protect him. When the foal is up and nursing, the mother will return to the herd.

About a week before the mare is expected to foal, begin to cut back on the amount of feed. Most breeders prefer to confine the mare where she can be observed and medically attended in case of an obstetrical emergency. The foaling quarters should be clean, dry, draft-free, and warm—preferably in familiar surroundings away from unfamiliar people and other distractions. A box stall is ideal, but a small, dry, grassy paddock can be equally satisfactory. A good light source is essential. The mare should be introduced to her foaling quarters at least two weeks before the expected date of delivery. If the mare is being moved to another farm to foal, it should be done one month prior to enable the mare to develop antibodies to viruses and bacteria in that environment, which will help protect the foal. The floor of the box stall should be covered with several inches of bedding. Clean straw provides good bedding and firm footing. Sawdust, wood shavings, and sand are poor bedding materials and have been associated with breeding complications after foaling. Sawdust and shavings may stick to the foal's eye, creating ulcers. Change the bedding at least once a day to maintain a clean, sanitary surface.

This is a good time to put together a foaling kit (see the table below)—items it will be handy to have at delivery. The equipment you will need includes a bucket of warm, soapy water, tail bandages, cotton towels, cloth strips for tying up the placenta, and 7 percent tincture of iodine for the navel stump. This kit should be stored in a place that's convenient to where foaling will occur but where it will be kept clean.

Foaling Kit

Bucket or case to hold everything

Index card with emergency number for veterinarian

7 percent tincture of iodine (not to be confused with milder iodine)

Dip cup: can be any small, clean container to put iodine in

Plastic disposable gloves to prevent iodine from staining your hands

Enema of buffered phosphate to help pass meconium stools

Hand wipes

Tail wrap: gauze wrap or veterinary wrap

Clock or stop watch, to record the time when the water breaks

Trash bag, to place the placenta in after it passes

String or cloth strips, to tie up placenta so the mare doesn't step on it and tear it

Clean towel or roll of paper towels

K-Y jelly or other lubricant (optional) to lubricate your hands and arms if the mare needs assistance

Cell phone and the telephone numbers of your veterinarian and an emergency clinic

When the mare approaches her foaling time, it is essential to check on her often. It's a good idea to have a comfortable observation post outside the stall. A mare about to foal should be checked on with a flashlight every 15 to 20 minutes during the evening and night, when most mares prefer to foal. Stall-mounted television monitors have been used successfully on large breeding farms. Foaling alarms are also available. Some strap around the abdomen to indicate the mare is lying down; others can be implanted in the vulva and detect when the water breaks.

SIGNS OF FOALING

About three weeks before delivery, the mare's udder will begin to enlarge, at first swelling at night and shrinking during the day. In the last two weeks before foaling, the mare's vulva swells, relaxes, and lengthens to enable her to expel the foal.

On the day before foaling, the udder remains full and tense. Clear to serumlike colostrum begins to drip from the udder. This colostrum dries to form a honey-colored bead at the end of each teat. This is called waxing. It usually indicates the mare will foal that night. However, it is not uncommon for udder distension and waxing to occur within a few days before foaling. When the wax falls from the ends of the teats, the mare may begin to drip white, opaque milk that is thick and sticky. When the white milk appears, the mare should foal in 8 to 12 hours. If the mare streams milk, she is losing large amounts of colostrum. The colostrum should be collected and frozen. Later, it can be thawed and given to the foal.

Another way to determine when a mare might foal is the milk calcium test. One milliliter of mare's milk is mixed with 6 ml of distilled water (it *must* be distilled water). A commercially available water hardness strip is dipped into the mixture. Results greater than 200 parts per million (ppm), *as determined by*

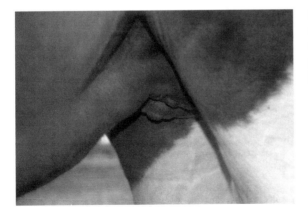

Close to delivery, the mare may exhibit edema or swelling from her udder extending under her tummy.

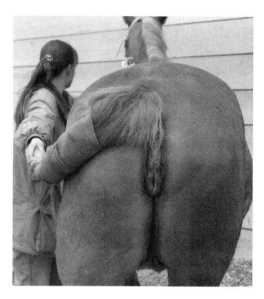

The mare's vulva relaxes, swells, and lengthens within two weeks of foaling.

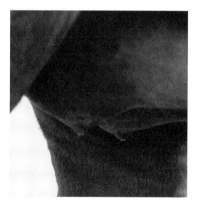

A honey-colored bead forms at the end of each teat the day before foaling; this is called waxing. Sometimes there is colostrum dripping.

the instructions with the strip, mean the mare will foal within 48 hours. If the result is 250 ppm or greater, the mare will usually foal within 12 hours.

Mares have some degree of control over the timing of delivery and prefer to foal at night. Eighty percent deliver between the hours of 10 p.m. and 4 a.m.

Normal Labor and Delivery

Although 90 percent of births occur without problems, it is important to be familiar with the normal sequence so you can recognize when something is wrong and either assist the delivery or summon your veterinarian. There are three stages of labor. Normal delivery may be preceded by several bouts of false labor.

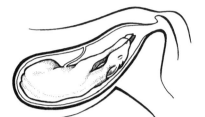

The foal is lying on its back before
the mare goes into labor.

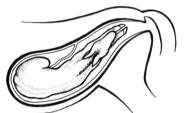

In the first stage of labor the foal
rotates with head and legs extended
in the birth canal.

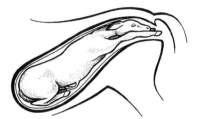

The nose and forelegs pass
through the birth canal with the pads
of the feet pointing down.

The position of the foal in the uterus during normal delivery.

First Stage of Labor

During the first stage of true labor (which lasts two to four hours), uterine contractions gradually dilate the cervix and shift the foal from the resting position into the orientation for delivery. The mare becomes noticeably more active and restless, paces in her stall, gets up and down several times, passes small amounts of urine and stool, looks and nips at her abdomen, and sweats and appears to have colic. Although these are the customary signs of first-stage labor, keep in mind that some mares pass through the first stage without giving strong indications.

Once you have determined the dam is in the first stage of labor, wrap her tail with a sterile gauze roll and wash her vulva and hindquarters with mild soap and water, as described in *Covering the Mare* (see page 471).

The end of the first stage is marked by the appearance of the bubblelike amnion protruding from the vulva. Within five minutes, this membrane ruptures, releasing yellow to chocolate-colored fluid, an event known as breaking the water. The amnion may rupture within the birth canal, in which case you will not see the bubble.

SECOND STAGE OF LABOR

Second-stage labor is typically brief, lasting 10 to 20 minutes. It begins when the water breaks and ends with the delivery of the foal. After the water breaks, the foal's forelegs should appear at the vaginal opening within 15 minutes.

Forceful contractions of the uterus and abdominal wall muscles during second-stage labor cause the placenta to separate from the wall of the uterus. In the horse, placental separation occurs rapidly, cutting off the oxygen supply to the foal. Although most foals are born within 20 minutes, a maximum of 40 to 60 minutes may pass between rupture of the amnion and delivery of the foal. *If there is no foal or progression within 15 minutes, call the veterinarian!* After that time, the foal is at serious risk of death. Accordingly, it is important to record the time when the water breaks, because from this point forward delivery is on a strict timetable.

After the water breaks, the mare usually lies down on her side with her legs extended. However, some mares get up and down frequently and others stand to deliver.

The normal fetal orientation in the birth canal is the anterior longitudinal presentation, in which the foal is aligned lengthwise with his spine parallel to the mother's spine, head tucked between extended forelegs, and pads of the feet pointing down. As the chest enters the birth canal, one leg is placed slightly in front of the other to allow the shoulders to pass through one at a time.

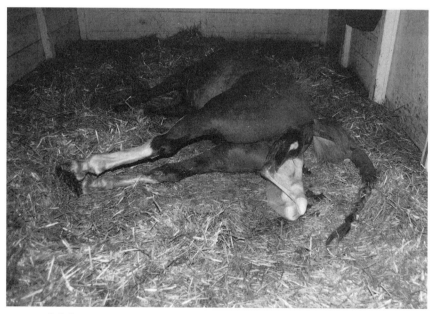

A normal delivery. The forelegs and head have passed through the birth canal.

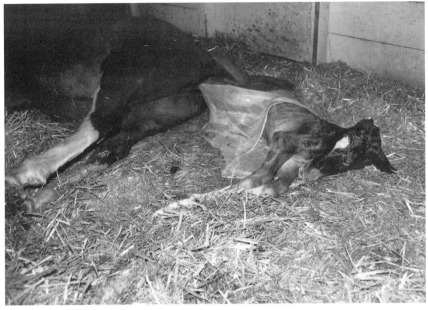

The amnion breaks, allowing the foal to breathe.

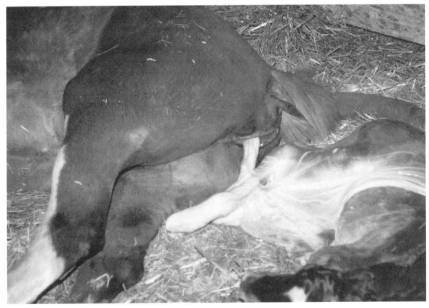

The foal rests. Note that the umbilical cord is still intact.

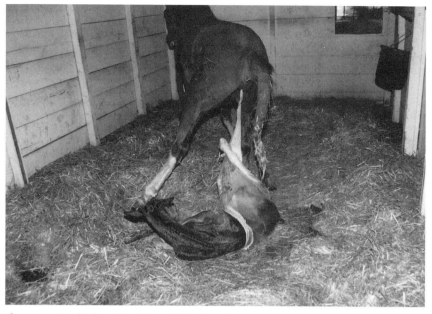

The mare stands, breaking the umbilical cord.

During passage through the pelvic opening, the amnion surrounding the foal will have ruptured in most cases. If, when the head is delivered, the nostrils are still covered with the amniotic sac, remove the membrane to allow the foal to breathe. If the mare stands to deliver, be prepared to catch the foal and lower him gently to the ground.

After the hips have been delivered, the foal usually rests with his hind legs in the mare's vagina for 10 to 20 minutes. *Resist the temptation to break the cord.* Allow this to happen naturally by the movements of the mare.

Once the cord separates, dip the navel stump in 7 percent tincture of iodine for 30 seconds. This step is important in preventing navel ill and neonatal sepsis. Tying off the cord is unnecessary and inadvisable, because it may cause cord infection. The stump will dry up naturally.

In the unlikely event that the cord does not break within 30 minutes, you should step in and break it by hand. Grasp the cord firmly 2 to 3 inches (5 to 7 cm) from the navel and pull the cord in the direction of the placenta until it tears. Don't cut the cord, as this may cause bleeding.

Once the cord has been severed, tie it in a knot above the mare's hocks to keep her from stepping on the end and tearing the placenta. A strip of cloth is helpful in tying up the cord and placenta.

How to revive a depressed foal is discussed on page 520.

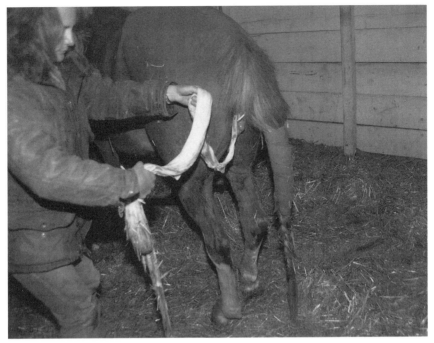

The placenta will pass spontaneously within three hours. Tie up the umbilical cord to prevent the mare from stepping on it.

THIRD STAGE OF LABOR

In the third stage, the placenta is expelled. This occurs in 30 minutes to 3 hours after foaling. Do not attempt to pull the placenta from the mare's uterus. This will damage the uterus or cause the placenta to tear. If the placenta tears, a piece will be retained. A piece of retained placenta can cause toxic uterine infection.

After the placenta has been expelled, examine both sides to be sure that no missing pieces remain in the uterus. Small tears can be detected by filling the placental sac with water and ballooning it out. An intact placenta resembles a pair of "Dutch britches," a configuration representing the two horns and body of the uterus.

If the placenta does not pass within three hours or there is a possibility of a retained fragment, the mare should be examined by a veterinarian at once (see *Retained Placenta*, page 535).

REVIVING A DEPRESSED FOAL

If a foal does not breathe within 60 seconds, he should be resuscitated at once. Extend the foal's head and remove secretions from his nostrils with a sterile gauze or a clean towel. Rub the foal vigorously all over with a clean towel. If this does not revive the foal, try to stimulate a cough reflex (which activates breathing) by tickling the inside of his nose with a blunt clamp or a piece of straw.

After a prolonged and difficult delivery, some foals are too weak or flaccid to breathe on their own, despite your efforts. You will need to administer mouth-to-nose resuscitation. Close one nostril with the flat of your hand to keep air from exiting. Enclose the other nostril with your mouth. Blow in with enough force to expand the chest. Release both nostrils to allow air to escape. Continue at a rate of 25 breaths per minute, pausing every 30 seconds to see if the foal is starting to breathe.

If the foal does not have a heartbeat, administer a brisk thump to the side of the chest behind the elbow. This may produce a heartbeat.

The use of prolonged cardiopulmonary resuscitation (CPR) has humane aspects to be considered. You can sometimes resuscitate a foal, but you must realize that if breathing cannot be established or the heart does not beat within the first few minutes, the outlook is grim. Cardiopulmonary arrest is usually secondary to systemic disease. If there is no chance of recovery, it would be inhumane to attempt any CPR. If the systemic disease has an unclear prognosis, the use of CPR is much harder to determine, but the results are usually death of the foal after heroic efforts. Resuscitation of foals should be discussed with your veterinarian well in advance of any need of such procedures.

New Foal Checklist

Make sure the foal is breathing.

Soak the umbilical stump in 7% iodine solution for 30 seconds.

Make sure the mare expels the afterbirth and check for completeness.

Make sure the foal nurses within three hours to receive colostrum.

Make sure the foal is protected against tetanus by colostrum or vaccination.

Give the foal an enema to ensure meconium passes.

Check the umbilical cord for several days for the presence of urine.

Check that the eyelids and lashes are turned out.

Get your veterinarian's advice about limb deformities or hernias.

Watch the mare for several days for signs of reproductive tract infection.

After the Delivery

The first few hours are critical in the development of a strong maternal bond between mare and foal. The mare will usually lie quietly, often licking her foal and nickering to him. As she starts to get up, make sure she does not tread on the foal.

Soon after delivery, the foal will roll up onto his chest and attempt to stand. It takes about an hour for a foal to gain enough coordination and strength to stand on his own. If the foal is not able to stand after two hours, consult your veterinarian.

As soon as the foal is able to stand, he will begin to search for a teat. This is a trial-and-error process and does not happen at once. Given time and assistance from his mother, the foal will find the teat and begin to nurse. If the foal is not nursing successfully within three hours of standing, something may be wrong and the foal should be checked.

It is good practice to examine the mare to be sure her teats are open and the nipples are well-formed and not inverted. It is essential that the foal receive the first milk of the mare, since it contains the all-important maternal antibodies that protect against newborn infections.

The first few hours of the foal's life present an excellent opportunity to imprint useful resistance-free behaviors on the new foal (see *Imprinting*, page 527). These behaviors help socialize the foal to humans and make him easier to handle and train later.

Resistance-free exercises include pressing down on the withers and lifting and stroking the girth. Repeat until resistance disappears. Other desensitizing exercises include rubbing the ears and head, examining the teeth and mouth, and taking the rectal temperature. Imprinting should be done gradually and

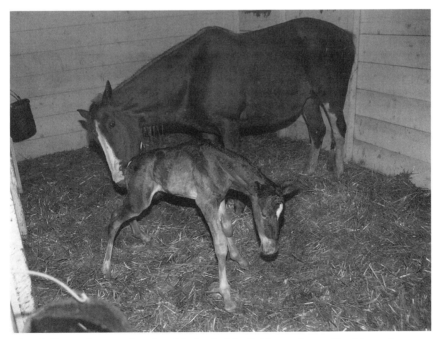

After delivery, the mare bonds with the foal by licking and nuzzling him as he attempts to stand.

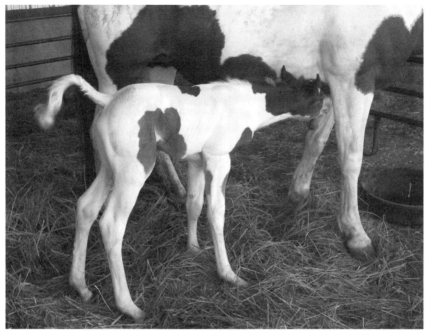

The foal may not always be successful looking for the udder. You must exhibit patience, allowing the foal time to find his dinner. If the foal has not successfully nursed within three hours of birth, there may be a problem; contact your veterinarian.

gently and with the acceptance of the mother. Do not separate mother and foal for resistance-free exercises. Repeat daily for three days.

Exercise is beneficial for both the mare and her foal. Begin on the first or second day by turning them out into an empty paddock or small field for 15 to 30 minutes twice a day. This amount of exercise will not tire the mare or the foal. Increase exercise gradually as weather permits. By two weeks, the mare and foal can be left out most of the day, unless the weather is very cold or wet. Foals cannot regulate their body temperature in extreme conditions until they are 4 to 6 weeks old. They should be separated from other horses until the foal is 3 to 4 weeks old.

WORMING AND VACCINATIONS

Twelve hours after foaling, the mare should be dewormed with ivermectin, which is effective against threadworms, ascarids, and large and small strongyles. In threadworm problem areas, treat the foal at three weeks of age. For routine deworming of foals, see chapter 2, "Parasites."

Foals at birth are capable of forming antibodies in response to vaccination, although the immune response is much weaker than it will be at 4 months of age. Tetanus antitoxin is no longer routinely administered, since it has been

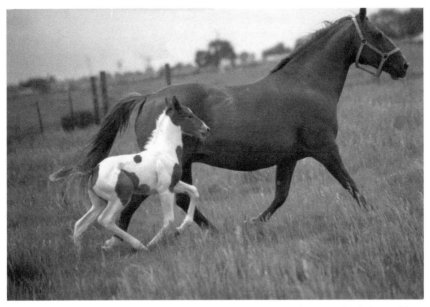

Exercise is good for the foal and the mare. By two weeks, they can be left outside most of the day, if weather permits.

associated with fatal cases of serum hepatitis. It is only indicated if the mother was not vaccinated against tetanus, in which case both tetanus antitoxin and tetanus toxoid should be given. For recommended vaccinations, see *Immunization Schedule* (page 100).

CARE OF THE MARE

The postpartum mare is susceptible to constipation and colic. To prevent these problems, cut back her feed by half. Gradually increase it over the next ten days until she is back on full ration.

As the uterus returns to its normal size, the mare will have a dark chocolate-colored vaginal discharge, which disappears by the seventh day. A persistent discharge, a yellow discharge, a heavy bloody discharge, or a foul-smelling, pus-like discharge is abnormal. The mare should be checked for delayed uterine involution, retained placenta, and postpartum metritis (see *Postpartum Problems*, page 534).

Note, however, that a foul discharge is not always present in cases of post-partum infection. Monitor the mare's temperature at frequent intervals throughout this period. A temperature above 101°F (38°C) indicates fever and infection.

Scaly skin and oily secretions tend to accumulate in the skin fold that divides the udder. Gently wash the mare's udder with warm water and Ivory soap to remove secretions. Repeat as necessary.

For the safety of the mare and to ensure that she is progressing on schedule, it is good practice to have your veterinarian examine her by rectal palpation one week after delivery. This is essential if you plan to breed her on the first postpartum heat (see *Breeding on the Foal Heat*, page 476).

MECONIUM COLIC

The foal should begin to pass meconium stools within the first 12 hours. Meconium is a greenish-brown to black material that accumulates in the foal's intestinal tract before birth. By the fourth day, meconium is replaced by the yellow feces of the normal neonatal foal.

When meconium is not passed, it becomes painfully impacted, usually in the small colon or rectum. Signs of meconium colic begin within 24 hours of birth. They include straining without passing meconium, restlessness, tail-switching, repeatedly getting up and down, rolling and thrashing, arching the back, and lying in an unusual position. The diagnosis is confirmed by digital rectal examination that reveals firm meconium within the rectum and pelvic colon.

Most foals with meconium colic respond to softening the stool. A prepackaged sodium phosphate enema or a soapy water enema will often relieve a simple impaction. The tip of the tube is carefully inserted its full length into

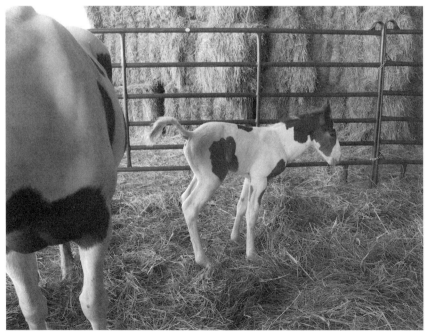

This newborn foal strains to pass meconium stool.

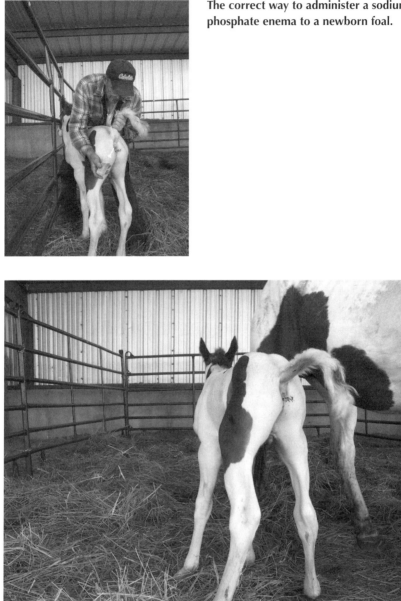

The correct way to administer a sodium phosphate enema to a newborn foal.

The foal successfully passes the meconium after his enema.

the foal's rectum and the enema administered without excessive pressure. Hold the tail down for a few minutes to prevent immediate return of the enema. If no response occurs within one hour, administer a second enema.

Your veterinarian may decide to give the foal a dose of mineral oil (250 ml) or a laxative such as milk of magnesia (8 ounces, 237 ml) by stomach tube to complete the flushing-out process. The mineral oil should pass in 24 hours. In unresponsive cases, surgery is required.

To prevent impaction, some people routinely give the foal a sodium phosphate enema after he is on his feet and has nursed. Meconium impactions may need to be treated by your veterinarian with a retention enema of acetylcysteine. This may resolve the problem without surgery.

It is important to note that your veterinarian must be called if two enemas have been given without successfully passing the meconium stool. *This is an emergency!*

Imprinting

The concept of imprinting was popularized more than 20 years ago by Robert Miller, DVM, after years of work and study with new foals. Many horse people are using some form of imprinting with great success. The idea is to handle the foal after birth when he is very impressionable, because this will make it far easier to handle and work with him in the future. Miller says imprinting should be done within 45 minutes of birth. Many horse owners are not lucky enough to be in attendance at birth, however. Imprinting is still effective later, but it needs to be done as soon as possible.

The basis of imprinting is to desensitize the baby to touching and handling by humans. This is accomplished by repeatedly rubbing or touching a foal in a specific spot until the foal relaxes and accepts the action without fear. You then repeat the rubbing and touching over the foal's whole body. It is extremely important to remember to touch both sides of the foal, because he needs to learn and accept the actions with both sides of his brain.

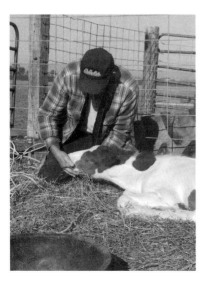

Imprinting the foal shortly after birth will help make later procedures, such as deworming, stress free.

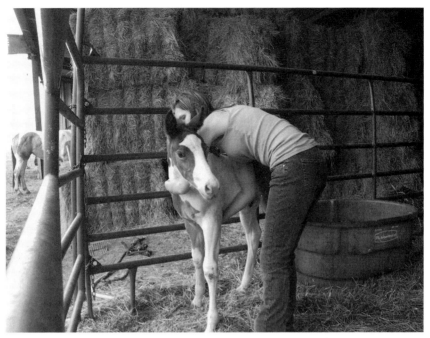

Imprinting this baby is stress free, and he is already learning to have pressure around his girth and to be restrained. From his eye level, the girl is above him, the way a rider will be when he is an adult.

Starting with the foal's head, stroke the entire face. Play with nostrils, even placing your fingers inside the cavity. Handle the colt's mouth, placing your fingers where the bit will someday lie. Stroke his ears inside and out. Once the foal accepts these actions—resistance free—move on to the neck and then the body.

Oftentimes, the underside of the foal is sensitive and he may be protective of his vital organs. The key is to continue rubbing or stroking until the foal relaxes. Put your arms around the girth area, squeeze and relax, simulating the feel of a saddle. Leaning down over the back of the foal while squeezing enables the colt to see you on his back in a nonthreatening way. After stroking the legs, pick up each foot, tapping on it lightly, similar to what a farrier will do.

For safety, the mare should be restrained so she does not get aggressive toward the person doing the imprinting. Studies have been done to see if imprinting affects the bonding between mare and foal. Although there do not seem to be any bonding problems, it does seem wise to allow the mare and foal a little time to acquaint themselves with each other before you begin imprinting exercises. If the colt does not rise right away, imprinting can be done with the foal lying on the ground; it does not need to be in a standing position.

If this process is repeated the first three days of the foal's life, it will reinforce this positive behavior even if the foal is turned out and not handled again until weaning. Imprinting reduces the stress of handling the foal in the future as he grows.

Dystocia (Prolonged Labor)

The prolongation of any stage of labor is called *dystocia*. Most cases of dystocia originate with the foal. Usually, the size or position of the foal creates a blockage in the birth canal that cannot be overcome by intense and forceful straining. In time, the mare becomes exhausted and the uterus is unable to contract, even after the blockage has been removed. This is called uterine inertia.

In horses, the length of the second stage of labor is critical. Once the water bag ruptures and the foal begins to descend, the placenta begins to detach and follow. If the foal is not born within 40 minutes, there is an increasing risk of fetal mortality. Accordingly, urgent veterinary assistance is needed if you suspect dystocia. A first suspicion would be if the forelegs do not appear at the vaginal opening 15 minutes after the water breaks.

Beyond risk to the foal, difficult and prolonged labor is associated with frequent complications in the mare. They include injuries to the birth canal, acute metritis, retained placenta, delayed uterine involution, rupture of the uterus, and prolapse of the uterus.

The most common causes of dystocia are discussed in this section. Other, less common causes of dystocia include hydrocephalus, contracted foal syndrome, torsion of the uterus, prolonged pregnancy with a large foal, hydrops amnion, ruptured prepubic tendon, and vaginal blockages caused by tumors or blood clots.

ABNORMAL PRESENTATIONS

Abnormal presentations are the most common cause of difficult or arrested labor. Presentation refers to the alignment of the long axis of the foal with the long axis of the dam. In a longitudinal presentation, the spine of the foal is parallel to the spine of the mother. In a transverse presentation, the two spines are at right angles. Presentation also refers to the part of the foal approaching the pelvic outlet (either head or tail).

Position is the relationship of the back of the foal to the four quadrants of the mare's pelvis: the sacrum, the right and left ileum, and the pubis. The normal position places the foal's back against the mare's sacrum. Thus, the normal orientation is called the anterior longitudinal presentation, dorsosacral position, with the head, neck, and forelimbs extended.

Abnormal presentations and positions prevent delivery by increasing the size of the presenting parts in relation to the fixed diameter of the pelvic canal. Suspect a problem delivery if:

- The two front feet do not appear at the vaginal opening within 15 minutes after the water breaks
- The feet appear but you do not see the nose and face following closely
- You see anything other than the head and nose between the two forelegs with the pads pointing down

The mare should be examined vaginally by your veterinarian as soon as possible to determine the cause of the problem.

The most common malpresentations are deviations of the head and neck. In the lateral deviation, the neck is bent to the side with the nose pointing toward the hind feet. In the ventral deviation, the head is bent down against the chest so the crown (instead of the nose) presents.

A common abnormal presentation is one in which one or both forelimbs are not extended. A leg can be bent at the elbow and caught in back of the pelvic brim, or folded under the foal with the feet pointing backward. You might see only one leg at the vaginal opening.

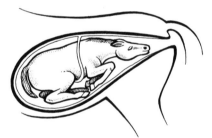

A common malpresentation with the forelegs folded. Push the foal back into the birth canal, then grasp and extend each leg.

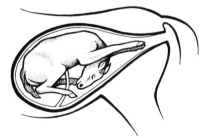

Ventral deviation of the head. Push the foal back into the birth canal, grasp the muzzle, and extend the head.

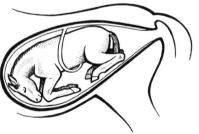

A posterior presentation. Under epidural anesthesia, it may be possible to draw out each back leg. Cesarean section is usually required.

Abnormal presentations of the foal.

A posterior or backward presentation is when the tail enters the birth canal instead of the head. You might see one or both rear legs protruding from the vulva. In a true breech, the back legs are tucked beneath the body and the rump is the presenting part. The posterior presentation is rare, occurring in 1 of 500 deliveries.

The most common malposition is one in which the foal does not rotate into the normal dorsosacral position. In this situation, the foal enters the birth canal on his side or on his back, with the pads of the feet pointing up.

Treatment: Abnormal presentations should be corrected as soon as possible. It is easier to do this before the foal becomes wedged tightly into the birth canal and the uterus is dry and contracted.

Regardless of the presentation or position, the legs of a full-term foal must be extended and the neck straightened out before the foal can pass through the birth canal. This is accomplished using a procedure called repulsion, in which the foal is pushed back into the uterus far enough to obtain room to grasp and pull out the legs or straighten the neck and extend the head.

The mare should be restrained and kept in a standing position, if possible. Epidural anesthesia is of great assistance. Intrauterine manipulation requires the use of sterile techniques and a long-arm obstetrical glove. Be advised that if an arm is caught between the foal and the wall of the uterus during a forceful contraction, it can easily be broken. Injuries to the birth canal also can occur during such attempts. Accordingly, intrauterine manipulation by a nonprofessional should be attempted only in a true emergency or when expert help is completely unavailable. One of the most effective things you can do while waiting for the veterinarian is to keep the mare on her feet and walking. This can retard labor for 30 to 60 minutes.

In addition to correcting an abnormal presentation by manipulating the foal's position, traction may be necessary. Obstetrical chains and blunt hooks are applied to parts of the foal to pull on him as the uterus contracts. Traction becomes less effective with the passage of time. The uterus contracts down around the foal, and the vaginal canal, initially well-lubricated by the ruptured sac, becomes very dry.

Although most abnormal presentations can be corrected by obstetric manipulation, cesarean section (see page 533) is occasionally necessary. It is indicated if there has been little or no progress after a reasonable attempt at obstetrical manipulation and the foal is alive with a chance for survival.

If the foal is already dead and cannot be delivered by repulsion and traction, your veterinarian may elect to remove it by fetotomy. The fetus is dismembered (using one or two incisions) and removed in parts. This is not without risk of lacerating the birth canal. If fetotomy cannot be performed with a minimum of dissection, it is safer to proceed to cesarean section.

OTHER CAUSES OF DYSTOCIA

Premature Separation of the Placenta (Red Bag Dystocia)

Separation of the placenta before the foal moves into the birth canal is rare. When it does happen, the placenta precedes the foal. Signs are those of difficult labor with the appearance of a red, basketball-like structure at the vulva. Behind the placenta is the intact water sac, which is prevented from entering the birth canal. The entire process arrests labor and must be immediately corrected to prevent asphyxiation of the foal.

Treatment: Rupture the protruding membrane using a pair of sharp scissors. Remove the placental membranes from the foal's nostrils to enable him to breathe. Labor should proceed quickly. Be prepared to revive a depressed foal (see page 520).

Small Pelvic Opening

A 2-year-old mare may be too immature to have developed an adequate pelvic outlet. A previously fractured pelvis is another cause of a narrow birth canal.

Treatment: Proceed to cesarean section. If the narrow pelvis is diagnosed before labor, C-section can be done electively. The size of the pelvic opening can be determined during the breeding soundness exam.

Twins

The presence of twins frequently prevents normal delivery because neither foal has room to enter the birth canal. The situation is further compounded if one or both of the foals are dead.

Treatment: This situation is difficult to correct if not recognized promptly. When both twins are in a normal anterior presentation, it may be possible to push one back into the uterus to allow the other room to come out. Once the first twin is delivered, the second follows without difficulty. An elective C-section should be considered when the diagnosis is made during pregnancy.

Uterine Inertia

Mechanical obstruction is the most common cause of uterine muscle fatigue. The uterus is so exhausted that it loses its ability to expel the foal even after a blockage has been corrected. Another cause of inertia is a weak uterine muscle. This can occur with age or chronic scarring.

Treatment: An inert uterus contracts tightly around the foal. This makes it even more difficult to complete the delivery. Cesarean section will be required.

WHEN TO CALL THE VETERINARIAN

Toward the end of the mare's gestation, call your veterinarian and discuss who will be available to cover for an emergency. Do not hesitate to call a veterinarian if you have any concern about the progress of labor. Most equine obstetrical emergencies are associated with impending or actual fetal distress. They will not correct with time. Someone must be prepared to step in quickly and save the life of the foal.

In summary, something is wrong when:

- The mare is in labor for more than four hours without rupture of the water bag.
- The water breaks but the front feet are not present at the vulva within 15 minutes.
- The foal is not delivered within 40 minutes.
- The foal presents in any orientation other than the normal anterior longitudinal presentation.
- A thick red membrane (instead of a shiny white one) appears at the vulva, indicating premature separation of the placenta.
- The placenta is not delivered within three hours after foaling.
- The placenta appears unhealthy or has pieces missing.
- The foal does not nurse within three hours after birth.

CESAREAN SECTION

Cesarean section is indicated to retrieve a live foal when arrested labor cannot be easily corrected by obstetrics. It is also indicated to remove a dead fetus that cannot be removed by fetotomy.

The operation is done through the flank or abdomen, with the mare recumbent and under anesthesia. The foal is removed and the incision in the uterus is closed with interlocking sutures to prevent postoperative bleeding. If the placenta does not separate easily at the time of surgery, it can be freed up and allowed to pass spontaneously in a few hours.

Proper operating room facilities must be available to perform a cesarean section. Elective and emergency C-sections can be done at equine veterinary hospitals and stud farms with operating facilities. Emergency C-sections in the field, away from anesthesia, padded operating tables, sterile instruments, and support facilities, cannot be done successfully.

Survival rates for mare and foal are good for elective C-sections. For emergency C-sections, they diminish rapidly with the length of labor. When used as a last resort, the prognosis for foal and mare survival is poor.

A disadvantage of a C-section is that it predisposes a mare to metritis and uterine scarring, which impairs future fertility.

Following a cesarean section, a mare may be too weak or exhausted to care for her foal. Due to failure of the recognition process, she may not bond with her foal or be willing to accept him. Accordingly, many C-section foals have to be raised as orphans.

Postpartum Problems

Problems that can affect the mare after delivery include postpartum hemorrhage, injuries to the birth canal, retained placenta, invagination of a uterine horn, acute metritis, and prolapsed uterus. Some mares may have problems with their milk supply, or develop mastitis and *edema* of the udder. A mare who refuses to accept and care for her foal is a difficult management problem.

HEMORRHAGE

Internal bleeding is a serious, often fatal complication caused by rupture of a large blood vessel in the pelvis or the wall of the uterus. Signs include severe pain in the abdomen, followed by weakness, staggering, pale mucous membranes, shock, and collapse. There is no external sign of bleeding.

External bleeding is apparent as bleeding through the birth canal. It is due to a laceration of the cervix, vagina, or perineum, generally caused by the foal's feet or by obstetrical manipulation. Bleeding from the wall of the uterus can occur if the placenta is torn prematurely in third-stage labor.

Treatment: Surgical intervention for internal bleeding in this situation is not successful. Confine the mare to a dark, quiet stall and keep her as calm as possible. Sedation is of benefit. The bleeding may stop spontaneously.

If you are able to see a bleeding artery, maintain pressure with a sterile dressing and call your veterinarian. The mare may need to be treated for shock and blood loss. Lacerations that do not stop bleeding should be sutured, if possible. When this is not technically feasible, the uterus and vagina can be packed with strips of gauze coated with petroleum jelly. Lacerations of the cervix should be repaired when uterine involution is complete—two to three weeks postpartum.

PERINEAL AND VULVAR LACERATIONS

Birth-related injuries to the vagina and vulva are common. A mare delivering her first foal is more likely to sustain such an injury, as are mares who go through difficult or prolonged labor.

Most perineal lacerations are caused by the feet of the foal. The feet can actually tear through the shelf between the vagina and the rectum and protrude through the anus. This happens most often with upside-down presentations.

Vulvar and vaginal bleeding occur from enlarged veins in the hymen area. The bleeding usually is not serious and stops spontaneously.

Treatment: Perineal lacerations should be repaired within a few hours, unless the tissue is swollen and hemorrhagic, in which case it is best to cleanse the wound and repair the injury in three to six weeks.

RETAINED PLACENTA

The placenta is normally expelled 30 minutes to 3 hours after foaling. Bacteria grow rapidly in the retained placenta and the uterus. After three hours, the placenta releases toxic by-products of this bacterial growth that initiate postpartum complications, including acute toxic metritis, laminitis, and blood poisoning. The frequency and severity of these problems depend on the amount of placental tissue retained and the length of time before it is removed.

Retained placenta is nearly always associated with arrested or difficult labor. It is seldom a problem after a normal, uncomplicated delivery.

If the intact placenta does not pass in three hours, or if examination reveals a tear or a missing piece, notify your veterinarian without delay.

Treatment: It involves the injection or infusion of oxytocin, which stimulates uterine contractions and aids in expulsion of the placenta. If the placenta is not expelled within two hours after a course of oxytocin, your veterinarian may infuse the uterus or the retained placenta itself with large volumes of warm, sterile water. In most cases, the placenta will be released using one or both of these methods. Antibiotics are indicated when the reproductive tract has been contaminated and when placental passage has been unduly prolonged.

DELAYED UTERINE INVOLUTION

Immediately after foaling, the uterus begins to shrink and return to its normal size and shape. This process is called *involution*. It occurs rapidly. By one week postpartum, the uterus is down to about twice the normal size. Some mares are ready to conceive and maintain a pregnancy by the 15th day after foaling. In others, the process takes longer (see *Breeding on the Foal Heat*, page 476).

Uterine involution is helped by nursing and exercise. Nursing releases oxytocin, which causes the uterus to contract. Exercise promotes uterine tone and strengthens the abdominal wall muscles.

Delayed involution is of concern because of the possibility that retained placental tissue is the cause of the delay. In addition, the slow progress of involution in mares who have had two or more foals and in older mares makes it unlikely that they can be bred on the foal heat.

Treatment: The size and shape of the uterus can be determined by rectal palpation. If your veterinarian finds that involution is not proceeding according to schedule, they may want to administer oxytocin to stimulate uterine contractions. If retained placental tissue is suspected, a uterine biopsy is helpful in confirming this diagnosis. Treat as described in *Retained Placenta* (see page 535).

POSTPARTUM METRITIS

This is an uncommon but serious infection of the entire uterine wall, characterized by the rapid onset of toxemia, blood poisoning, and laminitis. It tends to occur among mares who have had a prolonged or complicated labor, a retained placenta, or massive contamination of the uterus.

Signs of acute toxic metritis begin 12 to 36 hours after foaling. They include fever, increased pulse and respiration, and marked apathy and depression. The vaginal discharge is reddish-brown and foul-smelling. A pounding digital pulse signifies the onset of laminitis.

Treatment: It is directed at evacuating the uterus, which usually contains several gallons of infected blood and pus. This is best accomplished by inserting a large-bore stomach tube into the uterus and flushing it with large volumes of warm, sterile water until the recovered fluid is clear. Antibiotics are instilled when the uterus is empty. This procedure is repeated twice a day, as necessary, for several days. The mare is also given intravenous oxytocin and antibiotics.

Laminitis may occur at any time in a mare with acute metritis, and can be severe enough to cause sloughing of the hooves. Intravenous flunixin meglumine is given to prevent the circulatory disturbances associated with the development of laminitis. It is continued until the toxemia is controlled. Shortening the course of toxemia with early, vigorous treatment of the infected uterus reduces the likelihood of laminitis.

INVAGINATION OF THE UTERINE HORN

In mares with this condition, one horn of the uterus turns inside-out and projects into the body of the uterus, where it can be felt by intrauterine palpation. Invagination is often associated with a retained placenta in that horn, the invagination occurring as a result of traction during attempts to expel the placenta. Signs include colic and restlessness beyond the ordinary. The diagnosis is made on postpartum examination performed for colic that is unresponsive to analgesics.

Treatment: Before placing the horn back to its normal position, a placenta (if present) must be manually removed. The horn is then kneaded inward until it returns to its former position. Infusing of 1 or 2 gallons (3.8 to 7.5 l) of warm, sterile water into the uterus facilitates complete replacement. Aftercare is like that described for *Retained Placenta* (see page 535).

PROLAPSED UTERUS

This is an uncommon complication in which the uterus turns inside-out and protrudes through the vulva. Prolonged straining during and after a difficult delivery, and pulling on the umbilical cord in a misguided attempt to deliver a retained placenta, are two common causes.

The uterus must be replaced as soon as possible to prevent shock and further complications. This procedure is quite difficult and requires a veterinarian.

Treatment: While waiting for the veterinarian, wrap the prolapse in a clean towel or sheet moistened with warm water to protect the everted uterus from further contamination. Keep the mare on her feet and walking. This slows down contractions and keeps the mare from lacerating the uterus by backing up against sharp objects.

Before attempting to replace the uterus, the mare should be sedated to prevent straining. Sedation can be achieved using drugs, or by giving an epidural or general anesthetic. The uterus is carefully and thoroughly cleansed with disinfectant soap and then worked back through the pelvic opening until it is completely reduced. Antibiotics are placed into the uterine cavity and then the vulva is sutured. Intravenous oxytocin and antibiotics are administered to shrink the uterus and prevent postpartum metritis.

A mare who has had a uterine prolapse is apt to do so again on the next foaling.

MARES WHO REJECT OR INJURE THEIR FOALS

A mare learns to recognize and care for her offspring as the foal is born, cleaned, and begins to nurse. Hormonal changes during and after delivery sensitize the mare's central nervous system to the sight, sound, and especially the smell and taste of her newborn foal.

For various reasons, a mare's brain may not respond to the usual sensory stimuli and the imprinting process fails to take place. For example, if a mare has had a prolonged labor or a C-section, exhaustion combined with artificial conditions can derail normal behavior. Arabians have a higher incidence of foal rejection than other breeds. Studies suggest that many neglectful mothers were rejected foals themselves or were raised away from the companionship of other horses.

There are two main categories of foal rejection. Refusal to allow suckling is the most frequent and aggression toward the foal is the most dangerous. Refusal to allow suckling generally occurs in first-time mothers. Often, it is the pain of a distended udder that seems to cause this behavior. The foal can be injured during the mare's attempts to evade or escape suckling attempts.

Rarely, a mare attacks and savages her foal, usually biting him on the withers. Because this behavior is similar to that of the foal-savaging stallion, it has been suggested that it may be caused by masculinization of the mare's central nervous system by mechanisms unknown. Hormone therapy has been attempted, with inconsistent results.

Treatment: The mare who refuses to allow her foal to nurse should be adequately restrained while one or two handlers assist the foal in locating the teat. Once the mare realizes that suckling relieves udder distension and pain, she usually accepts the foal. If the mare continues to refuse suckling, she can be restrained in a stall divided by a horizontal bar at shoulder height. The bar is placed so that it holds the mare against a wall but the foal can go beneath the bar to nurse. Consult with your veterinarian for further help, if needed.

Tranquilizing the mare is an alternative. However, tranquilizers are passed in the milk and may tranquilize the foal, resulting in ineffective nursing.

The mare who attempts to physically injure her foal is a most difficult problem. Attempts to reunite the foal and dam usually prove futile. The mare and foal must be watched at all times to prevent injury to the foal. Keep in mind that a foal nurses every 15 to 20 minutes during the first week of life. If you do not have the resources to deal with this problem, it is best to remove the foal and raise him as an orphan (see page 542).

Lactation

The mare's udder is made of two separate milk sacs, which lie on either side of the midline between her back legs. Each milk sac has two mammary glands, or lobes. The milk ducts of the two lobes come together to form a common duct, which opens at the nipple or teat. Thus, although the mare has four mammary lobes, she has only two teats.

Milk letdown is controlled by oxytocin released from the pituitary gland during labor and delivery. Tactile stimulation of the teats (suckling or washing) helps trigger the release.

FEEDING DURING LACTATION

The mare's nutrient requirements during lactation are greater than at any other time in her life. A lactating mare produces three times her own weight in milk in five months of lactation. Nutrient requirements during the first three months of lactation are shown in the table on page 395. In essence, the lactating mare requires almost twice as much energy and more than twice as much protein, calcium, phosphorus, and vitamin A than a normal mare.

When good-quality grass hay or grass forage is being fed free-choice, a mare cannot consume enough feed to meet these requirements. However, if you are feeding unrestricted amounts of high-quality alfalfa or lush green legumes, she should be able to consume enough roughage to meet these nutritional needs—with the exception perhaps of phosphorus, which can be supplied free-choice by a salt-mineral mix such as monodicalcium phosphate (see the table on page 404). Hay or forage of this high quality is often not available, though, which means you will have to feed a grain supplement. Half hay and half grain, by weight, is suitable. Many good commercial diets are available for lactating mares. Vitamin A supplements (and supplemented feeds) are of greatest value when used during lactation. The lactating mare needs 30,000 IU of vitamin A per day. Alfalfa and legume hay stored for less than six months may meet these requirements. Corn is the only grain that contains significant amounts. In most cases, you'll need to add a supplement.

If you have been feeding a commercial ration as the sole source of feed, note that standard horse rations do not contain enough protein for the lactating mare and quite often are deficient in lysine, an amino acid essential for high-quality milk production and foal growth. A protein supplement such as soybean meal should be added to the diet. Soybean meal is an excellent source of both protein and lysine.

Some commercial grain supplements are designed to be fed to lactating mares along with hay or equivalent forage. These rations will meet protein and energy requirements when fed according to the directions. Foal *creep feeds* and mare and foal pellets, are examples.

Keep trace-mineralized salt available for free-choice consumption. A nursing mother requires a great deal of water and should have access to a fresh supply at all times. This often means an extra bucket in the stall, filled twice as often as usual.

NURSING PROBLEMS

One condition that originates with either the dam or the foal is the failure of *passive transfer* of maternal antibodies, which occurs if the foal does not nurse during the first 18 hours of life. Failure to receive colostrum, the first milk of the dam, is the single most important cause of neonatal infections. For more information, see *Lack of Colostrum* (page 549).

Agalactia (Insufficient Milk)

For the first two to three months of life, the foal's nutritional requirements are entirely met by his mother's milk. When the milk does not come in spontaneously after foaling, warm compresses to the udder and an injection of oxytocin may initiate the flow. If not, the problem is most likely due to inherent failure of the mammary glands to produce milk. The foal will have to be raised as an orphan.

Mares on tall fescue pastures in the southeastern United States experience a high incidence of agalactia because they often ingest a specific fungus that grows on the grass. The fungus produces an alkaloid that blocks pituitary prolactin. Prolactin is the hormone that stimulates milk production.

Insufficient production of milk is suggested by the appearance and behavior of the foal. A foal who is not getting enough milk is thin and nurses vigorously, but never seems to be satisfied.

The volume and composition of milk produced is not related to the mare's consumption of feed—at least not initially. A mare fed less energy than needed will make up the difference at the expense of her own weight and body stores. It is only after she uses up all her reserves and her weight drops to a body condition score of 4 or less (see *Weight Gain or Loss*, page 420) that her milk production begins to decline.

Treatment: A diet high in energy, protein, and other nutrients, sufficient to enable her to gain weight back to the ideal condition, will help prevent this problem from occurring. The mare also should be given unrestricted access to water and trace-mineralized salt. Mares exposed to fescue toxicity may be given domperidone to prevent the risk of lengthened gestation and also to stimulate milk production. Reserpine will also aid in normal milk production for mares who may have been exposed to fescue toxicity. If these measures are not successful, the mare most likely has an inherited defect in milk production. Begin supplementing the foal at an early age, as described in *The Orphan Foal* (see page 542).

Mastitis

Inflammation of one or more quarters of the mammary gland is called mastitis. It usually occurs a few weeks after foaling, but may occasionally occur before foaling. It is rare in mares.

The teat becomes warm, swollen, and painful. The swelling may extend to involve the undersurface of the abdomen. The mare may refuse to nurse or be unable to eject her milk. The milk from the infected gland appears curdled and usually contains blood. Laboratory examination of the milk will show bacteria; *Staphylococci* and *streptococci* are the most common.

Treatment: The foal should be temporarily removed and fed by hand, as described in *The Orphan Foal* (page 542). Empty the udders by hand to relieve pressure and continue milk production. Cold packs help reduce swelling. Antibiotics are started pending the results of bacteria culture. The infection responds rapidly to treatment. The foal can usually return to the mare in one week. However, if lactation has stopped, nothing can be done to restart the milk flow.

There is a type of noninfectious mastitis caused by eating the leaves, bark, or fruit of the avocado tree. In cases of avocado poisoning, milk production stops and there may be scarring of the milk-producing glands. If diagnosed early in the course of the disease, the mare can return to milk production within two weeks. When the glandular milk-producing tissues are extensively scarred, the mare may not recover or ever be able to produce milk again.

18

PEDIATRICS

Care of the newborn *foal* is discussed in *After the Delivery* (see page 521).

Feeding for the First Year
THE NEW FOAL

During the first two months of life, the foal receives all her nutrition from the milk of her mother, although she will begin to nibble on the mare's grain and hay when she is only a few days old. After 2 months of age, the foal's nutritional needs are increasing while the mother's milk supply is stable or decreasing. At or before 2 months of age, begin to feed a creep ration.

A creep ration is a concentrate mix composed of processed grain specifically formulated to meet the needs of the nursing foal. Studies have shown that after 2 months of age, foals who are fed a creep ration free-choice gain weight at a significantly faster rate than foals who nurse exclusively. Nursing foals who don't eat a creep ration may experience a compensatory growth spurt shortly after weaning, when placed on a weaning diet. This compensatory growth spurt greatly increases the risk of incurring a developmental orthopedic disease. Foals on a creep-feeding program, however, do not experience this growth spurt.

The National Research Council recommends that a *creep feed* contain 23 percent crude protein, 1.4 percent calcium, and 0.8 percent phosphorus, based on the total weight of the ration. Such creep feeds can be purchased from feed stores or formulated using grains and concentrates (using the online resource Nutrient Requirements of Horses, www.nap.edu/catalog).

Creep feeds are fed free-choice with all the hay or forage the nursing foal will eat. There is no need to restrict the amount of creep feed eaten by the foal until she is consuming 4 to 5 pounds (1.8 to 2.3 kg) a day. When this happens, start feeding one-half to three-quarters of a pound (227 to 340 g) per day, per 100 pounds (45 kg) body weight of the foal. If you do not restrict the creep ration this way, some foals will eat too much creep feed and be at increased risk for a developmental orthopedic disease.

The creep ration should be divided into equal portions and placed in the creep feeder at least twice daily. Remove moldy or wet feed. A creep feeding station can be designed by placing a feeder inside a fenced enclosure with an entrance just wide enough for a foal to go in, but too small for a *mare* to pass through. Alternately, you can place the ration in a feed box with bars across the top, spaced so that a foal (but not a mare) can put her nose through. A feeder can be placed in the corner of a stall and screened from the mare by bolting a strong board across the corner at a height that just allows the foal to go under.

Creep feeders in pastures should be placed in areas where the mare grazes. A foal won't use a creep feeder if it means being separated from her mother.

When several foals are using the same creep feeder, some may consume more grain than their daily allotment. It is best to separate and feed them individually. If this is not feasible, reduce the grain ration by half and make up the difference in weight using high-quality roughage, such as chopped alfalfa.

Keep trace-mineralized salt available at all times. Studies suggest that increasing the concentrations of copper and zinc in the creep feed to 50 mg per kilogram of body weight (on a dry matter basis) for copper and 60 mg per kilogram of body weight for zinc decreases the risk and incidence of developmental orthopedic disease. For more information, see *Trace Minerals* (page 405).

The Orphan Foal

A foal who is rejected by her mother or orphaned at birth can sometimes be raised by another lactating mare if one is available. Many breeding farms keep a nurse mare with foster mother qualities for this purpose. There may be a nurse mare farm in your area, and a mare can be ordered as needed. Your veterinarian or local school of veterinary medicine may know of a mare who may be available as a nurse. The process of getting a nurse mare to accept a foal can be dangerous and may require special restraint that may go on over a period of several days. When a newborn foal does not receive adequate colostrum from her true mother, follow the procedure described in *Lack of Colostrum* (see page 549).

Generally, most mares will accept an orphan foal within 12 to 72 hours if they are well enough restrained that the foal can nurse repeatedly without being injured. Tranquilization should be avoided because most tranquilizers are transferred in milk and may sedate the nursing foal. If it is necessary, it should be done only under strict guidance from your veterinarian. Methods for restraint are discussed in *Mares Who Reject or Injure Their Foal* (see page 537).

The first 30 minutes after birth is the best time to substitute a live foal for a stillbirth. Since mares rely primarily on their sense of smell for close-up identification, it is helpful to make the foal smell like the mare. You can smear the foal with amniotic fluid or coat the foal with the mare's sweat, milk, or feces. Occasionally, the stillborn placenta or stillborn skin can be used.

On some farms the use of a milk goat has been successful. Many nannies readily accept foals. The composition of goat's milk is different from mare's milk, but not enough to cause problems. The nanny (or nannies) may need to stand on a raised platform, but foals are very adept at learning to nurse from a nanny goat.

If a foster mother is not available, the foal can be raised by hand. This involves the use of a milk substitute and attention to feeding and hygiene. A good-quality commercial milk replacer, such as Foal-Lac, Mare's Match, or Mare's Milk Plus, is the most suitable substitute for mare's milk.

The dietary energy and water requirements of a young foal are extremely high. As a result, a large volume of milk must be consumed—14 quarts (13 l) per day for a newborn foal. Add 1 quart (1 l) per week until the foal is consuming 18 to 20 quarts (17 to 19 l) per day. Milk replacer is reconstituted with water according to the directions on the package. Also follow the manufacturer's instructions for frequency and amount to feed. In general, milk replacer is fed in four or more equal feedings. If the foal is less than 1 week old, often she will need to be feed every one to two hours, beginning with half the daily requirement during the first 24 hours and increasing to the full daily requirement thereafter. The purpose of starting slowly is to avoid digestive upset and diarrhea.

The milk replacer can be given by bottle or bucket. Bucket feeding is easier, safer, and faster than bottle feeding. Bucket feeding reduces the behavior problems resulting from the foal associating food with human contact. Start with a shallow pan, so the foal's nose can touch the bottom. Dip your fingers into the milk and allow the foal to suck on your fingers. If the foal does not suck well, move your fingers against her tongue and palate to stimulate a better suckling reflex. Once the foal begins to suck, encourage her to drink by lowering your fingers, along with her head, into the pan. It may take only a few minutes or up to two hours to teach a foal to drink from a pan, but with time and patience this is easily accomplished.

Once the foal learns to drink from the pan without submerging her nostrils, switch to a plastic bucket with a wide opening. Hang the bucket in a convenient location. Foals typically drink small amounts frequently both day and night. Clean all feeding equipment and change the buckets every 12 hours. Also provide continuous access to fresh water.

When the foal is several days old, begin feeding milk replacer (milk transition) pellets, which are available from feed stores. Start by putting pellets in the foal's mouth several times a day. Then put as many pellets in a bucket or creep feeder as the foal will eat and keep it refilled. Old pellets should be discarded twice a day.

After the foal is eating 2 to 3 pounds (1 to 1.4 kg) of pellets a day, add a high-quality creep feed ration, as described on page 541. As soon as the foal is eating 4 to 6 pounds (1.8 to 2.7 kg) of this creep feed and pelleted mixture a

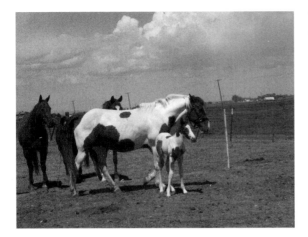

The foal should be introduced to the herd under supervision to avoid injury. Note how the mare keeps between the other horses and her foal. The other horses will be curious and the mare may kick out at them.

day, the pellets can be stopped. At 4 months of age, the orphan foal can be fed as a normal weanling.

Orphan foals are at risk of developing behavior problems later in life, especially if they are hand raised. It is best to find a nurse mare or at least a companion to provide a normal herd environment.

Inducing Lactation in a Nonpregnant Mare

This protocol, although experimental at this time, shows promise for the horse owner faced with an orphan foal and no lactating nurse mare. It requires a mare who has had at least one foal previously and nursed successfully. This experimental protocol originated with researchers in Belgium and was modified and simplified by a group at the Hagyard Equine Medical Institute in Lexington, Kentucky. In this revised protocol, nonpregnant mares were given progesterone and estradiol injections on days 1 through 7 of the protocol. On days 1 through 10, the mares received twice-daily intramuscular injections of sulpiride. On day 7, they received a single injection of lutalyse.

Starting on the first day of treatment, the orphan foal was put with the mare to provide suckle stimulus. Oxytocin was administered on a discretionary basis. Each foal was supplemented with mare's milk or milk replacement until the mare had enough milk to support the foal.

This revised protocol had an 80 percent success rate in inducing nonpregnant mares to lactate sufficiently to raise a foal.

THE WEANLING

Wild mares do not wean their foals until they are nearly 2 years old. This lengthy period of bonding and nursing is accompanied by increasing periods of independence, so that when the foal is finally weaned (usually because of a new foal), it occurs quite naturally and without physical or emotional trauma.

Artificially imposed weaning is stressful for both mare and foal. In foals, weaning-induced stress reduces feed intake and growth rate, depresses the immune system, and may cause disease. In her anxiety to return to her mother, the foal may incur injuries or the mare may injure herself. Most horse owners prefer to wean foals at 5 to 7 months of age, but foals can be weaned at 4 months of age without adverse effects on growth or development. However, foals younger than 4 months of age have yet to attain adult immune status, as indicated by levels of serum immunoglobulin (*IgG*). Accordingly, if there is no medical reason to wean early, it is probably best not to wean until a foal is at least 4 months old.

Before weaning, the foal should be in good health, on a vaccination and deworming program, and eating 1 pound (453 g) of creep ration daily for each month of age, as well as consuming some hay or pasture. Unless all of these conditions are met at least two weeks before weaning, do not wean. Five days before weaning, eliminate grain from the mare's ration to encourage her milk to dry up.

There are a number of weaning methods. The abrupt, complete separation of foal and mare works well for a herd of mares and foals. The selected mare is quietly led from the pasture while her foal is distracted. She is stabled or pastured completely out of sight and hearing of the herd. The foal is left in her former surroundings in the company of other mares and foals with whom she is familiar.

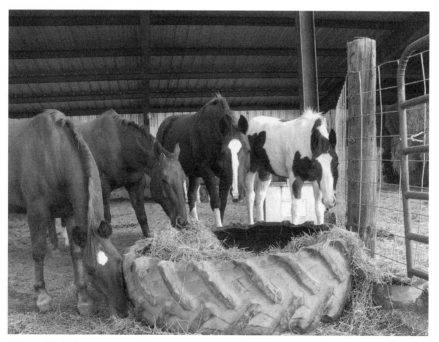

This foal is being prepared for eventual weaning. At 4 months of age, he is comfortably eating with familiar horses, temporarily separated from his mother.

A partial separation method seems to produce less anxiety, due to the reassuring presence of the mother. On the day of weaning, the mare is led into an adjacent pasture or paddock within sight and touch of her foal but separated by a secure fence that won't injure the foal but will prevent her from nursing. The fence can be made of chain link, small-weave mesh wire, or board with an electric wire.

If possible, leave the foal in her customary pasture and in the company of other horses or foals with whom she is familiar. Weaning is complete in one week, at which time the mare is removed entirely. To prevent the mare from coming back into milk, the mare and foal should remain separated for six weeks.

Feeding the Weanling

The nutrient requirements of the weanling foal at 6 months of age are shown in the table on page 395. Most weanlings will consume 2 to 2.3 percent of their body weight in feed per day. A 6-month-old weanling weighing 462 pounds (209 kg) will thus consume between 9.25 and 10.6 pounds (4.2 and 4.8 kg) of feed per day.

The daily ration of the average weanling (1,100 pounds, 500 kg, mature weight) should consist of 40 percent hay and 60 percent grain, by weight. As a rule of thumb, feed 1 pound (453 g) of grain for each month of age. At the same time, the weanling should consume at least 1 pound of good-quality roughage for every 100 pounds (45 kg) of body weight. If this amount is not being consumed, cut back on the amount of grain until it is consumed. Heavier breeds and larger horses should be fed slightly less, since they tend to grow more slowly than lighter horses.

An insufficient amount of calcium, phosphorus, or both will result in a mineral deficiency and resulting lameness and bone disease. These deficiencies can be prevented by making sure adequate amounts of both minerals are present in the weanling's diet (see the table on page 404). Of equal importance, the diet should contain more calcium than phosphorus to maintain a positive calcium-to-phosphorus ratio (ideally, 1.25:1). A properly formulated grain mix will contain adequate calcium and phosphorus to meet these mineral requirements. When feed sources are marginal, provide a supplemental mineral mix, as described in *Calcium and Phosphorus* (see page 404). Also make sure the diet consumed by the weanling (and the yearling) contains adequate concentrations of copper and zinc. For more information, see *Minerals* (page 400).

The table on page 402 shows the amount of commercial horse feed to provide along with good-quality hay or forage. Feeding instructions vary with the product. Feed commercial rations according to the guidelines provided by the manufacturer.

Overfeeding is a major problem in growing horses. Excessive weight gain and spurts of growth associated with overfeeding may cause or exacerbate developmental orthopedic diseases. Feeding more than 8 or 9 pounds (3.6 or 4 kg) of grain is not necessary or recommended unless hay quality is poor. When feeding a diet that is 60 percent grain concentrate mixture, the daily allotment of high-quality legume hay should be restricted to half a pound (226 g) per 100 pounds (45 kg) body weight of the mature horse. After 12 months of age, the amount of high-quality roughage consumed is no longer a concern.

Drying up the Mare

Immediately after removing her foal, stop feeding grain to the mare and reduce her daily hay or forage consumption to 1.5 to 2 pounds (680 to 907 g) per 100 pounds (45g) of body weight. The purpose of temporarily reducing feed and energy is to help stop milk production and excessive udder pressure and discomfort. Apply lanolin or hand lotion to the mare's udder, if necessary, to keep the skin from drying and cracking. However, do not milk out the mare. Milking stimulates and prolongs lactation. In addition, it is the buildup of pressure that stops the milk from forming.

Encourage the mare to exercise. Within one week the udder should be soft and flabby. When this happens, dietary restrictions are no longer needed.

If the newly weaned mare is in good condition, feed her a maintenance diet. If she is thin, feed additional forage and grain to increase her body weight and condition to moderately fleshy. If the mare is pregnant, see *Care and Feeding During Pregnancy* (page 504).

THE YEARLING

The average yearling achieves 65 to 70 percent of her mature weight by 12 months of age. Growth now slows and nutritional requirements do as well.

Diets for most yearlings should consist of 50 percent hay and 50 percent grain by weight. This is a lower grain ratio than for weanlings. Feed 1 pound (453 g) of grain mix concentrate per 100 pounds (45 kg) body weight of the horse per day, up to a maximum of 9 pounds (4 kg) of grain per day, until the horse reaches 90 percent of her anticipated adult weight. This occurs at about 2 years of age. Grain should be fed along with all the good-quality roughage the horse will eat.

A sample ration for feeding a yearling at 12 months of age using the online resource Nutrient Requirements of Horses, (www.nap.edu/catalog).

Preventive Medicine
VACCINATIONS

A foal who has received passive immunity through her mother's colostrum is protected from most infectious diseases for about five months. Although newborn foals are immune-competent and capable of forming antibodies in response to vaccination or natural infection, the immune response is weak in comparison to what it will be at five months of age, when the first vaccination series is usually given. During this transition period between maternal protection and vaccination-produced antibodies, the foal is most susceptible to infectious diseases. It is a good idea at this time to prevent unnecessary exposure to contagious diseases.

When, for a specific reason (such as obtaining a mare with unknown vaccination status in an area with a prevalent disease), early vaccination at 1 to 3 weeks of age is advisable, the vaccinations should repeated in two months, even though this will increase the number of vaccinations given. The recommended immunization schedule for foals and weanlings is listed in the table that begins on page 100.

At 1 year of age, administer annual booster vaccinations as shown in the table mentioned above.

Deworming

Most foals are infected very early in life with ascarids, threadworms, and pinworms. Foals also acquire other worm parasites, including strongyles and bots. Ascarids, threadworms, and the large and small strongyles, in particular, can cause delayed development and maturation, unthrifty appearance, and coughing. Even when foals show no signs, enough intestinal damage can occur to adversely affect feed use and growth.

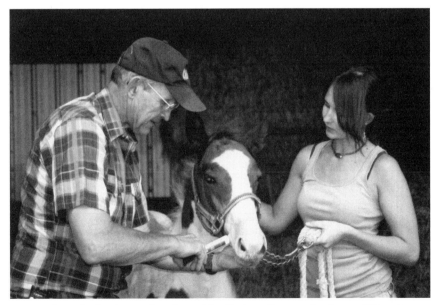

Deworming a foal at 2 months of age. Her first routine vaccinations will be given between 3 and 4 months old.

At 8 weeks of age, the foal should be started on a deworming schedule as described in *Interval Deworming* (see page 54). On this schedule, the foal is given a dewormer at 2 months of age and every other month until 12 months of age. The mature foal is then put on the same deworming schedule as an adult horse. On farms where threadworms are a problem, foals should be dewormed for threadworms at 1 week of age. At 1 year of age, the horse should be switched to an adult deworming schedule, as described in *Deworming Your Horse* (see page 51).

Do not use any dewormer that is not labeled for use in foals! This is especially true for moxidectin.

Diseases of the Foal

A number of diseases can affect the neonatal and growing foal. Although many of these diseases occur in adult horses as well, they do not pose the same threat to health and life as they do in foals.

Foals are especially susceptible to certain infections during the first few weeks of life, most notably foal septicemia, tetanus, rhinopneumonitis, equine influenza, and rotavirus infection. Signs of illness include listlessness, weakness, lack of vigorous suckling, nasal or eye discharge, coughing, lameness, swollen joints, and diarrhea.

Fever is a serious sign in a young foal and always merits examination by a veterinarian. The normal temperature of a foal is 99 to 102°F (37.2 to 38.9°C). If a foal is lethargic, depressed, or does not nurse normally, call your veterinarian immediately. If you suspect illness, take the foal's temperature and notify your veterinarian if the temperature does not fall within this range.

LACK OF COLOSTRUM (FAILURE OF PASSIVE TRANSFER)

Late in pregnancy, the mare produces a special milk that is high in fat, vitamins, minerals, and protein. This is the *colostrum* or first milk of the dam. The most important thing about colostrum is that it contains *immunoglobulins,* antibodies, and other immune substances that protect the foal from neonatal diseases.

In many species, including humans, the fetus receives protection against infection when antibodies and immunoglobulins (IgG) pass across the placenta. This does not happen in horses. The foal is born without circulating immunoglobulins and can acquire them only by ingesting colostrum during the first 18 to 24 hours after birth. Immediately after birth, through a special adaptation in the cells of the intestinal lining, antibodies from the colostrum are able cross the mucosal barrier and enter the foal's bloodstream. This is called *passive transfer.* By 24 hours, this barrier closes and antibodies are no longer absorbed. Failure of passive transfer of immunoglobulins from dam to foal is the single most important cause of neonatal infection and death during the first week of life.

Failure of passive transfer can occur for any number of reasons, including death of the dam, premature lactation before delivery, insufficient production due to maternal illness or advanced age, delay in suckling due to foal weakness or illness, and maternal rejection. Any mare who drips milk before foaling is losing colostrum. This should alert her attendants to the possibility of partial or complete failure of passive transfer. If possible, the milk should be collected and frozen. It can be thawed immediately after delivery in warm water (do not warm it in a microwave oven) and given to the foal in a nursing bottle.

The foal must ingest several pints of mare's colostrum to get adequate blood levels of IgG. When there is doubt about the quantity ingested by the foal, a rapid, simple IgG blood test can be run on the foal's serum by your veterinarian to determine if adequate colostrum has been ingested. The test should be run about six hours after birth to leave enough time to obtain a colostrum replacement. A low test at this time does not mean there is a failure of passive transfer. The test is not considered to be accurate until 12 to 24 hours after nursing begins. This test is unnecessary if failure of passive transfer is obvious (for example, maternal death or failure to suckle). As soon as a colostrum deficiency is diagnosed, colostrum replacement should be initiated without delay. Oral colostrum should be administered within the first 18 hours of life to ensure success.

Most breeding farms maintain a colostrum bank, obtained by milking 6 to 8 ounces (177 to 237 ml) of colostrum from postpartum mares and then pooling it and freezing it for use later. This volume is safe to collect without depriving the foal. Frozen colostrum should be thawed slowly in a warm, not hot, water bath. Do not microwave, as this destroys the immunoglobulins. If mare's colostrum is unavailable, the foal can be given bovine (cow) colostrum, equine blood plasma, or freeze-dried equine IgG. The best way to ensure that the foal receives the substitute colostrum is to give it by nursing bottle. IgG is better absorbed by bottle than by stomach tube.

After 24 hours, failure of passive transfer is treated by giving the foal 1 to 2 liters (34 to 68 ounces) of pooled equine plasma intravenously. The decision to treat, as well as the amount of plasma to give, depends on the level of circulating IgG as determined by blood testing, potential for exposure to foal septicemia, and other factors.

Newborn foals are dependent on colostrum to provide vitamin A. In the colostrum-deficient foal, vitamin A deficiency may be a concern and can be prevented by giving an intramuscular vitamin injection, as determined by your veterinarian.

FOAL SEPTICEMIA

Foal septicemia is a rapidly progressive, often fatal systemic infection that affects foals less than 7 days of age. It is the most common cause of severe illness and death in newborn foals. Rather than a specific bacterial infection, foal septicemia is a complex of symptoms caused by a number of different bacteria. The general signs and treatment of foal septicemia will be discussed in this section. Specific bacterial infections that cause foal septicemia will be discussed in the sections that follow.

The most significant predisposing factor in the development of foal septicemia is failure of passive transfer (see page 549). Other factors that predispose the foal to septicemia include premature birth, a complicated foaling, overcrowding, and the stress of cold or wet surroundings. Any foal who does not stand within two hours, does not suckle within two to three hours, or exhibits behavioral or physical abnormalities is at risk.

The actual source of the infection may be difficult to identify. Some bacteria are transmitted across the placenta and infect the foal before birth. Others are acquired during passage through the birth canal. Umbilical stump infection is a serious predisposing cause. Ingesting infected mother's milk or contaminated fodder are other possibilities. Still other infectious agents are airborne.

Signs of foal septicemia generally appear at about 2 to 4 days of age and are followed by rapid deterioration. Early signs include weakness, lethargy, and reluctance to nurse (often indicated by engorgement of the mare's udder). An indication of lethargy is an unusual amount of time sleeping or lying on the side. Cough or diarrhea can be the first sign in some infections. By the time the foal appears toxic and has difficulty breathing, swollen joints, shock, collapse, convulsions, or coma, the outlook for recovery is poor.

Treatment: Because foal septicemia progresses so rapidly, treatment must be started immediately, often without cultures to pinpoint the specific bacteria. There are few clues to distinguish septicemia caused by actinobacillus, for example, from that caused by salmonella or another organism. However, cultures should be obtained because they may modify treatment at a later stage.

Since many cases of foal septicemia are associated with partial or complete failure of passive transfer, serum immunoglobulin levels should be obtained routinely. If the IgG level is low, the foal can be transfused with 2 to 4 liters (68 to 135 ounces) of plasma. Broad-spectrum intramuscular or intravenous antibiotics are given to treat septicemia and to prevent complications. Vigorous fluid replacement is essential to prevent or treat dehydration and shock. X-rays and ultrasound studies may assist in localizing the site of infection.

Supportive therapy is absolutely necessary and often makes the difference between survival and death. Recumbent foals should be kept on a soft mattress, a waterbed, or a suitable protective surface, and kept in the sternal position. If this is not possible, turn the foal from side to side every two hours. Prevent chilling and hypothermia with blankets, heating pads, or radiant heat lamps. Intranasal oxygen will benefit foals with respiratory distress. Sterile eye lubricants should be applied several times a day to prevent surface drying and corneal ulceration. The perineum of foals with diarrhea must be kept clean and dry. Apply zinc oxide ointment to prevent skin scalds. The umbilical stump should be treated twice a day with tincture of iodine.

Nutrition is vital. If the foal is not strong enough to stand with assistance and suckle, the mare should be milked out and the milk given to the foal by nursing bottle. Mare milk replacer can be used if mother's milk is not available. If the foal is too weak to nurse, the feeding can be done by nasogastric tube.

If the foal survives the initial septicemia episode, localized infections may develop in various body cavities. Joint ill is a common sequel, as is panophthalmitis, an inflammation of all the inner structures of the eyes. Meningitis (inflammation of the brain) can cause seizures and coma.

Prevention: Prevent foal septicemia by quickly recognizing and treating failure of passive transfer. Provide clean, dry, sanitary foaling quarters, and using good hygienic techniques when handling the mother and foal during and after delivery.

ACTINOBACILLOSIS (SLEEPY FOAL SYNDROME)

The bacteria *Actinobacillus equuli* is a common cause of foal septicemia. Signs usually appear during the first 48 hours of life. However, sudden death can occur as early as six hours after birth. This bacteria may be present in the reproductive system of seemingly healthy mares without producing any illness. This may explain why some foals are infected at birth. Others apparently acquire the bacteria by ingesting contaminated material.

Infected foals are extremely weak and have difficulty standing and nursing. They appear to sleep all the time and may even be found in a coma. Diarrhea is common. Foals who survive the acute illness often develop septic joints and osteomyelitis.

Treatment: Treatment is like that for foal septicemia (see page 551).

UMBILICAL INFECTION (NAVEL ILL)

Navel ill is a serious and frequently fatal disease in newborn foals. It is caused by a bacterial infection of the umbilical structures, which include the artery, vein, and urachus. It is acquired either during foaling or from subsequent contamination of the healing stump. A number of bacteria can be involved, but *Streptococcus* is the most common.

There is a pus-like infected discharge from the navel. The navel stump is often hot, tender, and swollen. Ultrasound examination of the umbilical structures helps determine the extent of the infection and whether there is an umbilical stump *abscess*. The foal appears apathetic and stops nursing. In the septicemic form, the bacteria enter the bloodstream through the umbilical vessels and spread to the liver, the joints, and elsewhere. The foal may become markedly depressed, go into shock, and die within 12 to 24 hours. Alternately, the foal may not develop an overwhelming septicemia but develop instead the signs of joint ill (see page 553).

Treatment: Intravenous antibiotics should be started at the first signs of navel infection to prevent death and the effects of joint ill. All navel abscesses should be opened and drained, and the infected umbilical structures surgically removed. Supportive care is important. Keep the umbilical area clean and dry and apply a topical antiseptic twice a day. Change bedding frequently and keep the stall as clean as possible.

Prevention: Navel infection can be prevented by good management practices. These include providing a sanitary environment for foaling, applying tincture of iodine to the umbilical stump after the foal is born, and ensuring that the foal receives a sufficient amount of colostrum. Tincture of iodine is recommended because the irritation effects of tincture of iodine may prevent umbilical hernias.

SEPTIC ARTHRITIS AND OSTEOMYELITIS (JOINT ILL)

Any type of neonatal infection that causes septicemia can cause joint ill. In 25 percent of cases, navel infection is the predisposing cause. The infection begins when bacteria enter the bloodstream and invade the bone or synovial membranes of the joint. Septic arthritis occurs when bacteria are present in the foal's blood and the bacteria then invade joints or bone, or both. Osteomyelitis is a type of septic arthritis in which the bacteria are in the bone or growth plates of the bone.

Joint and bone infection can occur in older nursing and weanling foals, as well, apart from foal septicemia. Bacteria gain entrance through the digestive or respiratory tracts, but produce few (if any) signs until the foal exhibits a sudden lameness along with one or more hot, swollen joints, accompanied by a fever of 102 to 104°F (38.9 to 40°C), listlessness, and a loss of appetite. Any foal who has unexplained lameness should be examined by a veterinarian.

The diagnosis is confirmed by aspiration and analysis of joint fluid. Fluid should be submitted for bacterial culture and sensitivity testing. Arthroscopy may be helpful in some cases. *Ultrasonography* is useful in distinguishing between an abscess around a joint and infected fluid within a joint. Repeated x-rays are necessary to identify developing osteomyelitis.

Treatment: Treatment is most likely to be effective when it is started early in the course of the infection. Massive doses of antibiotics should be given for at least three weeks. Septic joints are irrigated every other day for several days, using large-bore needles to infuse and remove large volumes of fluid under pressure. If the infection has been present for more than one week, it is usually necessary to open the joint to remove pus and debris. A suction drain is inserted and the leg is immobilized by an occlusive dressing. (An occlusive dressing completely covers a wound and prevents all contact by air or water.)

Stall rest and physical therapy are important to a successful outcome. The prognosis depends on the number of joints involved, their location, and the duration and extent of infection. Foals with bone infection usually develop permanent arthritis.

Foal Pneumonia

Pneumonia is a serious and often fatal infection that attacks newborns and foals up to 8 months of age. In foals younger than 1 month, the most common causative bacteria are *Streptococcus equi* subspecies *zooepidemicus*. *Rhodococcus equi* is more common in foals older than 3 months old. *Rhodococcus equi*, found commonly in soil and the intestinal tract of horses, causes a particularly severe illness and may be associated with contagious outbreaks involving up to 50 percent of foals on a farm. Viral pneumonia generally is caused by either rhinopneumonitis (EHV-1) or an equine influenza virus.

Factors that predispose a foal to pneumonia include failure to receive colostrum, overcrowding, cold and damp quarters, soiled feed and bedding, an inadequate vaccination and/or deworming program, recent viral respiratory illness, transporting the foal (especially in hot weather), or any condition that weakens the foal's resistance. Most of these can be avoided by good management.

Bacterial infection in newborn foals follows the same course described for foal septicemia (see page 550). It may be difficult to determine whether the pneumonia preceded the septicemia or occurred as a result of it. *Streptococcus equi* subspecies *zooepidemicus* is the bacteria most frequently isolated in cases of neonatal respiratory infection. Newborn viral pneumonias can be acquired in utero. Shortly after birth, infected foals become progressively weak and lethargic and soon develop respiratory distress. Secondary bacterial infection occurs. The majority die in the first seven days. A vaccination program (as described in *Care and Feeding During Pregnancy*, page 504) will prevent most cases.

Pneumonia in foals 1 to 8 months of age usually starts insidiously with a lack of appetite, inactivity, and *depression*. Respiratory signs appear shortly thereafter. They include high fever, diarrhea, rapid pulse, difficulty breathing, watery eyes, cough, and nasal discharge. A thick nasal discharge containing pus is a sign of bacterial pneumonia.

Treatment: A penicillin antibiotic should be started as soon as possible, and can be changed if necessary, subject to culture and sensitivity tests. *Rhodococcus equi* responds dramatically to the combined use of oral erythromycin, azithromycin, and rifampin. Antibiotics should be continued throughout the course of the illness, and then one week longer. Failure to complete a full course of antibiotics is the chief cause of relapse and lung abscess.

Good nursing care, as described for foal septicemia (page 550), is essential. The foal should be kept in warm and dry quarters, treated for dehydration, and given anti-inflammatory drugs to reduce fever, if recommended by your veterinarian. Maintaining hydration is critical to liquefy secretions and promote their elimination.

Foals with lung abscesses require prolonged treatment.

Tyzzer's Disease

This rare and rapidly fatal disease occurs in foals under 6 weeks of age. It is caused by an infection of the liver. The causative bacterium is *Bacillus piliformis*. It is not known how this disease is spread, but it is picked up from the environment.

The onset is sudden, with high fever, diarrhea, collapse, and seizures—all occurring within a matter of hours. In most cases, the foal is found dead or in a coma.

Treatment: Treatment is directed at supporting the foal with intravenous fluids, antibiotics, and anticonvulsants. Unfortunately, the rapidity of the disease makes it difficult to initiate treatment in time to save the life of the foal. The diagnosis is often made at autopsy.

Prevention: No vaccinations are available. Maintaining good farm and stall sanitary conditions are the best prevention.

Foal Diarrhea

Diarrhea is the most common problem affecting foals. Although foal heat diarrhea is mild and inconsequential, infectious enteritis is serious and often fatal. Familiarity with diarrhea illnesses will help you determine when to seek help from your veterinarian.

Foal Heat Diarrhea

Foal heat, or "ninth-day diarrhea" (which actually occurs from days 6 to 14), affects nearly all newborn foals. The stool is soft, pasty yellow, and not profuse. The foal appears unaffected, remains bright and alert, and nurses at regular intervals. The diarrhea is characteristically self-limiting, lasting fewer than seven days.

Since the diarrhea coincidentally occurs when the mare enters her first heat after foaling, it was believed that hormones in the mare's milk caused the diarrhea. In fact, the same diarrhea also occurs in orphan foals. Often infestation with threadworms is the cause. Newborn foals normally eat manure and feedstuffs such as grain and hay. It appears that ingesting these substances may upset the flora of the foal's immature intestinal tract and cause the temporary diarrhea.

Treatment: Diarrhea of short duration associated with the mare's foal heat requires little treatment. If the foal was dewormed at 1 week for threadworms, it may help prevent foal heat diarrhea. Keep her dry and clean around her tail and perineum. Apply zinc oxide ointment to prevent scalding. If the diarrhea persists longer than expected, you can give bismuth subsalicylate (Pepto-Bismol or Kaopectate) or a kaolin and pectin suspension (20 ml per 100 pounds, 45 kg, body weight) by syringe or tablespoon two to three times a day for one to two days. Restrain the foal and insert the medicine into the corner of her mouth. Do not use a laxative or an intestinal purgative, because this will make the diarrhea worse. Your veterinarian may also recommend Imodium (loperamide), but caution must be taken to avoid constipation.

Nutritional Diarrhea

A common type of mild diarrhea is associated with ingesting too much milk. It occurs when the mother is a heavy milk producer. Additionally, a temporary lactase deficiency resulting in lactose intolerance may occur in some neonates who are either hand-fed or recovering from viral enteritis.

Treatment: Diarrhea caused by too much milk can be helped by milking out the mare two or three times a day. The foal should not be restricted from nursing because the milk is her only source of water. As the foal grows, her nutritional needs will increase and she will need more milk. This corrects the problem. A temporary lactase deficiency can be treated by giving an oral over-the-counter medicine (OTC) for lactose intolerance, such as Lactaid. Give your foal Lactaid Ultra using one package of the powdered form or crushing one tablet (6,000 units). Administer four times a day for four days.

Parasitic Diarrhea

Threadworms are the first intestinal parasites to mature in the foal, but large numbers are required to cause symptoms. The worms are transmitted to the foal in the mother's milk. Diarrhea caused by threadworms can appear during the first two weeks of life; thus, threadworm diarrhea often overlaps foal heat diarrhea.

The diarrhea caused by large strongyle infection is associated with severe *colic* and often constipation. It usually affects foals 1 to 4 months of age.

A heavy roundworm infestation causes diarrhea, colic, poor growth and body condition, nasal discharge, and cough. It usually affects foals 3 to 6 months of age.

Treatment: This includes careful deworming to avoid a worm bolus, and supportive care. Zinc oxide ointment is useful to prevent skin scalding. Observe the foal for dehydration. Your veterinarian may ask if the foal is urinating, if the urine looks dark in color, and if the foal is lethargic.

Prevention: Parasitic infestations can be prevented by following a deworming schedule, as described on page 54.

Protozoal Diarrhea

Cryptosporidiosis causes a protozoal diarrhea only in foals. Usually the disease is mild and self-limited, consisting of a watery diarrhea that persists for two weeks. However, in Arabian foals with combined immunodeficiency disease and in neonatal foals with failure of passive transfer, the disease is serious. The diagnosis is made by identifying the organism in the stool. *Cryptosporidiosis* can be *zoonotic*, so take precautions to protect yourself with good hand washing.

Treatment: Treatment involves oral and intravenous fluid replacement. There are no effective antibiotics. Disinfect contaminated areas using ammonia (5 percent), bleach, or 10 percent formalin.

Bacterial Enteritis

Enteritis is inflammation of the small intestines. A number of bacteria species produce severe and often fatal infection of the large and small intestine of newborn foals. Failure of passive transfer of colostral antibodies is involved in a high percentage of cases.

Salmonellosis. Salmonella infection is a leading cause of newborn septicemia. This bacteria often settles in other systems including the lungs, joints, eyes, kidneys, and brain. Several species of *Salmonella* cause infectious enteritis in foals 1 to 4 months of age. Signs include fever, weakness, and profuse, watery diarrhea that contains blood. The foal becomes depressed, stops suckling, and quickly dehydrates. Take precautions to protect yourself, as this infection can be *zoonotic*.

Clostridial infection. Both *Clostridium perfringens* and *Clostridium difficile* produce highly lethal infectious diarrhea in newborn foals. The diarrhea is bloody, foul-smelling, profuse, and associated with severe colic. It is unusual for a neonatal foal with clostridial diarrhea to live more than 48 hours. In fact, the foal may be found dead before the diarrhea develops. *Clostridia* are normal inhabitants of the horse's colon. Therefore, recovery of the bacteria does not necessarily prove a causal relationship. Finding the *exotoxin* in the foal's stool or serum is more accurate for a diagnosis. Take precautions to protect yourself, as this infection can be zoonotic.

Vaccinating pregnant mares with *Clostridium perfringens* toxoid has been advocated on farms with a history of clostridial foal infections. However, the safety and effectiveness of this vaccine is not yet established. Good sanitation and hygiene are imperative to prevent potential infection in humans.

E. coli infection. *Escherichia coli* is the most common bacteria isolated from blood cultures in septicemic foals. This bacterium tends to seed multiple organ systems. Diarrhea is a late and often terminal symptom. *E. coli* is an infrequent cause of diarrhea in older foals.

Treatment: Regardless of the causative bacteria, rapid correction of dehydration using large volumes of intravenous fluid is the top priority. Plasma is given to replace protein losses. Salmonella species rapidly develop resistance to antibiotics, which renders antibiotics less effective for salmonellosis than for other types of bacterial enteritis. However, antibiotics are given in all bacterial diarrheas to contain symptoms and prevent seeding of organs. Supportive treatment, as described in *Foal Septicemia* (see page 550) is of great importance.

Proliferative Enteropathy

This diarrheic disease is caused by the bacteria *Lawsonia intracellularis*, which lives within the intestinal cells. The time of incubation from ingestion to symptoms is usually two to three weeks. The organism is found in many wild species, but pigs are the most often infected domestic animal. Although individual foals may be infected, the disease may also affect many foals on a single farm. Foals show diarrhea at any age from 3 months up to 1 year. The stress of weaning markedly increases the incidence of this disease in foals from 4 to 8 months. Besides soft, dark, or watery diarrhea, fever, depression, loss of appetite, and marked weight loss are seen. Diagnosis is made by ultrasonography, blood tests, and polymerase chain reaction (PCR) analysis of the stool.

Treatment: Treatment relies on rapid diagnosis of the causative organism and the antibiotic erythromycin estolate, which may be combined with rifampin, or azithromycin may be given alone. Treatment is required for at least three weeks. Prevention is based on isolating sick foals to prevent the spread of the illness and using quaternary ammonium or iodine disinfectants in stalls. A vaccine used in pigs may be used on affected horse farms, but only on the advice of your veterinarian.

Rotavirus Infection (Viral Enteritis)

Rotavirus is a highly contagious enteritis that attacks foals up to 6 months of age. Most cases occur in 2-month-olds. This correlates with the interval during which the foal's maternal antibody levels are in natural decline. Adult horses usually do not develop the disease, but they may serve as a reservoir.

Rotavirus is found worldwide. Annual spring epidemics can involve up to 70 percent of foals on a single farm. The virus is shed in the stool by infected and convalescent foals, and by exposed asymptomatic adults. The virus is rapidly transmitted through contact with contaminated feed, water, bedding, human hands, grooming utensils, and other sources.

Following an incubation period of 18 to 24 hours, the illness begins with pronounced apathy and high fever. The severity of the diarrhea varies. Some foals have a few stools of cow pie consistency, nurse lethargically for one or two days, and then recover. In others the diarrhea is explosive, with the stool appearing watery green to gray. In foals with the acute form of the infection, a profuse diarrhea may last five to seven days, and results in significant fluid and *electrolyte* losses. The illness is most severe in foals under 1 week of age. These neonates dehydrate rapidly.

During the acute infection phase, the rotavirus destroys the intestinal brush border cells lining the upper intestinal tract. These cells produce lactase and also are responsible for nutrient absorption. The degree of injury varies. Regeneration may occur within a few days, but some foals sustain a prolonged lactase deficiency and an impaired ability to absorb nutrients. The malabsorption and lactase deficiency can be the cause of another diarrhea, which persists long after the first is eliminated.

Treatment: Administer bismuth subsalicylate (Pepto-Bismol or Kaopectate), or a kaolin and pectin suspension, and/or loperamide (Imodium) at 20 ml per 100 pounds (45 kg) body weight three to four times a day to control diarrhea and protect the lining of the intestines. Zinc oxide ointment is recommended for skin scalds involving the perineum and hind legs. A severely dehydrated foal requires intravenous fluids and hospitalization. Diarrhea associated with a lactase deficiency is managed by switching to solid feeds and weaning the foal as soon as possible (see *The Weanling,* page 544).

Prevention: Sick foals should be isolated to prevent the spread of disease. Thoroughly disinfect the premises and equipment. Formaldehyde or a phenol disinfectant such as Pine-Sol, used in a strong solution, are effective. In an outbreak, sanitation of the premises cannot be emphasized enough. Contaminated stall waste must be composted for months, far away from possible exposure to other foals on the farm.

A vaccine for pregnant mares is safe and effective, and decreases the severity and incidence of the disease. Mares vaccinated at eight, nine, and ten months gestation will have antibodies present in their colostrum. These antibodies will protect the foal during the first three months. If you are considering the rotavirus vaccine, contact your veterinarian.

ULCERS IN FOALS

Ulcer disease is common in foals. In fact, it has been estimated that up to 50 percent of foals will develop an ulcer during the first four months of life. These ulcers occur in the stomach, or just beyond the outlet of the stomach in the duodenum, which are the first few feet of the small intestine. The majority of ulcers do not produce symptoms and disappear with age.

Among horses, stress appears to play a major role in causing ulcers. Stress affects foals in the neonatal period in association with septic diarrhea and other infections. It also occurs at 2 months when maternally acquired immunity begins to wane, and again at 4 to 5 months in association with weaning.

Symptoms develop in a minority of foals. Symptoms include abdominal pain, grinding of the teeth (called bruxism), frothy salivation, poor appetite, diarrhea of varying frequency, poor growth, rough haircoat, potbellied appearance, and tendency to frequently lie on the back. The best way to make the diagnosis of gastric ulcers and determine the number, location, and size is to examine the stomach interior by *gastroscopy.*

Severe complications can occur. The most common is scarring. When this occurs near the outlet of the stomach or in the duodenum, a stricture can develop that partially or completely prevents the stomach from emptying. Affected foals are reluctant to eat and may experience regurgitation and aspiration pneumonia. Ulcers can perforate the stomach or duodenum, spilling intestinal contents into the abdomen and causing fatal peritonitis. The diagnosis can be confirmed by the veterinarian performing an abdominocentesis—tapping the abdomen with a needle and recovering ingested feed. This result indicates that the gastrointestinal tract has perforated.

Treatment: The most important step is to treat precipitating illnesses and remove all causes of stress. Medical management using anti-ulcer drugs such as omeprazole is very effective. Foals with strictures that prevent gastric emptying can be treated successfully with surgery.

Gastrointestinal rupture cannot be treated and the foal must be euthanized.

Prevention: Any severely ill foal should receive omeprazole as a preventive. The risk of ulcers is extremely high with the use any anti-inflammatory drug, so these medications must be used with great care.

NEONATAL MALADJUSTMENT SYNDROME (HYPOXIC ISCHEMIC ENCEPHALOPATHY)

The neonatal maladjustment syndrome (also called convulsive foal syndrome, barker, wanderer, or dummy foal syndrome) is believed to be caused by hypoxia (lack of oxygen) to the central nervous system during or after delivery. The reason for the oxygen deprivation is usually not apparent. All laboratory studies may be normal.

Typically, after a rapid, uncomplicated delivery, the foal appears normal, but then minutes or hours later loses her suckling reflex and begins to exhibit abnormal behavior. This behavior either gets progressively worse or fluctuates. Indications of brain involvement include seizures with jerking movements of the head and body, followed by spasms of the neck, limbs, and tail, and thrashing of the legs. These convulsions are accompanied by pronounced respiratory distress. The foal often emits a high-pitched whinnying or barking sound—this is called the barker stage of the disease.

Another characteristic feature of neonatal maladjustment syndrome is a loss of the righting reflex. This is a sign of spinal cord involvement. The foal is incapable of making the coordinated movements necessary to turn herself onto her sternum or to stand alone.

After the barker stage, the foal passes into the dummy stage. The foal is inert and recumbent, does not respond to stimuli, appears to be blind, and loses affinity for her mother. Later, she becomes extremely active and wanders about aimlessly, bumping into objects.

As a consequence of repeated convulsions, the foal may develop brain swelling as well as thermoregulatory, respiratory, and circulatory failure. This leads to death, which occurs in about half the cases.

Foals suffering from actinobacillosis (a bacterial infection), foal septicemia, and neonatal meningitis often exhibit symptoms like those of neonatal maladjustment syndrome. Accordingly, blood cultures and laboratory studies should be run on all foals exhibiting dummy or wanderer behavior, since some of these foals will have an infectious disease.

Treatment: Your veterinarian may recommend that the foal be treated at a hospital in an intensive care unit. The first priority is to control the convulsions. This frequently can be accomplished by simply turning the foal onto her sternum. Helping the foal to stand is also helpful. If convulsions persist, diazepam (Valium) or an anti-epileptic drug can be given by intravenous injection. Nasal oxygen is of value. DMSO may reduce brain swelling.

Prevent hypothermia by covering the foal with a woolen or electric blanket and raising the temperature of the stall. Provide a clean, well-padded surface for the foal to lie on.

Foals who are not able to suckle should be given 2 quarts (1.9 l) of mare's colostrum by nasopharyngeal catheter within 18 hours of birth. If this is not possible, see *Failure of Passive Transfer* (page 549). Maintain nutrition and water balance by feeding mother's milk and/or warm milk replacer via nasopharyngeal catheter every hour at a rate of 20 percent of body weight per day. Milk the mare, both to obtain milk and to prevent her from drying up.

Gastric ulcers are common in convulsive foals. Preventive anti-ulcer treatment is recommended (see *Ulcers in Foals*, page 559).

Foals surviving the convulsive phase have a favorable outlook. Reflexes return gradually over two to three days, but full recovery may take weeks. The suckling reflex is the last to return. Once coherent, the foal must be trained to walk, nurse, and follow her mother. Complete recovery with no residual neurological deficit is possible if the foal has adequate IgG levels, does not develop foal septicemia, and is able to stand and suckle within four days of birth. Many foals develop secondary complications, such as pneumonia.

SHAKER FOAL SYNDROME

The shaker foal syndrome is a paralytic disease caused by ingesting spores of the bacteria *Clostridium botulinum*, which may be present in hay and feeds. The spores grow in the intestinal tract of the foal, releasing a powerful neurotoxin that causes the paralytic signs. The syndrome occurs exclusively in the Mid-Atlantic states and is most common in Kentucky, where soils contain a high concentration of spores.

Foals 2 weeks to 8 months of age are most often affected. Symptoms appear one to four days after ingesting the spores. The first sign is a generalized weakness. The foal walks with a stiff, stilted gait or may be found lying down. When forced to stand, she trembles and shakes, then drops to the ground and rolls on her side. Paralysis of the swallowing mechanism causes drooling and protrusion of the tongue. Liquids may dribble from the foal's nose and mouth. Death by respiratory paralysis or aspiration pneumonia occurs in one to three days. The mortality rate is 90 percent.

Treatment: Treatment is like that described for *Botulism* (see page 431).

Prevention: Vaccinating pregnant mares with *Clostridium botulinum* type B toxoid offers some protection against the shaker foal syndrome. Note that there are three types of neurotoxin: Vaccination protects against only type B (the most common), but does not protect against types A and C. Vaccination should be considered in endemic and high-risk areas, especially on farms where the shaker foal syndrome has occurred before. The primary immunization series consists of three vaccinations at four-week intervals, with the last dose given two to four weeks before foaling. Boosters for adult horses are suggested annually. In immunized broodmares, administer the annual booster two to four weeks before foaling. The product is not labeled for the vaccination of foals.

Narcolepsy-Cataplexy (Fainting Foal Syndrome)

The fainting foal syndrome is a rare sleep disorder first reported in foals less than 6 months of age and subsequently seen in adult horses. A biochemical abnormality in the sleep-wake centers of the brainstem is thought to be the cause. Although many breeds are affected, it is most common in miniature horses, with a familial incidence among Suffolk and Shetland ponies.

Signs include excessive daytime sleepiness accompanied by rapid eye movements as if the horse were dreaming. The head is held close to the ground, the eyes are closed, and occasionally you will hear snoring. As the horse begins to fall asleep, her muscles relax. If the horse wakes before she falls, the condition is called narcolepsy. But if the horse actually collapses or "faints," it is called cataplexy. Recovery occurs in minutes to hours. Between attacks, the horse is normal.

These attacks are provoked by certain stimuli that are specific for each individual, such as eating food, being led from a stall, or being stroked or groomed. The diagnosis can be confirmed by giving a drug which brings on the attack, or giving a drug that eliminates attacks for several hours.

Treatment: Your veterinarian may prescribe an antidepressant drug. It acts on the sleep center to suppress the type of disorder associated with this syndrome. It must be given three times a day. Oral administration is less consistent than intravenous administration. The prognosis varies. In some foals and adult horses, several attacks may occur and then the condition disappears completely. In Shetland and Suffolk ponies, however, the disease is more likely to persist indefinitely.

Neonatal Isoerythrolysis

Neonatal isoerythrolysis results when the blood group of the dam is incompatible with that of the foal. It begins shortly after a foal ingests the mare's colostrum, which contains antibodies that attack the foal's red blood cells. This results in the destruction of the red blood cells of the foal. This disorder, also called hemolytic disease of the newborn, may result in a fatal anemia.

The antibodies are manufactured by the mare when fetal red blood cells of a type incompatible with her red cells cross the placenta and stimulate the mare to develop antibodies to the foreign protein. This generally occurs during a prior pregnancy but can happen during the current pregnancy. A blood transfusion containing incompatible red cells produces the same result.

The antibodies in the colostrum will not attack the foal's red cells if she inherits the same blood type as her mother. However, if the foal inherits her sire's blood type, and if this is the same type to which the mare was sensitized, then incompatibility exists and a hemolytic anemia may develop.

Only about 1 to 2 percent of mares are at risk to produce foals who develop neonatal isoerythrolysis. These include mares who lack the Aa and Qa antigens on their red blood cells—although other blood groups can also cause neonatal isoerythrolysis. (For more information on blood types, see *Equine Blood Types*, page 328.)

For neonatal isoerythrolysis to develop, a specific series of events must occur. First, a mare who is Aa or Qa negative (lacks the antigen) must be bred to a stallion who is Aa or Qa positive (has the antigen). The fetus will then inherit antigens from both parents. If the fetus inherits the Aa or Qa antigen from the stallion, she will have a different blood group than the mare. If the mare is exposed to her fetus's blood (which can occur late in the pregnancy or during foaling), she will produce antibodies directed against the Aa or Qa blood type. This is not a problem during the first exposure, because the mare does not have sufficient time to produce antibodies. However, in successive pregnancies, problems can arise. The mare has been creating antibodies against Aa and Qa blood and then accumulates them in her colostrum during later pregnancies. Any subsequent foal who is born Aa or Qa positive is now at risk. When the foal drinks the mare's colostrum, the antibodies are absorbed into the bloodstream from her digestive tract. They then attack and destroy the foal's red blood cells (hemolysis).

An affected foal is normal at birth, but 24 to 36 hours after suckling experiences weakness and lethargy that may progress to collapse. Heart rate and respiratory rate are increased. The foal often lies with her chin resting on the ground while gasping for air. The breakdown of red cells releases free hemoglobin, which turns the urine a dark tea color. The liver converts the hemoglobin to bilirubin, which turns the whites of the eyes and the gums yellow (jaundice). In a severe crisis, a foal may die before developing jaundice.

Your veterinarian can generally diagnose neonatal isoerythrolysis based on the clinical signs, followed up with laboratory tests on blood from the mare and foal or the mare's colostrum.

Treatment: The degree of hemolysis and attendant anemia depends on several factors, including the amount of colostrum ingested. If the disease is not suspected during the first 24 to 36 hours before the foal develops symptoms, there is no reason to stop nursing because the mare's milk no longer contains colostrum, and in any case maternal antibodies will no longer be absorbed from the foal's intestines.

If the hemolysis is severe, intravenous fluids may be needed to flush out hemoglobin before it damages the kidneys. Prophylactic antibiotics are a consideration to prevent secondary infections. Blood transfusions are required only if the anemia is life-threatening. The mare's own blood can be used, provided the serum is first siphoned off and the cells are washed. Otherwise, a different horse of acceptable blood type should be used as the donor. The prognosis is good if the anemia stabilizes and the foal does not develop a secondary infection.

Prevention: This is a completely preventable disease. If a mare has lost one or more foals shortly after birth, her blood should be tested to determine her blood type and if she is in the higher risk group (Aa or Qa negative). If a mare has had problems with incompatibility of the foal, it is recommended to only breed her to compatible stallions (those who are also Aa or Qa negative). The stallion must be typed before breeding.

When a pregnant mare is carrying a foal with the potential for neonatal isoerythrolysis, you can send a serum sample obtained in late pregnancy to a laboratory equipped to discover whether the mare's serum contains antibodies to foreign red cells. If antibodies are detected, the foal might develop hemolytic anemia—depending on her inherited blood type.

Since this cannot be determined until after birth, as a precaution do not allow the foal to suckle for the first 24 to 36 hours and provide an alternate source of colostrum (see *Failure of Passive Transfer*, page 549). Strip the mare's udder every two hours for two days to remove all colostrum. Leave the foal with her mother but do not allow her to nurse. Provide an alternate source of milk for the first 24 to 36 hours.

Congenital Disorders

Any disorder that is present at birth is *congenital*. Some are genetically determined while others are caused by accidents during labor and delivery. The more common congenital disorders will be discussed here.

Ruptured Bladder

This occurs in somewhat less than 1 percent of newborns. It is caused by developmental weakness in the wall of the bladder, along with bladder compression during delivery. One cause of bladder weakness is urachal infection. (The urachus is a tube in the umbilical cord that connects the foal's bladder to her mother's placenta.) Dystocia, and possibly compression during delivery, increases the risk of rupture.

Signs appear within 36 hours. The foal appears depressed, stops suckling, and makes frequent unsuccessful attempts to urinate or passes urine in small amounts. Shortly thereafter, the foal's abdomen fills up with urine and she has difficulty breathing, suffers seizures, or goes into a coma, and develops a number of metabolic abnormalities, including heart arrhythmias.

Treatment: The bladder can be surgically repaired if the rupture is recognized within three to four days. Before surgery, the foal requires medical treatment to drain the urine from her abdomen, correct the metabolic abnormalities, and treat any infection, if present.

PATENT URACHUS

This is a common congenital *anomaly*. The *urachus* is a tube in the umbilical cord that connects the foal's bladder to her mother's placenta. This channel normally closes at birth when the cord is severed. When the urachus fails to close spontaneously, urine dribbles from the umbilicus and scalds the skin around the navel. The inflamed, macerated skin is an excellent medium for bacterial growth. Infection may ascend into the abdomen via the urachus and cause peritonitis or foal septicemia (see *Umbilical Infection*, page 552).

Treatment: Keep the area as clean as possible and apply a topical antiseptic. Treat urine scalds with zinc oxide ointment. Infected skin requires topical antibiotics or, occasionally, oral antibiotics. The urachus can often be made to close by chemically cauterizing the opening and about 2 inches (5 cm) along the urachus, twice daily with silver nitrate sticks. If this is not successful within several days, surgical closure is required.

BROKEN RIB

Ribs can be broken during passage through the birth canal, especially in Thoroughbred females. The signs are those of respiratory difficulty, with a characteristic grunt heard as the foal breathes in. Pneumothorax (collapse of the lung) will occur if the sharp edges of a broken rib puncture the lung. Pneumothorax usually is fatal.

Treatment: If a newborn has difficulty breathing, notify your veterinarian immediately. Do not attempt to pick up or restrain the foal by grasping her chest. There is no treatment for broken ribs. However, your veterinarian will check for collapse or displacement.

HERNIA

A hernia is a protrusion of an organ, or part of an organ, through an opening in the abdominal wall that would normally close in the course of fetal development. Hernias present at birth or shortly thereafter have a hereditary basis.

There is a genetic predisposition for delayed closure of the abdominal ring (openings in the abdominal wall for the inlet and outlet of the inguinal canal) in most cases. Hernias occur in both sexes. Horses with congenital hernias should not be bred.

If a hernia can be pushed back into the abdomen, it is said to be reducible. If it cannot, it is said to be incarcerated. Incarcerated hernias are associated with colic and signs of intestinal obstruction. Strangulation and death of a segment of bowel occurs if its blood supply becomes pinched off by the abdominal ring or by adhesions. *Incarceration* and strangulation are surgical emergencies.

Inguinal Hernia

In horses with this condition, the hernia sac (containing fat or a loop of intestine) comes through the abdominal ring and into the inguinal canal. If it descends further, it enters the scrotum. Inguinal hernias usually occur in foals, but can occur in stallions as a consequence of trauma, breeding, or physical exertion. Adult-onset hernias are not considered congenital.

Inguinal hernias are detected by palpating over the inguinal canal and feeling for a bulge or swelling. In some stallions, the hernia is detected by rectal palpation.

Treatment: Usually the hernia can be reduced by pushing the bulge back up through the abdominal ring into the belly. Small inguinal hernias tend to correct spontaneously as the foal grows older. It may be necessary to reduce the hernia several times before this occurs.

Scrotal Hernia

Scrotal hernias are large inguinal hernias that descend into the scrotum and produce an obvious swelling around the testicle. In stallions, they can occur quite suddenly after strenuous breeding activity. Scrotal hernias usually produce signs of intestinal obstruction.

Treatment: Rapid surgical correction is necessary. This involves closure of the ring and removal of the testicle on the side of the hernia.

Umbilical Hernia

Ligation of the umbilical cord, manual breaking of the cord, and cord infection with abscesses are predisposing causes of umbilical hernia, in which the intestines or omentum protrude through the muscles of the abdomen. A strangulated umbilical hernia can be recognized by a hard, painful swelling at the navel that does not reduce with applied pressure.

Treatment: Most umbilical hernias close spontaneously by the time the colt or *filly* is 1 year of age. For a strangulated umbilical hernia, rapid surgical correction is imperative.

Prevention: Dipping the umbilical cord at birth in 7 percent tincture of iodine may prevent umbilical herniation.

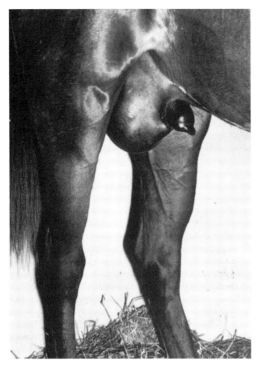

This scrotal swelling is associated with a large inguinal hernia.

Nutritional Myopathy (White Muscle Disease)

Nutritional myopathy is a disease of foals from birth to 1 year of age. It is caused by selenium deficiency. Foals are selenium-deficient because the mare does not get enough selenium during pregnancy and lactation. One function of selenium is to enhance vitamin E uptake from the gut. Therefore, vitamin E deficiency may also be a problem.

Foals with acute selenium deficiency often show a lack of appetite and diarrhea, muscle pain, and stiffness. In a severe case the foal may develop respiratory insufficiency, heart failure, and death. Post-mortem examination of muscle discloses abnormal fibers that appear white on close inspection. Thus, the disorder has been called white muscle disease.

Treatment: Selenium and vitamin E injections are used, and supportive care may be necessary.

Prevention: In areas where selenium deficiency has previously occurred, add a selenium supplement to the mare's diet as described in *Selenium* (see page 405). A selenium injection during the last trimester of pregnancy is recommended, although it may not prevent the deficiency in all foals. It is also important to treat the foal with a selenium injection shortly after birth. It may not be necessary to repeat the injection, as long as the foal's creep and weanling diets contain adequate amounts of selenium and vitamin E.

Myotonia

Myotonia is a rare congenital muscle disorder affecting foals 3 weeks and older. These foals appear overmuscled. In fact, under the microscope individual muscle fibers appear twice the normal size.

The muscles of the limbs contract rigidly and relax slowly. The first few steps are taken rigidly, but as the foal warms up, she moves more freely.

Treatment: An effective treatment has not been established. A similar condition in humans has been treated using quininelike medications.

Contracted Foal Syndrome

The contracted foal syndrome encompasses a group of angular limb and/or spinal deformities in which the foal's bones and joints are permanently twisted into abnormal positions. These deformities occur during gestation and often result in fetal death and abortion.

If the mare carries the contracted foal to term, normal delivery is generally impossible because of the flexed position of the forelimbs and the increased diameter of the shoulders and chest. Either fetotomy or cesarean section will be required to relieve the blockage. When the foal can be delivered alive, she is seldom able to stand and nurse.

Treatment: Surgical correction is rarely successful. The most humane course is to euthanize the foal.

Limb Deformities

Angular limb deformities (knock-knees, bowlegs, and bucked knees) and flexural limb deformities (contracted digital flexor tendons and clubfoot) are frequently congenital in origin. Some are acquired after birth as a result of improper exercise and nutrition. Acquired deformities are discussed in *Developmental Orthopedic Diseases* (see page 261).

Treatment: When a foal is born with weak or crooked legs, this is not of immediate concern as long as the foal can stand and nurse. Many deviations correct themselves with time. If they do not, casting or bracing can be used to straighten limbs. Trimming the hooves may aid in straightening the affected limb. Based on x-rays, your veterinarian may offer advice on different treatment options before the growth plates seal.

Contracted tendons are often treated with oxytetracycline within the first few days of life. Surgery for angular limb deformities includes periosteal stripping and transphyseal bridging.

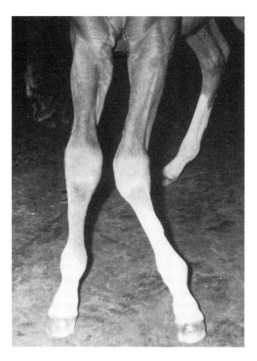

Angular limb deformities, such as knock-knees (shown here), may correct spontaneously.

Eye Diseases

Entropion is a birth defect in which the foal's eyelids roll inward, causing the eyelashes to rub against the surface of the eye. *Ectropion* is the opposite condition, in which the eyelids are everted, exposing the eye to excessive drying. Both conditions should be treated to prevent permanent eye damage.

Congenital cataracts are present at birth and are the most common cause of blindness in foals. Because of the hereditary nature of this condition, a horse affected with congenital cataracts should not be bred.

A foal can be born with one or both eyes smaller than normal. In some cases there is an almost complete absence of an eye. A small eye is often associated with a congenital cataract. Occasionally, a foal may be born without a normal eye globe.

Congenital night blindness is a hereditary condition found primarily in Appaloosas, but it also affects Standardbreds, Thoroughbred, Paso Finos, and Quarter Horses.

For more information on these disorders, see chapter 5, "The Eyes."

Cleft Palate

The hard and soft palates separate the nasal and oral cavities. When these structures do not form completely, there is a cleft in the roof of the mouth and an opening between the two cavities at the back of the palate. This condition is rare in foals.

Affected foals find it impossible to suckle. They cough, choke, gag, and are unable to swallow milk. The milk comes out the nose when the foal's head is down. A fatal aspiration pneumonia (when a foreign substance is inhaled into the lungs) may result.

Treatment: Surgical correction can be attempted. The results are best when the defect is small and involves the soft palate only. Foals with large defects are usually poor surgical candidates.

ABSENCE OF THE ANUS

Absence of the anus (anal *atresia*) is a relatively common congenital defect and may occur in association with anomalies of the urinary and reproductive systems. The entire anus may fail to develop or the rectum may extend down to a well-developed sphincter with a dimple at the site of the anal opening. The second type can be corrected surgically. Often the first sign is straining or not defecating, and may be discovered when you are trying to give an enema after birth.

Treatment: When the rectum extends down to a sphincter with a dimple at the site of the anal opening, the defect can be corrected surgically. Absence of part or the entire large colon is rare and surgical repair is difficult.

OVERO LETHAL WHITE SYNDROME

In foals with overo lethal white syndrome (OLWS), the ganglion nerve plexus in the wall of the bowel fails to develop. Lacking this plexus, the colon remains somewhat paralyzed and contracts poorly. This leads to bowel obstruction. This condition is genetic, and is linked to the same gene that causes the overo white pattern (frame overo). Both parents must have the defective gene.

The defective gene has been found in American Paint Horses, American Miniature Horses, Half-Arabians, Thoroughbreds, and cropout Quarter Horses (foals born to registered Quarter Horse parents who have too much white to qualify for registration with the American Quarter Horse Association).

OLWS foals have blue eyes and are completely or almost completely white at birth. These foals initially appear normal. After a varying period of time, signs of colic emerge due to the foal's inability to pass feces.

Treatment: Surgical correction is not possible. The foal will die within 72 hours after birth, and euthanasia is usually the most humane course of action.

Prevention: Genetic testing has been developed to help breeders and veterinarians identify carriers of this disease (see *Genetic Testing*, page 462).

HEART DEFECTS

Heart defects are not common in foals. Mild defects may be asymptomatic and compatible with a normal life span. Signs of moderate to severe heart disease include poor growth, lethargy, exercise intolerance, rapid heavy breathing, cyanosis (blue color to mucous membranes of nose, lips, and gums), and collapse. For more information, see *Congenital Heart Disease*, page 322.

NEONATAL HYPOTHYROIDISM

Hypothyroidism in newborn foals begins in utero, and generally is caused by feeding kelp or a diet with too much iodine to the pregnant mare. Less frequently, it is caused by grazing or consuming plants containing chemicals that block the activity of the thyroid. In either case, the foal does not manufacture or release enough thyroid hormone.

The most characteristic sign of the disease is enlargement of the thyroid gland (goiter). Thyroid enlargement is a compensatory effort to boost thyroid production by increasing the size of the gland. The enlarged thyroid in the neck may or may not be visible, depending on its size.

Newborn hypothyroid foals are weak and lethargic. They exhibit incoordination and poor righting and suckling reflexes, and are often hypothermic. Some foals are asymptomatic when born but develop skeletal problems at 2 weeks of age, including angular limb deformities and contracted tendons. The diagnosis is made by thyroid function tests.

Treatment: Thyroid hormone replacement corrects most of the symptoms. However, any skeletal defects are permanent.

COMBINED IMMUNODEFICIENCY DISEASE

Combined immunodeficiency disease is a fatal inherited disease of Arabian horses that is characterized by a deficiency of B and T cell lymphocytes. These specialized cells are essential to the immune system. Affected foals are highly susceptible to infections such as adenovirus pneumonia and, once infected, succumb rapidly. The diagnosis is made by a blood sample revealing a lymphocyte count of less than 1,000 per ml.

Treatment: Currently there is no treatment. Genetic testing is available for this disease (see *Genetic Testing*, page 462).

CEREBELLAR ABIOTROPHY

Incomplete neurological development of the cerebellum is an uncommon disease that occurs almost exclusively in horses of Arabian ancestry, although a similar disorder has been described in Gotland ponies and Oldenburg horses. It tends to occur in individuals from inbred lines. The disease is characterized by a decrease in the number and distribution of specialized neurotransmitter (Purkinje) cells in the cerebellum.

Signs are occasionally present at birth, but usually appear suddenly after 6 months of age. Head tremors, incoordination, and staggering gait are characteristic. Often there is a peculiar type of gait called "goose-stepping," which is most pronounced in the front legs. The foal may buckle in the rear or fall over backward.

Treatment: There is no effective treatment. Many mild to moderately affected foals appear to function normally as adults, presumably by learning to compensate.

OCCIPITOATLANTOAXIAL MALFORMATION

Occipitoatlantoaxial malformation is a developmental malformation involving the bone socket at the base of the skull and the first and second cervical vertebrae. The effect of the malformation is to narrow the spinal canal and compress the spinal cord. The disease occurs most often in Arabians and less frequently in Morgans and Standardbreds. It is inherited as a recessive trait.

Some affected foals are born dead. In others, symptoms develop within the first few months of life. Signs include weakness, spasticity, uncoordinated gait, and limb paralysis. The neck is held in a stiff, characteristically erect position, like a "weather vane horse." Bending the neck to nurse can increase cord compression and cause the foal to collapse. A few foals develop a deviation of the head and neck without signs of brain or spinal disease. The head and neck are extended and a deformity with decreased movement can sometimes be felt.

Treatment: Medical treatment is not effective. Surgical decompression (dorsal laminectomy), as described *Wobbler Syndrome* (see page 352), stabilizes or improves symptoms in some foals. The surgery should be performed before the cord is damaged.

HYDROCEPHALUS

Hydrocephalus begins in utero. It is caused by a blockage in the circulation of cerebrospinal fluid in the brain. The fluid is formed more rapidly than it can be removed. The increased pressure around the brain causes the development of a large, dome-shaped skull. The skull is often too large to pass through the birth canal, resulting in the necessity for cesarean section or fetotomy to deliver the foal.

Treatment: Surgery to shunt the fluid off the brain has met with limited success in horses.

Junctional Epidermolysis Bullosa

Also known as red foot disease, junctional epidermolysis bullosa causes moderate to severe blistering of the epithelial cells of the skin and mouth, and sloughing of the hooves in newborn foals. The condition worsens with time until the foal develops secondary infections or has to be euthanized. Found in Belgian Draft Horses, it is a recessive gene so an animal must inherit the gene from both parents to develop the disease. A horse with only one copy of the defective gene will be a carrier. Affected foals are always the product of mating two carriers, since foals with this condition will not survive to breeding age.

Treatment: There is currently no treatment.

Prevention: Genetic testing has been developed to help breeders and veterinarians identify carriers of this disease (see *Genetic Testing*, page 462).

Glycogen Branching Enzyme Deficiency

Glycogen branching enzyme deficiency is a fatal condition occurring in newborns. Lacking the enzyme necessary to store glycogen, heart, brain, and skeletal muscles are unable to function. Occasionally, this birth defect causes late-term abortion.

Abortion or stillbirth of a foal may be the first sign of glycogen branching enzyme deficiency. If the foal is born alive, there will be overall weakness, inability to stand, and low body temperature at birth. Bottle feeding or feeding milk via a stomach tube and helping her to stand and suckle regularly will help the foal gain strength. Other signs include sudden death on pasture from cardiac arrest or seizures, due to low blood sugar. There may be a high respiratory rate and weakness of the muscles used to breathe, and contracted tendons in all four legs.

Your veterinarian may run lab tests to differentiate glycogen branching enzyme deficiency from other birth defects.

Treatment: There is no treatment. Foals usually die within the first few days.

Prevention: Genetic testing has been developed to help breeders and veterinarians identify carriers of this disease (see *Genetic Testing*, page 462).

Lavender Foal Syndrome

This condition occurs in Arabian foals. They are born with an unusually colored coat and severe neurological symptoms. This lethal genetic disorder is not gender-specific. Research is ongoing to isolate the gene or genes responsible, so that a genetic test can be performed to determine if the parents are carriers.

Treatment: There is no treatment. Foals usually die within the first few days.

Neonatal Epilepsy

This condition occurs more frequently in Arabian foals than in other breeds. In Arabians, it is called idiopathic or benign epilepsy. Affected foals exhibit a form of intermittent spasm in which the head and heels are bent backward and the body is bowed forward, with paddling of the hooves. Although there is no abnormal coloring or color dilution, as seen in the lavender foal syndrome, research may prove that the genetics are linked.

Treatment: See *Seizures*, page 358.

19

GERIATRICS

Horses do not age at the same rate. An "old" horse is not defined by chronological age, but rather by functional age. Functional age is determined by the use of the horse. Thus, an old racehorse is simply a young hunter. *Broodmares* must be reproductively functional, so 16 may be old for a broodmare but a prime age for a dressage equine athlete.

A horse's biological age and expected life span depend on his genetic inheritance, nutrition, state of health, and lifetime sum of environmental stresses. Of greatest importance is the care the horse has received throughout his life. Well-cared-for horses suffer fewer infirmities as they grow older. When nutrition, immunizations, parasite control, hoof care, and attention to dental problems are neglected, the aging process is accelerated.

There is no fixed point in life at which a horse becomes a geriatric. As a rule, a horse approaching 20 years of age can be considered old, although many horses live well beyond 20—some even into their 30s. Preventive management of the older horse is key to a good quality of life.

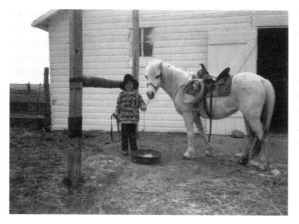

This little horse remained active and functional well into her late 30s, despite being blind in one eye and losing many teeth. A senior formulated feed, plus high-quality chopped alfalfa, helped her maintain her condition.

Physical Changes

The horse's physical appearance changes only slowly as he approaches this period of his life. One of the most visible changes is a sagging in the back, giving a swaybacked curvature to the spine. The slight indentation above the eyes, the supraorbital fossa, becomes deeper and more pronounced. The lower lip sinks and becomes droopy.

The Musculoskeletal System

The geriatric horse may still enjoy performing the various skills he was called upon to perform in his youth. Pleasure riding, showing, trail rides, and other moderate physical activities are well within an older horse's capability, but he will not be as quick or as fast as he was when he was young. There is a gradual decline in *condition*, and the horse will fatigue sooner and require longer rest periods between events.

Degenerative changes in the muscles may lead to stiffness and intermittent lameness that improves with activity.

Moderate exercise helps keep joints supple and should be encouraged. However, an old horse should not be asked to exert himself beyond his level of comfort. A specific condition (such as heart disease) may require that exercise be restricted.

When the horse begins to show signs of arthritis—chronic lameness, stiffness of gait, bony enlargements around the joints—there are medications to manage and treat these maladies (see *Osteoarthritis*, page 268). Your veterinarian may use intramuscular polysulfated glycosaminoglycans or intravenous hyaluronic acid. Oral *nutraceuticals* such as glucosamines have been reported to provide relief to joint pain. Nutraceuticals have been reported to have protective qualities, but it should be noted that their effectiveness is unproven. *Acupuncture* (see page 614) may be helpful in providing relief from musculoskeletal pain.

Older horses may have trouble rising due to hock pain or arthritis in general. Consequently, these horses are reluctant to lie down and may fall. Injecting hyaluronic acid directly into the hock may provide relief. If the horse is spending long periods lying down or having constant trouble rising, euthanasia should be considered (see page 587).

The Feet

To minimize stress on joints and hoof structures, routine farrier care every six to eight weeks should be included in the older horse's preventive management.

If the horse has difficulty standing with his limbs flexed for any length of time, phenylbutazone, a nonsteroidal anti-inflammatory drug (*NSAID*), may be administered on the morning of the scheduled foot work.

THE SKIN

Older horses are more likely to develop tumors, and this is certainly true for the skin. Regular grooming, which promotes good skin health and circulation, is an excellent opportunity to look for any unusual lumps or bumps on or beneath the skin. On old gray horses, be sure to check beneath the tail, as this is a common site for melanomas.

THE HEART

Coronary artery disease does not occur in horses. However, valvular heart disease (see page 320) exists in many older horses and may limit cardiovascular fitness in some. Although congestive heart failure (see page 322) can occur in older horses, it is related to acquired heart disease and not simply to aging.

THE LUNGS

Recurrent airway obstruction (RAO, see page 303) becomes more symptomatic with time. However, RAO, like heart disease, is an acquired condition. Horses who have spent most of their lives outdoors or lived in well-ventilated barns and stables usually do not develop RAO as they age.

THE KIDNEYS

Because of scarring acquired throughout the horse's life from various diseases, and general loss of kidney function, many old horses must put out large amounts of urine to eliminate nitrogen and the wastes of metabolism. Therefore, if these horses do not drink frequently, they are likely to become chronically dehydrated. One of the important side effects of dehydration is increased dryness of the manure. The stool becomes hard and difficult to pass, which contributes to bouts of *colic* and constipation—painful for the horse and difficult to treat. The painful abdomen may lead to anorexia and, ultimately, significant weight loss.

If kidney disease is suspected, your veterinarian may wish to run some lab tests. These may include, but are not limited to, *electrolytes* (sodium, potassium, and chloride), BUN, calcium, and creatinine.

As always, it is important to ensure that the horse has good access to a supply of fresh, clear water. This may mean relocating a water tank from a steep hillside or a far corner of the property to a site closer to the horse's hayrack and shelter. Otherwise, the geriatric horse may simply find it too difficult to make several trips a day just to get a drink of water.

THE LIVER

The liver performs a large number of metabolic functions and has a large regenerative capacity (meaning that, to some extent, it can "regrow").

Signs of liver failure are nonspecific and can vary a great deal, depending on the extent and duration of the disease. Seventy-five percent of the liver must be involved before signs are obvious; often the onset is sudden. Liver failure is associated with weight loss, jaundice, malaise, and decreased appetite. Less common signs may include photosensitivity, diarrhea, laryngeal paralysis, and bleeding disorders.

The two most consistent signs of liver failure are weight loss and failure to thrive. Chronic liver disease may be present without weight loss. Weight loss, in the case of liver disease, is due to anorexia and loss of liver metabolic activities. Weight loss and anorexia are also two common conditions seen in geriatric horses. It is important, therefore, especially with vague symptoms, to consult your veterinarian. Your veterinarian may wish to run some lab work, including but not limited to liver enzyme tests (such as alkaline phosphatase or AST), total protein, albumin, bilirubin, triglyceride, and cholesterol, to better pinpoint the problem.

There are also certain plants such as cestrum, lantana, and sencio that are hepatotoxic, meaning they are toxic to the liver (see *Forage Toxicities*, page 427). It is important to be aware of the plants your horse may have access to.

Bacterial hepatitis in the mature horse is usually secondary to another infection caused by bile stones or inflammation of the intestines. If the infection is resolved, the disease does not progress or get worse. However, if the infection is not resolved, chronic liver disease will occur.

To treat liver disease, the cause must be diagnosed and supportive treatment should be given. Protein and fat should be restricted in the diet. Vitamins B and C are synthesized in the liver, and with decreased liver function, they must be supplemented (see chapter 15, "Nutrition and Feeding," for more information on vitamin supplements).

THE INTESTINES

As your horse progresses into advancing age, certain intestinal disorders may become apparent. Among the most serious can be *colic*, either occasionally or frequently. In the older horse, improperly chewed food or decreased water consumption or a combination of both may cause impactions in the colon or even constipation. This is another reason to have your veterinarian perform frequent dental examinations. Making sure the food you give your horse is properly chewed can help prevent colic problems. Remember, in colder climates you should encourage winter water consumption by keeping the water at least 45°F (7.25°C).

In some areas of the United States, especially California, geriatric horses are prone to developing stones, called enteroliths, inside of the intestines. A diet of alfalfa hay may contribute to stone formation, and Arabian horses may be predisposed.

THE TEETH

The shape of the jaw changes and the incisors and molars wear down as the horse ages. These changes cause chewing problems, particularly loss of the ability to grind coarse feeds. In turn, this results in inadequate digestion of feed, loss of weight and body *condition*, and increased risk of colic and constipation.

The horse's incisors may become so worn down that he can no longer graze on pasture or eat long-stemmed hay. Many horses with worn incisors can continue to graze, but the worn incisors may be a clue to worn molars, which are definitely more of a problem. Points on the cheek teeth, more likely to form at this age, become a major concern. If chewing becomes too painful, the horse will simply stop eating so the wear on the molars needs to be monitored.

Accordingly, routine dental care for old horses is absolutely essential. They need a thorough dental exam twice a year. A mash or gruel may be indicated if a horse does not have enough teeth or if the teeth are not long enough for him to eat. The mash can be made by soaking complete feed pellets, beet pulp pellets, or both in enough water to soften them.

Periodontal disease (see page 195) is defined as the presence of disease and loss of tissue surrounding the teeth. Signs of periodontal disease include excess saliva, sensitivity to cold water, halitosis, and improperly digested food in the feces. It is important to detect these changes to prevent irreversible damage.

WEIGHT

Old horses are much more likely to experience rapid weight changes. Visual inspection for body condition is not as accurate in geriatric horses as it is in younger individuals. A better way to judge body condition is to feel the horse's ribs. Each rib should be felt distinctly, with a slight indentation on either side. If the indentation is deep, the horse is too thin. If the indentation is absent (especially if the ribs can't be felt), the horse is too fat. See *Weight*

Gain and Loss (page 420) for more information on how to estimate body condition.

A horse gains weight when he is fed a diet meant for an active horse but does not exercise regularly. Obesity is highly undesirable in geriatric horses. It increases the cardiovascular workload and imposes additional stresses on the bones and joints. Obesity may predispose the horse to insulin resistance and may indicate Cushing's disease. A horse loses weight when he does not get enough feed to meet his energy needs. In old horses, this is usually caused by dental disease or a low spot in the pecking order at the feeding station. Kidney failure should always be considered, as well, since it is another cause of unexplained weight loss in old horses. Liver disease, heart disease, and infectious diseases are uncommon causes. Cancer is an uncommon cause of weight loss. If your horse is losing weight, ask your veterinarian to run some blood tests to screen for these diseases and Cushing's disease. To reverse weight gain or loss, see *Weight Gain and Loss* (page 420). Weight changes in geriatric horses should proceed slowly. Any sudden change in weight may impose a severe stress on the body. When weight loss is accompanied by protein deficiency (as determined by serum protein levels), a protein supplement such as soybean or linseed meal can be added to the daily ration.

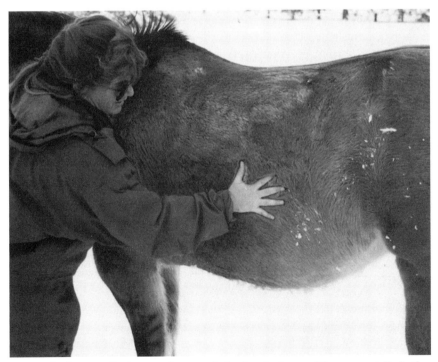

Feeling the horse's ribs is a good way to judge her body condition, especially in the winter when her coat is long.

THE SENSES

The vision and hearing of older horses does not decline with age, as they do with people. Blindness and deafness result from diseases that are acquired at all stages of life. Even when there is a loss of eyesight or hearing, however, the horse compensates well by relying on his other senses.

However, loss of taste is a function of aging. This is one more reason why it is important to feed a palatable, high-quality diet, as described in *Diet and Nutrition* (see page 584).

Behavioral Changes

Older horses are more sedentary, less energetic, and more restricted in their scope of activity. They adjust more slowly to changes in diet, activity, and routine. They are less eager to please and more inconvenienced by work. However, the training and discipline a horse has received in his younger years is not lost. With just a little more patience and effort, the geriatric horse will continue to perform well.

An older horse may no longer dominate in a social hierarchy at the level he enjoyed during his prime. Younger, more aggressive horses often displace the geriatric individual, who is driven from the feed trough. This leaves the coarser, less nutritious feed for the older horse. Clearly, in this situation the geriatric horse should be fed separately.

Temporary boarding and hospitalization are poorly tolerated in old age, because geriatric horses tend to be anxious in an unfamiliar environment. If possible, keep the horse at home. Arrange for a friend or a paid attendant to drop by daily and tend to the horse's needs.

Equine Cushing's Disease

Equine Cushing's Disease (ECD) commonly occurs in horses over 20 years of age. Occasionally, younger horses may be affected but this is predominately a disease of geriatric horses. There does not seem to be a predilection due to the sex of the horse; both sexes are almost equally affected. Morgan Horses, and to a lesser extent, ponies, are the breeds most commonly seen with ECD.

ECD is caused by a malfunction of the pituitary gland, which is located at the base of the brain. This causes increased stimulation of the adrenal glands, which lie under the backbone just forward of the kidneys. The adrenal glands produce the body's steroids, and overactive adrenals produce marked hormonal imbalances in the horse and account for the clinical signs. This disease is also sometimes called pituitary pars intermedia dysfunction.

The most common sign is hirsutism—growth of a shaggy, long haircoat that does not shed in the spring and lasts through the summer. Profuse sweating on the shoulders and neck are commonly seen. Loss of muscle tissue in the rump and along the back are often found when a thorough examination is performed. This may go unnoticed because the ECD horse has increased fat deposits over the tail head, in the penile sheath of male horses, and most noticeably, a thick pad of fat along the top of the neck.

Laminitis is frequently found in horses with ECD and is caused by the excessive production of corticosteroids by the adrenal glands. The corticosteroids react to stress and inflammation in the normal horse. In horses with Cushing's disease, they are responsible for muscle loss, laminitis due to changes in blood flow to the hooves, and recurrent foot abscesses.

The adrenal glands also produce increased amounts of mineralocorticoids. These hormones cause the increased urination and water consumption noted in ECD horses.

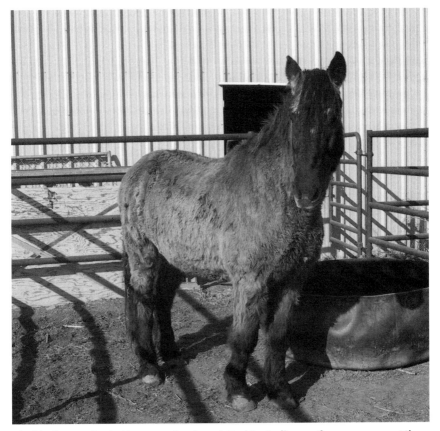

Blackjack, a geriatric Mustang, developed Cushing's disease three years ago. His owners shave him each summer for his comfort. This picture was taken in early fall and his hair has not completely grown back in.

The diagnosis of equine Cushing's disease is based on hirsutism, muscle loss, and a dexamethasone suppression test (DST). In one such test protocol, a blood sample is taken from the horse and tested for cortisol. After the initial blood sample is drawn, a specific dose of the corticosteroid dexamethasone is given to the horse. Twenty-four hours later, a second blood cortisol level is sampled. If the second blood sample's cortisol level falls below the first, the horse probably does not have Cushing's disease. If the second blood cortisol level stays markedly above the first sample's level, the diagnosis of equine Cushing's disease is definitive.

Treatment: Once your horse has been diagnosed with ECD, drug therapy is available using cyproheptadine or pergolide (which is available for horses from your veterinarian through compounding pharmacies). Most veterinarians have found that pergolide is the most effective, adding up to five years to the life of the geriatric horse. However, pergolide has to be given daily and it does have a moderate monthly cost. Additionally, blood work performed by your veterinarian is essential. If treatment is stopped, the ECD horse will quickly start showing symptoms within a few weeks.

Horses with hirsutism are often quite uncomfortable in the summer. Shaving their hair short for the summer can increase their comfort level.

Caring for the Geriatric Horse

Care of the teeth is the single most important consideration in the physical well-being of the older horse. The teeth of older horses should be examined by a veterinarian every six months. It is most important to file the cheek teeth to prevent sharp points from lacerating the cheeks and gums, causing a painful stomatitis and reluctance to eat and chew. Old teeth that become cracked or loose often do not fall out because they are tightly held in place by adjacent teeth. These loose teeth should be removed to promote better chewing and prevent root infections.

The geriatric horse should continue to receive good foot and hoof care. Even though the horse will not be ridden as often, it is still of paramount importance to trim the feet at least every six to eight weeks to maintain good hoof condition and pastern axis. Geriatric horses are less tolerant of musculoskeletal stresses imposed by a long toe, splayed-out foot, or overgrown frog, and are more likely to develop injuries and lameness when the hooves are neglected.

Shelter becomes quite important for the geriatric horse, since he is less able to regulate his body temperature on his own. A pasture or corral with a three-sided shelter for inclement weather allows the horse to move, which eases the aches and pains of arthritis, while still having a place to warm up. An outdoor environment also minimizes respiratory irritants, such as mold and ammonia, which build up in stalls. Additional bedding in the horse's shelter or stall will add significantly to his comfort.

During cold weather, when impactions are most common, it is important to check the temperature of your horse's water supply to be sure the water is not unduly cold or frozen solid. Horses do not like to drink water at temperatures near freezing. Old horses, in particular, may not drink enough cold water to maintain an optimal state of hydration. Install a water heater to ensure that the temperature in the tank is at least 45°F (7.2°C).

DIET AND NUTRITION

Most geriatric horses require fewer calories than younger horses need. Their caloric requirements are close to those of the mature horse at maintenance, (shown in the table on page 395). Overfeeding will result in weight gain. Controlling obesity is one of the most important considerations in keeping an old horse healthy.

The geriatric horse may have difficulty consuming a diet that contains adequate amounts of roughage, because of the condition of his teeth. Compensate by feeding him high-quality hay. Hay for old horses should be fine-stemmed and leafy. Large-stemmed hay is coarse, less palatable, more difficult to chew, and may lead to colic. Poor-quality hay is tasteless, dirty, and contributes to a loss of appetite and condition.

Alfalfa may be used if the horse does not have chronic kidney failure. In a horse with kidney failure, the protein and calcium contents of alfalfa are too high, adding to the problems of uremia (see page 338). A ration containing grass hay and corn is more appropriate for a uremic horse, since it is also low in phosphorus (which has been shown to accelerate the progress of kidney failure).

When alfalfa is not available or should not be used, you can switch to pelleted or cubed feeds. These feeds are easier for the horse to chew and digest. Note that feeding small dry pellets to older horses may lead to choking. This is because old horses do not produce as much saliva or their teeth are in poor condition, and therefore the feed is swallowed in a drier state. To prevent choking, moisten the pellets with water to a gruel-like consistency.

Commercial rations are now available that meet all the nutrient and roughage requirements of the old horse. These products are labeled specifically for senior horses. Commercial products are convenient to feed, providing a correct balance of calories, fiber, vitamins, and minerals, and are available in a semi-moist pelleted form, which helps prevent choking.

Old horses need more vitamins and minerals, because their ability to absorb vitamins through the intestinal tract diminishes as they age. In addition, B vitamins are lost in the urine of horses with reduced kidney function. If you are feeding your horse a complete commercial ration, you should not need to add vitamin supplements. However, if there is a question about the quality of the horse's diet, or if the horse suffers from kidney or liver disease, it is a good idea to provide supplemental vitamin A and B-complex vitamins. Mineral supplements should not be given unless prescribed by a veterinarian. The horse's kidney function should always be investigated before giving supplemental calcium or phosphorus.

The correct amount of feed is important to maintain body condition, so consider feeding the older horse separately if he is in a mixed-age group. This reduces competition for food.

Geriatric horses are more sensitive to extremes of temperature and weather. In hot humid weather, it is important to feed slightly less and provide shade or a cool shelter. In cold rainy weather, energy requirements are greater than normal. Because older horses may have difficulty meeting these needs by simply eating more food, these energy requirements can be met by giving vegetable oil (see *Fat and Oil Supplements,* page 417). Vegetable oils provide a high density of energy in a small volume. Moreover, they are palatable and readily consumed. Depending on the horse's weight and need for additional energy, add 1 to 3 cups (236 to 711 ml) of corn oil or another vegetable oil to the daily ration. One cup provides approximately 2,000 calories of digestible energy.

Managing Chronic Pain

Nonsteroidal anti-inflammatory drugs (*NSAIDs*) are effective pain therapy for horses. However, the side effects may be amplified in the geriatric horse. These side effects can include oral, gastric, and duodenal ulceration, kidney failure, and others. Additional therapies that may help optimize the athletic function of the geriatric horse may include steroids, *chondroprotective* agents, nutraceuticals, oral supplementation, topical treatments, acupuncture, massage, and chiropractic, all of which are discussed in chapter 21, "Alternative Therapies."

Drugs that may be injected into the joint include steroids and chondroprotective agents. Steroids are effective in decreasing the joint inflammation, but a significant side effect is that they also break down cartilage. Chondroprotective agents appear to modify the progression of osteoarthritis by preventing further breakdown of cartilage. The benefits of these agents, such hyaluronic acid and polysulfated glycosaminoglycan, are unpredictable, although they are commonly used. There are no known side effects, they have some analgesic properties, and they provide *viscosupplementation* (supplementation of the joint fluid). It is unknown whether these medications have any protective or reparative properties. There is danger of infection if these medications are injected directly into the joints, so they are often administered intramuscularly.

Other chondroprotective agents are nutraceuticals—products that lie somewhere between a nutrient and a drug. Nutraceuticals are believed to have medical value based on subjective evidence of their effectiveness, although clinical evidence based on controlled studies is lacking for many of these treatments. Unlike drugs, nutraceuticals do not undergo an approval process and are not regulated by a federal agency.

Most nutraceuticals used to treat osteoarthritis contain glucosamine, polysulfated glycosaminoglycans, and chondroitin sulfates—compounds known to be involved in the synthesis and repair of joint cartilage. There is a decrease in joint lubrication with age, and glucosamine and chondroitin are the building blocks for the synthesis of glycosaminoglycan (GAGs), an important component of connective tissues. These compounds are given orally and can be considered as follow-up therapy after intramuscular injections, or in any condition in which joint damage is anticipated or expected, such as trauma, surgery, or degenerative joint disease.

Other oral supplements include manganese, copper, vitamin C, yucca perna mussel, MSM (methyl sulfonyl methane), and a derivative of DMSO (dimethyl sulfoxide). A commonly used commercial supplement is Cosequin, which is a combination of glucosamine hydrochloride, chondroitin sulfate, manganese, and vitamin C. A variety of products are available that contain various combinations of these ingredients. You'll need to use any product for at least three months to see if it is effective for your horse.

An herb called devil's claw (*Harpogophytum procumbens*) provides pain relief and is an anti-inflammatory. It is available in several different forms. Its effectiveness has not been proven in clinical trials, but there is a large body of anecdotal evidence to support its efficacy. However, use devil's claw with extreme care, because this herb causes abortions in pregnant mares.

Capsaicin, made from hot peppers, is a topical ointment used for musculoskeletal pain. It reduces pain by reducing the neurotransmissions that send pain messages from the body to the brain.

Acupuncture, massage therapy, and chiropractics are three other therapies that may be used in conjunction with the supplements just described. Acupuncture manages pain hypersensitivity, balances energy flow, and causes the body to release natural opioids. Massage therapy aides in increasing the circulation, releasing scar tissue, balancing muscle function, and promoting relaxation. Chiropractic is a physical manipulation that is based on neurologic mechanisms and the biomechanics of the spine. Each modality treats the entire horse to improve function and comfort. They should be done only by individuals with specialized training in that discipline. For more information on all these modalities, see chapter 21, "Alternative Therapies."

An effective chronic pain management plan includes a veterinary evaluation. At this time, a plan for the use of NSAIDs, chondroprotective anti-inflammatory agents, regular exercise, stretching, massage, acupuncture, chiropractics, and oral supplements can be determined and implemented.

Euthanasia

The time may come when you are faced with the prospect of having to end your horse's life. This is a difficult decision to make—both for you and for your veterinarian. Many old and infirm horses can be made quite comfortable with just a little more thoughtfulness and extra tender loving care. Old horses can still enjoy months or years of happiness in the company of loved ones.

When it is clear that comfort is no longer possible, it is time for euthanasia. Discuss the options with your veterinarian to make sure this is the best choice for your horse. Your veterinarian can also explain the procedure; an intravenous injection of an anesthetic agent in sufficient amount to cause immediate loss of consciousness and cardiac arrest. Usually, a catheter is placed in the neck vein to make it easier to give the drugs. A mild sedative may be given at first, but the horse will die from an injection of a strong barbiturate.

There will be no physical pain associated with this injection. Once it is given, the horse may continue to stand for several seconds before collapsing. He may move his legs and take several deep breaths, and his eyes may move back and forth and remain open after death. Generally there is no blood and the horse will urinate or defecate within minutes. The horse is completely unaware of what is happening.

The death of your horse may be difficult to watch. Your veterinarian will respect your decision, and will give you time for good-byes.

There are companion animal loss hotlines available and grief counselors are now better equipped to deal with this kind of loss. Your veterinarian can provide these resources for you, if needed.

No one wants to imagine that they need to plan ahead, and yet planning can prevent a lot of distress if the time does come when you must euthanize your equine friend.

A FINAL MEMORIAL

Ideally, you need to think about how to handle the body before your horse has died. Burial is the choice of some families, although local laws may prohibit this in your area. Cremation may not be locally available, and if it is, it can be expensive for a horse. Your veterinarian can advise you about this option. You can also engage a rendering company.

There are many ways to memorialize your horse. A clay impression of the horse's hoof and hair from the mane or tail can become treasured keepsakes. Many families decide to make a donation in their horse's memory to a rescue group or to an equine health research fund. All of these are worthy causes and enable you to keep your horse's memory alive in a very positive way.

20

Drugs and Medications

The drugs and medications available to today's horse owners are varied and powerful. It is up to you to protect your horse by being knowledgeable about the medications your horse will receive. Take the initiative in communicating with your veterinarian. Help your horse by asking questions; you are her voice. Do not be afraid to say that you don't understand something and get clarification. Communication is the key to success.

- Do you understand what the medication is for?
- How is the medication to be administered?
- Are you comfortable with the method of administration, or does your veterinarian need to demonstrate how to give a pill or shot?
- What side effects should you watch for?
- How often are you to give the medication and for how long?
- Does this medication have special storage needs?
- Have you made your veterinarian aware of all supplements and any other medications you are giving your horse?

For a list of common medications your veterinarian may prescribe, see the online supplement to this volume at www.wiley.com/go/horsevethandbook.

Anesthetics and Tranquilizers

Anesthetics are drugs used to block the sensation of and reaction to pain. Anesthetics can be given as a local injection, intravenously as general anesthesia, or as inhaled gases administered through a tube placed in the windpipe.

Local anesthetics are used for procedures on the surface of the body, where they are injected locally into the tissue or into a regional nerve. They also may be applied topically to mucous membranes. Although local anesthetics (such as lidocaine) have the fewest risks and side effects, they are not suitable for most major surgery.

Intravenous sedation involves the use of tranquilizers. Tranquilizers are drugs used to relieve anxiety, to prepare a horse for surgery, and to calm a horse for handling and treatment. The exact mode of action of tranquilizers varies, depending on the specific drug. Some act on the brain to reduce anxiety, others achieve their effect primarily by increasing the threshold for pain—which is known as sedation. The dose that produces sedation in the standing horse is often close to the dose that causes stumbling and collapse. Accordingly, intravenous sedation drugs are usually started at a low dose and incrementally increased to achieve the desired effect.

Acepromazine, diazepam (Valium), and other tranquilizers are generally safe and effective when used as directed and in the correct situation. Horses can still strike or kick without warning even when properly tranquilized. Use the same precautions as you would around a horse who is not sedated.

Xylazine (Rompun), romifidine (Sedivet), and detomidine combine both tranquilization and pain control. They are useful for short procedures, such as floating the teeth. They are also effective in relieving the pain of *colic*. The effects of both drugs can be reversed with yohimbine or tolazoline—a valuable consideration if there is an overdose.

To further enhance analgesia while minimizing side effects, tranquilizers and narcotic analgesics can be combined. The combination of acepromazine with butorphanol is used most often. Drug combinations allow some painful procedures to be done under intravenous sedation that would otherwise have to be done under general anesthesia.

General anesthesia renders the horse unconscious. Isoflurane gas is used for longer procedures, such as those on the bones and joints, or within the abdomen. The dose of all anesthetics is computed by the weight of the horse. Nonetheless, susceptibility varies greatly, even among horses of the same weight. Therefore, anesthetics require the services of a trained professional to monitor and control the degree of sedation.

The horse removes anesthetic agents from the body by the lungs, liver, or kidneys, depending on the specific agent. Impaired function of these organs can cause anesthetic complications. To make sure the horse is in good health before surgery, a complete checkup, including appropriate laboratory tests, is advisable. This becomes even more important for older horses.

If a horse is going to be given a general anesthetic, hay and grain should be withheld for 12 to 24 hours before surgery. This is done to decrease the amount of material in the gastrointestinal tract so it does not press on the diaphragm and restrict breathing when the horse is asleep or placed on her back or her side. Allow access to water. Horses on a high-concentrate diet should be weaned to a low-concentrate diet during the preceding week. Horses do not need excessive energy food during convalescence; the recovery period will require stall rest. The most common post-anesthetic complication is myopathy of prolonged *recumbency* (see page 283).

Anti-Inflammatory Drugs and Analgesics

Analgesics are used to relieve pain; anti-inflammatories reduce inflammation. Often, as with the case of *NSAIDs*, a particular drug does both.

Morphine, pentazocine (Talwin), and butorphanol are narcotic analgesics; therefore, they are subject to federal regulation and must be purchased by prescription. The effect of narcotics on horses is unpredictable. They can produce excitation, apprehension, and increased muscular activity rather than analgesia and sedation. They are not suitable for home veterinary use.

CORTICOSTEROIDS

Corticosteroids are among the most powerful anti-inflammatory agents. The anti-inflammatory properties of cortisone derive from the ability of the drug to enter the cell and alter functions associated with the inflammatory response. However, the suppressive effects are not selective. This means cell functions associated with cellular immunity and wound healing are likewise suppressed by cortisone. This can delay wound healing for up to a year. The likelihood of wound infection is also increased. All these risks are proportional to the length of steroid usage. They are unlikely to occur when ultra-short-acting steroids are used for only a few days.

Cortisone injections into and around joints are commonly used to reduce swelling and inflammation. These injections can be beneficial when administered under veterinary supervision and when accompanied by adequate rest. Too often, however, cortisone masks the pain and lameness associated with the injury, and the horse is returned to exercise or training too soon, with the result that the injury is further aggravated.

Injectable corticosteroids have a limited but real potential for producing acute laminitis. This makes nonsteroidal drugs less risky and a better choice for treating the pain and swelling associated with the majority of musculoskeletal injuries.

Multiple injections into the same joint may produce a condition called steroid arthropathy, an accelerated form of degenerative arthritis. One other risk of any injection into a joint is the potential for septic arthritis (joint infection).

A further risk of long-term cortisone usage is adrenal insufficiency. The adrenal gland stops making cortisone because the hormone is being supplied by the medication. Once the medicine is stopped, the horse has no readily available source of cortisone and may suffer from a shocklike condition called an Addisonian crisis, although this is rare.

Corticosteroids are often combined with antibiotics, particularly in topical preparations for use in the eyes. In some eye conditions, particularly those associated with a virus, secondary effects on the cornea can lead to perforation and blindness. Accordingly, it is important that eye preparations containing steroids be used only with veterinary approval.

NONSTEROIDAL ANTI-INFLAMMATORY DRUGS

Nonsteroidal anti-inflammatory drugs (*NSAIDs*) are the most commonly used and the safest pain relievers for horses. These drugs interfere with prostaglandin synthesis and the production of undesirable inflammatory products and enzymes.

All NSAIDs, including phenylbutazone (Butazolidin), have the potential for toxicity at high levels. Toxicity can occur when NSAIDs are used for a prolonged period of time, when an NSAID is given at twice the recommended dose, or when two or more NSAIDs are given at the same time (the effects are cumulative). The gastrointestinal tract and kidneys are the target organs for drug-induced toxicity. NSAIDs have different levels of risk for causing complications.

Ulcers in the mouth, stomach, and large colon occur with long-term use. The signs include loss of appetite, weight loss, gastrointestinal bleeding, and diarrhea. Kidney damage leads to protein losses in the urine, followed by *edema* of the limbs, chest, and abdominal wall. Death can occur from colon ulceration or kidney failure. Treatment involves stopping the drug, replenishing protein and *electrolyte* losses with intravenous fluids and plasma, and administering anti-ulcer medications.

The NSAIDs described here are currently used in equine practice.

- **Flunixin meglumine (Banamine).** This NSAID has a rapid onset of action, making it the agent of choice in the initial treatment of tendonitis, colic pain, and many musculoskeletal injuries. Banamine is also a cyclooxygenase inhibitor, which means it prevents the unwanted circulatory and vascular effects of bacterial *endotoxins* and *exotoxins*. Accordingly, it is used to treat the *endotoxemia* associated with acute laminitis, acute colitis, and acute septic metritis.
- **Firocoxib (Equioxx).** This is a new NSAID used to treat pain and inflammation. It is said to have fewer side effects.
- **Diclofenac sodium (Surpass).** This topical NSAID is used to control inflammation and pain.
- **Carprofen and eltenac.** These NSAIDs are both very effective analgesics as well as anti-inflammatories.

- **Ketoprofen.** This NSAID has a wide spectrum of activity with a relatively low risk of toxicity.

- **Naproxen (Equiproxen).** This drug is perhaps the most effective NSAID for treating muscle pain and soft tissue injury. It is not as effective in treating joint injuries.

- **Phenylbutazone (Butazolidin).** "Bute" is the most widely used anti-inflammatory painkiller in horses. It is especially effective for injuries involving bone, joint, tendon, and muscle. It can be administered by tablet, paste, powder, or injection, which gives it great versatility. Butazolidin is preferred for long-term maintenance because of its longer-lasting effects and low cost. However, long-term use of Butazolidin has been associated with stomach ulcers and kidney failure.

- **Salicylates (aspirin).** The short duration of action of aspirin, plus the high dosage required in horses, makes aspirin generally impractical for pain relief. However, aspirin in small doses (10 to 20 mg per kilogram of body weight) is used to inhibit platelet aggregation in horses with acute laminitis and other illnesses associated with intravascular clotting. Thiosalicylate is an injectable salicylate with a longer duration that has been used for its analgesic effect.

OTHER ANTI-INFLAMMATORY DRUGS
Dimethyl Sulfoxide

Dimethyl sulfoxide (DMSO) is a powerful free-radical scavenger that helps remove many of the harmful by-products of inflammation. It has great membrane permeability and passes readily through the skin. It also has the ability to carry other topical drugs along with it, and it is frequently used for this purpose along with topical corticosteroids. It should not be used on open wounds.

DMSO rapidly absorbs moisture and becomes diluted with water if left open to the air. When applied to the skin, it draws moisture from the deeper tissue, which explains why it is effective in treating swelling caused by contusions and hematomas. It is not an antibacterial and should not be used to treat cellulitis.

There are several ways to apply topical DMSO. The choice depends on the location of the injury and the reasons for using it. It is best to seek directions from your veterinarian.

Because DMSO carries other agents along with it, it should be used with caution on skin that has already been treated with antiseptics, antibacterials, and other chemicals. In addition, wear rubber gloves when handling DMSO to prevent skin contact. Signs of toxicity in humans caused by DMSO absorption include headache, dizziness, dermatitis, and an oysterlike taste in the mouth.

DMSO as a 10 percent solution is used intravenously to treat a number of acute disorders, including tendonitis, *colic*, endotoxemic states, and brain and spinal cord injuries. Higher concentrations, particularly when given rapidly, have been associated with the rapid destruction of red cells (hemolysis).

CHONDROPROTECTANTS
Hyaluronic Acid

Hyaluronic acid (HA) is a naturally occurring constituent of the synovial fluid in joints and tendon sheaths. HA prevents destructive enzymes from breaking down cartilage and causing inflammatory adhesions and scars. It can be injected intravenously or into the joints, and has proven to be beneficial in horses with joint and tendon ailments not accompanied on X-rays by bony destruction. Injection into the tendon sheath to treat tendonitis has given good results.

Polysulfated Glycosaminoglycan (Adequan)

Polysulfated glycosaminoglycan (PSGAG), like hyaluronic acid, occurs naturally in synovial fluid and protects cartilage from stress-induced damage. There is evidence that PSGAG can partially restore cartilage that has suffered some degree of structural damage. Although usually injected directly into a joint, PSGAG is also available orally and intramuscularly, which has the advantage of treating more than one joint.

Antibiotics

Antibiotics are extracts of rudimentary plants such as molds and fungi. They are capable of destroying some microorganisms that cause disease. Today, many antibiotics are made synthetically from basic chemical structures.

Antibiotics fall into two general categories. Those that are *bacteriostatic* (or fungistatic) inhibit the growth of microorganisms but do not kill them. *Bactericidal* and fungicidal drugs destroy the microorganisms outright.

Bacteria also are classified according to their ability to cause disease. Pathogenic bacteria are capable of producing a particular illness or infection. Nonpathogenic bacteria live on (or within) the horse, but don't cause illness under normal conditions. These bacteria are referred to as normal flora. Some actually produce substances that are necessary to the well-being of the host. For example, bacteria in the bowel synthesize vitamin K and the B-complex vitamins, which most animals cannot do for themselves.

For a list of antibiotics, antifungals, and antiprotozoals your veterinarian may prescribe, see the online supplement to this book at www.wiley.com/go/horsevethandbook.

Why Antibiotics May Not Be Effective
Misdiagnosis of Infection

Signs of inflammation (such as heat, redness, and swelling) can exist without infection. A severe bruise is a good example. To be certain of infection, one should see inflammation and *purulent* discharge (*pus*). The discharge may have an offensive odor. Other indications of infection include fever and elevated white cell count.

Inappropriate Selection

An antibiotic must be effective against the specific microorganism that is causing the infection. The best way to confirm that effectiveness is to recover the organism, culture it, and then identify it. Antibiotic discs are then applied to the culture plate to see which discs inhibit the growth of the bacteria. The results are graded according to whether the microorganism is sensitive or resistant to a particular antibiotic. Much of the effectiveness also depends on the location of the infection and the ability of the antibiotic to reach the site of infection.

If an infection is suspected, preliminary tests may be done to confirm, such as a cytology test or gram stain (where presumed infected material is applied to a microscope slide, stained, and looked at microscopically for bacteria and white cells). A culture takes at least 24 hours and a sensitivity test requires an additional 24 hours before the most appropriate antibiotic can be determined. Many times, the veterinarian will start the horse on one antibiotic based on preliminary findings and switch later, when the culture and sensitivity tests are complete. (For more information, see *Culture and Sensitivity*, page 632.)

Although laboratory findings do not invariably correlate with the results of treatment, culture and antibiotic sensitivity testing are still the surest way of selecting the most effective antibiotic.

Inadequate Wound Care

Antibiotics enter the bloodstream and are carried to the source of the infection. Abscesses, wounds containing devitalized tissue, and foreign bodies such as dirt and splinters are resistant areas, meaning the antibiotics are unable to get to the source of infection. Accordingly, it is important to drain abscesses, irrigate and cleanse dirty wounds, removing foreign bodies, diseased bone, and tissue.

Route of Administration

The effectiveness of an antibiotic diminishes if it is given by the wrong route. In equine practice, most antibiotics are given intramuscularly. Some are given intravenously and a few are given orally. The choice depends on the type of antibiotic, the type of infection, the severity of the illness, and whether the gastrointestinal tract is functioning normally. A horse with colic or diarrhea will not absorb antibiotics well and will not maintain adequate blood levels.

Dosage and Frequency of Administration

The total daily dose is computed by estimating the weight of the horse, then dividing the dose into equal parts and giving each part at a specified time. When the total dose is too low or a dose is skipped, the horse does not maintain a drug level high enough to kill all organisms, which can lead to drug resistance by the organism.

Factors that have to be taken into account when computing the daily dose include the severity of the infection, the condition of the horse's kidneys and liver, and whether the horse is taking another antibiotic.

COMPLICATIONS OF ANTIBIOTICS

All drugs should be viewed as poisons. The toxic effects of a drug can be more dangerous than the disease. Antibiotics should never be given without justifiable indications. Common complications of antibiotics are discussed.

Allergy

Antibiotics, more so than other classes of drugs, can cause allergic reactions, including *hives*. An immediate life-threatening allergic reaction can occur when a horse is exposed to an antibiotic to which she has developed hypersensitivity through prior exposure. See *Anaphylactic Shock* (page 28).

Toxicity

There is a margin of safety between a therapeutic dose and a toxic dose. Toxicity can be caused by overdose, prolonged use, or impaired elimination from the body. Drugs are removed by the liver and kidneys. If these organs are failing, the antibiotic is not broken down and excreted rapidly enough to prevent toxic buildup.

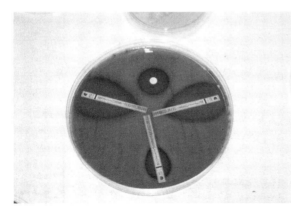

For an antibiotic sensitivity test, strips impregnated with antibiotics on an agar plate show which antibiotics inhibit growth of the bacteria cultured. The clear areas are the areas where the growth of the bacteria is suppressed.

Toxicity can affect one or more systems. Signs of toxicity are difficult to recognize in horses. Thus, they can be far advanced before they come to your attention.

- **Ears.** Damage to the optic nerves leads to hearing loss and deafness. The loss can be permanent.
- **Liver.** Toxicity can lead to jaundice and liver failure.
- **Kidneys.** Toxicity causes nitrogen retention, uremia, and kidney failure.
- **Bone marrow.** Toxicity depresses the production of red cells, white cells, and platelets. These effects may be irreversible.

Secondary Infection

Antibiotics alter the normal flora that serves as a protective barrier to infection. Pathogenic bacteria are thus freed to multiply and cause disease. The best example of this is the severe enterocolitis that can follow the use of antibiotics that change the normal flora of the bowel.

Emergence of Resistant Strains

Strains of bacteria that exhibit resistance to antibiotics evolve when antibiotics are used for a long time, in too low a dose, and/or when the antibiotic is bacteriostatic. Microorganisms that develop resistance to one antibiotic may be resistant to others of the same class.

Use During Pregnancy

Certain antibiotics can affect the growth and development of unborn or newborn foals. Tetracycline and griseofulvin are two examples. They should not be used during pregnancy.

How to Give Medications

For a list of common medications for veterinary use, see the online supplement to this book at www.wiley.com/go/horsevethandbook. How to medicate the eyes is discussed on page 146. How to medicate the ears is discussed on page 170.

CAPSULES AND TABLETS

The most common way of medicating your horse is to dose her with ground pills or capsules. Since equine tablets are usually quite large, grinding the tablet gives an option of presenting it in something sweet or in a syringe. It is important to thoroughly crush the pills so there are no chunks that can be spit out. Pills may be ground with a mortar and pestle or an automatic coffee grinder. Not many people have a mortar and pestle handy, but if you use a coffee grinder, it should not be used for anything else.

Pills such as Butazolidin and trimethoprim-sulfonamide combinations can be dissolved in water and given by syringe, as described for pastes (see below), or broken up and mixed with feed or molasses. If mixed with feed, a good choice is rolled corn or oats. Add 2 tablespoons (30 ml) of water to a quart of grain. This should be sufficient to get the powder to stick to the grain but not create a mush. The horse must be observed to make sure she eats all of her medicated

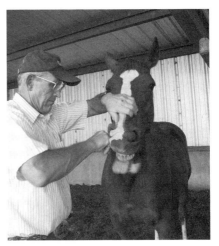

Some horses look forward to their applesauce with crushed pills.

grain. Other mixtures may include applesauce, honey, peanut butter, or mashed carrots.

Not all horses will eat medicine "treats," and some simply don't like the "off" taste. An irrigation syringe with a catheter style end works well for the difficult-to-doctor equine. Mix powdered medication with water or Kool-Aid, shake it up, load the syringe, and shoot the liquid into the back of the horse's throat like a paste wormer. If mixed with molasses, the powder can be put into a 60-ml syringe along with 2 ounces (56 g) of sorghum molasses and delivered like a paste. Molasses is sweet and most horses will readily swallow it. It is important to hold the horse's head up until she has swallowed.

PASTES

Many horse dewormers and some medications come conveniently packaged in disposable syringes with markings on the syringe to show the number of milliliters of paste to deliver per pound weight of the horse. Remove all feed before giving the paste. It is easier for the horse to spit out the medication if there is food in her mouth to go along with it. Insert the end of the syringe into the horse's mouth through the space between the teeth. Depress the plunger. The horse's head should be restrained to prevent her from pulling back and injuring her mouth.

LIQUIDS

Liquid medications and *electrolyte* solutions can be given by large-dose syringe, drenching bottle, or stomach tube. The syringe is used as described for pastes, but with a drenching bottle it is important to raise the horse's chin so her nose is parallel to the ground. This will prevent the liquid from running out of her mouth.

Mineral oil (and other oils) should never be given by syringe or drenching bottle. Mineral oil, in particular, has no taste and therefore is difficult to swallow. As a result, the horse could inhale the oil, resulting in fatal aspiration pneumonia. Accordingly, all oils must be given by stomach tube.

STOMACH TUBE

A stomach tube is a plastic or rubber tube about 10 feet (3 m) long. The tube is introduced through the horse's nose and gently advanced into the esophagus. As the tube passes down toward the stomach, you can often follow its progress as a ripple down the side of the horse's neck next to the jugular vein.

Once the end of the tube is just above the stomach, the medication is flushed down the tube with a large-dose syringe or a hand pump. The tube should then be flushed with water to deliver any residual medication in the tube.

Improper placement of the stomach tube (into the trachea) is a potential hazard. The horse may cough as the tube enters the larynx, but this does not always happen. If the medicine is delivered into the lungs, the horse will aspirate and possibly drown. For this reason, a stomach tube should be passed by a veterinarian or an individual trained in its use.

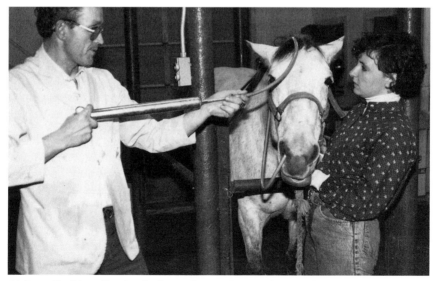

Giving a liquid medication by large-dose syringe and stomach tube.

Injections

Some injections are given under the skin (subcutaneous), some into the muscle (intramuscular), and others directly into a vein (intravenous). The directions with the product will indicate the correct route. Have your veterinarian demonstrate the correct procedures for giving injections if you have any questions.

The injection itself usually is not painful to the horse, but inserting the needle may be painful for a moment. If this occurs unexpectedly, the horse may shy or kick. For this reason, horses should be restrained for injections. An assistant in control of the halter and lead is adequate restraint for most well-trained horses who are used to being handled and treated. If the horse is high-spirited or not used to being handled, a more secure restraint may be necessary (see *Handling and Restraint,* page 2).

Draw the medicine into the syringe and point the needle up while pressing the plunger to expel air. Then detach the needle from the syringe.

Select the site for injection. The three best sites for intramuscular injection are the side of the neck, the buttocks, and the back of the thigh (see the photos on pages 600 and 601). The skin along the side of the neck is a good place for subcutaneous injections. Here the skin is loose and readily forms a fold when pinched. Intravenous injections are given into the jugular vein. Experience is necessary to locate this vein and penetrate it with a hypodermic needle.

To give an intramuscular injection, swab the skin with an alcohol sponge. Angle the needle so that it is at a right angle to the surface of the body. Insert the needle up to the hub with a quick jab. If the horse jerks back, wait a few seconds until she settles down. Attach the syringe to the needle. Draw back on the plunger and look for blood. The presence of blood indicates that the point of the needle has entered a vein. If that happens, do not give the injection. Withdraw the syringe and start again. Once you see that the injection can be given safely, depress the plunger. Withdraw the needle and rub the skin for a few seconds to disperse the medication. Injections into bones, nerves, and joints can be avoided by giving the shot in the locations illustrated on pages 600 and 601.

For a subcutaneous injection, grasp a fold of skin to form a ridge. Swab the skin with alcohol. Remove the needle from the syringe. Firmly push the needle through the skin fold into the subcutaneous fat. The angle of insertion should be somewhat parallel to the surface of the body to prevent the needle from either going into the muscle or coming out the other side of the skin fold. Attach the syringe to the needle. Draw back on the plunger and look for blood. The presence of blood indicates that the point of the needle has entered a vein. If that happens, do not give the injection. Withdraw the syringe and start again. Once you see that the injection can be given safely, depress the plunger. Withdraw the needle and rub the skin for a few seconds to disperse the medication.

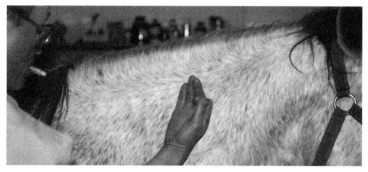

Giving an injection. First alert the horse by tapping the injection site with the back of your hand.

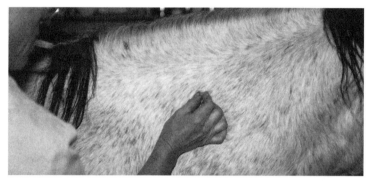

For an intramuscular injection, insert the needle vertically before connecting the syringe. This way, if the horse startles the needle will not break off.

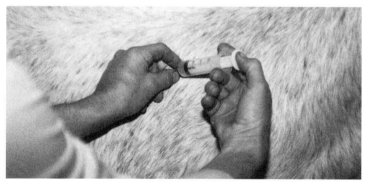

Aspirate for blood and inject the medicine.

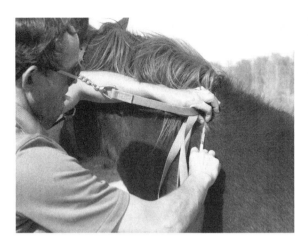

The neck is a good location for subcutaneous injections. Grasp a fold of skin to form a ridge.

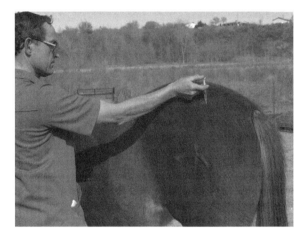

The correct site for giving injections into the buttocks. Feel for bone and inject well away from it into the bulging muscle.

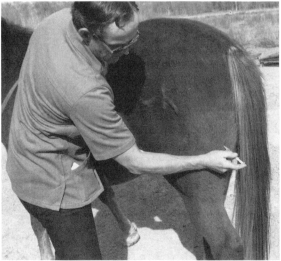

An injection can be given into the muscle at the back of the thigh.

ENEMAS

Enemas are used to treat rectal impactions. They are not prescribed for routine use; there are better ways to treat chronic constipation (see *Constipation*, page 388). If the horse has colic, enemas are contraindicated because they may rupture the colon.

Sodium phosphate enemas and soapy water enemas are often given to newborn foals with impacted meconium or to prevent impaction. How to give these enemas is discussed in *Meconium Colic* (see page 525). The procedure for giving a soapy water enema to an adult horse is described in *Rectal Impactions* (see page 378).

21

ALTERNATIVE THERAPIES

As is the case with changes in human medicine, therapeutic procedures have progressed in equine medicine. Along with remarkable advances in surgical techniques and drug therapies for a wide range of diseases, alternative therapies for the treatment of certain diseases of the horse have emerged as new frontiers in everyday clinical medicine.

Holistic veterinary medicine offers a complete approach to the care of your horse by drawing on all disciplines of health care. Holistic is defined as treatment for the whole animal and complete systems, rather than just treating a single body part or system. It combines conventional diagnostic and therapeutic medicine with alternative therapies.

Among these alternative therapies are herbal medications, *nutraceuticals*, manual therapies (which include chiropractic procedures, physical therapy and massage therapy), and *acupuncture* for the horse. These therapies have been used as a sole treatment for a disease, as an additional treatment to complement medical and surgical procedures, and as a last resort when a horse fails to respond to traditional Western medicine. Sometimes, these methods are successful when traditional medicine or traditional drug therapy cannot be used.

The authors do not endorse or disparage any particular alternative therapy, simply because each illness or disease process is unique to the individual patient. Consultation with your veterinarian, who knows your horse and his condition, will be more productive than any particular treatment regimen discussed in this book.

We cannot stress enough that you should consult only professionals with advanced training. A proper understanding of your horse's anatomy and potential medical issues is necessary to diagnose and effectively plan treatment. Many veterinarians are also trained in herbal medicine, massage therapy, acupuncture, and chiropractic therapy. It is important to tell your veterinarian about any herbal formulas that you are giving your horse, because these are potent treatments and may interfere with or amplify the effects of any medication that is prescribed, or mask any symptoms necessary for a diagnosis. Remember, many modern medications had their start as herbal supplements.

Nutraceuticals

Nutraceuticals are nutritional supplements, micronutrients (nutrients that are needed in tiny amounts but are crucial to health because they enable the body to produce enzymes, hormones and other substances essential for proper growth and development), and macronutrients (nutrients that are required in relatively large amounts) that are used to provide a health benefit or a protection against some particular disease. The desired substance is added to or fed as part of the horse's diet.

Two of the most familiar products in the nutraceutical category are chondroitin and glucosamine. Chondroitin is a component of tendons, cartilage, and bone tissue. Chondroitin sulfate, the therapeutic form of this nutraceutical, is derived from sharks, pork products, and the windpipes of cattle.

Glucosamine is the basic building block of connective tissues and fluids. Glucosamine sulfate can be manufactured from a chemical process involving the simple sugar glucose and an amino acid, or it can be derived from shellfish such as the shells of shrimp, crabs, and lobsters. It is important to note that although there are other types of glucosamine (N-acetyl-glucosamine and glucosamine HCL) found in different supplements, they are not the same as glucosamine sulfate and are not very effective. Chondroitin sulfate and glucosamine sulfate are used to treat osteoarthritis, joint diseases, and tendon and cartilage injuries.

There are nutraceuticals available to treat a variety of conditions, including stress and nerves, ulcers, chronic bleeding, insect bites, Lyme disease, and the lactic acid buildup of tying-up syndrome. Further in-depth research is needed to verify the benefits and best uses for these products, because most of the information at this time is based on anecdotal and personal experiences of the users. These products should be used only as part of a complete health plan developed to prevent any harm to your horse.

It is important to note that many of the manufacturers do not list the active ingredients in their product, nor is there scientific data available to provide assurance of potency. The safety, effectiveness, or purity of these products has neither been established nor proven. The manufacturing standards for nutraceuticals usually have not been established, so it is entirely possible that the dosage of the active ingredient in the product may vary enough from manufacturer to manufacturer to be toxic or entirely ineffective for your horse.

These products are not regulated the way drugs are, and so have not had the objective comparative trials and testing that is required of all drugs.

Indeed, potential side effects may not be known, especially when some nutraceuticals are used for a long time. Often these treatments have been recommended by someone whose horse seemed to benefit, but may have improved in any case, with or without treatment.

INDICATIONS FOR USE

Nutraceuticals are frequently used to treat arthritis and tendon injuries, and there is some evidence, based on studies, that glucosamine and chondroitin are effective. Cosequin and Adequan are two of the well-known brands that are made for horses and whose formulations are consistent and safe. The effectiveness for other uses remains to be proven.

CONTRAINDICATIONS FOR USE

None are known at this time.

Herbal Medicine

Naturopathy and herbology use natural substances such as plants and minerals to provide a source of medicines to treat disease. Herbs and naturally occurring plant products have been used to treat a variety of conditions, including musculoskeletal diseases such as arthritis and muscle pain. An example is the plant devil's claw. It has been used in place of nonsteroidal anti-inflammatory drugs (NSAIDs). However, devil's claw should not be used if your horse has a gastric ulcer, heart problems, or is pregnant, as it has known abortive properties.

Most herbs used to treat horses are selected by the owner or recommended by another horse owner. Creative, persuasive advertising may also lure the owner to use herbal formulas. The veterinarian is often not included in diagnosis and treatment options, which allows for overuse and incorrect use of herbs. "A little is good, so a lot is better" is often practiced by ill-informed owners. But herbs are potent drugs, and overdosing can have serious consequences.

Even if you are consulting a qualified herbalist, remember that herbalists are often not trained in understanding disease processes or the unique equine systems. What works for people may not work for horses. Many veterinary practitioners are affiliated with the American Holistic Veterinary Medical Association (www.ahvma.org) or the Veterinary Botanical Medicine Association (www.vbma.org).

As the interest in herbs is growing, the field of zoopharmacognosy—the study of how animals self-select plants and minerals to address disease or discomfort—is growing. This is a multifaceted discipline that includes animal behaviorists, ecologists, pharmacologists, anthropologists, and parasitologists.

Many studies have been done, but it is interesting to note that there is a huge difference between wild animals and domestic animals in the way they consume or self-select plants to treat disease. You cannot expect your own horse to be able to select what is good for him or to avoid what is bad.

Drug Testing and Herbs

The United States Equestrian Federation (USEF) lists a number of herbs that are prohibited in competition in the United States. USEF guidelines state, "Any product is forbidden if it contains an ingredient that is a forbidden substance, or is a drug that might affect the performance of a horse/or pony as a stimulant, depressant, tranquilizer, local anesthetic, psychotropic (mood or behavior altering) substance, or might interfere with drug testing procedures." The chart (below) lists only a few of these banned substances.

Herbs Specifically Prohibited in Competition in the United States

Common Name	Scientific Name
Arnica, leopard's bane, wolf's bane	*Arnica montana*
Cayenne (capsaicin and derivatives)	*Capsicum annuum*
Chamomile (species not specified in regulations)	*Matricaria spp., Ormenis mixta/multicola, Anthemis nobilis*
Comfrey	*Symphytum officinale*
Devil's claw	*Harpagophytum procumbens*
Hops	*Humulus lupulus*
Kava kava	*Piper methysticum*
Laurel	*Laurus nobiles*
Lavender	*Lavandula spp.*
Lemon balm	*Melissa officinalis*
Nightshade	*Solanum spp.*
Passionflower	*Passiflora incarnate*
Rauwolfia	*Rauwolfia serpentine*
Red poppy	*Papaver rhoeas, Papaver somniferum*
Skullcap	*Scutelleria lateriflora*
Valerian	*Valeriana officinalis*
Vervain	*Verbena officinalis*

Some herbs used topically, such as peppermint, menthol, and rosemary, may be licked by the horse; these are considered masking agents for illegal drugs, and therefore are also banned.

Some Chinese herbs that may be forbidden in the racing community in the United States include (but are not limited to) ephedra (ephedrine), papaver (morphine), strychnos (strychnine), daura (atropine), and acacia (theophylline).

In Australia, prohibited herbs include white willow, kola, kava kava, guarana, and valerian, but other herbs may be tested for.

INDICATIONS FOR USE

Horses are herbivores and are designed to eat raw herbs. The horse's cecum effectively breaks down plant fibers. There are no studies that have looked at the most effective form of using herbs for horses—dried, fresh, extract, or tincture. Topical herbs are well tolerated by most horses, although their use should be discontinued if the horse's skin peels or becomes irritated.

Historically, herbs have been used to improve health after a serious illness has resolved. Today, healthy horses are fed large quantities of herbs for extended periods, with the idea of promoting general health or preventing disease. In nature, all plants become scarce during the winter, giving the body a break from them. This rest period is important.

The following are some common equine conditions for which there may be a variety of herbal formulas.

Arthritis or chronic degenerative joint disease (DJD) is one of the most common conditions that limits a horse's performance, and many different herbal formulas are available to treat it. Different horses respond differently to each treatment. Although one horse may respond well to devil's claw or meadowsweet, the next horse may have no response.

Colic in the acute form is rarely treated with herbs, because they simply don't work fast enough. However, chronic colic may be treated with such formulas as chamomile and valerian or a combination of comfrey, marshmallow, slippery elm, licorice, and valerian.

Ulcers in the horse must be treated with measures that include changing the lifestyle. Distilled aloe as a single herb has also been used.

Moonblindness or recurrent uveitis has been treated with bilberry and echinacea. An eyewash can be made of calendula, but undiluted it may sting, making the horse difficult to treat.

Laminitis is a complex disease that is not easily treated with herbs. However, herbs are used as an anti-inflammatory to support other treatment therapies.

Anxiety and nerves are among the most common conditions for which modern horse owners use herbal remedies. However, many horses with this condition spend too much time in their stall, have inadequate exercise, and eat too many carbohydrates. Many formulas are advertised to "calm" a horse. The results vary.

Recurrent airway obstruction may be associated with a dry cough, which can be treated with asparagus root, licorice, borage leaf, and yarrow.

Traumas, bruises, and sprains are often treated topically with wolf's bane (also called mountain arnica), lavender, comfrey, witch hazel, yucca, white willow bark, and rue.

Parasites may be treated with herbal anthelmintic formulations, but many are relatively toxic to the horse and should be used with care.

CONTRAINDICATIONS FOR USE

The current popularity of these products has had some unfortunate results. As with nutraceuticals, the potency and purity of herbal products varies. There have been instances of herbal supplements and nutraceuticals being contaminated with or naturally containing toxic metals or other drugs. Veterinarians and horse owners should only use products from a reputable company with a strong dedication to research, quality control, and ethical harvesting. In the United States, you can contact the National Animal Supplement Council, which is an alliance of companies dedicated to quality control and self-regulation.

In addition, although there is a tendency to assume "natural" means "safe," these medicines can have potent effects and should only be used with the advice of trained practitioners. Some of these medications may be toxic if proper dosage regimens are not followed.

There is a potential for adverse reaction and no database is widely available on adverse events related to herbal medicine in horses. Consultation with an experienced equine herbalist may be useful.

It is important to mention the use of any herbal preparation to your veterinarian. Herbs have the potential to alter a horse's response to a drug and to cause serious adverse reactions.

A number of herbs are contraindicated during pregnancy due to the potential of causing uterine contractions, altering hormones that could be a risk to the pregnancy, or causing birth defects.

Homeopathy

Homeopathy is the practice of using a potent chemical that in large doses causes the signs of a specific disease, but in small doses is said to cure that disease. These remedies are extracted from plants, animals, and minerals, including wild hops (bryonia), nightshade (belladonna), flint, sulfur, sepia (cuttlefish ink), and apis (the body of the honey bee). There is no scientific evidence for the efficacy of homeopathic remedies, and their effectiveness is based only on anecdotal reports.

Many practitioners are associated with the American Holistic Veterinary Medical Association (www.ahvma.org).

Manual Therapies

The manual therapies include massage, physical therapy, and chiropractic. These techniques have gained many proponents in the past decade and they do have some practical applications. Your veterinarian may be able to guide your selection of the proper therapy, after your horse has a thorough and complete diagnostic work-up.

MASSAGE

Massage is the application of the practitioner's hands and body to manipulate the muscles of the horse. This technique focuses on promoting the return of blood flow from affected muscles, which causes relaxation of the targeted muscles. It is one technique in the physical therapy toolbox.

Several techniques are used in massage therapy, each with a specific purpose: to relieve inflammation and prevent adhesions, to restore posture, to help drain lymphatic fluid, to massage points of tension, to massage acupuncture points, to stretch skin, and to provide deep muscle massage.

Two supplementary tools used by equine massage therapists are electrotherapy and therapeutic ultrasound. Electrotherapy involves the application of low, medium, or high frequency electric current. The benefits include vasodilatation, reabsorption of *edema*, sedation, and muscle stimulation. Therapeutic ultrasound is discussed in the next section.

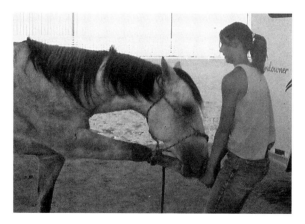

Mobilizing and stretching, protractions of the forelimb. Note how relaxed the horse is throughout the procedure.

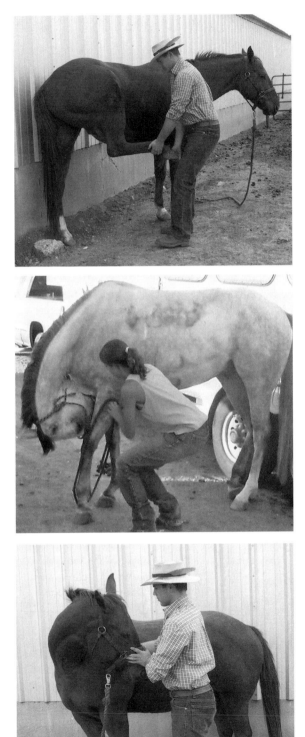

This is the basic position for implementing all the movements of the hind leg.

Flexion the caudal section of the neck.

Lateral flexion aids in the overall flexibility of the equine athlete.

Indications for Use

The goals of massage are:

- Reduce or improve pain management
- Treat inflammation
- Promote healing
- Keep the equine athlete active
- Prevent exercise-related injuries
- Prevent or manage problems secondary to the horse's athletic protocol

Contraindications for Use

The therapist must take care not to overstretch muscles or hyperextend joints, which can further irritate already injured tissues.

THERAPEUTIC ULTRASOUND

Therapeutic ultrasound (similar to diagnostic ultrasonography, which is used to detect pregnancy and diagnose ligament and tendon injuries) is capable of causing a significant rise in temperature of the deep tissues without increasing the skin temperature. Because of its penetrating nature, it can selectively heat certain tissues, such as muscles or ligaments, without heating the skin. Heating increases the metabolic activity of the cells, which increases oxygen demand, causing vasodilation, bringing more oxygen and nutrients while increasing waste removal. Waste includes products of injury, including prostaglandins and histamines, which are implicated in pain. Therapeutic ultrasound also aids in the breakdown of scar tissue fibers and acts as an analgesic by reducing the speed of conductivity of the nerves.

It is extremely important that only properly trained persons administer therapeutic ultrasound because the difference between therapeutic healing and ultrasound damage is just 9°F (5°C).

Contraindications for Use
- Do not use on or around the eyes; causes irreversible damage
- Do not use on the uterus of a pregnant mare; may damage the pregnancy
- Do not use over or near the growth plates in the long bones; disrupts normal bone growth
- Do not use on healing fractures; delays calcification and retards healing
- Do not use on inflamed blood vessels; can dislodge a clot
- Do not use in cases of cellulitis; may exacerbate an infection
- Do not use on any injured area immediately after exercise; increases irritation

Physical Therapy

Physical therapy is a scientifically based health care modality directed at evaluating, restoring, and maintaining physical function and movement. Physical therapy is an adjunct to recovery from some physical trauma in the horse's life. This therapy is still in its infancy for horses, but it is growing in popularity.

Sports medicine can be used extensively to aid the equine athlete who is training for a specialized discipline. In most of the training regimens, the same muscles and joints are used repeatedly and this may lead to damage of a young horse's bones and joints. Proper preparation for athletic endeavors is the key to preventing injury. The horse should stretch and flex, and the trainer must pay strict attention to muscle fatigue.

The goals of physical therapy include reducing pain, restoring range of motion, restoring strength, and preventing re-injury. Besides massage, other physical therapy techniques include stretching and warming up muscles (this is a key activity) and heat or cold therapy. Cold therapy slows down chemical reactions in *acute* injuries and inhibits enzyme activity, thus decreasing inflammation. It must be initiated in the acute stage and there is a limited time for benefit. Heat facilitates healing by increasing metabolic activity in the cells, thereby increasing vasodilatation and encouraging oxygen consumption and waste removal.

There is a need to further study, evaluate, and apply various physical therapy approaches to the recovery of injured horses. This applies not only to the original injury but also to the problems created by the horse compensating in various ways for the injury. Any horse in physical therapy must begin with a complete medical work-up and diagnosis, followed by a carefully structured program designed by practitioners who have had many hours of education and experience in rehabilitating injured horses. Many are associated with veterinary schools.

Chiropractic

Chiropractic focuses on disorders of the musculoskeletal system and the nervous system, and the effects of these disorders on general health. The equine chiropractor uses adjustments, primarily of the spinal column and directed to specific points in the horse's body, to create changes in nerve reactions, muscles, and joint structures. Chiropractic uses high-speed, low-force movements to restore motion to joints and vertebrae that have been damaged as a result of repetitive motion, muscle stiffness, or trauma. The chiropractor relieves the pressure on nerves that travel from the spine and carry information to all body parts.

As the person responsible for your horse's health, you must select an equine chiropractic practitioner who has extensive postgraduate education in equine anatomy, equine chiropractic techniques, and general chiropractic principals. Unfortunately, there are many lay personnel who have only a general knowledge of this therapeutic discipline but lack knowledge of equine anatomy, pathology, or physiology. At best, the untrained layperson will do no harm to your horse, but will not provide any particular benefit. At worst, inadequate treatment may cloud or cover up a particular disease process and delay a favorable outcome for your horse.

There are many veterinarians and other practitioners who have the advanced training and knowledge to obtain a proper history and do a thorough musculoskeletal examination and a clinical workup, as well as a complete neurological examination—all necessary to ensure the success of a chiropractic treatment. Veterinary practitioners are certified by the American Veterinary Chiropractic Association (www.animalchiropractic.org) or visit www.avcadoctors.com to search for an AVCA-certified practitioner.

Indications for Use

One application of chiropractic therapy is to treat back pain that results from exertion or a poor fitting saddle, and neck pain from falling over backward. Signs that may suggest a need for a chiropractic treatment include:

- Abnormal posture
- Discomfort when saddled or riding
- Extending the head and neck
- Hollowing out the back
- Stiffness in the neck or back
- Wringing the tail, pinning the ears
- Poor performance
- Abnormal behavior
- Facial expression of fear or apprehension
- Sensitivity to touch
- Unusual gait
- Muscle wasting

Contraindications for Use

A complete medical work-up and diagnosis must be done before chiropractic therapy begins, to avoid masking injures. Avoid chiropractic treatment if there's a chance that there is a fracture, because movement will exacerbate the injury. If there is a fresh injury, especially with a wound, any chiropractic treatment may be painful because of bruising and muscle or tissue damage.

Acupuncture

Acupuncture is the insertion of very fine needles (sometimes in conjunction with electrical stimulus) into specific points on the body's surface in order to influence the physiological functioning of the body. The purpose of the needles is to stimulate the specific points, which then causes a release of many physiological and biochemical processes to create a desired outcome. The aim is to aid the body in repairing itself. Acupuncture is a medical discipline that has been practiced for many millennia by doctors in Asia, and is part of a holistic system known as Traditional Chinese Medicine (TCM).

Unlike some alternative therapies, veterinary acupuncture has been shown to have more than an empirical effect on the horse. Many biochemical and physiological responses produced by the patient's body can be measured and quantitatively assayed to show alterations in response to acupuncture. Acupuncture has therefore attracted great interest in the veterinary world as a very useful addition to the treatment of disease. Its usefulness is especially apparent in the relief of pain, and a single treatment may last for much longer periods of time than the conventional drug therapy. As an important benefit, the horse does not become refractory to the treatment, as may happen with other types of pain-relief medications. Acupuncture usually will not have any toxic side effects.

Acupuncture can repair abnormally functioning tissues and organs by stimulating the neurological and endocrine systems. It stimulates the nervous system to release neurotransmitters, which are chemicals that carry information across nerve synapses. It also stimulates the endocrine system for pain relief.

The specific locations where the needles are inserted into the patient are called acupoints. Other techniques may also be used by the veterinary acupuncturist such as injecting liquids into an acupoint (aquapuncture), heating the needle (warm needling or moxibustion), firm massage of an acupoint (acupressure), bleeding of certain acupoints, applying a mild electric current to the needles (electroacupuncture), injecting air into the acupoint (pneumoacupuncture), and implants of metal or catgut. The implants and heated needles are used for long-term relief of pain associated with chronic conditions.

In the past, acupuncture was thought to have only a placebo effect—that is, it worked by "mind over matter." Since patients expected to see an improvement after a treatment, they did. Animals, however, don't know that it's supposed to work. It either does or it doesn't, and there are no psychological effects. TCM practitioners says acupuncture works by stimulating the flow of *qi*, the energy force within the body that flows along specific pathways, called meridians. However, the scientific community has researched and studied acupuncture, trying to find a more scientific answer for how and why it works.

There are five theories as to why acupuncture works. There are no hard facts and, in truth, the reason it works is perhaps a combination of all five.

The first theory is that acupuncture blocks pain signals to the brain. This blockage decreases the pain at the site. The second theory is by increasing the

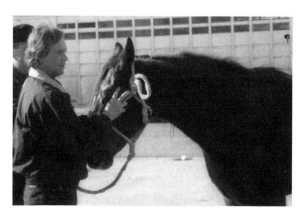

A good acupuncturist starts with a comprehensive physical examination.

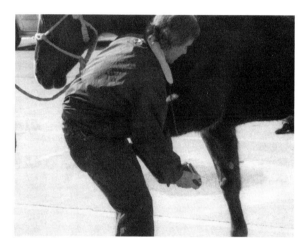

A lameness examination was in order for this sore mare before the acupuncture treatment began.

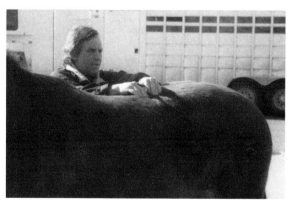

A physical exam demonstrates a sore back that will benefit from acupuncture.

blood supply in a specific area, acupuncture relaxes muscles and relieves local pain. Next is the humeral theory that endorphins are produced in response to the needle placement. Endorphins are chemicals that inhibit pain and produce a feeling of euphoria. The fourth theory is that the nervous system is stimulated by acupuncture and consequently produces an enzyme in the adrenal gland (called AMP) that increases blood flow and decreases inflammation. The fifth theory is needling near the site of pain activates a local mechanism to decrease pain and increase healing. Conversely, needling away from the site of pain activates pain relief in the whole body by circulating neurohormones.

Acupuncture shows great potential to treat certain equine conditions, especially in pain management and for a return to athletic function. It is important to work with a practitioner who has the many hours of education and

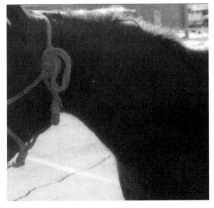

Look carefully for the three fine needles inserted into the acupoints in the neck (the third is not easy to see). These have a sedative effect.

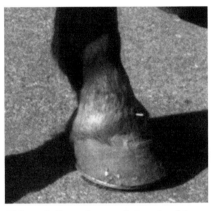

Although the pain was determined to be caused from hip and back stress, needles are placed into different meridians to stimulate the flow of *qi*.

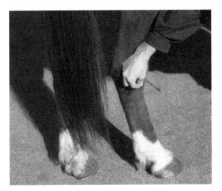

Needles for back pain are also placed in the lower leg.

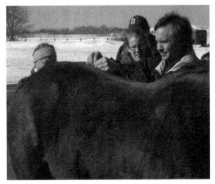

Finally, acupuncture needles are placed ahead of the hip to treat this mare's back pain. At the end of this session, the mare had visible relief from her back pain.

extensive continuing education necessary to be proficient in this medical discipline. Certified veterinary acupuncturists can be found through the American Academy of Veterinary Acupuncture (www.aava.org) or the International Veterinary Acupuncture Society (www.ivas.org).

INDICATIONS FOR USE

Acupuncture has been found to be effective in relieving pain from osteoarthritis, hip and hind leg pain, pain from colic, and pain resulting from surgical procedures. Geriatric horses who do not tolerate NSAIDs might benefit from acupuncture for relief of pain of any origin. All factors leading to musculoskeletal problems must be considered, including environment, use, shoeing, rider, and saddle fit.

The following are some conditions that can be treated with acupuncture.

- Caudal heel pain, navicular syndrome. These conditions respond well to acupuncture. Hoof balance and shoeing are integral to continued success.
- Laminitis. Acupuncture is effective in decreasing the pain of acute laminitis within minutes. Conventional treatment is important to prevent permanent lameness and injury.
- Arthritis. This is a good treatment for pain management.
- Stifles. In addition to relieving pain, acupuncture seems to promote muscle tone and stabilize the stifle joint.
- Tendonitis. Relief from pain and inflammation may be aided by acupuncture in conjunction with cold compressions.
- Thorocolumbar pain or pain in the lower back. This pain is often caused by a poorly fitting saddle; acupuncture may help with the initial pain but the cause needs to be addressed.

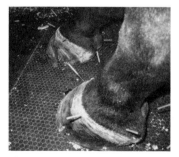

This Thoroughbred mare is being treated for laminitis and associated pain.

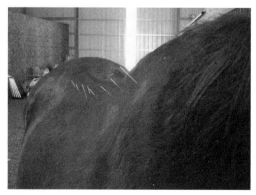

This high-level dressage horse is receiving an acupuncture treatment for chronic back pain that is interfering with performance.

- Cervical pain. Acupuncture may eliminate pain in the neck. This area is one where it is vital that a properly trained veterinarian do any acupuncture or chiropractic therapy.
- Temporomandibular joint pain. Acupuncture can relieve pain in the jaw. However, pain in this area is usually secondary to dental problems. Often, the teeth need floating.
- Neurological conditions. Problems that may benefit from acupuncture in conjunction with veterinary care and treatment include wobbler syndrome, facial paralysis, and nerve paralysis.
- Respiratory problems. Conditions that may benefit from acupuncture in conjunction with veterinary care and treatment include heaves or recurrent airway obstruction, and exercise-induced pulmonary hemorrhage.
- Reproductive problems. Conditions that may benefit from acupuncture in conjunction with veterinary care and treatment include poor uterine tone and decreased libido due to pain.
- Immunological problems. Acupuncture enhances the immune system. It should be used in conjunction with veterinary care and treatment.
- Dermatological problems. These are often caused by a depressed immune system. Acupuncture should be used to enhance immune function, in conjunction with veterinary care and treatment.
- Colic. Acupuncture is not meant to replace traditional care, but it can control pain and normalize gut motility.
- Postoperative ileus. As an adjunct therapy, sometimes only a single treatment is needed to alleviate the problem.
- Gastric ulcers. Reactivity of the acupuncture points is used to suggest the presence of ulcers. Lifestyle changes still must be made.
- Poor appetite. The proper acupuncture points can stimulate a horse's appetite.

CONTRAINDICATIONS FOR USE

Misapplication of acupoints may hide pain. Therefore, it is important to have a good medical history before any therapy is done, to avoid masking injuries. Sudden overuse of acupuncture may create a new injury. Acupuncture should not be performed on a horse who is receiving systemic corticosteroids, as the drug interferes with the positive effects of acupuncture. It should also not be performed on the pregnant *mare*, because it may induce labor or cause *abortion*.

NORMAL PHYSIOLOGICAL DATA

Normal ranges are just that—ranges. They will vary from horse to horse. It is important to know what is normal for your horse. A good practice is to periodically check your horse when he is healthy to know his normal range. Do not wait until the horse is ill to do this. Knowing how he is when he is feeling good will increase your ability to recognize when something is not right. Being able to communicate your horse's vital signs to your veterinarian will enable them to know how serious the problem is and formulate the best response.

Body Temperature

Foals are not very effective at regulating their body temperature until about 2 months of age. An adult horse's temperature can vary during the temperature extremes of different seasons. In winter, a horse's temperature may drop to 97°F (36°C). Intense competition or summer heat may raise a horse's temperature, so take into consideration what your horse was doing before you took his temperature. The real worry is a temperature rise seen with infection. If your horse's temperature is above 102° F (38.9°C), call your veterinarian.

Adult horse (mares and stallions): 99.5 to 101°F (37.5 to 38.3°C)

Foal: 99 to 102°F (37.2 to 38.9°C)

HOW TO TAKE YOUR HORSE'S TEMPERATURE

The only effective way to take your horse's temperature is by using a rectal thermometer. Bulb and digital thermometers are equally suitable. If you're using a bulb thermometer, shake it down until the bulb registers 96°F (35.5°C). Lubricate the bulb with petroleum jelly. Stand to the side of the horse to avoid being kicked. Raise the horse's tail and hold it firmly; then gently insert the bulb into the anal canal with a twisting motion. Insert the thermometer 2 to 3 inches (51 to 76 mm).

Hold the thermometer in place for three minutes. Remove the thermometer, wipe it clean, and read the temperature by the height of the silver column of mercury on the thermometer scale. If you're using a digital thermometer, follow the directions of the manufacturer. The speed read digital thermometers are especially handy for foals and difficult mares.

It's important to clean the thermometer with alcohol to prevent the transfer of diseases and bacteria.

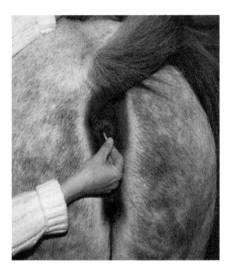

Lubricate the thermometer and insert it 2 to 3 inches (51 to 76 mm) into the anal canal.

Heart Rate

The horse's pulse is the rate at which his heart is beating. The normal pulse rate is most often taken by listening to the heart on the left side of the chest, just behind the elbow. Fit horses may have a pulse rate as low as 28 beats per minute. If the rate is above 40, the horse should be evaluated by a veterinarian. Rates of 40 to 60 beats per minute are serious, and are often accompanied by elevated temperatures. Rates over 80 are critical.

These rates apply only to the horse at rest. Exercise and excitement will temporarily elevate the pulse. Reasons for a persistently raised pulse rate include:

- Pain
- Fever
- Heat exhaustion
- Shock
- Heart disease

> Adult horse: 30 to 45 beats per minute at rest
>
> Nursing foal (1 month of age): 70 to 90 beats per minute

To learn how to take your horse's pulse, see *Pulse*, page 313.

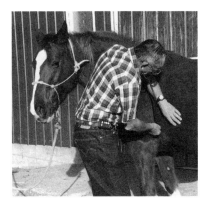

You can listen to the heart rate and time the beat with a stethoscope; this is best accomplished behind the horse's left shoulder.

Respiratory Rate

There are many factors that determine whether the horse's breathing is abnormal. It is important to observe and note anything other than quiet easy breathing. Observe his breathing for anything out of the ordinary, including:

- Deep breathing
- Breathing with an extra abdominal effort
- Abnormal breath noises
- Labored breathing
- Gasping

Determine the respiratory rate by observing and counting the movements of the horse's nostrils or flanks.

> Adult horse: 10 to 20 breaths per minute
>
> Average: 12 breaths per minute at rest
>
> Foal: First 15 minutes of life, 60 to 80 breaths per minute; then 20 to 40 breaths per minutes until 4 to 6 months of age.

Mucous Membrane Color

Check the gums for mucous membrane color. In a normal horse, the membranes are pink. Some abnormal conditions and their corresponding mucous membrane color include:

- Pale pink: low perfusion (fluid passing through the blood vessels), indicating shock
- Deep red: also a shock condition, usually with toxicity
- Purple or blue: low oxygen levels or serious toxicosis
- Yellowish: some yellow may be normal, but very yellow (the whites of the eyes may also look yellow) may indicate jaundice

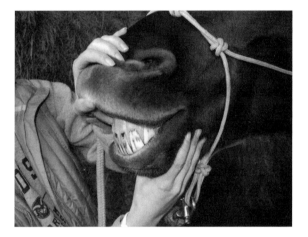

Checking the color of the gums is as easy as curling up the horse's lip.

CAPILLARY REFILL TIME

When you use a finger to apply firm pressure on the gums, the area should blanch. When released, color should return in one to two seconds. A delay of three seconds or more indicates poor perfusion and is often associated with serious dehydration or shock.

Borborygmus

Borborygmus is the gut sounds of a horse digesting his feed. There should be a normal gurgling on both sides of the abdomen near the flanks. You should definitely listen to this sound while the horse is healthy so you can establish what is normal for your horse. The sounds are best heard with a stethoscope. There should be two long rolls, followed by several small gurgles over a period of about one minute. Absence of sounds or fast sounds are abnormal.

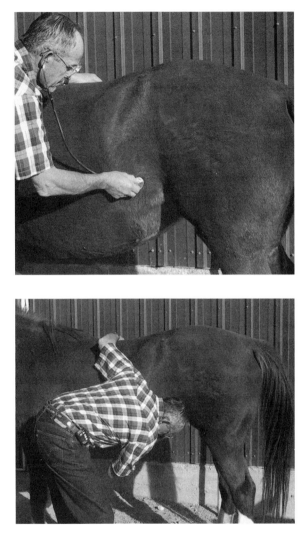

Listening to gut sounds with a stethoscope in the flank area is the best way to hear gut sounds—or lack of sounds.

If a stethoscope is unavailable, or if it's an emergency, before calling the vet you can press your ear to the horse's flank area and listen.

Hydration

The best way to determine a horse's state of hydration is through blood tests. However, a skin turgor test, in which the skin over the shoulder is pinched, can be used as a quick guide. If the skin snaps back quickly, the horse is adequately hydrated. Any delay means the horse needs further evaluation. Older horses will have more relaxed skin.

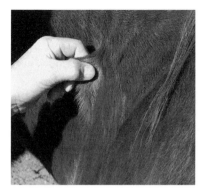

Pinching the skin over the horse's shoulder is a quick test for hydration. The skin should quickly snap back into place.

Reproductive Data

Reproductive maturity (mares and stallions): 36 months

Natural breeding season (northern hemisphere): April to September

Length of estrous cycle: 21 to 23 days during natural breeding season

Length of estrus (heat): 4 to 8 days

Length of gestation (pregnancy): 320 to 370 days; average is 340 days

LABORATORY TESTS

Laboratory tests are a common way to determine what disease process is going on with your horse, to rule out certain illnesses or possibilities, or to monitor an ongoing condition. Usually, a combination of different tests will guide the veterinarian to a diagnosis. The most common tests done on the blood, urine, and stool are discussed here. Blood samples are normally taken from your horse's jugular vein in the neck. Fasting is recommended before some blood tests, and your veterinarian will let you know if your horse should be fasting.

Complete Blood Count (CBC) or Hemogram

A complete blood count tests the different cell types in your horse's blood.

RBC DATA

Red blood cells (RBCs) carry oxygen in the blood. Hemoglobin is the protein in RBCs that binds the oxygen to the red blood cells. The packed cell volume (PCV), or hematocrit, measures of the number of red cells in the blood as a percentage of the whole blood volume. If a horse does not have enough RBCs or hemoglobin, she is said to be anemic. Blood loss, either acute from trauma or chronic from an ulcer, dysfunctional bone marrow, or certain medications may all decrease the packed cell volume. Too many red blood cells can indicate dehydration.

WBC DATA

White blood cells (WBCs) have several functions. The main function is to fight infection, and they accomplish this in two ways. First, they actually "eat" the bacteria or virus—meaning they engulf and dissolve it. Second, they produce antibodies in response to the infection. Different kinds of white cells are produced depending on whether there is a bacterial infection, viral infection, or parasites.

White cells that fight infections or cellular invaders include neutrophils, basophils, and monocytes. Eosinophils fight parasite infestations and are involved in allergic reactions. Lymphocytes produce antibodies in response to an immune challenge.

Normally, white blood cell counts rise with bacterial infections, but if the infection is winning the battle, counts may be lower than expected. Viruses may also lower the white blood cell count. The number of white blood cells may be increased or decreased in horses with certain cancers.

PLATELETS

Platelets are cells that initiate clotting and coagulation. Platelet numbers can be low in horses with certain immune disorders, some cancers, bleeding disorders, disseminated intravascular coagulation, equine infectious anemia, and equine ehrlichiosis.

Coagulation Testing

Coagulation times can be prolonged in horses with rodenticide poisoning, clotting factor deficiency, and disseminated intravascular coagulation. Some of the tests frequently used to evaluate the coagulation ability of the horse include:

- APTT: activated partial thromboplastin time
- PT: prothrombin time (evaluated in conjunction with platelets and fibrinogen)
- FDP: fibrin degradation products
- Fibrinogen: tests the serum levels of fibrinogen, a protein produced by the liver that helps blood clots form; increased levels indicate an inflammation process

Blood Chemistry Panel

A blood chemistry panel evaluates the enzymes that are important to many organ functions and also looks at certain proteins and electrolytes that are important for normal body functions. Some of the blood chemistry tests include:

Albumin. A blood protein produced by the liver, albumin binds and transports other proteins, hormones, and drugs. Levels decrease with certain types of liver and kidney damage or with intestinal problems, and can increase in dehydration and malnutrition.

ALK. Alkaline phosphatase is an enzyme that may increase with liver or bone disease, or along with steroid use or Cushing's disease.

Pregnancy and the bone growth experienced by the young horse can elevate ALK. Phenobarbital, used to control seizures, may also increase the levels of this enzyme.

Amylase. This is an enzyme manufactured primarily by the pancreas and released into the digestive tract to help digest starch and glycogen. It may be elevated in a horse with pancreatic necrosis or intestinal obstruction.

AST. Aspartate aminotransferase is an enzyme present in most cells. Although the test is commonly used as a measure of liver function, any disruption of soft tissue will lead to an increase in the enzyme, as will tying-up syndrome. This test is primarily used to differentiate between muscle disease and liver disease.

Bilirubin. Bilirubin is made in the liver from by the breakdown of dead red blood cells. This value may increase in horses with liver problems or with diseases that destroy red blood cells. Accumulation of this pigment in the body may cause a yellow coloring or jaundice that can be noted in the whites of the eyes.

BUN. Blood urea nitrogen is protein waste material made by the liver and eliminated via the kidneys. A low BUN may indicate liver disease or a low protein diet, and a high BUN may indicate kidney disease or dehydration.

Calcium. Calcium is a very important mineral for muscle and nerve action as well as bone development. Changes can occur after exercise; therefore, it is important to obtain the blood sample after rest. Increases of calcium may indicate primary hyperparathyroidism, too much vitamin D, certain cancers, or chronic renal disease. Decreases of calcium may indicate hyperparathyroidism, vitamin D deficiency, acute pancreatitis, lactation tetany, or acute renal failure.

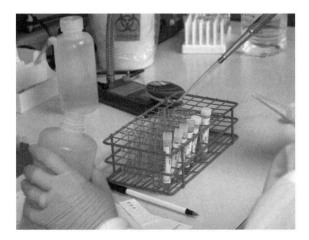

Although many laboratory tests are automated, some tests still require manual dilutions.

Chloride. An extracellular electrolyte, chloride is important to the function of nerves, muscles, and cells. Chloride is regulated by the kidneys and adrenal glands, and is usually associated with a high or low sodium or potassium level. Loss of gastric hydrochloride in small intestine obstruction results in decreased chloride levels.

Cholesterol. The concentration of blood cholesterol is related to lipid metabolism. Cholesterol is a building block for brain and nerve cells, and for the production of some hormones. It can increase with starvation; as adipose or fat tissue reserves are mobilized, the cholesterol and triglyceride levels will increase. Increased cholesterol may be seen in horses with hypothyroidism, Cushing's disease, and biliary obstruction. A decrease may be associated with liver damage, severe infection, or cortisol therapy. In the horse, cholesterol is not a predictor of heart disease.

Creatinine. Creatinine is a waste product of muscles and is normally removed by the kidneys. An increase can indicate kidney disease or dehydration.

CK. Creatinine kinase is a muscle enzyme that increases with muscle damage, including damage to the heart muscle. This will also be elevated in a horse following unaccustomed exercise, as seen with tying-up syndrome or geriatric horses who have been recumbent.

Glucose. Glucose is blood sugar. Increased levels may occur in horses with equine metabolic syndrome, Cushing's disease, or a pancreatic cancer. A decreased level may also indicate a pancreatic malfunction, malabsorption syndrome, or extreme exercise.

GGT. Gamma glutamyl transferase is an enzyme that can be used to very accurately measure liver tissue.

Potassium. Potassium is an electrolyte found inside the cells. Its major role is to maintain water balance in the cells and help in the transmission of nerve impulses. Potassium is very important for muscle and nerve functions and for proper regulation of the heart. Kidney failure, an obstructed bladder, hyperkalemic periodic paralysis in Quarter Horses, and Addison's disease can all increase potassium levels. A decrease in potassium level may indicate inadequate potassium intake, excessive loss fluid from the gastrointestinal tract, excessive sweating, or kidney failure.

Sodium. Sodium is an important electrolyte that is necessary for normal muscle and nerve function and is regulated by the kidneys and the adrenal glands. Dehydration or excessive saline therapy may cause an increase in sodium. Chronic renal disease and gastrointestinal fluid loss (diarrhea) may lower sodium levels.

Total protein. This is a measure of the proteins in the blood, including albumin and globulins (which are associated with infections and inflammation). It is useful in evaluating overall health and nutrition.

High levels can occur in horses with dehydration or immune stimulation. Low levels may indicate liver problems, renal disease, or gastrointestinal disease.

Triglyceride. A product of fat metabolism, triglyceride acts as a major form of stored energy. This biochemical marker is useful to characterize metabolic alterations such are found in horses with equine metabolic syndrome or Cushing's disease.

Reference Laboratory Values

Reference laboratory values are normal laboratory values, sometimes ranges, as determined by the reference lab. Each lab will establish its own set of normal ranges based on population and testing methodology. Your test results must be compared to the testing lab ranges to be meaningful.

When you request laboratory tests, the lab you use will provide a set of values applicable to their methodology—which will vary from lab to lab. For a list of sample reference laboratory values, see the online supplement to this book at www.wiley.com/go/horsevethandbook.

Urinalysis

Urinalysis is the laboratory analysis of urine, which offers an assessment of the urinary system and can be used to evaluate other body systems, as well. Urine is a filtrate of plasma formed by forcing blood through the kidneys, which act as filters. Urine is secreted by the kidneys, stored in the bladder, and discharged by the urethra. Healthy horses produce .5 to 3 gallons (2 to 11 l) of urine a day, which is amber in color.

There are a number of pathologies associated with urination and the urinary system: polyuria is an increase in the volume of urine produced; oliguria is a decrease in the volume of urine produced; *dysuria* is painful urination.

Urine samples may be collected when a horse is voiding or by using a catheter inserted directly into the bladder. The second method is preferred if an infection is suspected because the sample is sterile and any bacteria cultured will be clinically significant.

Urine is evaluated for chemical and cellular constituents, as well as concentration, color, clarity. Abnormal matter found in the urine may include acetone, albumin, bile, blood, glucose, hemoglobin, fat, white cells, or epithelial cells. Specific gravity is another parameter to consider; it measures how concentrated or diluted a urine specimen is.

Fecal Tests

Fecal tests are laboratory examination of feces. Feces are the excrement discharged from the bowel, which consist of bacteria, cellular matter, secretions, and food residue. The specimen may be manually evacuated from the rectum by hand, or picked up when the horses passes stool. To be of value, the fecal material must be fresh.

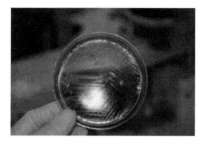

A culture plate with special agar (Hektoen) that inhibits many of the enteric bacteria (those found in the intestinal tract) and enables the lab to recover Salmonella.

Tests that may be performed on feces include:

Fecal blood. This is a simple test to detect the presence of blood in the stool. The presence of blood can indicate a parasite infestation, gastric ulceration, enteritis, colitis, or drugs (such as an *NSAID*) that are causing gastrointestinal bleeding.

Parasite examination. A qualitative and quantitative analyses for parasites and their eggs can be used to monitor the effectiveness of a parasite control program.

Stool culture. Diarrhea in the adult horse can be caused by *Salmonella, Ehrlichia risticii, Clostridium difficile,* and *Lawsonia intracellularis.* Salmonellosis is the most commonly diagnosed cause of diarrhea in adult horses and is easily cultured. *Clostridium difficile* is a frequent cause of gastrointestinal disease associated with the use of anti-microbials. Difficult to culture, the test of choice is polymerase chain reaction (PCR), which is specific, sensitive, and rapid. *Lawsonia intracellularis* is the causative agent of ileitis in horses. Culture detection is difficult. Currently, there is no serological test for *L. intracellularis.* PCR is useful in both tissue and fecal specimens.

Serologic Tests

Serology is a blood test to detect the presence of antibodies targeted against a specific microorganism. Certain microorganisms (antigens) stimulate the body to produce antibodies during an active infection. In the laboratory, the antibodies, if present, react with antigens in specific ways to confirm the identity of the specific microorganism. Some of the techniques for serological tests include, but are not limited to, agglutination, precipitation, complement fixation, fluorescent antibodies, and polymerase chain reaction (PCR).

In a normal horse there are no antibodies present. Exposure to an antigen will initially cause a small rise in antibody production. As the disease progresses, the number of antibodies increases. If a disease is suspected, a second test may be done looking for the rise in antibody numbers (called a *titer*).

These are some of the diseases that can be detected by serologic tests.

> **Babesiosis.** The complement fixation test detects this disease. This test looks for evidence of infection by testing for the presence of a specific antibody or antigen.
>
> **Borrelia burgdorferi (Lyme disease).** Direct immunofluorescence detects this disease. This test uses antibodies tagged with a special dye to detect the presence of other antibodies.
>
> **Eastern/Western encephalitis.** Enzyme-linked immunoassay (ELISA) detects this disease. ELISA detects an enzyme that is linked to a specific antibody or antigen.
>
> **Ehrlichiosis.** The serology, indirect fluorescent antibody test, indicates only that the horse was exposed to the rickettsial organism but does not confirm the disease. The indirect fluorescent antibody test uses antibodies tagged with a special dye.
>
> **Equine infectious anemia.** There are two tests available: agar gel immunodiffusion (as known as a Coggins test; it tests for equine infectious anemia antibodies in the blood) and competitive enzyme–linked immunoabsorbent assay (C-ELISA).
>
> **Equine protozoal myelitis (*Sarcocystis neurona* infection).** This test is looking for the protozoal parasite *Sarcocystis neurona* that causes EPM. The Western blot is used to test serum and spinal fluid. (The Western blot test can detect one specific protein in a mixture of proteins.) PCR tests are used to find protozoal DNA in spinal fluid.
>
> **Equine viral arteritis.** The test most commonly used is serum neutralization.
>
> **Influenza.** A nasal swab can be cultured for the virus or tested by ELISA for the viral antigen. PCR can be performed on either a blood specimen or a nasopharyngeal swab.
>
> **Potomac horse fever.** The antibody to *Ehrlichia risticii* is measured by indirect fluorescent antibody testing.

Cytology Tests

Cytology is the study of cells. Cells are naturally shed from mucous membranes, organs, and skin lesions, and can easily be collected for examination. Cytology exams can be performed relatively quickly, are inexpensive, and provide a great deal of information.

The site of collection determines the method of collection. A skin or lesion test may involve nothing more than scraping the surface or pressing a glass microscope slide against the lesion. Mucous membranes such as are found in the digestive, respiratory, and reproductive tracts may be collected with a sterile swab or washing.

A wash can be collected using a catheter or a fiber-optic endoscope to flush the area with a small amount of sterile saline. This fluid or wash is examined for cells or microorganisms.

Needle aspiration collects cells or fluid from joints, closed cavities, or lesions to diagnose the cause of fluid accumulation (for example, inflammation or infection) and to determine the next step in treatment.

BIOPSY

A *biopsy* is a surgical collection of a solid piece of tissue. The tissue is preserved, stained, and examined microscopically by a pathologist. Normal and abnormal cells are analyzed. Some tumor cells can be classified or graded to determine malignancy or aggressiveness of the tumor.

Culture and Sensitivity

Samples are taken from an infected area with a swab, in a syringe of aspirated material, or as pieces of tissue. These samples are then cultured, which means that they are spread across the surface of a jellylike medium called agar, contained in a petri dish. The agar and petri dish together are called a culture plate. There are many kinds of agars that help in differentiating the various kinds of bacteria.

Depending on the site of culture, whether it is from a sample that is normally sterile (such as blood or spinal fluid) or skin (which normally has bacteria present), the microbiologist looks for pathogens or the bacteria causing the infection.

The organism will grow on the agar for 24 hours or more, each organism grows into a colony, which shows up as a small bump on the agar. The organisms can be isolated and identified by a battery of additional tests. Once identified, the next step is to check the organism for antibiotic sensitivity—the antibiotic that this organism is most sensitive to.

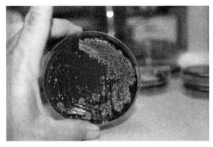

Blood agar is used to culture samples from many different sites. This culture plate has many organisms growing; each dot represents a colony.

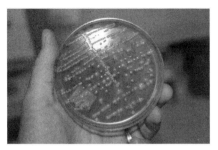

This agar is selective for bacteria that commonly cause urinary tract infections. Urine is normally sterile, meaning there should be no bacteria present. This culture indicates a pure culture because all the colonies are the same. Different kinds of bacteria would look different on the agar.

SENSITIVITY

The susceptibility of bacteria to anti-biotics is called antibiotic sensitivity. Antibiotic sensitivity tests are used to determine which antibiotic will be most successful in treating a bacterial infection. Minimum inhibitory concentration (MIC) in microbiology refers to the lowest concentration of an antimicrobial that inhibits the visible growth of a microorganism. MIC is determined by either agar or broth dilution methods. The agar method of Kirby Bauer sensitivity consists of placing small wafers containing known amounts of antibiotics on an agar plate on which the bacteria are growing. If the bacteria are sensitive, a clear ring is seen around the wafer, indicating poor growth.

The broth dilution method consists of wells of broth with varying concentrations of antibiotics. A measured amount of bacteria is inserted into each well. After incubation overnight, the amount of growth or lack of it is measured.

MIC determines not only the concentration but also the type of antibiotic and its effectiveness, and is based on the location of the infection, the ability of the antibiotic to reach the site of infection, and whether the bacteria can resist the antibiotic's action.

There is a danger of the bacteria becoming resistant to antimicrobial drugs. Therefore, antibiotics must be used carefully. Some of the most dangerous bacteria are those for which there is no effective antibiotic.

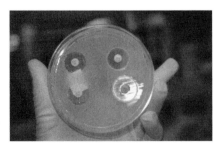

The tiny disks on this plate are infused with antibiotics. The clear areas represent the space where bacteria will not grow due to inhibition by the antibiotics.

GLOSSARY

Words in italics are defined elsewhere in the Glossary.

Abortion   Death of a fetus after organ development (28 days), followed by expulsion of the products of conception.

Abscess   A collection of pus in a cavity. It may be beneath the skin, in an organ, or in a body space.

Acidosis   A buildup of acids in the blood, resulting in a lower pH than normal.

Acupuncture   Puncturing the body with needles at specific points to cure disease or to relieve pain.

Acute   Occurring suddenly. Often indicates the early stage of a disease, when symptoms are most pronounced. Acute symptoms are usually short term.

Aerobic   Bacteria that only grow in the presence of oxygen.

Allergen   Any substance that is capable of causing an allergic reaction. Drugs, insect toxins, pollens, molds, dust mites, foods, and vaccinations are common allergens.

Anaerobic   Bacteria that grow without the presence of oxygen.

Analgesia   Pain relief.

Anaphylaxis   An unusual or exaggerated reaction to foreign protein or other substances.

Anemia   A reduction in the number of red blood cells to below normal levels.

Anestrus   The stage of the estrous cycle in which there is little, if any, ovarian activity. The length of this phase varies, being seasonally cyclic, during spring, summer, and early autumn, regulated by the effects of light on the pituitary gland, on average 21 days.

Aneurysm   The sac formed by the dilation of the walls of the arteries or veins and filled with blood.

Anomaly   Out of the ordinary; a condition that departs from the normal.

Anorectal   Anatomically, the area encompassed by the anus, anal canal, and rectum.

Anorexia   Loss of appetite and failure to eat.

Anthelmintic   A medication that acts to dispel or destroy parasitic intestinal worms. An agent that is destructive to worms is an anthelmic.

Antibody   A protein substance produced by the immune system to neutralize the effects of an *antigen*.

Antigen   A substance recognized by the immune system as foreign to the body. The immune system develops antibodies that bind the antigen and prevent it from harming the animal or causing disease.

Antiserum   A serum that contains antibodies. It may be obtained from an animal who has been subjected to the action of an antigen by injecting it into the tissues or blood.

Antitoxin   The antibody to the toxin of a microorganism, usually the bacterial exotoxins.

Arrhythmia   An abnormal heart rhythm. It may be inconsequential, or serious enough to cause cardiac arrest.

Arthritis   Inflammation of a joint.

Ascarids   Roundworms.

Ascites   An abnormal accumulation of fluid in the *peritoneal cavity*. Congestive heart failure and liver failure are the most common causes.

Assay   Testing the *serum* to determine the relative proportion of a substance, such as the concentration of an *antigen* or *antibody*.

Ataxia   Incoordination; an inability to coordinate voluntary muscle movements that is symptomatic of some central nervous system disorders and injuries and is not due to muscle weakness. The adjective is *ataxic*.

Atresia   Failure of a channel or passage to open in the course of fetal development.

Atrophy   Shrinkage in the size of an organ or tissue due to disuse or death of cells.

Auditory nerve   Nerves related to the sense of hearing.

Autoimmune disease   A disease resulting from *auto-antibodies* targeting host tissue.

Azoturia   Excess of urea or other nitrogen compounds in the urine.

Bacterial sensitivity   Testing bacteria for sensitivity to antibiotics.

Bactericidal   Capable of killing bacteria, as opposed to just inhibiting their growth.

Bacteriostatic   Inhibiting the growth or multiplication of bacteria.

Basal   Pertaining to a base condition or rate.

Benign   An abnormal growth that is not a malignant cancer. Benign growths are usually not life threatening and do not spread to other areas of the body.

Bezoars   Foreign bodies in the stomach composed of hair and other ingested materials that form hard concretions too large to pass out of the stomach or intestines.

Bilateral   On both sides.

Biopsy   The removal of tissue for microscopic examination and diagnosis.

Blepharospasm   Spasms of the obicularis oculi muscle usually producing complete closure of the eyelids.

Boil   A small skin *abscess*, usually at the site of a hair follicle.

Borborygmus   The sounds produced by the horse's bowels while digesting food.

Broad spectrum   A chemical agent that is effective against multiple organisms.

Bronchitis   Inflammation of the air passages.

Bronchoscopy   A procedure in which an *endoscope* is passed into the trachea and bronchi to directly visualize the interior of the respiratory tract.

Brood mare   A mare used for breeding and producing foals.

Cancer   A tumor on the surface of the body or within an organ that has the potential to destroy tissue and kill the animal through local growth and/or spread to distant parts.

Capillary refill time   The time it takes for the gums to pink up after being firmly pressed with a finger—normally one to two seconds or less. A measure of the quality of the circulation.

Cardiac massage   Compression of the heart, resulting in temporary support of the circulation.

Castrate   To remove the testicles of a male horse, often referred to as *gelding*.

Cellulitis   Infection of all layers of the skin along with inflammation of the connective tissue, characterized by redness, swelling, tenderness, and increased warmth. Usually very painful.

Cerebral edema   Swelling of the brain following injury or a period of oxygen deprivation.

Chemotherapy   The use of drugs that are cellular poisons to attack and kill cancer cells, or to suppress the immune system in the treatment of autoimmune diseases.

Chondroprotective   Compounds that protect joint cartilage from the destructive effects of degenerative joint disease.

Choroid   A layer of blood vessels that nourish the retina.

Chromosome The collection of DNA proteins that are organized into genes and aligned to provide genetic information to the body.

Chronic Present for a long period. Often indicates that stage of a disease in which symptoms persist in a milder form.

Cilia Hairlike projections on cells in the respiratory tract.

Ciliary body Pertaining to or resembling the eyelashes.

CK Creatine kinase, an enzyme found in muscle tissue that is released when there is muscle injury or disease.

Cochlea The essential organ of hearing that forms part of the inner ear.

Colic Acute abdominal pain.

Colostrum The first milk of the mare, containing the all-important maternal antibodies that protect the foal from common diseases for the first three months of life.

Colt A young male horse who has not reached sexual maturity.

Condition (of the body) A subjective term that refers to overall health as shown by the coat, general appearance, body weight, and musculature.

Conformation How the various angles, shapes, and parts of the horse's body conform to the breed standard.

Congenital A condition that exists at birth, although it is not always clinically evident until later in life. Congenital conditions can be either genetically determined or acquired before or during delivery.

Cornea The large transparent part of the front of the eye.

Corpus luteum A growth that forms in the ovary at the site of ovulation. The corpus luteum manufactures progesterone, essential to supporting pregnancy. The plural is corpora lutea.

CPR Cardiopulmonary resuscitation; the combination of mouth-to-nose resuscitation and cardiac massage.

Creep feed A supplemental feed given to foals before they are weaned.

Crib A bad habit in which the horse grasps a firm object in his mouth and sucks in a large quantity of air.

Crossmatch Determination of the compatibility of the blood of a donor and that of a recipient.

Cryotherapy A procedure in which tissue is destroyed by freezing it with liquid nitrogen.

Cryptorchid A male with one or both testicles retained in the abdomen or the inguinal area instead of in the scrotum.

CT scan   Computerized tomography, a diagnostic x-ray procedure that produces cross-sectional views of a body structure. CT scans may be available only at veterinary referral centers. Sometimes called CAT scan, an acronym for computer-assisted tomography.

Culture   Growing microorganisms in special media.

Cyanosis   A bluish discoloration of the gums and tongue due to inadequate oxygen in the blood.

Cystitis   Inflammation of the urinary bladder.

Cytology   The microscopic examination of cells to determine the cause of a disease.

Depigmentation   Loss of dark color in the skin caused by destruction of *melanin*-producing cells. Depigmented areas are shades of white.

Depression   A marked decrease in activity in which the horse withdraws, spends most of his time lying down, is disinterested in his surroundings, and exhibits little or no interest in eating.

Dermis   The sensitive connective tissue layer of the skin located below the epidermis.

DODs   Developmental orthopedic diseases.

Dominant   A gene is dominant if it alone is capable of determining the expression of a particular trait.

Donkey   The domestic ass.

Duodenum   The first part of the small intestines, after the stomach.

Dysfunction   Abnormal performance of an organ or system.

Dysphagia   Painful and/or difficult swallowing.

Dyspnea   Difficult or labored breathing.

Dystocia   The prolongation of any stage of labor.

Dysuria   Painful and/or difficult urination.

Early embryonic loss   Loss of the products of conception before 42 days of gestation, often by internal reabsorption so that no external evidence of the loss is found.

ECG   Electrocardiogram; the readings from an electrocardiograph, which measures the changes in electrical currents associated with heart activity. An ECG is used to measure heart function and detect abnormalities. Sometimes called EKG.

Echocardiogram   A test that uses plain and Doppler ultrasound (high-frequency soundwaves) to create a computerized image of structures within the heart and a detail of blood flow. The procedure that uses an echocardiogram to diagnose heart disease is called echocardiography.

Ectropion   The outward turning of the eyelid.

Edema   The accumulation of fluid beneath the skin.

Electrolytes   Sodium, chloride, potassium, bicarbonate, calcium, phosphorus, and other minerals required for organ functioning.

ELISA   Enzyme-Linked Immunosorbent Assay, a *serologic* test used to detect antibodies to a protein, such as those associated with a bacteria or virus.

Embolus   A blood clot that develops at another site and travels through the circulatory system to a smaller vessel, where it becomes lodged and interrupts blood flow.

Embryo   A *conceptus* younger than 14 days of gestation, before the stage of organ development.

Empyema   Accumulation of pus in a pouch in the body.

Encapsulated   Surrounded by a capsule that creates a distinct boundary between two tissue planes.

Encephalitis   Inflammation and/or infection of the brain.

Encephalomyelitis   Inflammation and/or infection of the brain and spinal cord, commonly associated with viral diseases.

Endemic   Dwelling in or native to a particular population or region.

Endometrial cups   The hormone-producing cells that attach the placenta to the uterus.

Endometritis   Inflammation of the mucus coat of the uterus.

Endometrium   A layer of glandular tissue lining the cavity of the uterus.

Endoscope   An instrument that uses lights and fiber optics or a miniaturized video camera to view the interior of a body cavity. The procedure of using an endoscope to visualize the interior of a body cavity is called endoscopy.

Endotoxemia   Disease caused by the release of *endotoxins*.

Endotoxins   Toxins that are part of the outer cell wall of bacteria and are released when the cell membranes rupture.

Enophthalmos   Abnormal protraction of the eyeball into the orbit.

Enteritis   Inflammation of the lining of the intestines, caused by bacterial, parasitic, or viral infection as well as *immune-mediated* diseases.

Entropion   The inward turning of the eyelid.

Eosinophil   A type of white blood cell that is often associated with diseases that have an allergic component or with parasites.

Epididymis   The coiled tube on top of the testicle that stores the sperm.

Epistaxis   Nosebleed.

Epithelium   A layer of nonliving cells that forms the surface of the skin, mucous membranes, and cornea.

Equid or equidae   A family of mammals that includes horses, donkeys, mules, and zebras.

Erosion   An area where a body surface has been destroyed by trauma or inflammation.

Erythrocytes   Red blood cells; the cells that carry oxygen and carbon dioxide.

Estrous cycle   The entire reproductive cycle, as determined from one ovulation to the next, normally occurring about every 21 days.

Estrus   Same as *heat*. The phase of the *estrous cycle*, during which the mare is receptive to the stallion; lasts on average seven days.

Etiology   Cause of the disease.

Euthanasia   The humane process of giving an animal a fatal, painless injection to end her suffering.

Excision   The surgical removal of a *tumor* or *lesion*.

Excoriation   A deep scratch or abrasion of the skin.

Exophthalmos   Abnormal protrusion of the eyeball.

Exotoxins   Toxic proteins produced by the bacteria and released into their environment.

Exudate   A liquid discharge that contains pus and bacteria.

FDA   Food and Drug Administration; licenses the use of human and veterinary drugs.

Febrile   Having a fever.

Fertility   In stallions, the ability to impregnate the mare. In broodmare, the ability to conceive and carry a foal.

Fetus   A *conceptus* older than 14 days of gestation, generally after the stage of organ development.

Fiber-optic cystoscopy   The use of an endoscope to view the inside of the urethra and urinary bladder.

Fibrosis   The replacement of normal tissue by scar tissue.

Filly   A female horse less than 4 years old.

Foal   A young horse, less than 4 months of age.

Foaling   Birth of a *foal*.

Follicle   A growth within the ovary that contains an egg. Also, the cells in the skin from which hairs grow.

Forage   Food horses eat by grazing.

Fresh semen *Semen* that is artificially inseminated into the mare within a few hours of collection.

FSH Follicle-stimulating hormone; produced by the pituitary gland. It causes the ovaries to produce egg *follicles*.

Galvayne's groove A groove on the surface of the tooth that only appears in the two upper corner incisors and is often used to gauge the age of a horse.

Gastroesophageal junction The anatomical area formed by the junction of the esophagus and the stomach.

Gastroscopy A procedure that uses an *endoscope* to view the interior of the esophagus, stomach, and duodenum.

Gelding A *castrated* or gelded male horse.

Gene The basic unit of heredity. Each gene contains the code that produces a specific protein or molecule.

Gestation Length of pregnancy; the period from conception to birth. In horses the average is 340 days, with a range of 320 to 370.

GI An abbreviation for gastrointestinal.

Glomerulus The capillary network that produces the urine in the kidneys by filtering waste products from the blood.

Gn-RH Gonadotrophin-releasing hormone; triggers the release of FSH and LH from the pituitary gland.

Gonadotropins Hormones released from the pituitary gland or placenta, acting on the ovaries or testicles to cause them to manufacture and release the sex hormones.

Head-pressing Pressing the head against a wall or solid structure without apparent purpose.

Heat See *estrus*.

Hemagglutination Clumping together of red blood cells, caused by *antibodies*.

Hematocrit The percentage of red blood cells in whole blood.

Hematoma A collection of clotted blood beneath the skin at the site of an injury.

Hematuria The passage of blood in the urine, recognized by red-colored urine or blood clots in the urine. Microscopic hematuria is the presence of red cells on microscopic exam.

Hemoglobin The oxygen-carrying pigment of red blood cells.

Hemoglobinuria Presence of hemoglobin pigment in urine.

Hemolysis Destruction of red blood cells.

Hemolytic anemia The disease that results when red blood cells are destroyed in the circulation.

Hernia A protrusion of an organ, or part of an organ, through an opening in the abdominal wall that would normally close in the course of fetal development.

Heterozygous Possessing a different set of genes in regard to a given characteristic.

Hives Small, raised, red, pruritic areas, generally caused by an allergic reaction.

Homozygous Possessing the same set of genes in regards to a given characteristic.

Hypoxia Lack of oxygen in the blood and tissues. If untreated, it results in coma and death.

Iatrogenic An unintended disease that results from a medical treatment or procedure.

Idiopathic A disease or condition for which no cause is known.

IgG A class of antibody that can cross the placenta or be present in the mother's milk.

IM Abbreviation for intramuscular; an injection given into the muscle.

Immune-mediated A process in the body in which proteins in the immune system lead the body to destroy its own cells. This can happen for unknown reasons (*idiopathic*) or due to a secondary cause such as infection, parasites, cancer, or drug reaction.

Immunoglobulin An antibody.

In utero Occurring in the uterus.

Incarceration Trapping an organ or part of an organ within a closed space. Most commonly refers to intestine trapped in a hernia.

Infarction Death of tissue as a consequence of an interruption in the blood supply.

Infection Disease caused by a bacteria or a virus.

Infertility Absence of *fertility*. A mare who can't conceive or a stud who can't sire a foal.

Infestation The presence of parasites in numbers that may be sufficient to cause an infection.

Intact An animal who has not been *spayed* or *gelded*.

Intra-articular Within a joint.

Intranasal Within the nose.

Intubation　Placing a breathing tube into the trachea to establish an airway for assisted breathing.

Intussusception　Telescoping of one section of bowel into another section of bowel.

Involution　The process by which the uterus empties and returns to normal size after *foaling*.

IV　Abbreviation for intravenous; an injection given into a vein.

Jaundice　A yellow discoloration in the whites of the eyes and mucous membranes of the mouth, caused by an accumulation of bile pigments in the *serum* and tissues. Usually associated with liver disease or the destruction of red blood cells.

Keratitis　Inflammation of the *cornea*.

Killed vaccine　A vaccine made from killed bacteria or virus particles. Killed vaccines are generally safe, but may not be as effective as *modified live vaccines* (MLV).

Labryrinthitis　Inflammation of the internal ear.

Labyrinth　The system of intercommunicating cavities that consist of the internal ear.

Lacrimal gland　Gland that produces tears.

Laparoscopy　A surgical procedure in which an endoscope and surgical instruments are inserted into the abdomen through several small incisions.

Lavage　Flushing out a wound or cavity with large amounts of irrigating solution.

Legume　A group of feed plants containing nitrogen-fixing bacteria in the roots, most common would be clovers and alfalfa.

Lesion　Damage to tissue caused by an injury or a specific disease.

LH　Luteinizing hormone, produced by the pituitary gland. It causes ovarian follicles to mature and ovulate.

Ligation　Tying off a vessel.

Lolling　A condition in which the paralyzed tongue hangs from the mouth.

Luxation　The displacement of a bone from its normal position within a joint.

Lymphadenopathy　The enlargement of one or more lymph nodes as the result of inflammation or cancer.

Malignant　A growth that is a cancer, which is likely to spread throughout the body and may be life threatening.

Mare　Mature female horse.

Mastitis   Inflammation of one or more quarters of the mammary gland.

Melanin   Naturally occurring dark pigment.

Meniscus   A cushioning pad of cartilage interposed between two bones.

Metastasize   The spread of a cancer from its site of origin to another part of the body.

MLV   Modified live virus vaccine; a vaccine made from live bacteria or viruses that have been treated so that they cannot cause disease.

Monorchid   Having only one testicle. True monorchids are unusual. Also see *cryptorchid*.

MRI   Magnetic resonance imaging, a diagnostic procedure that uses a nuclear magnetic spectrometer to produce computerized images of body structures. Usually available only at veterinary referral centers.

Mucociliary blanket   The mucosal lining of the upper respiratory tract that contains cells with *cilia* that are capable of propelling inhaled irritants into the back of the throat.

Mucopurulent   A discharge containing mucus and pus.

Mucosa   The inner layer of mucus-producing cells that lines the respiratory, gastrointestinal, and genitourinary tracts.

Mucus   The slippery substance that is secreted as a protective coating by cells and glands of the mucosa. The adjective is mucoid.

Mule   The offspring of a male donkey and a mare.

Multiparity   Having had two or more pregnancies that resulted in live offspring.

Mutation   An alteration in a gene causing a change in some bodily function that is perpetuated in all the cells that descend from the original mutant cell.

Mycotoxins   Toxins produced by fungi.

Myelitis   An infection or inflammation of the spinal cord.

Myeloencephalitis   Inflammation of the spinal cord and brain.

Myelogram   A spinal tap in which dye is introduced into the spinal canal for x-ray studies looking for signs of spinal cord compression.

Myoglobin   The iron-containing pigment in muscle that contributes color and acts as oxygen storage.

Myopathy   A disease of muscle or muscle tissue.

Nebulizer   A device for generating a spray.

Necropsy   Examination of a body after death. The animal equivalent of an autopsy.

Necrosis   The death of a cell or group of cells that are in contact with living tissue.

Nephritis   Inflammation of the kidney.

Nephron   The basic working unit of the kidney, composed of a glomerulus that filters urine and a system of tubules that concentrates the urine and reabsorbs water and *electrolytes*.

Neutering   Removing both testicles in the male or both ovaries in the female.

Nictitating membrane   The third eyelid; a membrane at the inner corner of the eye that comes out across the eye in response to eye pain and other conditions.

NSAID   Nonsteroidal anti-inflammatory drug.

Nutraceutical   A nutritional supplement that may have disease-modifying effects.

Nystagmus   A rhythmic movement of the eyeballs in which the eyes slowly wander a few degrees in one direction and then jerk back. Seen in horse with diseases of the inner ear, brain, and occasionally sleeping sickness.

Occlusion   An obstruction or closure of a passageway or vessel.

Occult   Not evident by clinical signs.

Off-label   Using a medication in a horse that is not approved by the FDA for use in horses. This may be a drug that is in common use for another species and it simply is not financially viable for a company to go through FDA testing.

Orbicularis oculi   The ring of muscles around the eyelids.

Organisms   Living members of the animal or plant kingdom; microorganisms usually refers to bacteria, viruses, and other small one-celled beings.

Ossicles   The small bones of the middle ear.

Osteomyelitis   Inflammation of a bone.

OTC   Over-the-counter; refers to drugs.

Otitis   Inflammation of the ear.

Oviduct   The tube that carries the egg from the ovary to the uterus.

Ovulation   The process during which the egg *follicle* releases the egg into the *oviduct*.

Palpation   Feeling, pressing on, and examining the body with the hands.

Parasite   An organism that lives upon or within another organism, at whose expense it obtains advantage without compensation.

Passive transfer   Transfer of the mare's antibodies through her milk to the foal.

Pathogenic   Having the potential to cause disease.

Pathogens   Agents such as bacteria, viruses, and fungi that are capable of causing disease.

PCR   Polymerase chain reaction is a laboratory test where parts of DNA strands are compared to a known value.

Perianal   The glands and skin structures surrounding the anal opening.

Perineum   The area extending from the anus to the bottom of the vulva in the female, and to the scrotum in the male.

Peristalsis   Rhythmic contractions that propel ingested foods and liquids from the mouth to the anus.

Peritoneal cavity   The abdominal cavity, containing organs of the intestinal, urinary, and reproductive tracts.

Peritonitis   Inflammation or infection of the peritoneal or abdominal cavity.

PHF   Potomac horse fever.

Pinna   The projecting part of the horse's ear, lying outside of the head.

Placentitis   Inflammation of the placenta, usually caused by bacteria that ascend into the uterus through the cervix.

Pleura   The membrane lining of the thoracic or chest cavity, as well as the lining covering the lungs.

Pleural effusion   An accumulation of fluid in the chest cavity caused by right-side heart failure, infection, or *tumor*.

Pleuritis   A painful inflammation of the membrane that lines the chest cavity.

PMN   Polymorphonuclear leukocyte; inflammatory cells that make up pus.

Pneumothorax   Air in the chest caused by a tear in the lung or a wound in the chest wall. The lung collapses, resulting in respiratory distress.

Polyuria   The passage of large amounts of urine, usually recognized by more frequent voiding.

Postpartum   After giving birth; the period after *foaling* that lasts four to six weeks.

Premature foal   A foal born before 320 days of gestation.

Prepuce   The foreskin; the sheath that surrounds the glans or head of the penis.

Productive cough   One that brings up a quantity of phlegm. Also known as a moist cough.

Progesterone   The pregnancy hormone, produced by the ovaries (corpora lutea).

Prognosis   A forecast based on the probable outcome of the disease.

Prolapse   Protrusion of an organ through a body opening.

Prophylactic   A medication or a procedure used as a preventive.

Prophylaxis   Preventive treatment.

Protrusion   Extending beyond the normal location, such as a protruding eyeball.

Pulmonary edema   The accumulation of fluid in the lungs, usually caused by congestive heart failure.

Purulent   Puslike; a discharge containing *pus*.

Pus   A discharge that contains *serum*, inflammatory cells, and sometimes bacteria and dead tissue.

Pustule   A small bump on the surface of the skin that contains pus.

Pyelonephritis   Inflammation of the kidney and its pelvis.

Pyoderma   A *purulent* skin infection including *pustules*, *boils*, *abscesses*, *cellulitis*, and infected scabs.

Quidding   Dropping partially chewed food from the mouth.

Radiograph   The use of x-rays to take an image of the inside of the body; commonly referred to as x-ray.

Recessive   A *gene* that expresses a trait only when it is combined with another recessive gene.

Recombinant vaccine   A vaccine made by splicing gene-sized fragments of DNA from one organism (a virus or bacteria) and transferring them to another organism (the horse), where they stimulate the production of antibodies.

Recumbency   Lying down.

Reflux   A reversal in the normal direction of flow.

Regurgitation   The passive expulsion of esophageal contents without conscious effort.

Remission   The period during which the horse remains free of symptoms.

Renal   Referring to the kidneys.

Renal pelvis   The funnel that collects the urine excreted by the kidney. It tapers and becomes the ureter.

Renal tubule   The filtering mechanism that concentrates the urine.

Resection   Removing *malignant,* dead, or unwanted tissue by surgically cutting it out.

Retina   A layer of photoreceptor cells at the back of the eye, which converts light into nerve impulses that pass via the optic nerve to the brain.

Retrobulbar abscess   An abscess between the bony orbit and the eyeball.

Sarcoid   A viral induced tumor of the skin.

Sarcoma   A cancer that arises from muscle, bone, or other connective tissue.

Scaly   Shedding flakes of skin.

Sclera   The white membrane surrounding the cornea of the eye.

Scrotum   The bag of skin and connective tissue that surrounds and supports the testicles.

Semen   The contents of the ejaculate, containing sperm cells, gel, and the secretions of the accessory sex glands.

Senile   An age-related decline in physical and mental faculties.

Sepsis   The presence of infection, often accompanied by fever and other signs of illness, such as vomiting and diarrhea. The adjective is septic.

Septicemia   The stage of *sepsis* in which microorganisms and/or their toxins are found in the blood.

Seroconversion   The production of specific antibodies in response to an antigen such as bacteria or virus.

Seronegative   Showing negative antibody reaction on a blood examination.

Seropositive   Showing a positive antibody reaction on a blood examination.

Serum   The clear fluid component of the blood. The adjective is serous. Serologic refers to blood tests that evaluate or measure antibody responses.

Soundness   Mental and physical health when all the organs and systems are functioning as intended.

Spermatogenesis   The production of sperm by the testicles.

Spinal tap   A procedure in which a needle is inserted into the spinal canal to remove cerebrospinal fluid for laboratory analysis.

Sporadic   Isolated, occasional, or infrequent.

SQ   Abbreviation for subcutaneous; an injection given beneath the skin. Also sometimes called SC or sub-Q.

Stallion   An intact male horse kept for breeding.

Stenosis   Constriction or narrowing, especially of a channel or passage. The adjective is stenotic.

Stillbirth   A full-term foal who is born dead.

Strabismus Deviation of the eye.

Strangulated The compression or pinching off of the blood supply to an abdominal organ, such as a segment of bowel. Leads to death of tissue.

Sternal position To lay upright on the sternum, not on the side.

Stridor A high-pitched, raspy sound caused by air passing through a narrowed larynx.

Stud Stallion.

Subclinical A stage of illness in which infection occurs without apparent signs.

Subluxation A partial dislocation, in which the bone is partly out of the joint.

Superinfection The development of a second infection on top of (or following) the first infection.

Synovial fluid analysis A procedure in which a needle is inserted into a joint to remove fluid for chemical and microscopic examination.

Systemic Into the system; used in reference to widespread dissemination of infection or cancer, or a drug given orally, intramuscularly, intravenously, or subcutaneously.

Tapetum lucidum Special layer of cells that acts like a mirror, reflecting light back onto the retina and producing a double exposure of photoreceptor cells.

Teratogenic That which causes developmental malformations in the fetus.

Testosterone The male hormone, produced by the testicles.

Thromboembolism The process by which a blood clot forms in a vein or artery and then moves up or down in the circulatory system, where it causes further clotting.

Titer The concentration of a measured substance in the *serum*.

Torsion The twisting of an organ and its blood supply, resulting in insufficient blood flow and death of that organ.

Toxemia A state of shock induced by the absorption of bacterial toxins from an infected area in the body.

Tracheobronchitis A viral or bacterial infection of the cells lining the trachea and bronchi.

Transtracheal washings Cells obtained by flushing the trachea with saline; used to diagnose the causes of upper respiratory infections.

Trichiasis Ingrowing of the eyelash.

Tumor Any growth or swelling (such as an *abscess*). A cancerous growth is called a neoplasm.

Tympanic membrane The membrane separating the middle ear from the external ear.

Ulcer A defect on the surface of an organ or tissue. A skin ulcer is an open sore with an inflamed base, involving the outer layer of the skin and often the dermis. A gastrointestinal ulcer is an open sore in the lining of the stomach or intestines. A corneal ulcer is on the clear surface of the eye.

Ultrasonography A diagnostic procedure that uses high-frequency sound waves to map a picture of an organ or structure inside the body.

Unilateral On one side only (as opposed to bilateral—on both sides).

Urachus A tube in the umbilical cord that connects the foal's bladder to its mother's placenta.

Ureter The tubes that carry the urine from the kidney to the bladder.

Urethra The tube that conveys urine from the bladder to outside the body.

Urethritis The inflammation of the urethra.

Urinalysis Chemical or microscopic analysis of urine.

Uveitis Inflammation of the iris and internal structures of the eye.

Ventricle A cavity or chamber. Ventricles within the brain contain cerebrospinal fluid. Within the heart, the ventricles are the larger chambers on both sides of the heart.

Vesicle A small skin blister filled with clear fluid.

Viscosupplementation The addition of substances to increase the lubricating fluids in the joint capsule.

Vulva The labia (lips) of the vagina.

Wheal An intensely itchy, raised patch of skin with a white center and a red rim. Varies in size from a pinhead to several inches. Often transient.

Zoonosis A disease that is communicable from humans to animals and vice versa under natural conditions. The adjective is zoonotic.

ABOUT THE AUTHORS

Tom Gore, DVM

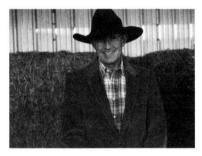 Tom Gore received his veterinary medical degree from Colorado State University School of Veterinary Medicine. He has been practicing veterinary medicine for more than 30 years. Growing up on a cattle ranch in the mountains of western Colorado, he has been caring for and caring about horses all his life. He is an active member of the American Veterinary Medical Association, Colorado Veterinary Medical Association, and the National Association of Federal Veterinarians. Tom spent years officiating at sanctioned events for competitive endurance rides. Horses remain an integral part of his life, including breeding, training, and riding his own small herd. Western Colorado and the family ranch are still favorite places to ride. Tom and his wife, daughter, and son live in Delta, Colorado.

Paula Gore, MT, ASCP, BB

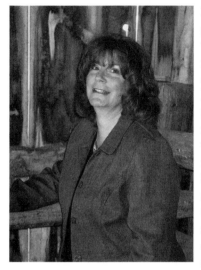

Paula Gore is a medical technologist; she graduated from Colorado State University with a degree in medical technology/microbiology. Paula is an active member of the American Society of Clinical Pathologists and has her blood bank certification. She has a lifetime of horse experience, and began training colts at 15 years of age. Her equine experiences include racetrack work, an Arabian breeding facility, showing in both English and Western disciplines, competing in team penning, and cattle work. She loves riding in the mountains with her family, especially in the places where the family says, "When I was a kid, there was a good trail here!" She makes her home with her husband and kids in Delta, Colorado.

James M. Giffin, MD

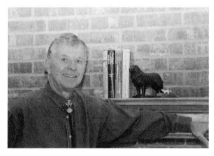

Jim Giffin graduated from Amherst College and received his medical degree from Yale University School of Medicine. After years of private surgery practice in Missouri and Colorado, Jim was called to active duty during Operation Desert Storm, serving as chief of surgery at military hospitals in Alabama, Korea, and Texas.

Jim had lifelong experience with cats, dogs, and horses. His interest in horses began with his daughter Kate's first horse, and continued through 4-H and various horse shows in the western United States.

In 1969, he established a Great Pyrenees kennel and became active in breeding, showing, and judging dogs. He was the coauthor of the award-winning books *The Complete Great Pyrenees*, *Dog Owner's Home Veterinary Handbook*, *Cat Owner's Home Veterinary Handbook*, and *Veterinary Guide to Horse Breeding*.

Until his death in 2000, he lived in western Colorado.

TECHNICAL REVIEWERS

Lauren Gnagey, DVM, received her Doctor of Veterinary Medicine degree, as well as a BS in Animal Science, from Michigan State University. Her main interests are equine medicine and nutrition. She is involved with the Michigan State Animal Response Team, is a member of American Association of Equine Practitioners, American Veterinary Medical Association, Michigan Veterinary Medical Association, and Michigan Equine Practitioners Association. Lauren practices at Kern Road Veterinary Clinic in Fowlerville, Michigan. She shares her free time with her husband, Ryan; cat, Shanny; and Corgi, Hooch.

Christina Kobe, DVM, attended Michigan State University to receive a Bachelor of Science degree in Animal Science, and then Michigan State's College of Veterinary Medicine. She now practices general equine medicine and surgery in an ambulatory setting at Kern Road Veterinary Clinic in Fowlerville, Michigan. She has special interests in ophthalmology and wound healing. Lameness and imaging are also primary interests. Christina is an active member of American Association of Equine Practitioners, American Veterinary Medical Association, and Michigan Equine Practitioners Association.

LIST OF TABLES

GENERAL INDEX

NOTE: *Page number shown in boldface contain detailed coverage of the item.*

NOTES

NOTES

NOTES

NOTES

NOTES

ART CREDITS

Unless otherwise noted here, photographs have been provided by the authors.

Molly Borman: 169, 331

Stephenie Carpenter, Academy of Equine Dentistry, Glenns Ferry, Idaho: 193, 194

Countryside Veterinary Clinic, Greely, Colorado, Doug Jergens: 188

Equine Medicine and Surgery, American Veterinary Publications: 46, 72, 129, 136, 151, 156, 261, 267, 294, 567, 569

Equine Medicine and Surgery, American Veterinary Publications, Courtesy of Dr. J.A. Auer: 265

Eric Ervin: 204

Rose Floyd: 233, 234

Mona Frazier: 147, 252, 272

James Giffin, MD: 652 (bottom)

Katie Gore: 161, 651, 652 (top)

Timothy Holt: 617

Lameness in Horses, 4th ed., Lea and Febiger: 198, 199, 219, 225, 242, 245, 246, 256

Nancy Mahoney: 609, 610 (middle)

Susan Stamilio: 1, 30, 141, 180, 181, 183, 185, 186, 200, 209, 214, 226, 231, 248, 250, 286, 311, 361, 442, 516, 530

We appreciate the publishers of *Adams' Lameness in Horses,* Edition IV, 1987 (Lea & Febinger) and *Equine Medicine and Surgery,* 1982 (American Veterinary Publications) for giving permission to use photographs and illustrations.